Clinical Manual
of Urology

Third Edition

D0684689

NOTICE

Medicine is an ever-changing science. As new research and clinical experience broaden our knowledge, changes in treatment and drug therapy are required. The author(s) and the publisher of this work have checked with sources believed to be reliable in their efforts to provide information that is complete and generally in accord with the standards accepted at the time of publication. However, in view of the possibility of human error or changes in medical sciences, neither the author(s) nor the publisher nor any other party who has been involved in the preparation or publication of this work warrants that the information contained herein is in every respect accurate or complete, and they are not responsible for any errors or omissions or for the results obtained from use of such information. Readers are encouraged to confirm the information contained herein with other sources. For example and in particular, readers are advised to check the product information sheet included in the package of each drug they plan to administer to be certain that the information contained in this book is accurate and that changes have not been made in the recommended dose or in the contraindications for administration. This recommendation is of particular importance in connection with new or infrequently used drugs.

Clinical Manual of Urology

Third Edition

Editors

Philip Hanno, MD
Division of Urology
University of Pennsylvania School of Medicine
Medical Director
Clinical Effectiveness and Quality
University of Pennsylvania Health System

S. Bruce Malkowicz, MD
Associate Professor
Division of Urology
Co-Director Urology Oncology Program
University of Pennsylvania School of Medicine

Alan J. Wein, MD
Chief, Division of Urology
University of Pennsylvania Medical Center
Professor and Chairman
Division of Urology
University of Pennsylvania School of Medicine

McGRAW-HILL
Medical Publishing Division
New York   Chicago   San Francisco   Lisbon   London   Madrid
Mexico City   Milan   New Delhi   San Juan   Seoul   Singapore
Sydney   Toronto

CLINICAL MANUAL OF UROLOGY

1234567890 DOCDOC 0987654321

ISBN 0-07-136201-0

This book was set in Times Roman by Carlisle Communications;
The editors were Martin J. Wonsiewicz, Susan R. Noujaim and
Barbara Holton;
The production supervisor was Richard Ruzycka;
The indexer was Deborah Tourtlotte;
R.R. Donnelley & Sons Company was printer and binder.

Library of Congress Cataloging-in-Publication Data

Clinical manual of urology / editors, Philip M. Hanno, Alan J. Wein,
S. Bruce Malkowicz.—3rd ed.
    p. ; cm.
   Includes bibliographical references and index.
   ISBN 0-07-136201-0
   1. Urology—Handbooks, manuals, etc.2. Urinary organs—Diseases—
Handbooks, manuals, etc. I. Hanno, Philip M. II. Wein, Alan J. III.
Malkowicz, S. Bruce.
   [DNLM: 1. Urologic Diseases—diagnosis—Handbooks.
2. Urologic Diseases—therapy—Handbooks. WJ 39 C641 2001]
RC872.9 .C57 2001
616.6—dc21   00-048068

DEDICATION

For our wives; Linda, Noele, and Denise. Their remarkable support
and encouragement is deeply appreciated.

For the medical students and residents who have inspired and encouraged us in this endeavor.

Table of Contents

Contributors

Mark P. Banner, MD [3, 4]
Professor, Radiology and Radiology in Surgery (Urology)
University of Pennsylvania School of Medicine
Director, Uroradiology
University of Pennsylvania Medical Center
Philadelphia, Pennsylvania

Ashok Batra, MD, FRCS, FACS [20, 31]
Adjunct Professor, Urology
Upstate Medical Center
Syracuse, New York
Medical Officer, FDA
Rockville, Maryland

Roy D. Bloom, MD [16]
Assistant Professor, Renal, Electrolyte & Hypertension Division
University of Pennsylvania
Philadelphia, Pennsylvania

Stephen B. Brandes, MD [11, 12]
Assistant Professor, Division of Urologic Surgery
Washington University School of Medicine
Chief of Urology, St. Louis VA Medical Center
St. Louis, Missouri

Douglas A. Canning, MD [30]
Associate Professor, Department of Urology in Surgery
The University of Pennsylvania School of Medicine
Director, Pediatric Urology
The Children's Hospital of Philadelphia
Philadelphia, Pennsylvania

Jeffrey P. Carpenter, MD [26]
Associate Professor of Surgery
University of Pennsylvania School of Medicine
Director Vascular Laboratory
Hospital of the University of Pennsylvania
Philadelphia, Pennsylvania

Numbers in brackets refer to chapter(s) authored or
co-authored by contributor

Michael C. Carr, MD, PhD [28]
Assistant Professor, Urology
University of Pennsylvania
Attending Surgeon, Children's Hospital of Philadelphia
Philadelphia, Pennsylvania

Gregory E. Dean, MD [29]
Assistant Professor, Urology and Pediatrics
Temple University
Philadelphia, Pennsylvania
Assistant Professor, Urology and Pediatrics
University of Medicine & Dentistry of New Jersey—The Robert
Wood Johnson School
Attending Staff, Temple Children's Hospital
Philadelphia, Pennsylvania
Attending Staff, Cooper Medical Center
Camden, New Jersey

Robert A. Grossman, MD [16]
Professor of Medicine and Surgery
Medical Director, Kidney Transplant Program
University of Pennsylvania School of Medicine
Philadelphia, Pennsylvania

Philip M. Hanno, MD [5, 7]
Division of Urology
Hospital of the University of Pennsylvania
Medical Director, Clinical Effectiveness & Quality
University of Pennsylvania Health System
Philadelphia, Pennsylvania

Ira Kohn, MD [8]
Scranton, Pennsylvania

Tanmay Lal, MD [25]
Transplant Fellow
University of Pennsylvania School of Medicine
Philadelphia, Pennsylvania

S. Bruce Malkowicz, MD [17, 18]
Associate Professor, Urology
Co-Director, Urology Oncology Program
University of Pennsylvania School of Medicine
Philadelphia, Pennsylvania

Ali Najay, MD, PhD [25, 26]
Professor of Surgery
University of Pennsylvania School of Medicine
Philadelphia, Pennsylvania

David M. Nudell, MD [21]
Clinical Instructor and Fellow, Male Reproductive Medicine & Surgery
Scott Department of Urology
Baylor College of Medicine
Houston, Texas

John J. Pahira, MD [9]
Professor, Department of Surgery, Division of Urology
Medical Director, Center for Kidney Stone Disease & Lithotripsy Unit
Georgetown University Medical Center
Washington, DC

Christopher K. Payne, MD [10]
Assistant Professor, Department of Urology
Director, Female Urology & Neurourology
Stanford University Medical Center
Stanford, California

Michel A. Pontari, MD [6, 22]
Associate Professor, Urology
Temple University School of Medicine
Philadelphia, Pennsylvania

Amir A. Razack, MD [9]
Renal Fellow, Department of Medicine, Division of Nephrology
Georgetown University Medical Center
Washington, DC

John F. Redman, MD [1]
Professor of Urology and Pediatrics
University of Arkansas College of Medicine
Little Rock, Arkansas

Eric S. Rovner, MD [13, 14, 15]
Assistant Professor of Urology
Hospital of the University of Pennsylvania
Philadelphia, Pennsylvania

E. James Seidmon, MD [23]
Professor of Urology and Diagnostic Imaging
Temple University School of Medicine
Philadelphia, Pennsylvania

Heather C. Selman, MD [6]
Clinical Instructor, Department of Urology
Temple University Hospital
Philadelphia, Pennsylvania

Rajesh Shinghal, MD [10]
Senior Resident, Department of Urology
Stanford University School of Medicine
Stanford, California

Howard M. Snyder III, MD   [27, 28, 30]
Professor, Department of Urology
University of Pennsylvania School of Medicine
Associate Director, Pediatric Urology
Children's Hospital of Philadelphia
Philadelphia, Pennsylvania

William F. Tarry, MD, FACS, FAAP [30]
Associate Professor, Urology and Pediatrics
Director, Renal Transplantation
West Virginia University School of Medicine
Morgantown, West Virginia

JC Trussell, MD [20]
Chief Resident, Department of Urology
Upstate Medical University
Syracuse, New York

Paul J. Turek, MD [21]
Associate Professor, Department of Urology, Obstetrics &
Gynecology, and Reproductive Services
University of California at San Francisco
San Francisco, California

Keith N. Van Arsdalen, MD [2]
Professor, Surgery (Urology) and Radiology
University of Pennsylvania Health System
Philadelphia, Pennsylvania

E. Darracott Vaughan Jr, MD [24]
Chairman, Department of Urology
New York Presbyterian - Weill Medical College
New York, New York

Alan J. Wein, MD [14, 15, 17]
Professor and Chair, Division of Urology
University of Pennsylvania School of Medicine
Chief of Urology, University of Pennsylvania Health System
Philadelphia, Pennsylvania

Jeffrey P. Weiss, MD [8]
Clinical Adjunct, Assistant Professor
Weill/Cornell University Medical College
New York, New York

Richard Whittington, MD [19]
Associate Professor, Department of Radiation Oncology
University of Pennsylvania
Philadelphia, Pennsylvania

Michael K. Yu, MD [21]
Chief Resident, Division of Urologic Surgery
Washington University School of Medicine
St. Louis, Missouri

Stephen A. Zderic, MD [27]
Associate Professor of Urology
University of Pennsylvania School of Medicine
Children's Hospital of Philadelphia
Philadelphia, Pennsylvania

Preface

Clinical Manual of Urology
Third Edition

The third edition of this introductory text in urology has tried to remain consistent with the goals of the initial endeavor 15 years ago: to present a publication that could serve as a basic, portable reference for the busy medical student and house officer rotating on the urology service, to enable program directors to use the information presented as a framework on which to present their particular management styles and strategies, and to serve as a ready-reference for the primary care physician, who often times is the first person to see the patient with what ultimately proves to be a urologic problem.

We are pleased to welcome a new editor, Dr. Bruce Malkowicz, to the Clinical Manual of Urology. Dr. Malkowicz is an erudite and valued colleague whose suggestions and contributions to the third edition have been much appreciated. We thank the many urologists who have found the previous editions to be a useful addition to their library and/or teaching practice, and have taken the time to send us comments meant to improve future editions. In this new edition all chapters have been updated to reflect the many changes in urology practice that have evolved over the last several years. The cancer section has been expanded considerably. A new section on adrenal pathology has been contributed by Dr. Darracott Vaughan. Each chapter now includes not only references for those seeking further information, but also self-assessment questions and discussion points to test comprehension of the material presented.

We hope that you, the reader, will find the text useful in your practice or as a part of your education. We thank our contributors and our publisher for making this volume possible. We trust that even in this world of information technology and computers, you will find this manual that still fits in your pocket to be a trusted resource and ready-reference.

Philip Hanno
Alan Wein
Bruce Malcowicz

Preface to the Second Edition

In the first edition of this introductory urology text, we tried to construct a publication that would allow program directors to use the information presented as a basis on which to present their particular management styles and strategies to house staff and medical students rotating on urology. We hope this open-ended type of format will again be evident, as we have tried to avoid a dogmatic approach, recognizing that the philosophy of management differs among institutions.

We are grateful for the widespread acceptance of *A Clinical Manual of Urology* and the many helpful suggestions that we received from urologists around the country after publication of the first edition. We recognize that some sections were academically "lighter" than they should have been and have made efforts not only to update all of the material presented, but also to improve the areas that needed a fuller presentation.

We hope that this new edition will continue to present the basic body of urologic material in a way that is applicable to the many different styles of patient management throughout the country. We have tried to keep the size of the volume reasonable so that it can be easily available for reference and have encouraged our contributors to list important suggested readings for those interested in pursuing individual topics.

We thank our many contributors, our editors, and our new publisher for their helpful suggestions and patience throughout the many months of preparation of the manuscript.

Philip M. Hanno
Alan J. Wein

Preface to the First Edition

This book is intended primarily for the busy student and house officer rotating on the urology service. The purpose of this text is not to provide a heavily referenced compendium of urologic practice complete with controversies and "the answer" to each. Rather, we have tried to concisely summarize agreed upon (for the most part) material in such a way that pathophysiology, presentation, evaluation, and treatment referable to a given problem can be easily understood. While "answers" may vary from institution to institution, we hope they will be consistent with the content presented. Although the practices and philosophy of the University of Pennsylvania staff may be evident, more so in some sections than in others, we have tried to keep "dogma" to a minimum, allowing others to add their input without the intellectual disruption (to the reader) of major disagreements.

We hope students, nonurologists, and first-year urology residents find this text a readily accessible, quickly read, and portable initial reference and starting point for more in-depth reading. Each author has been encouraged to carefully select and list suggested references at the end of each section rather than to use exhaustive citations throughout.

Our thanks are due to the contributors for trying to inform rather than persuade, and to the editors for their encouragement and forebearance.

Philip Hanno
Alan Wein
July 1986

CHAPTER 1

Anatomy of the Urogenital Tract

John F. Redman

An understanding of function, either normal or abnormal, must be preceded by an understanding of structure. The study of the anatomy of the genitourinary system involves knowledge of not only the organs and collecting structures of that system but also the innervation, vasculature, and lymphatic associations. Because urology is a subspecialty of surgery, anatomy, as it applies to urology, encompasses more than just the genitourinary tract itself; it also includes the surrounding structures that must be incised to gain operative access.

I. SKELETAL ANATOMY

Knowledge of the bony skeleton forms the basis for the comprehension of the muscular anatomy. Of interest to the urologist are the thoracic, lumbar, and sacral vertebrae; the lower ribs; and the bony pelvis (Fig. 1-1).

A. Vertebrae

The vertebrae of interest to the urologist are the lower thoracic, lumbar, and sacrococcygeal. The thoracic and lumbar vertebrae have in common a large ventral body that is separated by an intervertebral disk and supports dorsally the vertebral arch. The vertebral arch is formed dorsally by the pedicle and lamina of the vertebra, which, respectively, support transverse and spinous processes. The opening formed by the vertebral arch overlying the body is the vertebral foramen through which runs the spinal cord. Between each pedicle is found the intervertebral foramen through which proceeds a spinal nerve. The sacrum is formed by the coalescence of the five sacral vertebrae with fusion of the transverse processes and intervertebral spaces. On the ventrum are found the pelvic sacral foramina, which provide for egress of the ventral rami of the pelvic nerves. The sacrum bulges into the

1

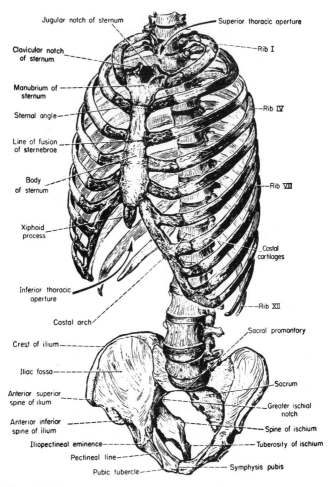

Figure 1-1 Bony and cartilaginous structures of chest, abdomen, and pelvis. (*Reproduced from Woodburne RT: Essentials of Human Anatomy, 6th ed, 1978, Fig. 243, p 305.*)

pelvis at its juncture with the lumbar vertebrae and is termed the sacral promontory.

B. Ribs

The lower five or six ribs are commonly encountered by urologists. Of significance is knowledge that the eleventh and twelfth ribs are tipped with cartilage ventrally and are not joined by their tips to the cartilaginous costal arch as are the sixth through tenth ribs. Of note is the costal groove on the inner inferior surface of the ribs that supports the intercostal vessels and nerve.

C. Pelvis

1. The bony pelvis is formed by four bones: the paired innominates (coxae), sacrum, and coccyx. The innominates are composed of three parts: the ilium, ischium, and pubis. The pubic bones are joined in the midline by a cartilaginous bridge, the symphysis pubis.

2. The pelvis has a cranial, bowl-shaped portion, the greater or false pelvis. Caudally, it has a ringshaped configuration termed the lesser or true pelvis. The two portions are separated by the linea terminalis, which runs from the pectineal line to the pubis to the arcuate line of the ilium to the sacral promontory.

3. The pelvis has two foramina in the bone and four foramina formed by ligaments. The obturator foramina are large foramina in the caudal aspect of the coxal bones. The sacrotuberous ligament, extending from the ischial tuberosity to the lateral aspect of the sacrum and coccyx, and the sacrospinous ligament, extending from the ischial spine to the dorsolateral aspect of the sacrum, form two foramina, the greater and lesser sciatic foramina in the space between the sacrum and the innominate bone.

4. Two other so-called pelvic ligaments are the inguinal ligament, which is the free edge of the external oblique aponeurosis extending from the pubic tubercle to the anterior superior iliac spine, and Cooper's ligament, which is the periosteum covering the pectineal line of the pubis.

II. MUSCULAR ANATOMY

Of interest to the urologist is the musculature of the lower thoracic region, the abdomen and pelvis. The abdominal musculature may be considered as anterior, anterolateral, and posterolateral.

A. Lower Thoracic Musculature

When making thoracic incisions, urologists may encounter the external abdominis oblique, latissimus dorsi, serratus anterior, intercostals, levators costarum, and serratus posterior inferior (Fig. 1-2). The description of the external oblique appears with the anterolateral abdominal muscles. The latissimus dorsi and serratus posterior inferior are described with the muscles of the posterior abdominal wall.

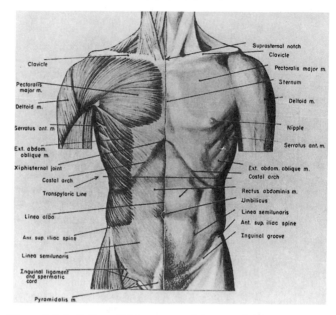

Figure 1-2 Left: Superficial anatomy; right: superficial anterior abdominal wall musculature. (*Reproduced from Crafts RC: A Textbook of Human Anatomy, 2d ed, 1979, p 61.*)

1. The serratus anterior is encountered at its lower four fleshy digitations, which mesh with the digitations of the external oblique over the lateral aspects of the fifth to ninth ribs.

2. The intercostal muscles are the external and internal intercostals, which may be thought of as a thoracic equivalent of the external and internal abdominis oblique muscles, respectively (Fig. 1-3). The fibers of the internal intercostals course obliquely downward and at the costochondral junction are replaced by a thin fibrous tissue, the external intercostal membrane. In similar fashion the fibers of the internal intercostal course obliquely upward and are represented from the angle of the ribs laterally by an internal intercostal membrane.

3. The levators costarum originate from the ends of the transverse processes and extend obliquely downward to insert on the cranial aspect of the next rib at its angle.

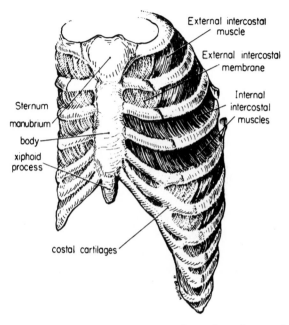

Figure 1-3 External and internal intercostal muscles and external intercostal membrane. (*Reproduced from Woodburne RT: Essentials of Human Anatomy, 6th ed, 1978, Fig. 249, p 310.*)

B. Abdominal Wall Musculature

1. Anterior abdominal wall The primary musculature of the anterior abdominal wall is the rectus abdominis muscles (Fig. 1-4). These are paired, segmented muscles that extend from the pubic crest to insertions on the fifth, sixth, and seventh ribs. The muscles are divided into segments by tendinous intersections. As regards the surface anatomy, the lateral aspect of the rectus abdominis muscles can be identified in leaner individuals as a vertical depression in the midclavicular line known as the linea semilunaris. The rectus abdominis muscles are encased in a fibrous tissue envelope, the rectus sheath (Fig. 1-5). The fibrous investments represent continuations of the anterolateral abdominal musculature and its aponeuroses: the external abdominis oblique, internal abdominis oblique, and transversus abdominis. The most ventral portion of the rectus sheath is formed from the aponeurosis of the external oblique muscle. Dorsal

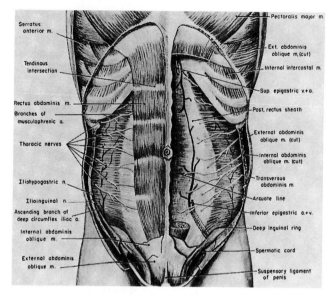

Figure 1-4 Anatomy of the anterior abdominal wall after reflection of external and internal abdominis oblique musculature. (*Reproduced from Crafts RC: A Textbook of Human anatomy, 2d ed, 1979, p 104.*)

to this investment is the aponeurosis of the internal oblique muscle, which splits at the lateral edge of the rectus muscle, the ventral portion melding with the external oblique aponeurosis and the dorsal portion melding with the aponeurosis of the transversus abdominis muscle. At a variable position halfway between the umbilicus and the pubis all of the aponeuroses pass dorsal to the rectus abdominis muscles. This arched termination of the heavy fascial sheath is known as the arcuate line. In the midline the recti are separated by the dense joining of these fascial layers known as the linea alba, which varies in thickness.

2. Anterolateral abdominal wall

The anterolateral abdominal musculature is comprised of the external abdominis oblique, internal abdominis oblique, and transversus abdominis oblique (Fig. 1-6).

a. The external abdominis oblique originates from the fifth to twelfth ribs and interdigitates with the origin of the serratus anterior and latissimus dorsi muscles. The fibers are oriented in a caudal and medial direction. The muscle per se inserts into the outer anterior

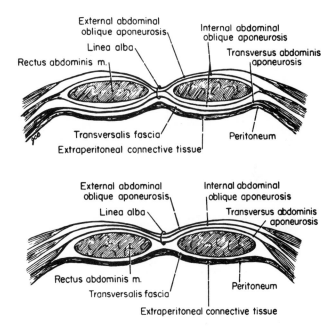

Figure 1-5 Rectus sheath. Top: Configuration cranial to the arcuate line. Bottom: Configuration below the arcuate line. (*Reproduced from Woodburne RT: Essentials of Human Anatomy, 6th ed, 1978, Fig. 302, p 373.*)

half of the iliac crest. Its aponeurosis inserts by the anterior rectus sheath to the xiphoid linea alba and symphysis pubis. The caudal free edge bridging between the anterosuperior iliac spine and the pubic tubercle is termed the inguinal ligament. At the level of the pubic tubercle the aponeurosis is thinned for the penetration of the spermatic cord and is known as the superficial inguinal ring. A thin continuation of the fascia continues over the cord as the external spermatic fascia.

b. The internal abdominis oblique arises from the posterior lamina of the lumbodorsal fascia, the anterior two-thirds of the iliac crest, and the iliopsoas fascia. The upper half of the fibers courses in an oblique and cranial direction, inserting into the inferior borders of the cartilage of the last three or four ribs. The lower half of the fibers courses almost horizontally to terminate by their aponeuroses in the anterior or posterior

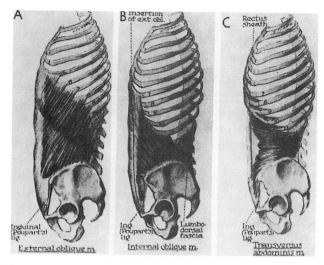

Figure 1-6 A: External oblique, **B:** Internal oblique, **C:** Transversus abdominis. (*Reproduced from Thorek P: Anatomy in Surgery, 2d ed, 1962, Fig. 275, p 36; Fig. 279, p 363; Fig. 280, p 364.*)

rectus sheath, ultimately inserting into the linea alba. A continuation of the internal oblique is the cremaster muscle, which extends caudally and with its fascia invests the spermatic cord.

The transversus abdominis muscle arises from the costal cartilages of the lower six ribs, the anterior lamina of the lumbodorsal fascia, and the anterior two thirds of the iliac crest. The fibers course transversely and insert by their aponeurosis, which forms a portion of the anterior and posterior rectus sheath cranial to the arcuate line and the posterior sheath caudally.

3. Posterolateral abdominal wall

The musculature of the posterior abdominal wall for consideration may be assigned to three groups: superficial, intermediate, and deep.

a. The superficial group includes the external oblique and latissimus dorsi muscles (Fig. 1-7). The external oblique is described with the anterolateral abdominal wall musculature. The latissimus dorsi is a large triangle-shaped muscle that covers most of the lower back. Its origin is from the posterior lamina of the

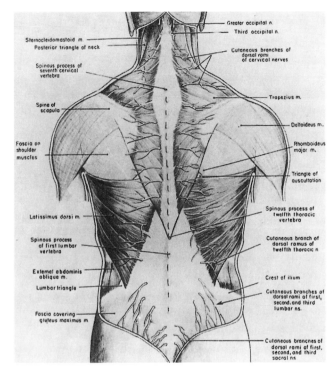

Figure 1-7 Posterolateral abdominal wall showing position of the latissimus dorsi. (*Reproduced from Crafts RC: A Textbook of Human Anatomy, 2d ed, 1979, p 61.*)

lumbodorsal fascia and the iliac crest with insertion into the humerus.

b. The intermediate group includes the internal oblique, serratus posterior inferior, and sacrospinalis or erector spinae (Fig. 1-8). The internal oblique is described with the musculature of the anterolateral abdominal wall.

1. The serratus posterior inferior arises from the spinous processes of the Tll to L2 vertebrae and, following an upward lateral course, inserts into the outer inferior border of the last four ribs just lateral to their angles.

2. The sacrospinalis or erector spinae muscle is large and complex and lies in the groove formed by the spinous and transverse processes of the lumbar

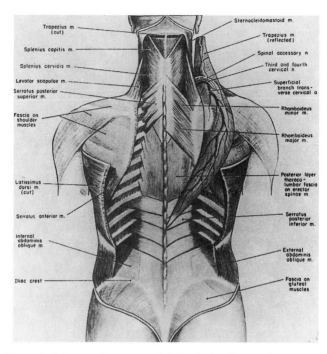

Figure 1-8 Intermediate group of abdominal wall musculature. (*Reproduced from Crafts RC: A Textbook of Human Anatomy, 2d ed, 1979, p 65.*)

and thoracic vertebrae, being covered by the posterior layer of the lumbar part of the lumbodorsal fascia. It originates caudally by a thick, wide tendon from the sacrum, iliac crest, and lumbar spinous processes. In the upper lumbar region it divides into three columns of muscles with the lateral-most portion inserting into the ribs and the more medial portion inserting into the spinous processes of the thoracic vertebrae. The deep group comprises the transversus abdominis, quadratus lumborum, psoas, and diaphragm (Fig. 1-9). The transversus abdominis has been described with the musculature of the anterolateral abdomen.

   i. The quadratus lumborum arises from the posterior iliac crest and, coursing obliquely upward, inserts into the transverse processes of the first four lumbar vertebrae and the medial half of the inferior border of the twelfth rib.

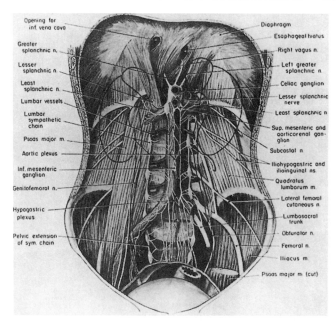

Opening for
int. vena cava

Greater
splanchnic n.

Lesser
splanchnic n.

Least
splanchnic n.

Lumbar vessels

Lumbar
sympathetic
chain

Psoas major m.

Aortic plexus

Inf. mesenteric
ganglion

Genitofemoral n.

Hypogastric
plexus

Pelvic extension
of sym. chain

Diaphragm

Esophageal hiatus

Right vagus n.

Left greater
splanchnic n.

Celiac ganglion

Lesser splanchnic
nerve

Least splanchnic n

Sup. mesenteric and
aorticorenal gan-
glion

Subcostal n

Iliohypogastric and
ilioinguinal ns.

Quadratus
lumborum m.

Lateral femoral
cutaneous n.

Lumbosacral
trunk

Obturator n.

Femoral n.

Iliacus m.

Psoas major m. (cut)

Figure 1-9 Deep group of anterior abdominal wall musculature. (*Reproduced from Crafts RC: A Textbook of Human Anatomy, 2d ed, 1979, p 261.*)

    ii. The psoas major lies ventral to the quadratus lumborum and, as it passes caudally into the pelvis, passes ventral to and on the medial aspect of the iliacus muscle whose tendon it joins enroute to its insertion into the lesser trochanter of the femur. The origin of the psoas is from the T12 to L5 vertebrae.

3. The diaphragm is a dome-shaped, fibromuscular structure separating the abdominal and thoracic cavities. The origin of the muscle is from its periphery, that is, the lower ribs, sternum, and lumbocostal arcs. The lumbocostal arcs are distinctive landmarks for the retroperitoneal surgeon to identify the margins of the diaphragm, with the lateral lumbocostal arc crossing over the quadratus and laterally over the transversus abdominis and the medial lumbocostal arc bridging over the psoas. The two crura of the diaphragm arising from the anterolateral aspects of the upper lumbar vertebrae form a median arc over the aorta. The diaphragm inserts into a large fibrous central tendon.

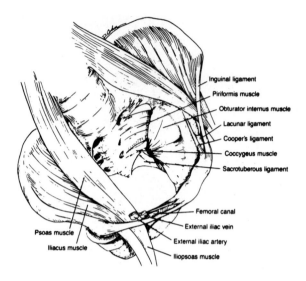

Figure 1-10 Pelvic musculature. (*Reproduced from Burnett LS: Anatomy, in Novak's Textbook of Gynecology, 11th ed., 1988, Fig. 2.3, p 44.*)

4. Pelvic musculature

Six muscles cover the floor and wall of the pelvis. Four of these muscles (the iliacus, psoas, piriformis, and obturator internis) either originate from or pass through the pelvis before inserting into the femur (Fig. 1-10). The remaining muscles of the pelvis are the levator ani and coccygeus (Fig. 1-11)

The iliacus covers the iliac fossa and is covered medially by the psoas muscle with which it joins caudally. For most pelvic operative procedures much of the pelvic musculature is not directly visualized. However, as the pelvic viscera are swept away from the pelvic sidewall, the obturator internis and levator ani are clearly seen. The greater part of the obturator internis is covered on its medial aspect by the levator ani. The levator arises by a thickening of the obturator internis fascia, termed the arcus tendinous, which bridges from the ischial spine to the superior pubic ramus.

For the most part, the pelvic floor or diaphragm is formed by the levator ani muscles through which pass the urethra, vagina, and rectum. The three component parts are the anteriorly located puborectalis and pubo-

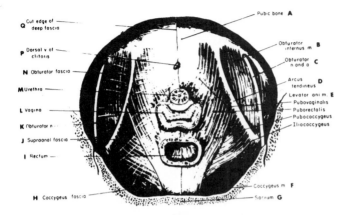

Figure 1-11 Musculature of female pelvis as viewed from above.
(*Reproduced from Crafts RC: Abdominopelvic Cavity and Perineum,
in Textbook of Human Anatomy, 3d ed, 1985, Fig. 5-65, p 327.*)

coccygeus and the posterolateral part, the ileococcygeus.
The levator ani arises from the arcus tendinous and pubis
and inserts into the anorectal raphe and coccyx.

III. VASCULAR ANATOMY

The vasculature of most interest to urologists is that of the posterior abdominal wall and pelvis, which is the outflow from the
aorta and the internal iliacs, respectively, with the venous return being via the branches of the internal iliacs and vena cava.

A. Arteries

1. Abdominal aortic branches. The significant branches of
   the aorta from the median arc of the diaphragm to the bifurcation are the paired inferior phrenics (which give
   rise to the superior suprarenal arteries), midline celiac
   trunk, paired suprarenals, midline superior mesenteric,
   paired renals followed by the paired gonadals, and inferior mesenteric (Fig. 1-12). Lumbar arteries, four pairs,
   course from the dorsolateral aspect of the aorta.
2. *Common iliac branches.* The arterial vasculature of the
   pelvis derives primarily from the branches of the common iliac artery, with the exception of the middle sacral,
   which arises from the bifurcation of the aorta, and
   branches of the inferior mesenteric artery, which vascu-
   larize the rectum (Fig. 1-13). The primary branch of the
   common iliac is the internal iliac (hypogastric), which

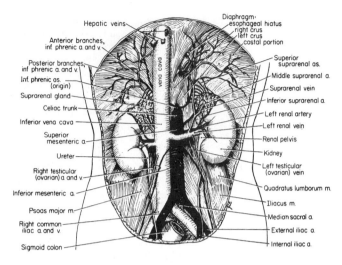

Figure 1-12 Abdominal aorta and vena cava with their important branches and tributaries. (*Reproduced from Woodburne RT: Essentials of Human Anatomy, 6th ed, 1978, Fig. 362, p 443.*)

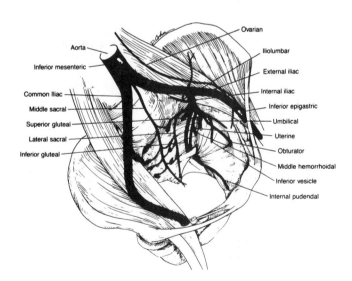

Figure 1-13 Arterial vasculature of the female pelvis. (*Reproduced from Burnett LS: Anatomy. In: Novak's Textbook of Gynecology, 11th ed, 1988, Fig. 2.7, p 47.*)

occurs at the level of the juncture of the sacrum and L5 vertebra. The external iliac, which is a direct extension of the common iliac, courses caudally and laterally along the medial aspect of the psoas and, passing beneath the inguinal ligament, becomes the femoral artery.

a. *External iliac branches.* The external iliac has two primary branches that occur just caudal to the inguinal ligament, the inferior epigastric medially and deep circumflex iliac laterally.

b. *Internal iliac (hypogastric) branches.* The majority of the vasculature of the pelvis is supplied by the branches of the internal iliac artery. Just caudal to its origin from the common iliac, the internal iliac divides into major branches, the posterior and anterior divisions.

The posterior division branches are the iliolumbar, lateral sacral, and superior gluteal. The superior gluteal supplies major vasculature to the gluteal muscles. Therefore, the admonition regarding ligation of the internal iliac to control pelvic hemorrhage, is to ligate distal to the posterior division of the internal iliac.

The branches of the anterior division may be divided for consideration into parietal and visceral branches. The parietal branches are the inferior gluteal, obturator, and internal pudendal, whereas the visceral branches are the umbilical, inferior vesical, middle hemorrhoidal, uterine, and vaginal arteries. The internal pudendal, which is the terminal branch of the anterior division, leaves the pelvis and courses through a fascial sheath on the medial surface of the obturator internis muscle (Alcock's canal) to provide the primary vasculature of the perineum.

B. Veins

The venous drainage of interest to urologists is that which occurs through veins that terminate in the vena cava and the vena cava itself (Fig. 1-12).

1. The vena cava in the abdomen is longer than the aorta. Just at the diaphragmatic hiatus of the vena cava are located the inferior phrenic veins and just caudal to them, the anteriorly positioned hepatic veins. Just caudal to the liver on the right side and just above the right renal artery the short right adrenal vein is found. The paired renal veins exit just caudal to the superior mesenteric artery. The long left renal vein is unique in that it receives the left adrenal and left gonadal veins entering, respectively, cranially and caudally opposite each other. Occasionally a lumbar vein also is found dorsally entering the left renal

vein just to the left of the aorta. Caudal to the right renal vein is the site of entrance of the right gonadal vein. Approximately four pairs of lumbar veins enter the vena cava dorsolaterally.

2. At its bifurcation the vena cava receives the common iliac veins, which drain the lower extremities via the femorals, and the internal iliacs, which provide the primary venous drainage of the pelvis. The pelvic venous drainage system is unique in that, although the veins generally follow the course of the arteries, they are multiple. The pelvic organs are further surrounded by plexuses of veins, the most pronounced of which are the vesical, prostatic, uterine, vaginal, and rectal.

IV. LYMPHATIC ANATOMY

Of interest to the urologist are the retroperitoneal or parietal lymphatics, which, like lymphatics in general, follow the vasculature (Fig. 1-14). The lymph node chains of the retroperitoneum are referred to by the name of the vessels that they accompany. Primary chains are the preaortic nodes, which include those of the celiac and superior and inferior mesenteric; the right and left lumbar chains; and the common, external, and internal iliac chains. The right lumbar chain or trunk lies on each side and behind the vena cava, whereas the left lumbar chain is found to the left of the aorta. Posterior to the great vessels at about L1 to L2, the lumbar trunks join in a variable dilatation termed the cisterna chyli, which drains to the thoracic duct.

The superficial inguinal lymph nodes are located external to the fascia lata of the anterior thigh and accompany the superficial epigastric and circumflex iliacs and external pudendal vessels. The deep inguinals accompany the femoral vessels just caudal to the inguinal ligament.

V. NEUROANATOMY

The abdomen and pelvis receive innervation from somatic and visceral nerves.

A. Somatic Nerves

The anterolateral musculature of the abdomen and superficial back is innervated by the sixth to twelfth intercostal nerves and their lateral and anterior cutaneous branches. The deep musculature of the back and pelvis is innervated by the branches of the lumbosacral plexus (Fig. 1-15).

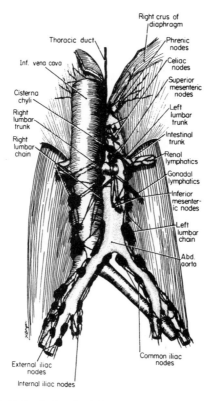

Figure 1-14 Abdominal and pelvic lymphatics. (*Reproduced from Woodburne R'T: Essentials of Human Anatomy, 6th ed, 1978, Fig. 365, p 448.*)

The lumbar plexus formed from the ventral rami of the L1–L4 nerves lies within the psoas muscle and gives off six branches of surgical interest: the iliohypogastric, which supplies sensory innervation to the skin of the thigh, pubis, and anterior scrotum and labia majora, and motor function to the lower abdominal muscles; the ilioinguinal nerve, which courses parallel and ventral to the iliohypogastric with a similar pattern of innervation; the lateral femoral cutaneous nerve, which supplies sensory innervation to the lateral thigh; the large femoral nerve and the genitofemoral nerve, which supplies sensory innervation to the cord, scrotum, labia, and skin of the anterior thigh.

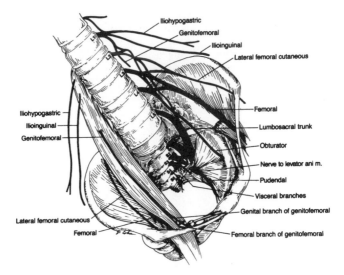

Figure 1-15 Lumbosacral plexus and its branches. (*Reproduced from Burnett LS: Novak's Textbook of Gynecology, 11th ed, 1988, Fig. 2.11, p 52.*)

The sacral plexus is formed from the ventral rami of the L4 and L5 and S1–S3 nerves and courses over the piriformis muscle in the pelvis. Twelve branches of the sacral plexus occur. Three are of interest to the urologist: the posterior femoral cutaneous nerve, which at the caudal border of the gluteus maximus gives rise to a perineal branch that innervates the skin of the scrotum and vulva; the pelvic splanchnic nerve (nervi erigentes), which carries preganglionic parasympathetic fibers and sensory fibers and joins the inferior hypogastric plexus to supply all of the pelvis and perineal viscera; and the pudendal nerve, which is the primary innervation of the perineum via the inferior hemorrhoidal, perineal, and dorsal nerves of the penis and clitoris.

B. Visceral Nerves

The autonomic innervation of the abdominal viscera is via sympathetic and parasympathetic nerves that are interspersed with ganglia and pass along innervation to the plexuses and ganglia along the ventrum of the aorta and sacrum.

1. Autonomic nerves
   a. The sympathetic nerves consist of the thoracic splanchnic nerves, which arise from the thoracic ganglia and terminate in the celiac and aortorenal ganglia overlying the ventrum of the aorta, and the lumbar sympathetic trunks, which connect with the lumbar nerves by white and gray rami communicantes and give rise to the lumbar splanchnic nerves that communicate with the mesenteric plexuses over the aorta and sacrum to innervate the pelvic viscera.
   b. The parasympathetic nerves are the anterior and posterior vagal trunks arising from the esophageal plexus, the posterior trunk supplying fibers to the kidney via the celiac and aortorenal plexus, and the pelvic splanchnic nerve, which is described with the sacral plexus.
2. Plexuses and ganglia
The autonomic innervation of the abdominal and pelvic viscera is carried through plexuses and ganglia located over the abdominal aorta, sacrum, and lateral aspects of the rectum (Fig. 1-16). In one instance, a plexus is referred to as a nerve (hypogastric nerve). Cranially to caudally, the plexuses and ganglia include the celiac ganglion adjacent to the celiac trunk; the superior mesenteric ganglion and plexus surrounding the superior mesenteric artery; the inferior mesenteric ganglion and plexus adjacent to the vessel of the same name; the superior hypogastric plexus overlying the sacral promontory; the left and right hypogastric nerves, which are actually plexuses connecting the superior hypogastric plexus with the inferior hypogastric plexus, which lies on either side of the rectum; and the inferior hypogastric plexus, which is formed by the hypogastric nerve and the pelvic splanchnic nerve. The inferior hypogastric plexus gives rise to the vesical–prostatic plexuses. The prostatic plexus located on the dorsolateral aspect of the prostate continues through the urogenital diaphragm as the cavernous nerve of the penis. In the female the inferior hypogastric plexus gives rise to the ureterovaginal (Frankenhauser's) plexus.

VI. RETROPERITONEAL CONNECTIVE TISSUE AND PERITONEUM

Familiarity with the retroperitoneal connective tissue is an adjunct to dissection of that area. A useful concept is to consider that the retroperitoneal connective tissue consists of three

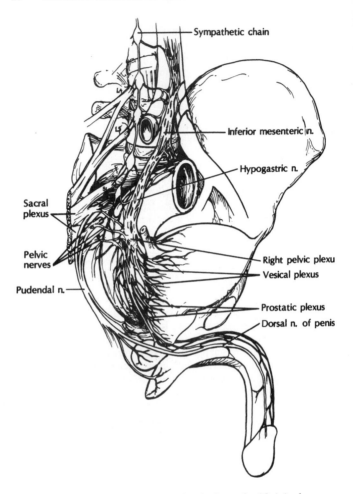

Figure 1-16 Pelvic visceral innervation in the male. (*Original drawing by Christine Young, redrawn from Toldt C: An Atlas of Human Anatomy, vol. 1, 1948, Fig. 1333, p 890.*)

layers or strata: outer, intermediate, and inner (Fig. 1-17). The outer stratum is the investing fascia (transversalis fascia) of the abdominal and pelvic walls. The inner stratum is the supporting connective tissue of the peritoneum. The intermediate stratum (at times termed endopelvic fascia in the pelvis) is the fatty connective tissue that surrounds the retroperitoneal viscera and lies between the inner and outer strata. Gerota's fascia sur-

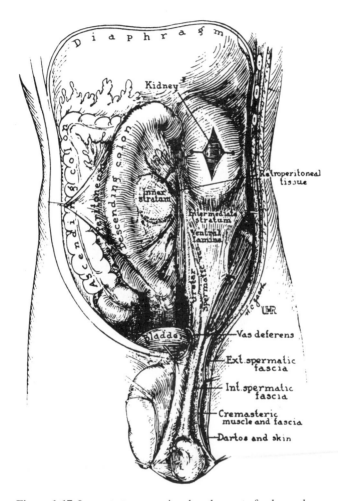

Figure 1-17 Inner stratum covering dorsal aspect of colon and mesentery. Intermediate stratum containing kidney, ureter, and gonadal vessels and extending through the internal ring into the scrotum. (*Reproduced from Tobin CE, Benjamin JA, Wells JC: Surg Gynecol Obstet 83:586, 1946.*)

rounding the kidney and the periureteric sheath are specializations of the layer. Fibrous condensations of the intermediate stratum form "ligaments" and pedicles, such as the uterosacral, cardinal, pubocervical, and pubourethral ligaments in the female and the puboprostatics in the male, and the lateral vesical pedicles.

A further useful concept is that of the fusion fascial planes, which occur where serosal surfaces once apposed each other developmentally, such as where the colon overlies the kidney, ureter, and gonadal vessels or between the rectum and bladder. These planes are readily developed planes of dissection.

VII. SPECIAL REGIONS OF SURGICAL INTEREST

Three anatomic regions of interest to urologists are the perineum, inguinal canal, and femoral triangle.

A. The Perineum

The perineum is generally described as a diamond-shaped area covering the caudal outlet of the bony pelvis with the reference points being the pubis, coccyx, and ischial tuberosities. The diamond, if sectioned along the ischial tuberosities, creates an anterior urogenital and posterior anal triangle.

1. *Urogenital triangle.* The urogenital triangle is marked by the genitalia, which are attached or penetrate it, and, is divided into superficial and deep spaces. The superficial space is the area between the superficial membranous fascia and inferior fascia of the urogenital diaphragm and contains, in the male, the corpus spongiosum, covered by the bulbospongiosus muscle, and the corpora cavernosa, covered by the ischiocavernosus muscle, along with the perineal vessels and nerves. In the female the homologous structures are found. The deep space contains the deep transverse perineal muscles and the sphincter urethrae along with Cowper's glands.

2. *Anal triangle.* The anal triangle is marked by the centrally located anus surrounded by the external anal sphincter, which connects to the central body of the perineum anteriorly, which is located midway between the ischial tuberosities.

B. Inguinal Canal

The inguinal canal, which in the male is traversed by the spermatic cord and in the female by the round ligament, on cross section is noted to have three sides: an anterior side formed by the external oblique aponeurosis, which in the medial third is replaced by the external spermatic fascia; a posterior side formed by the transversus aponeurosis and transversalis fascia; and an inferior side formed by the inguinal ligament. The posterior side or transversalis fascia is reinforced by three fibrous structures: the iliopubic tract, transversus aponeurosis, and Henle's ligament (Fig. 1-18).

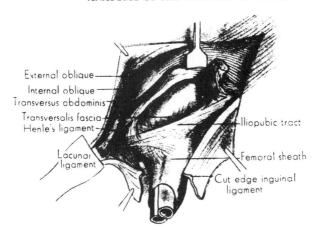

Figure 1-18 Floor of the inguinal canal. (*Reproduced from Clark JF, Hashimoto EI: Utilization of Henles ligament: Iliopubic tract, aponeurosis transversus abdominis and Coopers ligament in inguinal herniorrhaphy. Surg Gynecol Obstet 82, 1946, Fig. 5, p 482.*)

The iliopubic tract is a fibrous thickening of the transversalis fascia. which parallels the inguinal ligament. Henle's ligament is a thin, lateral expansion of the rectus sheath.

1. *The femoral triangle.* Familiarity with the femoral or Scarpa's triangle is a requisite for performing superficial and deep inguinal node dissections (Fig. 1-19). The boundaries are a base formed by the inguinal ligament, a lateral side formed by the sartorius muscle, and a medial side formed by the abductor longus. The floor is formed from medial to lateral by the pectineus, psoas, and iliacus muscles. The femoral vein, artery, and nerve are, from medial to lateral, found on the floor of the femoral triangle emerging from under the inguinal ligament enroute to the lower extremity. The vessels are encased in the fibrous femoral sheath, which is contiguous with the transversalis fascia above. The femoral triangle is covered by the fascia lata, which is fenestrated by the fossa ovalis, through which the superficial external pudendal, superficial inferior epigastric, and superficial circumflex iliac arteries emerge and through which the greater saphenous and superficial veins enter. The lymph nodes deep to the fascia lata are termed the deep inguinals, whereas those superficial to the fascia are the

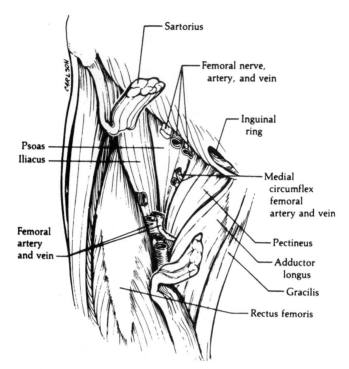

Figure 1-19 Floor of the femoral triangle. (*Reproduced from Johnson DE, Ames FC: Groin Dissection, 1985, Fig. 1-3, p 6.*)

superficial nodes. The highest deep inguinal node, located medial to the femoral vein, is Cloquet's node.

VIII. ADRENAL GLAND
A. Gross Structure
The adrenal glands are thin, cadmium yellow structures located above the kidneys bilaterally. They are contained within the intermediate stratum of retroperitoneal connective tissue surrounded by its specialization of Gerota's fascia. The right adrenal gland has a triangular appearance, whereas the left adrenal gland has a more elongated, leaf-like appearance (Fig. 1-20).
B. Microscopic Anatomy
The adrenal glands are composed of two distinct sections: the outer adrenal cortex, which makes up the bulk of the gland; and the inner adrenal medulla.

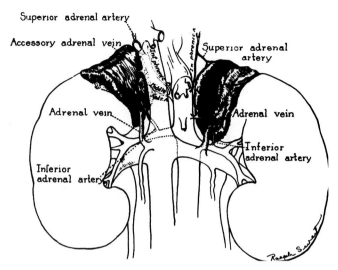

Figure 1-20 Position and morphology of the adrenal glands.
(*Reproduced from Hinman F: Principles and Practice of Urology,
1935, Fig. 127, p 250.*)

Each gland is surrounded by a thin, fibrous capsule. The
adrenal cortex is composed of three distinct layers: an outer
zona glomerulosa, a middle zona fasciculata, and an inner
zona reticularis. The centrally located medulla consists primarily of chromaffin cells.

C. Blood Supply
The adrenal gland is supplied generally by three arteries
that, adjacent to the gland, subdivide into as many as 50
small vessels. An adrenal artery from the renal artery (inferior suprarenal) supplies the lower portion, whereas the
medial aspect is supplied by a branch from the aorta (middle suprarenal). A superior artery derives from the inferior
phrenic artery (superior suprarenal). The venous drainage
on the left side is via the left adrenal vein, which empties
into the left renal artery. On the right side an extremely
short adrenal vein drains directly into the vena cava.

D. Innervation
The innervation of the adrenal gland is to the medulla only
and is by sympathetic outflow via the greater splanchnic
nerve and celiac and aortorenal plexuses.

E. Lymphatics

The lymphatics follow the venous drainage and drain into the lateral aortic lymph nodes.

IX. KIDNEY

A. Anatomy

1. The kidneys are paired, bean-shaped organs located retroperitoneally lateral to the psoas muscle. This position is somewhat oblique, with the lower pole of the kidney displaced lateral to the muscle. The kidney is a relatively large organ in the adult, measuring approximately 11.5 cm in length, 6 cm in width, and 2.5 to 3 cm in thickness. Near the center of the medial convex border of the kidney is a shallow depression, the hilum, through which the renal vasculature, nerves, lymphatics, and renal pelvis pass. The interior of the kidney is a space called the renal sinus and is occupied by the major renal collecting structures, minor calyces, major calyces, pelvis, the larger renal vasculature, and fat (Fig. 1-21).

2. The kidneys, along with the adrenal gland, are encased in retroperitoneal connective tissue (Fig. 1-17), which is thickened around the kidney to form Gerota's fascia. The fatty tissue that is external to Gerota's fascia is known as paranephric fat, whereas that within Gerota's fascia is known as perinephric fat. Posterior to the kidney the fatty layer is thick, whereas anterior to it, it is relatively thin. Although these coverings by other organs do not directly encroach on the kidneys, knowledge of the organ relationships to the kidneys is of clinical significance. The right lobe of the liver, the descending duodenum, and the hepatic flexure of the colon are in proximity to the right side of the kidney. The stomach, spleen, splenic flexure of the colon, pancreas, and jejunum are close to the left side of the kidney (Fig. 1-22).

3. If the kidney is sectioned sagittally, it will be noted that it is covered by a thick renal capsule that is penetrated by capsular vessels. The substance of the kidney as usually seen is divided into cortex and medulla. The cortical tissue that extends to the renal sinus between the pyramids is known as columns of Bertin (Fig. 1-21). The medulla is composed of pyramids that end in papillae that terminate in minor calyces or drain into the pelvis of the kidney itself.

B. Renal Blood Supply

1. Because the major function of the kidney is to regulate the composition and volume of the blood, the vasculature of the kidney is most important.

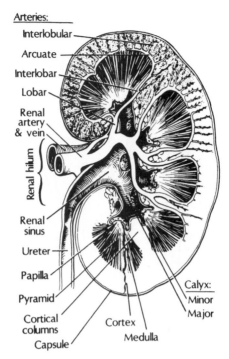

Arteries:
- Interlobular
- Arcuate
- Interlobar
- Lobar
- Renal artery & vein
- Renal hilum
- Renal sinus
- Ureter
- Papilla
- Pyramid
- Cortical columns
- Capsule
- Cortex
- Medulla

Calyx:
- Minor
- Major

Figure 1-21 Longitudinal section of left kidney showing major structural detail. (*Reproduced from Redman JF: Anatomy of the Genitourinary System. In: Adult and Pediatric Urology, 2d ed, vol. 1, 1991, Fig. 1-36, p 25.*)

2. Both renal arteries transport approximately one fourth of the total cardiac output. Although there may be great variation in renal vasculature, a general pattern is noted. It should be stated that renal arteries are end-arteries and the more proximal that a renal artery is occluded, the greater the amount of tissue that will be devascularized. Basically, the renal artery is a single, large artery, although there may be two or more arising from the lateral aspect of the aorta just caudal to the superior mesenteric artery. Prior to entering the renal hilum, the artery branches into anterior and posterior divisions. The arteries are found posterior to the renal vein and anterior to the renal pelvis. The posterior division of the renal artery generally does not branch until it enters the renal substance and supplies the posterior segment of the

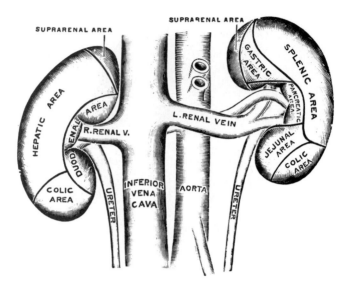

Figure 1-22 Position of visceral relationships of kidney. (*Reproduced from Gray H: Anatomy of the Human Body, 29th ed, 1973, Fig. 17-17, p 1279.*)

kidney. The anterior division divides into three or four branches and provides superior, anterior, and inferior segmental arteries and usually an apical artery. The kidney is thus considered to be divided into superior, anterior, inferior, and apical segments. Within the substance of the kidney, the arteries branch into interlobar, arcuate, and interlobular arteries.

3. The veins generally accompany the arteries. They differ from the arteries in that they intercommunicate; thus, if an intrarenal vein is ligated, the segment drained by the vein will drain through another venous channel. On the posterolateral surface of the kidney, a whitish depression known as Brodel's white line will be noted. This line does not represent a vascular plane but instead is the line of division between the anterior and posterior rows of pyramids. The left renal vein is unique in that two major branches enter it; cranially the venous drainage of the left adrenal and caudally the left ovarian or spermatic vein.

C. Microscopic Anatomy
1. In general, the cortex of the kidney is composed of nephrons, whereas the medulla is composed primarily

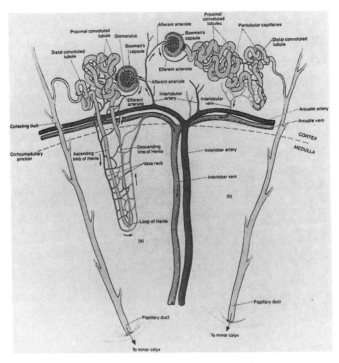

Figure 1-23 Schematic representation of the nephron and its vasculature. (*Reproduced from Woodburne RT: Essentials of Human Anatomy, 6th ed, 1978, Fig. 359, p 439.*)

of collecting ducts. The primary functioning unit of the kidney is the nephron, which consists of the renal corpuscle and the collecting tubules (Fig. 1-23). The renal corpuscle consists of Bowman's capsule and the glomerulus; the proximal tubule, which has convoluted and straight portions; the loop of Henle; a distal tubule, which has a straight portion with a specialized portion adjacent to the glomerulus called the macula densa and a convoluted portion; and a collecting duct.

2. The glomerulus or capillary tuft, which fits within Bowman's capsule, is fed by an afferent arteriole that arises from the interlobular artery. Blood is drained from the capillary tuft by an efferent arteriole that then supplies blood to the remainder of the nephron through peritubular capillaries. Long loops of vessels called the vasa recta also proceed alongside the loop of Henle. Peritubular capillaries eventually form interlobar veins,

draining through arcuate veins to the interlobar veins and then to the segmental veins. Bowman's capsule itself consists of two layers as if the balloon-shaped end of the nephron had been invaginated by the glomerular tuft (Fig. 1-24). The outer layer is called the parietal layer and is composed of simple squamous epithelium. The visceral layer consists of epithelial cells that are called podocytes. These foot processes give off smaller processes, termed pedicels, which cover the endothelial pores. The space between the visceral and parietal layers of epithelium is known as Bowman's space and is contiguous with the lumen of the proximal convoluted tubule.

3. The proximal convoluted tubule is the longest part of the nephron. Its wall consists of cuboidal epithelium that is covered by microvilli.

4. The descending, or thin, limb of Henle's loop descends into the medulla, proceeding in hairpin fashion. The ascending, or thick, limb of Henle's loop is thicker in diameter and consists of cuboidal and columnar epithelium.

5. The ascending limb becomes convoluted as it reaches the cortex and is known as the distal convoluted tubule, being lined by cuboidal epithelium. The distal tubule terminates in a straight collecting duct that passes through the renal pyramid and opens into the papillae in a terminal duct of Bellini.

6. Although the distal convoluted tubule is so termed because of its distance from Bowman's space, it also lies adjacent to the afferent arteriole. This particular closeness modifies cells of both the afferent arteriole and the distal convoluted tubule. The modified smooth muscle cells of the tunica media of the afferent arteriole are known as juxtaglomerular cells. A modification of the cells of the distal convoluted tubule is known as the macula densa. Together these modified cells are collectively known as the juxtaglomerular apparatus. There are two type of nephrons: cortical nephrons, in which the glomerulus and the remainder of the nephron are contained wholly within the cortex; and juxtamedullary nephrons, in which the glomerulus is close to the cortical medullar junction with the other parts of the nephron being found within the substance of the medulla.

D. Innervation

The renal nerve supply is derived from the renal plexus of the autonomic nervous system, which overlies the aorta just

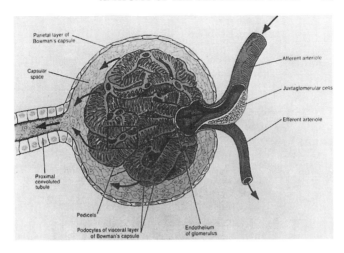

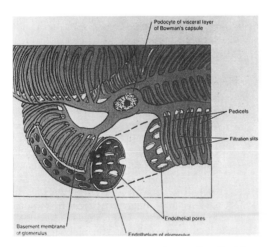

Figure 1-24 A. Anatomy of the glomerulus. B. Detail of Bowman's capsule. (Reproduced from Tortora GJ, Anagnostakos NP: Principles of Anatomy and Physiology 3d ed, 1981, Fig. 26-42, p 673.)

cranial to the renal arteries and originates as preganglionic fibers in the twelfth thoracic and upper lumbar segments. The nerves accompany the renal arteries and enter the kidney at the hilum and continue along the course of the vessels. The synapses occur in the renal ganglion. Parasympathetic innervation is from the vagus.

E. Lymphatics

The lymphatic vessels of the kidney are in the form of three plexuses located within the substance of the kidney, beneath the fibrous capsule, and in the perinephric fat. The latter two communicate freely. The lymphatics from the intrarenal plexus join to form larger lymphatic trunks that exit at the hilum and follow the course of the renal vasculature to drain into the para-aortic nodes.

X. CALYCES, RENAL PELVIS, AND URETER

A. Gross Structure

1. The major collecting structures of the urinary tract begin at the renal papillae. The collecting part itself is termed a minor calyx, which number from 7 to 13. Each calyx may enclose more than one papilla. The calyces are connected by necks, termed infundibula, to form two to three major calyces that coalesce to form the funnel-shaped renal pelvis.

2. The ureters are approximately 25 to 30 cm in length and extend from the renal pelvis to the bladder. For discussion, the ureter may be divided into abdominal and pelvic portions. The ureters from the renal pelvis to the bladder are contained within the intermediate stratum of retroperitoneal connective tissue. The pelvic portion of the ureter is located dorsal to the obliterated umbilical artery (medial umbilical ligament) and the vascular leash proceeding to the bladder. In females the uterine artery crosses ventral to the ureter, as does the vas deferens in the male. The three areas of relative narrowing of the ureter are the ureteropelvic junction, the site of crossing of the iliac vessels, and the ureterovesical junction.

B. Microscopic Anatomy

On cross-section, the ureter appears to be composed of three layers. The body of the ureter is surrounded by the intermediate stratum of retroperitoneal connective tissue and its specialized thickening, the periureteric sheath. The innermost portion of the ureter is mucosa that is composed of transitional epithelium. The bulk of the wall of the ureter is composed of muscularis that is generally said to be composed of inner longitudinal and outer circular layers. The differentiation between the two layers is not so pronounced because they tend to run obliquely and mesh together. In the terminal portion of the ureter the muscularis is primarily longitudinal. At the ureterovesical juncture itself the bladder musculature reflects onto the ureter and is separated from the ureteric musculature by loose connective tissue that has been termed Waldeyer's sheath.

C. **Blood Supply**

The ureteric blood supply is predominantly longitudinal but derives from several adjacent structures. The renal calyces, pelvis, and upper ureter derive their blood supply from the renal arteries. The midportion of the ureter may receive blood from the gonadal vessels. The more distal portions of the ureter are supplied from the aorta near its bifurcation, the common iliacs, internal iliacs, and ureteric branches of the superior and inferior vesical arteries. In the female, blood supply may be derived also from the uterine artery. The venous drainage accompanies the arterial supply.

D. **Innervation**

Innervation is autonomic and derives from the inferior mesenteric, testicular, and pelvic plexuses. The afferent supply of the ureter is contained in the thoracic nerves XI and XII and first lumbar nerves. Nerves basically follow the course of the blood vessels to the ureter.

E. **Lymphatics**

The lymphatic drainage of the ureter generally accompanies the arteries and thus drain to nodes adjacent to the renal artery in the upper portion. In the mid-portion, drainage is to the aortic nodes and in the terminal portion, to the internal iliac nodes.

XI. **BLADDER**

A. **General**

The urinary bladder is a hollow, tetrahedron-shaped, muscular organ that, when filled with urine, is spherical; its shape has great variability, however, depending on its degree of filling. In the adult it is basically a pelvic organ, whereas in the child, it occupies a more abdominal position. It is described as having four surfaces: superior, two inferolateral, and posterior or basal. The superior surface of the bladder is covered by peritoneum. The posterior surface of the bladder, or base of the bladder, lies on the ventral aspect of the rectum in the male and on the vagina in the female. The remainder of the bladder is surrounded by intermediate stratum of retroperitoneal connective tissue. The potential space between the ventral surface of the bladder and the pubis has been termed the retropubic or Retzius space. The apex of the bladder is connected to the umbilicus by a fibrous cord termed the urachus or median umbilical ligament. On either side of the median umbilical ligament are two other fibrous ligaments, called the medial umbilical ligaments, which are the obliterated umbilical arteries. In the male the base of the bladder is supported by the prostate and a condensation of intermediate stratum that bridges the pubis and bladder, termed the puboprostatic ligaments. A similar condensation of endopelvic fascia, termed the pubovesical or pubourethral ligament, is located in the female. In the male, the seminal vesicles lie between the base of the bladder and rectum and more medially, the ampulla of the vas deferens.

B. Gross Anatomy

In most general descriptions of gross anatomy of the bladder wall, three muscular layers are noted: outer longitudinal, middle circular, and inner longitudinal. It is probable that the arrangement most closely approaches a meshwork of musculature (Fig. 1-25). Although an internal sphincter is frequently spoken of, a ring of musculature as such does not exist (Fig. 1-26). Instead, a prominent detrusor band is noted that thickens toward the prostate as it progresses caudally where it divides and spreads around the neck of the bladder and base of the prostate. A further bundle of musculature that progresses from the anterior vesical neck posteriorly has been termed the bundle of Heiss. Over the inner musculature of the bladder is a well-developed mucosal layer that is composed primarily of transitional epithelium supported by a lamina propria. The trigone is the triangle-shaped internal base of the bladder. It is formed by the ureteric musculature as it both crosses the midline to blend with the ureteric muscle of the opposite side and spreads toward the vesical neck. The muscular band that forms the base of the trigone is termed the interureteric ridge. The ureteral orifices themselves appear slit-like, the appearance varying with the site of entrance of the ureter into the bladder.

C. Blood Supply

The arterial supply of the bladder is derived primarily from the internal iliac artery; it further branches to supply a superior artery and an inferior vesical artery. The upper portion of the bladder is supplied by the superior vesical artery, a branch of the umbilical artery, whereas the caudal portion of the bladder is supplied by the inferior vesical artery and at times the obturator or inferior gluteal arteries. In the female, uterine and vaginal arteries may also supply the bladder. The venous drainage does not follow the arteries but forms a complicated plexus primarily on the inferior surface and base of the bladder. The venous drainage terminates in the internal iliac veins.

D. Innervation

The bladder per se is innervated by the vesical plexus, which is a portion of the pelvic plexus located on the lateral aspects of the rectum. Sympathetic innervation is derived

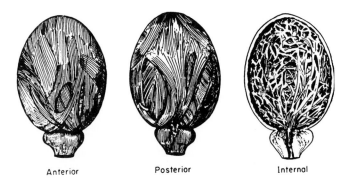

Anterior   Posterior   Internal

Figure 1-25 Detail of bladder musculature. (*Reproduced from Woodburne RT: J Urol 100, 1968, Fig. 6, p 479.*)

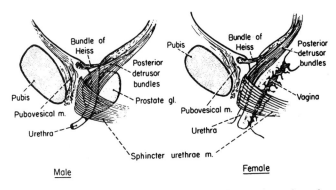

Male   Female

Figure 1-26 Detail of vesical neck and urethral musculature in males and females. (*Reproduced from Woodburne RT: J Urol 100, 1968, Fig. 10, p 482.*)

from the T10 to L2 cord segments, whereas parasympathetic innervation derived from the S2–S4 spinal cord segments reaches the pelvic plexus via the pelvic splanchnic nerves. The detrusor is primarily supplied by parasympathetic nerves, whereas the bladder neck receives sympathetic innervation in the male, in contrast to parasympathetic supply in the female. The urethral sphincter is supplied by the pelvic splanchnic nerves.

E. Lymphatics

The bladder wall is rich in lymphatics. The lymphatics intercommunicate and drain into the vesical, internal iliac, external iliac, and common iliac lymph nodes.

XII. PROSTATE

A. General

The prostate is a chestnut-shaped glandular structure that lies between the neck of the bladder and the external sphincter. It is traversed throughout its length by the posterior urethra and is fixed to the pelvic floor by investments of the transversalis fascia and intermediate stratum. Two dense condensations of the intermediate stratum that affix the prostate to the pubis are the puboprostatic ligaments. The prostate is encased in the intermediate stratum of retroperitoneal connective tissue that contains a rich plexus of veins that are received from the dorsal vein of the penis beneath the pubic symphysis. Posteriorly, the prostate is separated from the rectum by Denonvilliers' fascia.

B. Gross Anatomy

The prostate is covered by a firm fibrous capsule. It comprises of four glandular regions or zones that are more or less easily noted on ultrasonic examination of the prostate (Fig. 1-27). They include the peripheral, central, and transition zones and the periurethral region. The bulk of the gland is composed of the peripheral zone, which makes up 75 percent of the volume of the glandular prostate, whereas the central zone constitutes 25 percent. The posterior aspect of the prostate is traversed by the terminal portions of the vas deferens, which exit in the ejaculatory ducts in the posterior urethra. The posterior urethra, which traverses the prostate, houses a small mound on its dorsal aspect, termed the verumontanum. In the middle portion of the verumontanum is a small pit, the utricle. The ejaculatory ducts exit on the verumontanum.

C. Microscopic Anatomy

On cross-section, the prostate is encased in a fibrous capsule. Its glandular structure resembles a sponge with the major ducts of the gland exiting into the floor of the urethra. The glands, which are surrounded by fibromuscular stroma, are distributed into external and periurethral glands, of which the external glands are the predominant glandular structures of the prostate.

D. Blood Supply

Primary vascularization of the prostate is from the prostatic artery, which derives from the inferior vesical artery. Two main groups of arteries occur, capsular and urethral. Some accessory vessels to the prostate are supplied from the middle hemorrhoidal and internal pudendal arteries. The venous drainage of the prostate is through a prostatic

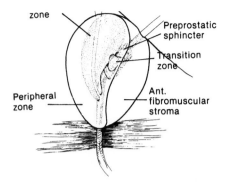

Figure 1-27 Schematic representation of prostatic zones. (*Reproduced from Tanagho EA: Anatomy and Surgical Approach to the Urogenital Tract. In: Campbell's Urology, 5th ed, vol. 1, 1986, Fig. 1-73, p 62.*)

plexus that joins the venous drainage of the penis in Santorini's plexus and then drains into the hypogastric veins. It is of note that the prostatic plexus connects with the prevertebral veins (Batson's plexus).

E. Innervation
Innervation of the prostate is via the pelvic plexus, with parasympathetic innervation deriving from the pelvic splanchnic nerves and sympathetics deriving from the hypogastric nerve.

F. Lymphatics
Prostatic lymphatics drain primarily to the internal thac nodal chains with posterior drainage to presacral lymph nodes.

XIII. URETHRA
A. Male Urethra
1. In the male the urethra runs from the vesical neck to the tip of the penis (Fig. 1-28). It is generally divided into two portions, posterior and anterior. The posterior urethra is that portion that transverses the prostate. The anterior urethra may be divided into three parts: bulbous, pendulous or penile, and glanular. The urethra itself is contained within an erectile body, termed the corpus spongiosum, which is held to the corpora cavernosa of the penis by Buck's fascia. Numerous mucous glands, the urethral glands, open into the lumen.

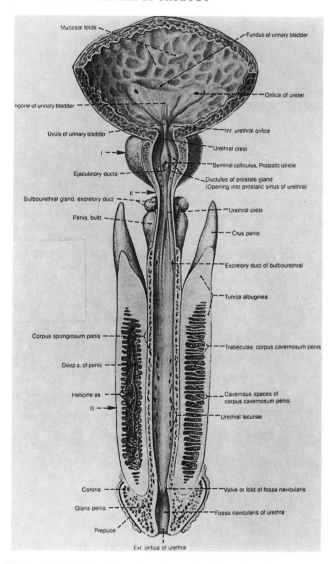

Figure 1-28 Relationships of urethra to bladder and penis. (*Reproduced from Ferner H, Staubesand J: Sobotta Atlas of Human Anatomy, vol. 2, 1983, p 193.*)

2. The posterior urethra is lined by transitional epithelium, whereas the major portion of the anterior urethra is lined by stratified columnar epithelium. As it passes through the glans, the urethra is dilated to form the fossa navicularis, which is lined by squamous epithelium.

3. The blood supply to the anterior urethra is from a branch of the pudendal artery, the bulbourethral artery.

4. The lymphatic drainage of the deep urethra is to the internal iliac lymph nodes. Drainage of the anterior urethra is to the superior and deep inguinal nodes and external iliac nodes.

B. Female Urethra

The female urethra is related on its dorsal aspect closely to the ventral aspect of the vagina. Its position in relation to the bladder is somewhat analogous to the posterior urethra in the male. It is also lined by transitional epithelium.

XIV. ENDOSCOPIC ANATOMY

Although endoscopy of body passages and cavities has burgeoned over the past several years, urology was one of the first fields to incorporate this examination modality. Although much of the urinary collecting structures can be negotiated and visualized, the most frequently visualized is the lower tract, which may be examined with a variety of rigid and flexible endoscopes.

On negotiation of the urethra from the meatus to the bladder neck, three fusiform dilatations of the urethra are noted. The most distal is the fossa navicularis as the scope passes through the glans penis. Within the fossa navicularis there are several small pits known as lacunae. The large one in the midline is known as lacuna magna. On the floor of the urethra are noted numerous small orifices that represent the orifices of the urethral or Littre's glands. The second dilatation of the urethra is the bulbous urethra. After negotiating the bulbous urethra, the bellows-like membranous portion of the urethra is noted. This represents the passage of the urethra through the urogenital diaphragm and marks the beginning of the posterior urethra. On the floor of the urethra and almost in its central portion is the verumontanum. In the central portion of the verumontanum is noted the pit-like utricle. On either side the ejaculatory ducts may varyingly be noted. The vesical neck is noted just ahead. With enlargement of the prostate, large lobes of hyperplasia may encroach laterally and a median lobe may be noticed that requires deflection of the endoscope upward to go over the lobe into the bladder. The trigone is noted on the floor of the bladder, with the orifices forming apices of the base of the triangle and the base itself being the interureteric ridge. The underlying detrusor under the mucosa gives a grid-like appearance to the wall of the bladder. With hypertrophy of the detrusor, frank trabeculations may be seen. With protrusion of the mucosa through these trabeculations, cellules or even diverticula may be formed.

XV. TESTIS AND EPIDIDYMIS
A. General

The testes are paired ovoid structures that measure 4.5 cm in length, 3 cm in width, and 2 cm in depth (Fig. 1-29). Adjacent to the testicle on its posterior aspect is an elongated structure, termed the epididymis. The testes reside dependently in the scrotum, which is divided into two compartments, with their long axis being vertical. The contents of the scrotum are comprised of investments of the testis and its epididymis. Immediately adjacent to the anterolateral aspects of the testis is the remnant of the patent processes vaginalis, termed the visceral and parietal layers of tunica vaginalis, which encompasses threefourths of the anterolateral aspects of the testis and epididymis. Surrounding these structures is the internal spermatic fascia, which is contiguous with the transversalis fascia of the abdominal wall. This is covered by the cremasteric muscle and fascia contiguous with the internal oblique musculature. This in turn is covered by the external spermatic fascia, which is contiguous with the investing fascia of the external oblique aponeurosis. The testicular and spermatic cord investments are covered by the dartos tunic of the scrotum, which is contiguous with the superficial membranous fascia (Scarpa's fascia of the anterior abdominal wall, Colles' fascia of the perineum, and the Dartos tunic of the penis).

B. Gross Anatomy

The testis is surrounded by a dense fibrous covering, the tunica albuginea. On longitudinal section the testis is seen to be divided by fibrous septa into approximately 250 lobules (Fig. 1-29). Each lobule contains one to three convoluted seminiferous tubules that coalesce to form straight seminiferous tubules that then join at the hilum of the testis to a network of tubules called the rete testis. The rete testis in turn drains into the efferent ductules in the epididymis and thus forms a single convoluted ductus of the epididymis that in turn forms the lumen of the ductus deferens. The cranial portion of the epididymis is known as the globus major or head of the epididymis. The caudal portion of the epididymis before it turns to become the vas deferens is known as the tail of the epididymis or globus minor. Vesti-

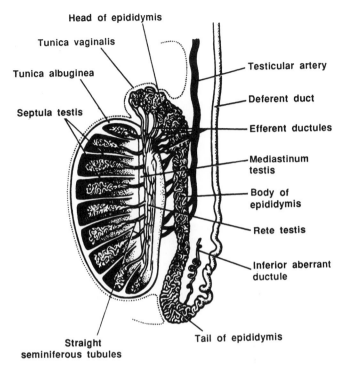

Figure 1-29 Schematic representation of longitudinal section of testis along with epididymis and vas deferens. (*Reproduced from Gray H: Gray's Anatomy, 36th British ed., 1980, Fig. 8.166, p 1411.*)

gial appendages are noted on the cranial aspect of the testis and head of the epididymis. These are known, respectively, as the appendix testis and appendix epididymis.

C. Microscopic Anatomy

The bulk of the testis is composed of the seminiferous tubules. The tubules consist of a basement membrane lined with a relatively thick layer of germinal cells that progress from primary spermatocytes to mature spermatozoa. Between the developing germ cells on the base of the tubule are Sertoli's (supporting) cells. Between the seminiferous tubules are clusters of Leydig's cells. The ductus epididymis is lined with a pseudo-stratified columnar epithelium. Its wall contains smooth muscle.

D. Blood Supply

Blood supply to the testicle is by the internal spermatic artery, which arises from the aorta near the ventral midline just caudal to the take-off of the renal arteries. The arteries pass through the retroperitoneal connective tissue, the internal ring, and down the inguinal canal to the testicle. Additional arterial supply to the testicle is by the vasal artery, which is derived from the superior vesical artery. Its return is by a plexus of veins, the pampiniform plexus, which coalesce to form a single gonadal vein. The gonadal vein on the right enters the vena cave obliquely, usually with a valve. On the left side the gonadal vein enters the left renal vein, usually without a valve.

E. Lymphatics

The lymphatic drainage of the testes accompanies the blood supply and drains to para-aortic lymph nodes that are located primarily between the renal vessels and the bifurcation of the aorta.

XVI. VAS DEFERENS AND SEMINAL VESICLES

From the internal ring the vas proceeds extraperitoneally, posteriorly, and medially. It passes between the ureter and behind the base of the bladder, where it becomes dilated and tortuous for several centimeters. This is termed the ampulla of the ductus deferens. The vas terminates in the ejaculatory ducts, which open into the prostatic urethra on either side of the utricle on the verumontanum. A large diverticulum, the seminal vesicle of the vas deferens, has its juncture adjacent to the ampulla of the vas near the ejaculatory ducts just above the base of the prostate (Fig. 1-30). Approximately 6 cm long, they are lobulated in appearance. Histologically, they are lined by pseudostratified epithelium. The wall is composed of thin circular longitudinal smooth muscle.

XVII. PENIS

A. Gross Structure

The penis is comprised of three erectile bodies: paired corpora cavernosa and the corpus spongiosum, which contains the urethra (Fig. 1-31). The cylindrical corpora cavernosa invaginate the glans distally. Proximally they diverge at the level of the pubic symphysis to end as the crura of the penis where they are attached to the inferior pubic rami by a fibrous extension of Buck's fascia, termed the suspensory ligament. The corpus spongiosum is in direct contact with the glans penis, and indeed the structures appear similar in composition. At the divergence of the corpora cavernosa, the corpus spongiosum becomes more dilated and is known

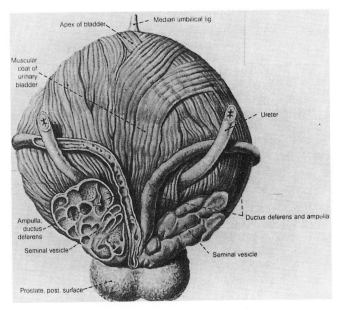

Apex of bladder
Median umbilical lig.
Muscular coat of urinary bladder
Ureter
Ampulla, ductus deferens
Ductus deferens and ampulla
Seminal vesicle
Seminal vesicle
Prostate, post. surface

Figure 1-30 Bladder and prostate viewed posteriorly showing relationships of seminal vesicles and ampulla of vas (*Reproduced from Ferner H, Staubesand J: Sobotta Atlas of Human Anatomy, vol. 2, 1983, p 189.*)

as the bulbous portion of the corpus spongiosum. On cross-section it will be noted that the corpora cavernosa and corpus spongiosum are held together as a single bundle by a dense fascia known as Buck's fascia. Covering Buck's fascia is the dartos tunic, which is in turn covered by skin.

B. Arterial Supply

The penis derives its blood supply from the internal pudendal artery, which branches at the bulb to form an artery to the bulb. The remainder of the penis is supplied by the deep artery of the penis, which runs the length of the corpora cavernosa through the center of the erectile body. The dorsal artery of the penis runs distally on the dorsum of the penis deep to Buck's fascia. Superficial blood supply to the penis is also supplied from the external pudendal artery. The venous drainage is by the deep dorsal vein that passes beneath the pubic arch and the cavernosal veins that drain from the proximal ends of the corpora cavernosa.

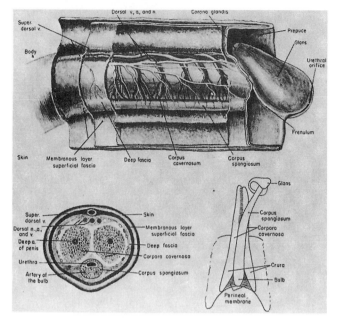

Figure 1-31 Gross anatomy of the penis. (*Reproduced from Crafts RC: A Textbook of Human Anatomy, 2d ed., 1979, p 324.*)

C. Innervation

The nerve supply generally accompanies the vessels. The innervation to the skin and fascia is by the dorsal nerve of the penis, which is a branch of the pudendal nerve. Branches of the perineal nerve, ilioinguinal nerve, and perineal branches of the posterior femoral cutaneous nerve of the thigh supply additional innervation. Sympathetic nerve supply is via the pelvic plexus supplies the corpora cavernosa.

D. Lymphatics

Superficial and deep groups of lymphatics drain to the superficial and deep inguinal lymph nodes and from there to the external iliac lymph nodes.

XVIII. APPLIED ANATOMY

The ultimate anatomic challenge for the clinical urologist is to accurately expose the structures of the genitourinary tract without inadvertent damage to any other structure of the body. Anatomy that seems so clear in illustrations may be hopelessly obfuscated through a small developing incision. In an effort to ease the transition from textbook anatomy to applied anatomy, the following short review of incisional anatomy is included.

A useful rule in selecting an incision is to carefully consider the area of surgical interest and plan for the center of interest to lie in the center of the ultimately fully developed incision. This requires a knowledge of bony and fascial landmarks and their relationship to the underlying structures. Actually marking landmarks on the skin and tracing the position of the underlying organs is a most useful way to accurately plan an incision.

A. Extraperitoneal Upper Abdominal and Flank Incisions

Upper abdominal incisions may be either transverse or oblique. Further, incisions may include the partial excision of a rib and its costal cartilage or may be cut between the ribs, even purposely incising the pleura. The most important decision to be made is whether or not to incise the intercostal nerves. The largest nerves to be encountered are the anterior cutaneous branches of the intercostal nerves which course, for the most part, transversly between the internal oblique and tranversus abdominis muscles. Markedly oblique incisions will undoubtedly result in damage to these nerves.

The identification of the layers of the oblique and transversus abdominis muscles is relatively easy, however, the separation of the transversalis fascia from the underlying intermediate stratum of retroperitoneal connective tissue requires care. Paying close attention to the interface and realizing that from the lateral border of the medial aponeurosis of the external oblique to the linea alba the peritoneum is only slightly separated from the transversalis fascia. A good dissection can be made by freeing the abdominal wall from the underlying viscera almost to the midline of the abdomen exposing a broad expanse of the retroperitoneum.

The peritoneum itself may be disected free from the underlying Gerota's fascia and from the gonadal vessels and ureter which are contained in the intermediate stratum of retroperitoneal connective tissue by persuing the fusion fascical plane. The plane is most easily approached by locating the lateral edge of the Gerota's fascia, which appears white against the fat of the colonic mesentery. An incision along this line in the overlying outer limiting membrane of the intermediate stratum is necessary to separate Gerota's fascia from the colonic mesentery. This plane, once developed, can be pursued over the renal vessels and over the anterior surface of the adrenal gland. A useful guide in the dissection caudal to the lower pole of the kidney is that the ureter and gonadal vessels will be encased in the fat that is being separated from the colon and the colonic mesentery. A further useful point is that dorsally the ureter will always be found in the dorsal aspects of the intermediate stratum of retroperitoneal connective tissue as it is being separated from the quadratus lumborum and psoas major muscles.

B. Anterior Transperitoneal Incisions

Transperitoneal incisions can be transverse, oblique or midline. Midline and transverse incisions will be the least damaging to the intercostal nerves. Access to the retroperitoneum involves an incision of the dorsal peritoneum which occurs along the peritoneal reflections. The most common approach to the kidney is to incise the peritoneum along the lateral borders of the ascending or descending colon (Toldt's white line). An incision on the right side along the root of the mesentery will allow for the elevation of all of the small bowel as well as the ascending colon for full exposure of the right side of the retroperitoneum. Similarly, an incision of the phrenicocolic ligament at the splenic flexure of the colon will allow for exposure of the left kidney and the retroperitoneum. Incision of the peritoneal reflections of the liver on the right side (triangular and coronary ligaments) will allow for medial reflection of the liver to visualize the adrenal gland and suprarenal vena cava.

C. Lower Abdominal Extraperitoneal Incisions

Lower abdominal incisions are developed as described for upper abdominal incisions. Transverse (Pfannenstiel) or midline incisions have in common an incision in the anterior rectus sheath followed by a separation of the rectus abdominis muscles. Dorsal to the rectus muscles the transversalis fascia is encountered caudal to the arcuate line, which may be reinforced, in many instances, almost to the symphysis pubis by investments from the transversus abdominis aponeurosis. In adults an incision in the transversalis fascia in the midline risks entrance into the peritoneum, and, therefore, an incision made near the lateral border of the rectus muscles will usually provide an easier separation of the transversalis fascia from the intermediate stratum, which gives good exposure of the pelvic side wall. Separation of the peritoneum from the spermatic cord or severance of the round ligament at the level of the internal ring allows the peritoneum and its contents to be completely swept cranially from the iliac vessels and lateral aspects of the bladder and pelvic side walls.

D. Extraperitoneal Exposure of the Terminal One Fourth of the Ureter

The terminal one fourth of the ureter is not immediately visualized in the pelvis, however, it can be quickly visualized if the surgeon remembers that the ureter lies immediately dorsal to the origin of the umbilical artery. The guide to the umbilical artery is the obliterated umbilical artery or medial umbilical ligament. The ligament may be ligated or simply identified and the underlying outer limiting membrane of the intermediate stratum of retroperitoneal connective tissue incised. The bladder and the peritoneum are then rolled medially and the ureter is identified along the peritoneum or lateral wall of the bladder.

E. Inguinal Incisions

The inguinal canal may be approached through an oblique or transverse incision. It is useful to remember that the inguinal canal lies just lateral and cranial to the pubic tubercle and just above the inguinal crease. Continuation of the incision of the external oblique aponeurosis through the external ring and also the external spermatic fascia will ultimately allow for the testes to be introduced into the canal by traction on the cord.

BIBLIOGRAPHY

Crafts RC: *Textbook of Human Anatomy,* 2d ed. New York: Wiley, 1979.

Ferner H, Staubesand J, eds: *Sobotta Atlas of Human Anatomy,* vol. 2. Baltimore: Urban and Schwartzenberg, 1983.

Goss CM, ed: *Anatomy of the Human Body,* 29th ed. Philadelphia: Lea & Febiger, 1973.

Tobin CE, Benjamin JA, Wells JC: Continuity of the fasciae lining the abdomen, pelvis, and spermatic cord. *Surg Gynecol Obstet* 83:586, 1946.

Woodburne RT: *Essentials of Human Anatomy,* 6th ed. New York: Oxford University Press, 1978.

SELF-ASSESSMENT QUESTIONS

1. Describe the composition of the anterior and posterior rectus sheath, cranial and caudal to the arcuate line.
2. Name and identify the position of the zones of the prostate.
3. Give the boundaries of the anterior femoral triangle.
4. Name the three strata of retroperitoneal connective tissue and describe them.
5. Give the divisions and their branches of the internal iliac (hypogastric) artery.
6. Give the ureteric blood supply.
7. Describe the musculature of the posterior and lateral abdominal wall. Give major groups and individual muscles.
8. Describe the blood supply of the penis.

CHAPTER 2

Signs and Symptoms: The Initial Examination

Keith N. Van Arsdalen

I. BACKGROUND

A. Definition

Urology is a surgical specialty devoted to the study and treatment of disorders of the genitourinary tract of the male and the urinary tract of the female. In addition to the surgical correction of acquired and congenital abnormalities, the urologist is often involved with the diagnosis and treatment of many "medical" disorders of the genitourinary tract.

B. Importance to Other Branches of Medicine

1. Approximately 15 percent of patients initially presenting to a physician will have a urologic complaint or abnormality.
2. There is a wide overlap with other specialties and frequent interaction with other physicians, including family practitioners, internists, pediatricians, geriatricians, endocrinologists, nephrologists, neurologists, obstetricians and gynecologists, and general, vascular, and trauma surgeons.
3. It is important that all physicians be aware of the specific diagnostic and therapeutic measures that are available within this specialty.

II. UROLOGIC MANIFESTATIONS OF DISEASE

A. Direct

The most obvious manifestations of urologic disease are those signs and symptoms that are directly related to the urinary tract of the male and female or to the genitalia of the male. Hematuria and scrotal swelling are examples in this category.

B. Manifestations Referred to or from Other Organ Systems

1. Symptoms from the genitourinary tract may be referred to other areas within the genitourinary tract or to contiguous organ systems.

    a. A stone in the kidney or upper ureter may produce ipsilateral testicular pain.

    b. This same stone may be associated with symptoms of nausea and vomiting.

    c. The gastrointestinal tract is probably the most common site to manifest symptoms from primary urologic problems. This is most probably due to the common innervation of these systems as well as the close direct relationship between the various component organs.

2. Primary urologic disorders may also be manifest in different organ systems and by seemingly unrelated signs and symptoms. Bone pain and pathologic fractures secondary to metastatic carcinoma arising in the genitourinary tract are examples.

3. Similarly, primary disease in other organ systems may result in secondary urologic signs and symptoms that initially lead the patient to the urologist. Diabetes may be detected by finding glucosuria in a patient presenting with frequency and nocturia. Other signs and symptoms mimicking urologic disease are related to inflammatory or neoplastic processes arising in the:

    a. Lower lobes of the lungs

    b. Gastrointestinal tract

    c. Female internal genitalia

C. Systemic

Fever, weight loss, and malaise can be nonspecific systemic manifestations of acute and chronic inflammatory disorders, renal failure, and genitourinary carcinoma with or without metastases.

D. Asymptomatic

Finally, it should be remembered that extensive disease may exist within the genitourinary tract without any signs or symptoms being manifest. Large renal calculi or neoplasms may only be found incidentally during other examinations. Far-advanced renal deterioration may occur prior to the detection of silent reflux or obstruction.

III. HISTORY
A. Symptoms

1. A symptom is any departure from normal appearance, function, or sensation as experienced by the patient. Symptoms are reported to the physician or uncovered by careful history taking, with varying degrees of importance and/or significance attached to each symptom by both parties.

    a. The chief complaint, history of the present illness, and past medical history are delineated in a standard fashion.

    b. The character, onset, duration, and progression of the symptom are carefully defined. It is important to note what factors exacerbate or ameliorate the problem.

2. Urologic symptoms are generally related to:

    a. Pain and discomfort

    b. Alterations of micturition

    c. Changes in the gross appearance of the urine

    d. Abnormal appearance and/or function of the external genitalia

B. Pain

1. Pain within the genitourinary tract generally arises from distention or inflammation of a part or parts of the genitourinary system. Pain can be experienced directly in the involved organ or referred as noted above. Referred pain is a relatively common symptom of genitourinary disease.

2. Renal pain

    a. The kidney and its capsule are innervated by sensory fibers traveling to the TI0–LI aspect of the spinal cord.

    b. The etiology of renal pain may be due either to capsular distention or inflammation or to distention of the renal collecting system.

    c. Renal pain can be a dull, aching sensation felt primarily in the area of the costovertebral angle, or pain of a sharp colicky nature felt in the area of the flank, with radiation around the abdomen into the groin and ipsilateral testicle or labium. The latter is due to the common innervation.

    d. The nature of the primary disease process within the kidney often determines the type of sensation that is experienced and depends on the degree and rapidity of capsular and/or collecting system distention.

3. Ureteral pain

    a. The upper ureter is innervated in a similar fashion to that described above for the kidney. Therefore, upper ureteral pain has a similar distribution to that of renal pain.

    b. The lower ureter, however, sends sensory fibers to the cord through ganglia subserving the major pelvic organs. Therefore, pain derived from the lower ureter is generally felt in the suprapubic area, bladder, penis, or urethra.

    c. The most common etiologic mechanism for ureteral pain is sudden obstruction and ureteral distention.

    d. Acute renal and ureteral colic are among the most severe types of pain known to humankind.

4. Bladder pain
   a. Pain within the bladder may be derived from retention of urine and overdistention or from inflammatory processes.
   b. The pain of overdistention is generally felt within the suprapubic area, resulting in severe local discomfort.
   c. The pain due to bladder inflammation is generally felt as a sharp, burning pain that is often referred to the tip of the penile urethra in males and the entire urethra in females.

5. Prostate pain
   a. Sensory fibers from the prostate mostly enter the sacral aspect of the spinal cord.
   b. Prostate pain is most commonly due to acute inflammation and is generally perceived as discomfort in the lower back, rectum, and perineum.
   c. Irritative symptoms arising from the bladder may overshadow the purely prostate symptoms.

6. Penile pain
   a. Penile and urethral pain is generally directly related to a site of inflammation.

7. Scrotal pain
   a. Pain within the scrotum generally arises from disorders of the testis and/or epididymis.
   b. The most common etiologic factors include trauma, torsion of the spermatic cord, torsion of the appendix testis or appendix epididymis, and acute inflammation, particularly epididymitis. The pain in these cases is generally of rapid onset, if not sudden, and severe in nature.
   c. Hydroceles, varicoceles, and testicular tumors can also be associated with scrotal discomfort but are generally of a more insidious nature and less severe in most cases.

C. Alterations of Micturition

1. Definitions and problems
   a. A variety of specific terms have been developed to describe alterations related to the act of micturition. This section defines a variety of these terms.
   b. It must be emphasized that a variety of disease processes can result in similar symptoms at the level of the lower urinary tract, and although these terms are used to describe specific symptoms in this area, they do not necessarily pertain to specific etiologies.

2. Changes in urine volume
   a. *Anuria* and *oliguria* are terms that refer to the varying degrees of decreased urinary output that may be sec-

ondary to prerenal, renal. or postrenal factors. In all cases, it is essential to rule out urethral and/or ureteral obstruction as postrenal causes for these problems.

b. *Polyuria* refers to an increase in the volume of urine excreted on a daily basis. The etiologic mechanisms include increased fluid intake, exogenous or endogenous diuretics, and abnormal states of central or peripheral osmoregulation.

3. Irritative symptoms

a. *Dysuria* is a term that refers simply to painful or difficult urination. The burning sensation that occurs during micturition associated with either bladder, urethral, or prostatic inflammation is generally used synonymously. This discomfort is generally felt in the entire urethra in females and in the distal urethra in males.

b. *Strangury* is a subtype of dysuria in which intense discomfort accompanies frequent voiding of small amounts of urine.

c. *Frequency* refers to the increased number of times one feels the need to urinate. This can be secondary to a true decrease in bladder capacity from a loss of elasticity or edema due to inflammation or secondary to a decrease in the effective bladder capacity due to a failure of the bladder to empty completely with persistence of a large amount of residual urine.

d. *Nocturia* is essentially the nighttime equivalent of urinary frequency, that is, there is a decreased real or effective bladder capacity that forces the patient to arise at night to urinate.

e. *Nycturia* refers to the excretion of larger volumes of urine at night than during the day and is secondary to mobilization of dependent fluid that accumulated when the patient was in the upright position. Nycturia can result in nocturia even in the presence of a normal bladder capacity if large quantities of fluid are mobilized.

f. *Urgency* refers to the sudden, severe urge to void that may or may not be controllable.

g. The irritative symptoms noted above are most commonly associated with inflammation of the lower urinary tract, i.e., the bladder and prostate. Acute bacterial infections probably represent the most common etiologic mechanism. It should be noted, however, that the irritative symptoms may be secondary to the presence of a foreign body, nonspecific inflammation, radiation therapy or chemotherapy, neoplasms, and neurogenic bladder dysfunction.

4. Bladder outlet obstructive symptoms
   a. *Hesitancy* refers to the prolonged interval necessary to voluntarily initiate the urinary stream.
   b. *Straining* refers to the need to increase intra-abdominal pressure in order to initiate voiding.
   c. *Decreased force* and *caliber* of the urinary stream refer to the physical changes of the urinary stream that may be noted due to increased urethral resistance.
   d. *Terminal dribbling* refers to the prolonged dribbling of urine from the meatus after the completion of micturition.
   e. *Sense of residual urine* is the complaint of a sensation of incomplete emptying of the bladder that the patient recognizes after micturition.
   f. *Prostatism.* All of the above symptoms may be noted with any type of bladder outlet obstruction, that is, secondary to benign prostatic hypertrophy, prostate carcinoma, or urethral stricture disease. The most common cause of these symptoms, however, is benign prostatic enlargement, and hence this complex of symptoms has often been referred to as prostatism.
   g. *Urinary retention.* The retention of urine within the bladder may occur on a chronic, gradual basis due to progressive obstruction and bladder decompensation, and large amounts of urine may be retained with minor changes in symptomatology. Acute urinary retention may occur as a complication of chronic urinary retention or de novo. Sudden acute urinary retention may be associated with severe suprapubic discomfort.
   h. *Interruption* of the urinary stream. Sudden painful interruption of the urinary stream can be secondary to the presence of a bladder calculus that ball valves into the bladder neck causing abrupt blockage of the urinary flow.
   i. *Bifurcation* of the urinary stream. The symptom of a double stream or spraying of the urinary stream can be secondary to urethral stricture disease or can occur intermittently without any obvious pathology.
5. Incontinence
   a. *True* or *total incontinence* occurs when there is constant dribbling of urine from the bladder. It may be due to the configuration of the bladder, such as with extrophy or epispadias, to ectopia of the ureteral orifices distal to the bladder neck in females, or to a fistula, usually between the bladder and the vagina. The most common cause, however, is secondary to injury to the sphincter mechanisms of the bladder neck and urethra due to trauma, surgery, or childbirth. Neuro-

genic disorders affecting the bladder outlet can also have similar effects.

b. *False* or *overflow incontinence* is seen with total bladder decompensation where the bladder acts as a fixed reservoir and the only outflow of urine is an overflow phenomenon with constant dribbling through the bladder outlet.

c. *Urgency incontinence* results when the sensation of urgency becomes so severe that involuntary bladder emptying occurs. This is commonly secondary to severe inflammation of the urinary bladder. This type of incontinence can also be due to uninhibited bladder contractions.

d. *Stress incontinence* is secondary to distortion of the normal anatomic relationship between the bladder and the urethra such that sudden increases in intra-abdominal pressure (laughing, straining, etc.) are transmitted unequally to the bladder and the urethra, resulting in elevated bladder pressure without a concomitant rise in urethral pressure. Most commonly, this is related to laxity of the pelvic floor, particularly following childbirth, but it may also be noted in women who have not had children. It is also a frequent sequel of radical prostatectomy surgery for prostate cancer.

e. It is important to differentiate the various types of incontinence as each is treated differently. Historical factors are very important in separating these different entities.

6. *Enuresis* refers to involuntary urination and bed-wetting that occurs during sleep.

7. Quantification of voiding symptoms.

a. The AUA Symptom Index (internationally known as the IPSS) is a self-administered questionnaire consisting of seven questions relating to symptoms of prostatism (Table 2-1).

b. Symptoms are classified as mild (0–7), moderate (8–19), or severe (20–35).

c. The symptom score is an integral part of the clinical practice guidelines for treatment planning and follow-up for benign prostatic hypertrophy (BPH) management.

d. The symptom score is not specific for or diagnostic of BPH. It can be used in men and women for general assessment of voiding symptoms.

D. Changes in the Gross Appearance of the Urine

1. Cloudy urine

a. Cloudy urine is most commonly due to the benign process of precipitation of phosphates in an alkaline

Table 2-1 The AUA Symptom Index

QUESTION	NOT AT ALL	LESS THAN 1 TIME IN 5	LESS THAN HALF THE TIME	ABOUT HALF THE TIME	MORE THAN HALF THE TIME	ALMOST ALWAYS
1. During the last month or so, how often have you had a sensation of not emptying your bladder completely after you finished urinating?	0	1	2	3	4	5
2. During the last month or so, how often have you had to urinate again less than 2 hours after you finished urinating?	0	1	2	3	4	5
3. During the last month or so, how often have you found you stopped and standard again several times when you urinated?	0	1	2	3	4	5
4. During the last month or so, how often have you found it difficult to postpone urination?	0	1	2	3	4	5

	None	1 Time	2 Times	3 Times	4 Times	5 or More Times
5. During the last month or so, how often have you had a weak urinary stream?	0	1	2	3	4	5
6. During the last month or so, how often have you had to push or strain to begin urination?	0	1	2	3	4	5
7. During the last month, how many times did you most typically get up to urinate from the time you went to bed at night until the time you got up in the morning?	0	1	2	3	4	5

AUA symptom score = sum of questions 1 to 7.

urine *(phosphaturia)*. This may be noted after meals or after consumption of large quantities of milk and is generally intermittent in nature. Patients are otherwise asymptomatic. Acidification of the urine with acetic acid at the time of urinalysis causes prompt clearing of the specimen.

b. *Pyuria* is a urinary tract infection in which large quantities of white blood cells cause urine to have a cloudy appearance. Microscopic examination of the urine sample will demonstrate the inflammatory nature.

c. *Chyluria* refers to the presence of lymph fluid mixed with the urine. It is an unusual cause of cloudy urine.

2. *Pneumaturia* refers to the passage of gas along with urine while voiding. There may be associated pyuria or frank fecal contamination of the urine, as this phenomenon is almost exclusively due to the presence of a fistula between the gastrointestinal and urinary tracts. On occasion, the presence of a gas-forming infection within the urinary tract can produce similar symptoms, although this is very unusual.

3. Hematuria

a. The passage of bloody urine is always alarming, and generally makes the patient make a prompt visit to the physician. Prompt investigation is always warranted, including a properly performed urinalysis to be certain that the red discoloration of the urine is indeed secondary to the presence of blood. For a differential diagnosis of the causes of red urine, see the following section.

b. Although hematuria is always a danger signal, a clue to its significance may lie in whether there is associated pain or whether the bleeding is essentially painless. Pain that occurs in association with cystitis or passage of a urinary tract calculus may indicate that the bleeding is in fact benign in nature. Painless hematuria, however, is always felt to be secondary to a urinary tract neoplasm until proven otherwise. This differentiation is not infallible, and therefore all urinary tract bleeding warrants investigation to be certain that there is not an associated neoplasm in addition to the more obvious cause for painful bleeding.

c. The probable site of bleeding within the urinary tract may be ascertained by determining whether the bleeding is initial (at the beginning of the stream only), terminal (at the end of the stream only), or total (throughout the entire stream). Initial hematuria generally indicates some type of anterior urethral bleeding that is flushed out by the initial passage of the bladder urine through the urethra. Terminal hematuria is often secondary to posterior urethral, bladder neck, or trigone bleeding and is noted when the bladder finally compresses these areas at the end of micturition. Total hematuria indicates that the bleeding occurs at the level of the bladder or above, such that all of the urine is mixed with blood and is therefore bloody throughout the entire stream.

4. *Colored urine* may result from a variety of foods, medications, and medical disorders. The colors may range from almost clear to black, with all other colors of the spectrum noted in between. (See Table 2-4 for common causes of colorful urine.)

E. Abnormal Appearance and/or Function of the Male External Genitalia

1. Sexual dysfunction
2. Infertility
3. Penile problems
   a. *Cutaneous lesions.* A variety of exophytic and ulcerative lesions may be noted by the patient. The relationship of the onset of these lesions to recent sexual activity should be explored. The physical characteristics of these lesions should be noted at the time of physical examination. The combination of historical and physical factors, as well as associated physical findings such as adenopathy, will provide a working diagnosis for the treatment of these lesions.
   b. *Penile curvature.* Bending of the penis, particularly during erection, is noted in association with scarring and fibrosis of the tunica albuginea. These plaque-like structures may be noted on physical examination. The process is essentially idiopathic and has been referred to as Peyronie's disease.
   c. *Urethral discharge.* The character of the urethral discharge should be described as well as its onset in relation to sexual activity as noted above. The presence of the discharge should be confirmed on physical examination and a microscopic examination performed and a culture obtained.
   d. *Bloody ejaculate.* Like hematuria, this is also a frightening experience that usually causes the patient to seek prompt attention. This problem, however, is generally secondary to benign congestion and/or inflammation of the seminal vesicles. The process is usually self-limited or treatable with antibiotics and does not initially require an extensive evaluation.

Table 2-2 Causes of Scrotal Swelling

STRUCTURE INVOLVED	PATHOLOGY
Scrotal wall	Hematoma
	Urinary extravasation
	Edema from cardiac, hepatic, or renal failure
Testis	Carcinoma
	Torsion of testes or appendix testis
Epididymis	Epididymitis
	Tumor
	Torsion of appendix epididymis
Spermatic cord	Hydrocele surrounding testis of involving cord only
	Hematocele
	Hernia
	Varicocele
	Lipoma

4. Scrotal problems
    a. *Cutaneous lesions.* The hair-bearing skin of the scrotum is susceptible to the variety of skin diseases that can occur anywhere else on the body. Fungal infections and venereal warts may also be noted commonly.
    b. *Scrotal swelling and masses.* The presence of scrotal swelling and/or a scrotal mass may be noted incidentally by the patient while bathing or performing a self-examination or due to the presence of associated discomfort. A variety of lesions can produce unilateral or bilateral scrotal enlargement. These range from normal structures that are misinterpreted by the patient to testicular neoplasms. The differential diagnosis is as noted in Table 2-2. A combination of historical information, particularly with regard to onset of the mass, progression, and associated pain, and the physical examination is helpful in differentiating some of the more confusing lesions. (See section on physical examination and Table 2-3.)

IV. THE PHYSICAL EXAMINATION
A. General Information
1. The problems delineated in the history will determine how extensive the physical examination should be. A complete physical examination is obviously necessary for someone who will undergo some type of urologic

Table 2-3 Differential Diagnosis of Scrotal Discomfort and Solid Mass Lesions

	TORSION	EPIDIDYMITIS	TUMOR
Age	Birth to 20 years	Puberty to old age	15 to 35 years
Pain			
Onset	Sudden	Rapid	Gradual
Degree	Severe	Increasing severity	Mild or absent
Nausea and vomiting	Yes	No	No
Examination			
Testis	Swollen together and both tender	Normal early	Mass
Epididymis		Swollen, tender	Normal
Spermatic cord	Shortened	Thickened, often tender as high as inguinal canal	—
Urinalysis	Normal	Often infection	Normal

surgery; in most instances, however, a limited examination of the genitourinary tract is usually sufficient at the time of the initial examination.

2. The commonly taught techniques of physical examination, including inspection, palpation, percussion, and auscultation, are also used during the urologic examination. Each has varying degrees of usefulness depending on the organ being evaluated. The process of transillumination with a high-intensity, small-diameter light source is useful in evaluating pediatric abdominal masses as well as scrotal masses in the child and the adult. Particular aspects of the physical examination will be noted below.

B. Kidneys and Flanks

1. *Inspection.* Inspection of the flanks is best carried out with the patient in the sitting or standing position facing straight ahead and the examiner located behind the patient facing the area in question. Scoliosis may be evident in the patient with an inflammatory process directly or indirectly involving the psoas muscle with resultant spasm. Bulging of the flank may be noted if there is an underlying mass, although this is only evident in most cases if the mass is extremely large or if the patient is very thin. Edema of the flank may be noted if there is an underlying inflammatory process.

2. *Palpation and percussion.* A method of bimanual renal palpation has been described with the patient in the supine position (Fig. 2-1). The examiner lifts the flank by placing one hand beneath this area and subsequently palpates deeply beneath the ipsilateral costal margin anteriorally. This technique is successful in children and thin adults but generally yields little information under most other circumstances. A large mass may be palpable. Percussion is a useful technique, particularly in the area of the costovertebral angle, to elicit tenderness due to underlying capsular inflammation or distention (Fig. 2-2).

3. *Auscultation.* This technique is particularly useful in evaluating patients with possible renovascular hypertension. An underlying bruit may be noted in the area of the costovertebral angle due to renal artery stenosis, aneurysm formation, or arteriovenous malformation.

4. *Transillumination.* This technique, which may differentiate a solid from a cystic mass in neonates or infants, has largely been replaced by ultrasonography, which defines these lesions much more clearly.

C. Abdomen and Bladder

1. *Inspection.* The abdominal and bladder examinations are best carried out with the patient in the supine position.

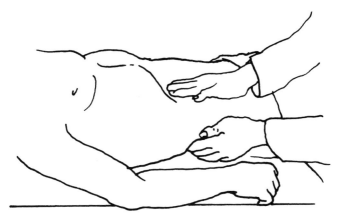

Figure 2-1 With the patient in the supine position, one hand is used to raise the flank while the abdominal hand palpates deeply beneath the costal margin.

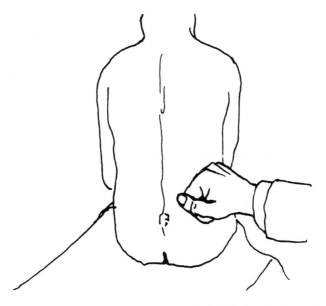

Figure 2-2 Gentle percussion with the heel of the hand in the angle between the lumbar vertebrae and the 12th rib is useful in eliciting underlying tenderness due to obstruction or inflammation.

The full or overdistended bladder may be visible on general inspection of the abdomen with the patient in this position.

2. *Palpation and percussion.* It is generally possible to palpate or percuss the bladder above the level of the symphysis pubis if it contains 150 mL or more of urine (Fig. 2-3). It should be remembered that in the child, the bladder *may* be percussible or palpable with much smaller volumes of urine relative to its size due to the fact that it is more of an intra-abdominal organ in the child than the true pelvic organ it is in the adult.

D. Penis

1. *Inspection.* Inspection of the penis will reveal obvious lesions of the skin and will define whether the patient has been circumcised. If the patient has been circumcised, the glans penis and meatus can be inspected directly. In the uncircumcised patient, the foreskin should be retracted and the glanular surface of the foreskin as well as the glans and meatus should then be inspected. The number and position of ulcerative and/or exophytic lesions should

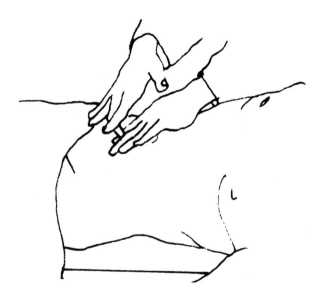

Figure 2-3 Percussion over the bladder can be particularly useful when palpation is difficult due either to obesity or failure of the patient to relax during the examination. The bladder can be percussed if it contains greater than 150 mL of urine in the adult.

be noted if they are present. The position and size of the urinary meatus should be defined.

   a. *Foreskin.* Phimosis is present when the orifice of the foreskin is constricted preventing retraction of the foreskin over the glans. Paraphimosis is present when the foreskin, once retracted over the glans, cannot be replaced to its normal position covering the glans.

   b. *Penile meatus.* The normal meatus should be located at the tip of the glans. Hypospadias is present when the meatus opens anywhere along the ventral aspect of the penis or in the perineum. Epispadias is present when the meatus is located on the dorsal aspect of the penis.

2. *Palpation.* Palpation of the penile shaft is important to identify and define the limits of areas of fibrous induration that may be found in patients with Peyronie's disease who complain of penile curvature during erection. The urethra should also be palpated for areas of induration that may be associated with periurethritis and urethral stricture disease. The urethra can also be "stripped" from the penile–scrotal junction toward the meatus to look for a urethral discharge that can then be collected for microscopic examination and culture.

E. Scrotum and Scrotal Contents

1. *Inspection.* The inspection of the scrotum and the remainder of this portion of the physical examination are best carried out with the patient initially in the standing position. Lesions of the scrotal skin are readily evident in this position. The examiner also generally notes that if two testicles are present, one usually hangs lower than the other. In most cases, the left testicle is lower than the right. In cases of congenital absence or failure of descent of one or both testicles, the involved side may demonstrate hypoplastic scrotal development. It is always important to note the presence or absence of the testes. Scrotal masses and the "bag of worms" appearance of an underlying large varicocele may be identified on initial inspection.

2. *Palpation.* The contents of each hemiscrotum should be palpated in an orderly fashion. First, the testes should be examined, then the epididymides, then the cord structures, and finally, the area of the external inguinal ring to check for the presence of an inguinal hernia (Fig. 2-4).

   a. Each testis should be in the dependent portion of the scrotum when the patient is relaxed and in a warm environment. The long axis of the testicle should be in a vertical direction and the size of the testis should be

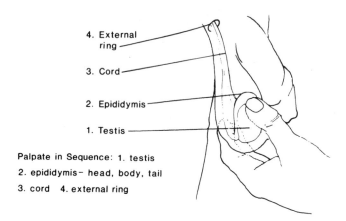

4. External ring

3. Cord

2. Epididymis

1. Testis

Palpate in Sequence: 1. testis
2. epididymis – head, body, tail
3. cord   4. external ring

Figure 2-4 Palpation of the scrotal contents should be carried out in an orderly, routine fashion. The examiner should begin palpating the testes, followed by the epididymides, the cord structures, and finally, the external rings. Palpating each structure from side to side is useful for detecting differences in testicular size and identifying varicoceles. All of the scrotal structures may be examined between the thumb and the index and middle fingers.

noted. The long axis of the testicle should normally be greater than or equal to 4 cm in adult males.

b. Each epididymis is adherent to the posterolateral aspect of the testicle. The head of the epididymis is noted to be near the superior pole of the testicle, the body of the epididymis near the middle portion of the testicle, and the tail of the epididymis represents the most inferior aspect of this structure. The examiner should palpate each portion of the epididymis looking primarily for areas of tenderness or induration.

c. The spermatic cord varies somewhat in thickness and often this depends on the presence or absence of what has been termed a "lipoma of the cord." The examiner should be particularly attentive to the presence or absence of enlarged venous structures (i.e., a varicocele, descending with the cord). If a varicocele is detected, the patient should also be examined in the supine position to be certain that the varicocele decompresses. If it does not, one must suspect inferior vena cava or renal vein obstruction. Changes in the size of the cord between the standing and the supine positions or when using the Valsalva maneuver with the patient in the upright position indicate the presence of a small varicocele. The vas deferens should be palpated. This structure normally has the thickness of a pencil lead and has a distinct, smooth firmness.

d. Finally, with the patient in the standing position, palpation of the inguinal canal may be carried out. Increasing intra-abdominal pressure by asking the patient to cough or by using the Valsalva maneuver will help to define the presence of an inguinal hernia.

3. Abnormal scrotal masses and transillumination (Figs. 2-5 and 2-6)

a. The presence of an abnormal mass within the scrotum is best defined by careful palpation. It should be noted whether the mass arises from the testicle, is contained within the testicle, arises from the epididymis, is located in the cord, or tends to surround most of the scrotal structures. It is important to note the character of the mass, that is, whether it is hard, firm, or cystic in nature.

b. All scrotal masses should be transilluminated and this can be accomplished with a small penlight. Any mass that radiates a reddish glow of light through the lesion represents a cystic, fluid-filled structure. Caution is advised in defining the benignity of these lesions, however, in that benign and malignant lesions can coexist. A hydrocele surrounding a testicular tumor is a not uncommon example.

c. See Table 2-3 for a differential diagnosis of scrotal masses.

F. The Rectum and Prostate

1. *Position.* A variety of positions have been described for performing a digital rectal examination (DRE). Having the patient lie on the examining table in the lateral decubitus position with the legs flexed at the hips and knees and the uppermost leg pulled higher toward the chest than the lowermost leg creates a comfortable position for the patient and the examiner (Fig. 2-7). Alternatively, the patient can bend over the examining table while in the standing position so that the weight of his upper body rests on his elbows. This lateral decubitus position typically allows for deeper penetration of the rectum to feel the prostate in obese patients or to feel the top of large glands. Probably more important than the position, however, is that the gloved examining finger be adequately lubricated and slow, gentle pressure be applied as the finger traverses the anal sphincter. A rectal examination can be an extremely painful or a painless experience depending

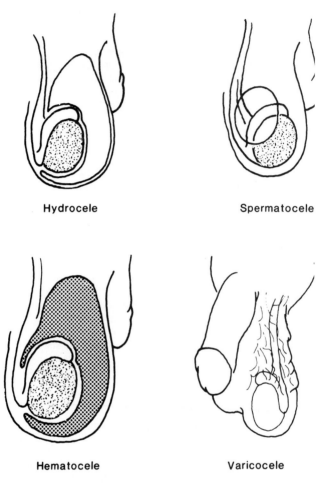

Figure 2-5 A variety of fluid-filled masses can develop within the scrotum. Hydroceles and spermatoceles (and occasionally bowel in a hernia sac) will transilluminate. Hydrocele fluid is contained within the tunica vaginalis and essentially surrounds the testicle. A spermatocele generally occurs above or adjacent to the upper pole of the testis and represents a cyst of the rete testis or epididymis. A hematocele is a collection of blood within the tunica vaginalis due usually to trauma or surgery. Occasionally, spontaneous bleeding will occur associated with bleeding disorders. A varicocele represents dilated veins of the pampiniform plexus. Hematoceles and varicoceles will not transilluminate.

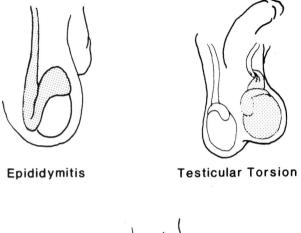

Epididymitis   **Testicular Torsion**

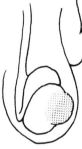

Testicular Tumor

Figure 2-6 Solid scrotal masses may be painful or painless and may involve the testis, epididymis, or both. Table 2-2 further differentiates the three lesions depicted in this figure.

on the skill and patience of the examiner. It is important at the time of the examination not only to palpate the prostate gland but to palpate the entire inside of the rectum in search of other abnormalities.

2. *Prostate.* During the rectal examination, the posterior aspect of the prostate is palpated (Fig. 2-8). The significance of this part of the general physical examination cannot be overemphasized. Most types of prostate carcinoma begin in the posterior lobe of the prostate, which is very accessible to the examining finger.

a. The prostate gland is normally a small, walnut-sized structure with a flattened, heart-shaped configuration.

Lying Position

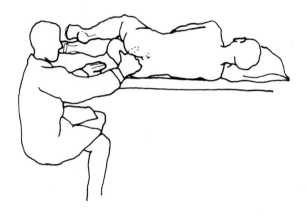

Standing Position

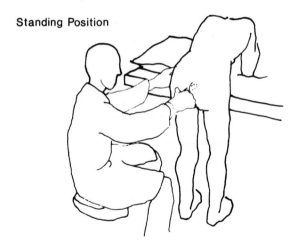

Figure 2-7 Two positions are illustrated for performing the digital rectal examination.

There is a median furrow, which runs down the longitudinal axis of the prostate. There are two lateral sulci, where the rectal mucosa folds back on itself after reflecting off the prostate. The consistency of the normal prostate is generally described as "rubbery" in nature and has been likened to the consistency of the

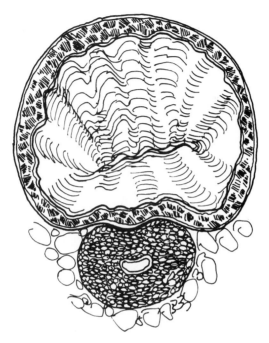

Figure 2-8 The posterior aspect of the prostate is palpable on rectal examination. The surface is normally smooth, rubbery, and approximately 4 × 4 cm in size. The median furrow may be lost with diffuse enlargement of the gland and the lateral sulci may be either accentuated or obscured. Deviations from normal contour, consistency, or size should be carefully described. Stating that an area is "hard" implies that one is suggesting the presence of carcinoma. The seminal vesicles are not normally palpable. *Remember:* check the entire rectum. Do not miss an occult rectal carcinoma. *(Redrawn, with modifications, from Smith DR: General Urology, 11 ed. Los Altos: Lange, 1984, p 40.)*

    thenar eminence when one opposes the thumb and fifth finger.

  b. Abnormal consistency of the prostate may be noted on rectal examination and includes nodular abnormalities that can be raised or within the substance of the prostate, areas of induration that can suggest malignancy, or areas of bogginess or fluctuance that can be associated with abscess formation.

c. Prostatic massage can be carried out in order to express prostatic secretions into the urethral lumen. These secretions may then be collected directly if they happen to drain through the penile meatus or by having the patient void a small amount of urine directly into a container immediately following the massage. Prostatic massage is generally carried out in a methodical fashion to strip the entire gland from a lateral to a medial aspect bilaterally.

3. *Seminal vesicles.* Under normal conditions, the seminal vesicles are not palpable. They can become evident on a rectal examination, however, if they are enlarged due to obstruction or inflammation.

G. The Vaginal Examination

1. *Inspection.* The vaginal examination is best performed with the patient in the relaxed lithotomy position. Inspection of the vulva may reveal a variety of venereal and nonvenereal lesions. The urinary meatus should be identified and its position and size noted. An erythematous tender lesion arising from the meatus may represent a benign urethral caruncle or possibly a urethral carcinoma. The character of the vaginal mucosa at the introitus should be noted. The examiner *may* also note the presence of a cystocele or a rectocele while examining the patient in this position. These structures may be accentuated with increases in intra-abdominal pressure such as occur with coughing or straining. In fact, this maneuver may elicit some leakage of urine in patients with stress urinary incontinence.

2. *Palpation.* Palpation of the urethra to the level of the bladder neck and trigone may be accomplished during examination of the anterior vaginal wall. Bimanual palpation is useful to define the internal genitalia and to define further the size and consistency of the urinary bladder.

V. THE URINALYSIS AND CULTURE

A. Collection

Proper collection and prompt examination of the urine is essential to gain the most information from the routinely collected specimen.

1. Males

a. A midstream urine collection is most commonly obtained in men for routine examination. With this technique, the male patient is instructed to retract the foreskin if he is uncircumcised and to gently cleanse the glans. He begins to urinate into the toilet, subsequently inserting a sterile glass container into the urinary stream to collect a urine sample. The container is then removed and the act of voiding is completed.

b. A variety of other collection techniques afford more information with regard to localization of infection within the urinary tract. Four such specimens may be obtained and analyzed separately by routine microscopic evaluation as well as culture techniques. These have been designated the VB-1, VB-2, EPS, and VB-3 specimens, according to Stamey. The VB-1 is the initial 5 to 10 mL of the stream, which contains bladder urine mixed with urethral contents that are initially washed from the urethra. The VB-2 specimen is essentially the midstream portion of the collection. The EPS specimen represents the expressed prostatic secretions following prostatic massage. Finally, the VB-3 specimen represents a small voided specimen that mixes bladder urine with the contents contained in the urethra immediately following the expression of prostatic secretions. This collection is particularly useful if inadequate amounts of secretion from the prostate are actually expressed during the prostatic massage. The value of these cultures for localization of urinary tract infection is that the VB-1 represents urethral flora, the VB-2 represents bladder flora, and the EPS and VB-3 represent prostatic flora.

2. Females

a. The midstream urine collection in females is somewhat more difficult to accomplish and is often considered to be inadequate for even the most routine examination. With this technique, the vulva is cleansed and the stream is initiated into the toilet with subsequent insertion of a collecting container as described above for the male. If this specimen is grossly contaminated or appears infected, then one of the collection methods noted below may be necessary to differentiate these two possibilities. However, if the collection has been done with reasonable care and the specimen is essentially negative on microscopic examination, then this technique is generally considered adequate.

b. A more proper method of midstream urine collection has been described in which the patient is placed in the lithotomy position and then asked to void. The nurse holds the labia apart to prevent contamination and collects a midstream specimen. This is often awkward, if not difficult, for both the patient and the nurse, however, this method of collection is not recommended.

c. If there is any question with regard to the problem of contamination versus infection of the midstream specimen as noted above, then catheterization to obtain a true bladder specimen is the preferred technique. An examiner should not hesitate to use this method to properly categorize a patient's problem.

3. Children
   a. Percutaneous suprapubic aspiration of urine from neonates and infants is a particularly useful method of obtaining a truly uncontaminated specimen of urine from the bladder. With this technique, the suprapubic area is cleansed with an antiseptic solution and percutaneous aspiration is performed with a fine-gauge needle. The specimen can then be examined for urinalysis and sent for culture.
   b. A variety of sterile plastic bags with adhesive collars are available that surround the male and female infant's genitalia. They are particularly useful for routine screening urinalysis, but, as with the collection of midstream specimens from women, it may be difficult at times to differentiate a truly infected urine from a contaminated specimen due to this collection technique.
   c. Older boys and girls may have urine collected in a fashion similar to that described above for their adult counterparts. One is generally quite hesitant, however, to catheterize young boys due to the possibility of urethral trauma. It is easier and safer to perform this in girls and may be used if necessary.

B. Physical Aspects of the Urine

1. *Color.* The color of the urine is generally a clear light yellow, but a wide range of colors has been described, as noted earlier. The changes in color can be secondary to foods and medications, as well as intrinsic disease processes. Table 2-4 describes the etiologic factors in relationship to abnormal urine color.

2. *pH.* The normal pH of urine ranges from 4.5 to 8.0. Urine is described as having an acid pH if it ranges between 4.5 and 5.5. It is referred to as having an alkaline pH if it ranges between 6.5 and 8.0.

3. *Specific gravity.* The specific gravity can be determined in the office by relatively simple techniques and gives some idea of the concentrating ability of the kidneys and their ability to excrete waste products. A variety of substances within the urine, such as intravenous contrast material, can detract from the value of this test. The osmolality of the urine is a better indicator of renal function but requires standard laboratory methods.

Table 2-4 Common Causes of Colorful Urine

Colorless	Very dilute urine
	Overhydration
Cloudy/milky	Phosphaturia
	Pyuria
	Chyluria
Red	Hematuria
	Hemoglobin/myoglobinuria
	Anthrocyanin in beets and blackberries
	Chronic lead and mercury poisoning
	Phenolphthalein (in bowel evacuants)
	Phenothiazines (Compazine, etc.)
	Rifampin
Orange	Dehydration
	Phenazopyridine (Pyridium)
	Sulfasalazine (Azulfadine)
Yellow	Normal
	Phenacetin
	Riboflavin
Green-blue	Biliverdin
	Indicanuria tryptophan indole metabolites)
	Amitriptyline (Elavil)
	Indigo carmine
	Methylene blue
	Phenols [IV cimetidine (Tagamet) IV promethanzine (Phenergan), etc.]
	Resorcinol
	Triampterene (Dyrenium)
Brown	Urobilinogen
	Porphyria
	Aloe, fava beans, and rhubarb
	Chloroquine and primaquine
	Furazolidone (Furoxone)
	Metronidazole (Flagyl)
	Nitrofurantoin (Furadantin)
Brown-black	Alcaptonuria (homogentisic acid)
	Hemorrhage
	Melanin
	Tyrosinosis (hydroxyphenylpyruvic acid)
	Cascara, senna (laxatives)
	Methocarbamol (Robaxin)
	Methyldopa (Aldomet)
	Sorbitol

C. Dipstick Tests

1. A variety of dipsticks are available to evaluate the urine sample. These consist of short plastic strips with small marker pads that are impregnated with a variety of reagents that react with abnormal substances within the urine.
2. In addition to determination of urinary pH, the most sophisticated dipsticks now contain reagents for the determination of the following:
   a. Protein
   b. Glucose
   c. Ketones
   d. Urobilinogen
   e. Bilirubin
   f. Blood
   g. Hemoglobin
   h. Leukocytes
   i. Nitrites

D. Microscopic Examination

1. A small portion of the collected urine sample is placed in a test tube and centrifuged at approximately 5000 rpm for 5 min. The supernate is then poured from the tube and the remaining sediment is resuspended in the small quantity of urine that drains back down the side of the tube to the sediment. A drop of the resuspended sediment is placed on a glass slide followed by a cover slip.
2. The wet specimen described above is then examined under low and high power for the presence and number of epithelial cells, red blood cells, white blood cells, bacteria, and casts.

E. Urine Culture

1. If a urine culture is desired, it should be promptly plated in the office or sent immediately to the laboratory to prevent overgrowth of bacteria and falsely elevated bacterial counts.
2. The value of localization cultures has been noted above.

VI. BLOOD TESTS

A. Panel 7 (or similar designation)

1. Serum electrolytes (Na, K, Cl, CO_2) are useful indicators of maintenance of homeostasis for which the kidney plays a significant role.
2. Glucose levels in the serum may be variable relative to the presence of glucosuria.
   a. Diabetes is a significant risk factor for voiding and sexual dysfunction.
3. BUN and creatinine are indicators of renal function.

B. PSA (Prostate Specific Antigen) Level
1. PSA is a protein kinase produced, essentially uniquely, by the prostatic epithelium.
   a. It is a normal component of the ejaculate responsible for liquification of the semen.
   b. Normally found in very low levels in serum (0–4.0 ng/mL).
2. Causes of PSA elevation
   a. Prostate cancer
   b. BPH
   c. Prostatitis (acute and chronic)
   d. Instrumentation (catheterization, cystoscopy, biopsy)
   e. Urinary retention
   f. Ejaculation
   g. Vigorous prostatic massage, probably little elevation for routine DRE
3. PSA as a tumor marker
   a. Limitations due to prostate organ specific but not cancer specific.
   b. Substantial overlap of values for men with prostate cancer and benign conditions (see above).
   c. Absolute value greater than 10 ng/mL has over 60 percent predictive risk of prostate cancer.
   d. Useful marker for following efficacy of treatment for prostate cancer.
4. Recommendations
   a. Yearly PSA and DRE for all men over 50 years old.
   b. Yearly PSA and DRE starting at 40 years old for blacks and all men with a positive family history of prostate cancer.

VII. DIAGNOSTIC INSTRUMENTATION
A. General Information
The instrumentation and procedures to be described below can be commonly performed in the office setting under local anesthesia. Some of these techniques, such as cystourethroscopy, placement of retrograde catheters, and biopsy of the prostate, may also be performed with regional or general anesthesia.

B. Urethral Catheters (Fig. 2-9)
1. *Straight catheters.* The standard straight, red, or Robinson catheter is useful for office catheterization when an indwelling catheter is not warranted. It is useful for collecting relatively uncontaminated specimens directly from the bladder as noted above.
2. *Standard balloon or Foley catheter.* This type of catheter has a double lumen that permits drainage of urine through

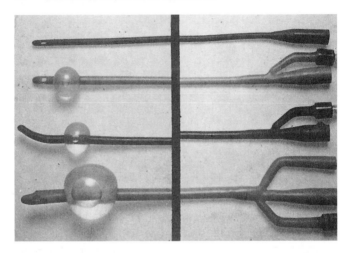

Figure 2-9 Four types of catheters. From top to bottom: Straight 14-F Robinson catheter, 18-F Foley catheter with 5-mL balloon, 18-F coudé tip catheter with 5-mL balloon, and 24-F three-way irrigating catheter with 30-mL balloon. (*Note: Catheters have been shortened for photography*)

the larger lumen and inflation of a balloon located at the tip of the catheter. This allows it to be retained within the urinary bladder. This type of catheter is useful following certain operative procedures on the urinary tract and for establishing temporary, constant urinary drainage to monitor urine output or for relief of bladder outlet obstruction. These catheters generally have 5- and 30-mL balloons, but the amount of water placed in these balloons is not precisely critical as each will hold significantly more than its stated volume.

3. *Coudé catheters.* Red Robinson catheters or balloon retention catheters may each be specially constructed to have a "coudé-tip configuration." This is essentially a curved tip that allows passage of the catheter beyond certain urethral, prostatic, or bladder neck impediments that may preclude passage of a straight catheter due to impingement of the catheter tip on these lesions.

4. *Three-way irrigation catheters.* This type of catheter has a triple lumen that has an irrigation port, a drainage port, and a port for inflating the balloon used for retention of the catheter within the bladder. Three-way irrigation catheters are particularly useful following transurethral

resection of the prostate and in cases of gross hematuria to irrigate the bladder and prevent formation and retention of clots.

5. *Technique of catheter insertion.* Insertion of a urethral catheter by the physician for either diagnostic or therapeutic reasons always involves sterile technique. Gloves should be applied and the glans and meatus of the male and the vulva and meatus of the female are then prepared with an antiseptic skin preparation solution. The catheter is then well-lubricated with sterile jelly and inserted gently into the meatus. Prior to inflation of the balloon, if a retention catheter is used, it must be certain that the tip of the catheter is within the urinary bladder and that urine is obtained. In cases in which urine does not flow freely from the end of the catheter, it is important to irrigate the catheter gently prior to inflation of the balloon to prevent inflation within the urethra. Hematuria and/or sepsis may be noted if this occurs. The catheter is then pulled gently to seat the balloon at the level of the bladder neck. It is then attached to a drainage bag with sterile technique.

C. Urethral Sounds and Filiforms and Followers

1. *General information.* These two types of instruments are often used to evaluate the urethra in cases of urethral stricture disease or for other reasons that preclude passage of a urethral catheter. They may be used in both a diagnostic and therapeutic fashion by the skilled urologist who is familiar with their use.

2. *Urethral sounds.* These metal objects come in a variety of sizes and shapes (Fig. 2-10). They must be passed carefully to prevent disruption of the lower urinary tract. They are never inserted with force and must pass smoothly into the urinary bladder, where rotation of the tip of the sound is confirmed with each passage.

3. *Filiforms and followers.* These instruments are also useful for establishing access to the urinary bladder and dilating urethral strictures (Fig. 2-11). The tiny filiform aspect of this set is used to gain access initially to the urinary bladder. These filiforms have different shapes at their tip that allow them to be manipulated through or around a variety of abnormal urethral configurations. It may be necessary to pass several filiforms simultaneously before access can be gained to the bladder. Once it is established that one of these filiforms has passed easily into the bladder, the follower can then be attached to the protruding threaded end and passed as a unit with the filiform into the bladder. Using serially larger followers, it is possible to dilate the urethra. Each follower has an eye in

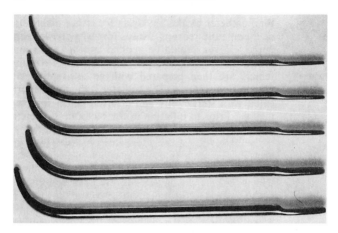

Figure 2-10 Van Buren urethral sounds. Five sounds are pictured ranging from 18 to 30 F in size.

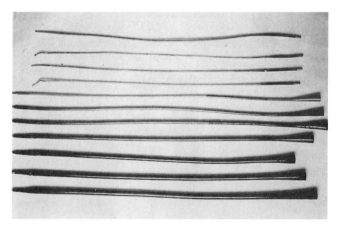

Figure 2-11 Filiforms and followers. Four small filiforms are shown at the top. Followers from 10 to 20 F are also shown.

the end and a hollow center so that urine can be obtained as the follower is passed. In cases of severe urethral stricture disease, it may be best to leave the follower in place prior to insertion of a Foley catheter. If the urethra dilates easily, the followers can be removed and a Foley catheter inserted immediately.

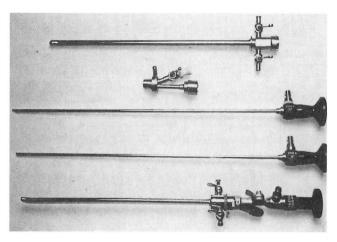

Figure 2-12 Cystoscope and components. The cystoscope consists of a sheath (*top*), a bridge (below sheath), and two interchangeable lenses with 30° and 70° viewing angles. The components of the Storz cystoscope are shown as is the assembled ACMI cystoscope *(bottom)*.

D. Cystourethroscopy and Associated Techniques

1. Equipment.

   a. The standard rigid cystourethroscope consists of a sheath, bridge, and lighted telescope for visualization (Fig. 2-12). An irrigation port is attached to the sheath that allows gravity-directed inflow of fluid to distend the urethra and bladder and aid in visualization. The bridge essentially attaches the telescope to the sheath and may contain a variety of working ports through which urethral catheters, biopsy forceps, and alligator forceps may be passed. The lighted telescopes generally have 30° and 70° viewing angles that allow complete inspection within the bladder.

   b. Flexible cystoscopes, like flexible endoscopes for GI endoscopy and bronchoscopy, consist of many tiny fiberoptic bundles organized with a deflection mechanism to allow movement of the tip. The flexible scope has an advantage for male patient comfort in that it conforms to, rather than straightens, the natural curves of the lower urinary tract. Its limitations relate to field of view and ease of working instrumentation.

2. Technique of insertion

   a. *Males.* Insertion of the cystourethroscope into the male is best performed under direct vision following antiseptic preparation and draping. The cystourethro-scope is assembled and a flow of fluid is obtained. The instrument is then introduced into the meatus and passed under direct vision through the anterior ure-thra. Some narrowing and voluntary constriction of the external sphincter may be noted, but this is passed with slow gentle pressure. With the patient in the lithotomy position, it is necessary to lower the eye-piece of the rigid scope to redirect the tip of the in-strument beneath the symphysis pubis, through the prostate and into the bladder. The bladder can then be emptied and inspected with both lenses. With the flex-ible cystoscope, the patient can remain supine and the tip directed by manipulation of the deflecting mecha-nism. Flexible cystoscopy can be performed at the bedside if necessary, such as in an ICU setting.

b. *Females.* The female patient is also placed in the lithot-omy position. After proper cleansing and draping, the cystourethroscope can be inserted into the bladder ei-ther under direct vision or with the obturator in the cy-toscope sheath taking care to follow the course of the urethra that may be deviated due to associated pathol-ogy such as a cystocele. Once again, the bladder is in-spected with both lenses and the urethra is inspected with the 30° lens.

3. Procedures

a. *Inspection.* In most cases, the urethra and bladder are merely inspected under local anesthesia with these en-doscopic techniques in the office setting. This allows the urologist to ascertain the presence or absence of urethral pathology, degree of anatomic obstruction, and state of the bladder mucosa and underlying mus-culature. It is also possible to note the presence or ab-sence of efflux from the ureteral orifices as well as judge their location and configuration. At the time of inspection of the bladder, bladder urine can be ob-tained for culture or cytology, The bladder can also be washed by barbotage techniques and the saline wash-ings sent for cytology.

b. *Bladder biopsies.* These may be taken under local anesthesia using cold cup biopsy forceps. Generally, however, there is some degree of associated discom-fort and if biopsies are necessary, they are usually best performed under regional or general anesthesia to en-sure an adequate specimen.

c. *Retrograde ureteral catheterization.* The placement of small (sizes 4 to 7 F) ureteral catheters may be per-formed without difficulty under local anesthesia.

These catheters can be passed just within the ureteral orifice for retrograde injection of contrast or to the level of the kidney for relief of obstruction within the ureter, to obtain renal washings or for the injection of contrast material for radiographic studies. They can be removed immediately or left temporarily in place.

d. A variety of resectoscopes and specialized endoscopes are available to perform more sophisticated procedures on the urethra, bladder, and prostate as well as the ureter and kidney. These are therapeutic rather than diagnostic procedures and require regional or general anesthesia. Their use is not considered further herein.

E. Ultrasound Evaluation of the Urinary Tract

1. *General information.* Small, portable utrasound machines are available from a number of manufacturers. These are increasingly being used in urologists' offices, in addition to radiology departments, to evaluate the urinary tract and to guide diagnostic procedures. Probes that have different frequencies and different configurations are designed to evaluate specific areas and aspects of the urinary tract.

2. *Renal ultrasonography.* The kidney can be evaluated for mass lesions, hydronephrosis, or the presence of stones or stone fragments.

3. *Abdominal ultrasonography.* Abdominal masses and the lower urinary tract, especially the bladder can be imaged. Built-in computer programs allow computation of ultrasound-determined residual urine volumes. This makes a determination of bladder emptying possible without catheterization.

4. *Ultrasonography of the external genitalia.* May be used to evaluate scrotal masses to determine whether they are cystic or solid and their relationship to the testicle and epididymis. Special Doppler probes are useful in evaluating penile blood flow in cases of erectile failure and in confirming the presence of venous reflux in suspected varicoceles.

5. *Transvaginal ultrasonography.* May be useful in evaluating the lower urinary tract in cases of incontinence and voiding dysfunction.

6. *Transrectal ultrasonography.* This technique is most frequently used to evaluate the prostate relative to carcinoma, although it may also be used to evaluate the benign prostate with regard to size and to look for abnormalities in cases of ejaculatory dysfunction. At this time, the indications for transrectal ultrasonography of the prostate are

in the assessment of prostate nodules that are palpable on the digital rectal examination, to look for abnormalities associated with elevated prostate specific antigen (PSA) levels, and for needle localization for biopsy of the prostate. It must be emphasized that there are no specific ultrasonographic findings that definitely differentiate carcinoma of the prostate from benign lesions.

F. Needle Biopsy of the Prostate

1. *General information.* Needle biopsy techniques are the most accurate means of determining whether a prostate nodule or other area of abnormality is benign or malignant.

2. *Techniques.* The prostate can be sampled by either a transrectal or transperineal approach. To be accurate, the tip of the needle must enter the area of concern. Localization may be by digital direction, but is now done most frequently by ultrasound guidance. Use of ultrasonography in combination with needles placed through a port in the probe has clearly improved the accuracy of this procedure and improved patient tolerance.

   a. Spring-loaded thin-core biopsy needles are available that may be passed directly through a channel or guide in the ultrasound probe such that the tip may be seen as it enters the lesion of concern. These cores are obtained for sectioning, and despite the use of a transrectal approach in most cases, there appears to be little risk of sepsis.

   b. Vim–Silverman and Tru-cut needles obtain cores of tissue for standard pathologic sectioning and examination. These are wide bore and, even with local anesthesia (transperineal route), are associated with significant patient discomfort. The transrectal route is more accurate and better tolerated but is associated with a higher rate of urosepsis. This method is used infrequently now.

   c. Skinny-needle aspiration obtains cells for cytologic evaluation and is well tolerated but lacks preservation of architecture and precise accuracy of sampling.

VIII. SUMMARY

The surgical subspecialty of urology deals with a well-defined organ system within the body. The urologist diagnoses and treats a wide variety of medical and surgical disorders that may have local or systemic ramifications for the patient. The history, physical examination, and urinalysis serve as the cornerstones of the initial evaluation of these patients. In addition, a variety of unique diagnostic and therapeutic instruments are available for use in the office or outpatient setting to aid in caring for those with urologic diseases. The frequency with which these problems are seen by generalists and other specialists necessitates that all practitioners have some familiarity with this field.

BIBLIOGRAPHY

Barry MJ, Fowler FJ Jr, O'Leary MP, et al: The American Urological Association symptom index for benign prostatic hyperplasia. *J Urol* 148:1549, 1992.

Brendler CB: Evaluation of the urologic patient: History, physical examination, and urinalysis. In: Walsh PC, Retik AB, Vaughn Jr. ED, Wein AJ, eds. *Campbell's Urology,* 7th ed. Philadelphia: Saunders, 1998, p. 131.

Carter HB: Instrumentation and endoscopy. In: Walsh PC, Retik AB, Vaughn Jr. ED, eds. *Campbell's Urology,* 7th ed. Philadelphia: Saunders, 1998, p. 159.

Polascik TJ, Oesterling JE, Partin AW: Prostate specific antigen: A decade of discovery—What we have learned and where we are going. *J Urol* 162:293, 1999.

Scott W, Burns P, Brown JL, Hammer L: Ultrasound evaluation of the urinary tract. In: Pollack HM, McClennan BL, eds. *Clinical Urography.* Philadelphia: Saunders, 2000, pp 388–472.

Stamey TA: *Pathogenesis and Treatment of Urinary Tract Infections.* Baltimore: Williams & Wilkins, 1980.

CHAPTER 3
Diagnostic Uroradiology

Marc P. Banner

I. OVERVIEW OF DIAGNOSTIC IMAGING

Radiology and endoscopy are the two major diagnostic pillars upon which the specialty of urology is built. Uroradiology constitutes that branch of radiology concerned with urinary tract imaging. All parts of the urinary tract may be visualized by one or more of the many available uroradiologic studies. Each study has a particular role and each will provide some knowledge not revealed by the others. Because there is a great deal of potential overlap in the information obtained, it is good to be familiar with the particular virtues and limitations of each method. A close working relationship between the urologist and uroradiologist is very beneficial for patient care and provides optimal utilization of resources within the radiology department.

II. EXCRETORY UROGRAPHY
A. Purpose

The excretory or intravenous urogram (IVU) is the basic diagnostic radiologic study of the urinary tract, visualizing the kidneys, ureters, and bladder in a noninstrumental fashion. No other radiologic or urologic examination currently surpasses urography as a screening procedure for the entire urinary tract. This study was previously referred to as an intravenous pyelogram (IVP).

B. Indications

1. At present, there are fewer indications for urography as a result of both the increasing availability of alternative methods of diagnostic imaging and a reassessment of the value (or lack of it) of the information provided by urography in many common urologic conditions. The latter include uncomplicated urinary tract infections, preoperative studies for various types of surgery (including prostatectomy), enuresis, scrotal pathology, infertility, renal insufficiency, multiorgan trauma, and hypertension.

Hypertension thought to be attributable to renovascular insufficiency or adrenal pathology is better evaluated with cross-sectional imaging. Hypertension due to reflux nephropathy, however, remains best diagnosed by urography in spite of highly sophisticated competitive radiologic studies.

2. Current indications include:
    a. Hematuria (macroscopic and microscopic)
    b. Suspected transitional cell carcinoma or papillary necrosis
    c. Surveillance protocol for patients with prior urothelial malignancy
    d. Preoperative evaluation for select endourological procedures
    e. Postoperative evaluation of urologic procedures
    f. Complicated or unusual urinary tract infections (including tuberculosis)
    g. Stone disease, often in conjunction with ultrasonography (US) and computed tomography (CT)

C. Contraindications

1. Absolute. Neither allergy, pregnancy, nor diabetes mellitus is an absolute contraindication to urography or the use of contrast media (CM) in the presence of compelling indications. Under certain circumstances, however, each may represent a relative contraindication.
2. Relative
    a. A documented allergic or idiosyncratic reaction to CM (including CM for oral cholecystography), excluding nausea, vomiting, or syncope. Such patients can receive contrast again, but the indication should be firm and the patients should be premedicated with corticosteroids and antihistamines and given low-osmolar contrast media (LOCM), as discussed below.
    b. *Multiple myeloma.* Patients with multiple myeloma may have transient oliguria after contrast administration, possibly secondary to the precipitation of protein-contrast aggregates in the renal tubules. This can be prevented by hydration before and immediately following the study and by using LOCM.
    c. *Renal insufficiency.* Patients with serum creatinine values higher than 2 mg/dL should be evaluated with alternative imaging modalities that do not employ radiographic CM. The diagnostic value of urography is compromised with azotemia, and the possibility of contrast nephrotoxicity increases. Alternative imaging modalities almost always provide the necessary diagnostic information. These include unenhanced computed tomography (CT), ultrasonography (US),

nuclear radiology, retrograde pyeloureterography (RPG), and magnetic resonance imaging (MRI).

d. *Fluid and electrolyte imbalance.* Severely dehydrated patients or those with marked electrolyte imbalance are at risk for posturographic oliguria. Such underlying disturbances should be corrected before CM is administered, especially if the patient also has associated congestive heart failure.

e. *Multiple consecutive contrast studies.* Patients who receive intravenous CM on two or more consecutive days are exposed to a risk of renal insult that is greater than the combined risk of two random contrast examinations. If studies such as CT, angiography, coronary arteriography, as well as urography, are all indicated, it is best to separate any two of these studies by at least 24 hours and preferably 48 hours, during which time the patient should be thoroughly hydrated. Once the body burden of CM has been eliminated, it is safe to continue with the next contrast study.

D. Basic Considerations

1. *Contrast agents.* Urographic contrast media (CM) consist of three atoms of iodine attached to a benzene ring. Those in most common usage are the sodium or methylglucamine salts of diatrizoate (Renografin, Hypaque) and iothalamate (Conray). Newer nonionic agents such as iohexol (Omnipaque) and ioversol (Optiray) offer a somewhat more pleasant examination to patients who are sensitive to the older contrast media, and produce fewer physiologic responses, although the rare life-threatening reactions are not eliminated by the use of these low-osmolality contrast media (LOCM). LOCM are more expensive than HOCM, making it difficult for most radiology departments to employ them exclusively. Accordingly, certain criteria for the use of LOCM prevail in most hospitals. These include any patient whose general condition appears fragile (e.g., cardiac decompensation, advanced age or debility, electrolyte imbalance); patients with renal functional impairment; and patients with a significant allergic history, including reactions to previously administered CM. Patients who have experienced prior anaphylactoid reactions to HOCM should be premedicated with steroids and antihistamines prior to repeat contrast exposure and examined with LOCM to minimize the chances of a repeat contrast reaction.

2. *Physiology.* The contrast molecules exist, for the most part, unbound in the plasma and are excreted almost entirely by glomerular filtration. Only a small amount is bound to serum albumin and excreted by the liver.

E. Technique

1. *Preparation.* A thorough bowel prep is desirable to eliminate overlying soft-tissue densities that may interfere with optimal visualization of the urinary tract. Vigorous dehydration is not necessary, but withholding of fluids overnight is advantageous for optimal renal concentration of the contrast medium. An empty stomach is also helpful in the event of vomiting after contrast administration.

2. *Plain film of the abdomen [scout film; preliminary film; kidneys, ureters, and bladder film (KUB); abdominal "flat plate"].* This is an essential component of every radiographic examination of the genitourinary (GU) tract. Important findings such as soft-tissue masses, calcifications, and bony changes will be disclosed on this study. Many urinary tract calculi are obscured by excreted CM and are seen only on the KUB. In addition, retained barium in the colon or even the presence of a fetal skeleton, if seen on the preliminary film, may contraindicate the injection of CM and justify postponing the urogram.

3. *Contrast administration.* CM is administered intravenously as a rapid bolus injection, slow, steady injection, or drip infusion. This is more often a question of individual preference rather than a matter of scientific selection. In the average-size adult, 100 mL of CM are usually administered. Larger and/or older patients with decreased glomerular filtration rates (GFR) often receive 150 mL of CM to optimize their urogram.

4. *Filming.* Immediately after the contrast has been injected, tomograms are made to visualize the renal parenchyma (nephrographic phase). Within 3 min, contrast is usually visible in the collecting systems and several films are taken to visualize the calyces, pelves, and ureters (pyelographic phase) (Fig. 3-1). Films of the bladder (often including a postvoiding film) conclude the examination.

5. Modifications of the urogram

   a. *Emergency urography.* This is usually performed for suspected renal colic or renal trauma. It is usually impossible to adequately prepare the patient's bowel, so the urogram is often not of the highest quality. Nonetheless, with careful attention to technique and appropriate filming, it is usually possible to identify acute ureteral obstruction or major renal injury, if present. In both of these circumstances, however, CT is replacing the IVU in most institutions.

   b. *Hydration (diuretic) urography.* This study is reserved for those patients suspected of having intermittent hydronephrosis in whom an initial (dehydrated) IVU revealed no obstruction. With forced diuresis, a borderline ureteropelvic junction or ureteral narrowing may

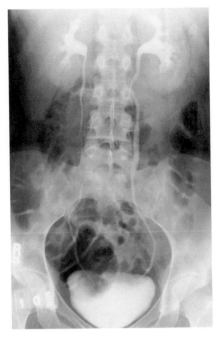

Figure 3-1 Normal intravenous urogram. A 10-min postinjection image from an IVU demonstrates visualization of both renal collecting systems, ureters, and urinary bladder. Although the renal parenchyma remains well opacified, it is better evaluated on images obtained earlier in the study.

become inadequate to carry the increased urine load and may result in hydronephrosis.

F. Complications
1. Immediate
   a. *Minor side effects.* These consist of nausea, vomiting, arm pain, and lightheadedness. Such reactions are fairly frequent but never serious, except for the possibility of aspiration following vomiting. These reactions are mitigated for the most part by the use of LOCM.
   b. *Allergic reaction.* Approximately 5 percent of patients demonstrate an allergic or histamine-type reaction to CM. This generally consists of erythema, urticaria, sneezing, or, in severe cases, severe vomiting, facial or glottic edema, or bronchospasm. In patients with a seafood or iodine sensitivity, the reaction rate is approximately 15 percent, with the majority of these

being mild. It is slightly higher yet in those who have a proven history of an allergic reaction to prior CM administration. Treatment is reserved for the more severe of these reactions and consists primarily of antihistamines. Steroids and/or epinephrine may be employed as needed. Prophylactic antihistamines and corticosteroids are strongly recommended in this group; they should also receive LOCM.

   c. *Chemotoxic or idiosyncratic reactions.* These are the most serious reactions but also the rarest. Manifestations include convulsions, pulmonary edema, cardiovascular collapse, thrombosis, thrombolysis, and cardiac arrest. They occur in perhaps 1 of every 7500 to 10,000 patients, of whom the majority are successfully managed with prompt effective treatment. The mortality rate for CM administration ranges from 1:50,000 to 1:100,000 patients. An allergic history is usually not obtained in patients experiencing this type of reaction, and there is little that can be done to anticipate which patients will experience this complication. They appear to be less prevalent with LOCM.

  2. *Delayed.* Although contrast agents are among the safest pharmaceuticals used in clinical medicine, they may aggravate preexisting renal disease in a small percentage of patients with underlying azotemia by a process not yet understood. Nephrotoxicity is extraordinarily low when kidney function is normal. Patients with diabetic nephropathy, especially if it began in childhood, and those whose creatinine levels are at or above 3 mg/dL appear to be the most vulnerable. This nephrotoxicity is usually reversible. LOCM offer significant protection against the development of contrast nephropathy.

III. RETROGRADE UROGRAPHY (RETROGRADE PYELOURETEROGRAPHY OR RPG)

A. Purpose and Indications

1. To investigate lesions of the ureter and renal collecting system that cannot be adequately defined by IVU.
2. To visualize the collecting systems and ureters when IVU is contraindicated (azotemia, severe prior contrast reaction).
3. To provide a "road map" to these structures to aid in manipulative procedures such as brush biopsy under fluoroscopic control (see Chapter 4).
4. To visualize the ureteral stump remaining after nephrectomy in a patient with hematuria or positive urinary cytology.

B. Contraindications

1. Untreated urinary tract infection.

2. Patients who cannot or should not be cystoscoped (e.g., patients recovering from recent bladder or urethral surgery).

3. RPG may be impossible in some patients such as those with very large prostates in whom the gland overlies the ureteral orifices preventing proper catheter placement. At times, even though the orifice is identifiable, it may not be possible to catheterize it, such as may occur with tortuous ureters or following ureteral reimplantation.

C. Technique

1. Preliminary cystoscopy is required.

2. A ureteral orifice is identified and catheterized with a small (usually 5 French) ureteral catheter. The catheter is advanced to the renal pelvis and contrast is instilled. The same contrast agents employed for IVU or CT are used for retrograde pyelography. Alternatively, when a catheter cannot or should not be passed, the ureter may be opacified by occluding its orifice and allowing contrast to fill it (and the renal collecting system) by gravity ("bulb" or occlusive tip retrograde).

3. Films

   a. A preliminary KUB film is essential. Following contrast injection, one or more films are obtained (Fig. 3-2) to delineate unopacified or poorly seen portions of the collecting system or ureter in question. If obstruction is suspect, a film several minutes after removal of the ureteral catheter is also obtained to ascertain the adequacy of ureteral peristalsis in draining the collecting system.

   b. The use of fluoroscopy is an important adjunct to RPG. In most hospital settings, however, this requires the placement of a ureteral catheter in the cystoscopy suite and the subsequent transport of the patient to the radiology department for catheter injection.

D. Complications

1. If anesthesia is used for cystoscopy, the patient is at risk for any of the complications of that anesthesia.

2. Instrumental perforation of the ureter is uncommon. When it does occur, there are usually no serious sequela and contrast extravasation outside the collecting system does not usually result in any harm. In some cases of perforation, diversion of urine may be required.

3. Because infected bladder urine may be carried to the upper urinary tract, pyelonephritis may, on rare occasions, complicate RPG. A too vigorous injection of contrast material in an infected urinary tract may disseminate bacteria

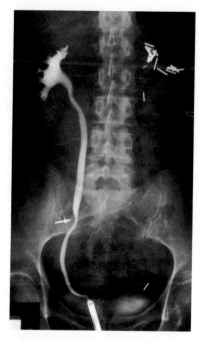

Figure 3-2 Normal right retrograde pyeloureterogram. Through a cystoscope, a ureteral catheter is positioned in the right ureteral orifice. By occluding the ureteral orifice, the right ureter and renal collecting system can be gravitationally filled with contrast (bulb retrograde). Note the normal extrinsic impression on the ureter by the right iliac artery (*arrow*). Metallic clips in the left renal fossa and left bony pelvis attest to prior nephroureterectomy for transitional cell carcinoma of the kidney.

throughout the bloodstream as well as the kidney. Fortunately, the normal antegrade flow of urine is usually enough to wash out any bacteria that may have been introduced. However, in the presence of a urinary tract obstruction, the risk increases.

4. Absorption of contrast agents from the upper urinary tract occurs regularly. As much as 10 to 15 percent of the injectate can be reabsorbed. In those patients truly sensitive to contrast media, therefore, the use of the retrograde approach does not confer immunity against a systemic contrast reaction, although reactions are much less common than after IV injection. Other drugs administered by this

route (e.g., antibiotics) will also undergo the same degree of reabsorption.

IV. ANTEGRADE PYELOGRAPHY

A. Purpose and Indications

1. To visualize the upper urinary tract when an IVU is unsatisfactory and RPG cannot be done.
2. To delineate the site or nature of upper urinary tract obstruction if retrograde pyelography has failed or alternative imaging techniques (US, CT, MRI) are not definitive.
3. To delineate the site or nature of upper urinary tract obstruction if RPG is impossible (e.g., ureteral diversion).
4. To ascertain whether a dilated collecting system is obstructed or not when azotemia and/or oliguria occurs after renal transplantation.
5. To perform upper urinary tract urodynamic testing (Whitaker test).

B. Contraindications

1. Bleeding diathesis.
2. Diffuse skin infection over the lumbar area (native kidney) or lower abdominal wall (renal transplant).
3. A nondilated collecting system is not a contraindication. Although it may sometimes be challenging to puncture a nondilated collecting system, it can usually be accomplished.

C. Technique

The renal pelvis is percutaneously punctured with a 20- or 21-gauge thin-walled needle from a posterior or posterolateral approach. Localization is provided by means of contrast excreted after an IV injection or, in the event of a nonvisualizing kidney, with US. The procedure is carried out and films are exposed under fluoroscopic control (Fig. 3-3).

D. Complications

1. Inadvertent puncture of neighboring structures may occur. Although puncture of the renal vein, kidney parenchyma, or liver and spleen is possible, few, if any, complications result because of the small size of the needle.
2. Some extravasation usually occurs with many antegrade pyelograms. However, the puncture site is very small and rapidly seals after the needle has been removed.
3. Localization of the renal pelvis is occasionally difficult and time consuming and, on rare occasions, may

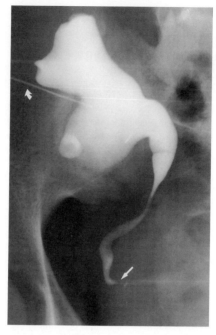

Figure 3-3 Antegrade pyeloureterogram. A thin needle (*curved arrow*) has been percutaneously inserted into the renal pelvis of a transplanted kidney and contrast material (CM) is being injected. The collecting system and proximal ureter are capacious, but not obstructed, as there is normal tapering of the ureter and flow of CM into the urinary bladder. An *arrow* points to the opening of the transplanted ureter in the urinary bladder.

fail completely, especially if the collecting system is not dilated.

V. CYSTOGRAPHY (STATIC CYSTOGRAM)
A. Purpose and Indications
1. To assess the size, position, and integrity of the urinary bladder by means of retrograde instillation of CM.
2. Suspected bladder trauma. Since the IVU is unreliable in such an evaluation, and even CT can miss some bladder ruptures, a properly performed cystogram, wherein a detrusor contraction is elicited, is indispensable in excluding a bladder rupture.

3. Evaluation of bladder diverticula. The ability of bladder diverticula to drain properly is best evaluated by cystography (alternatively with US).
4. Evaluation of fistulae beginning or terminating in the urinary bladder.
5. Evaluation of postoperative healing following open bladder or distal ureteral surgery.

B. Contraindications

Contraindications to passage of a urethral catheter may make attempts at cystography inadvisable, but there are no contraindications to cystography itself. When a patient has sustained pelvic trauma, the integrity of the urethra must first be established before blindly passing a urethral catheter. This may often require that retrograde urethrography precede cystography.

C. Technique

1. After a preliminary KUB, a urethral catheter is passed and CM is instilled into the bladder. Films of the filled bladder are made in multiple projections. The bladder is then allowed to empty through the catheter, after which a drainage film is obtained.
2. Cystography may also be performed from above (antegrade) through an existing cystostomy tube or via suprapubic puncture.

D. Complications

1. Complications of cystography are rare. Excessively forceful injection may result in bladder rupture or disruption of a fresh suture line.
2. The results of traumatic urethral catheterization must also be considered as potential complications.

E. Modifications of Cystography

Cystography can be tailored to specific clinical situations, such as stress incontinence, and altered to provide relevant information about the probable cause of the incontinence and the most rational approaches to its elimination. Findings sought in the incontinent patient include the degree of bladder neck descent on coughing or straining (sustained Valsalva maneuver), the level at which urine is held (both voluntarily and involuntarily), and whether the bladder neck remains competent or is open at rest (Fig. 3-4).

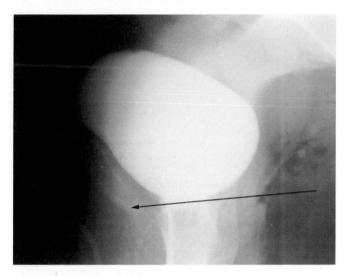

Figure 3-4 Stress or incontinence cystogram. The urinary bladder has been filled with 150 mL of CM through a urethral catheter (*arrowheads*). With the patient standing and turned into a lateral position, images of the bladder and urethra are obtained (**A**) at rest and (**B**) during a sustained Valsalva maneuver. The long black *arrow* connecting the inferior margin of the symphysis pubis and the coccyx represents the normal position of the pelvic floor. **A.** At rest, the bladder base is normally situated above the pelvic floor and the bladder neck is normally closed around the ureteral catheter.

VI. VOIDING CYSTOURETHROGRAPHY (VCUG OR ANTEGRADE URETHROGRAPHY

A. Purpose
1. To demonstrate the anatomy of the lower urinary tract during the physiologic act of micturition.
2. To establish the presence or absence of vesicoureteral reflux.

B. Indications
1. Recurrent urinary tract infections, especially in children, in whom reflux is not uncommon.
2. Evaluation of the posterior urethra in the male and the entire urethra in the female. By means of VCUG, posterior urethral pathology may be demonstrated. VCUG is especially valuable in evaluating urethral stricture disease,

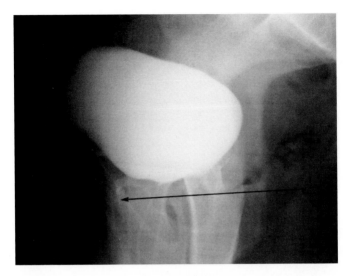

Figure 3-4 (*continued*)   **B.** With abdominal straining, the bladder base descends to a position below the normal pelvic floor (pelvic floor relaxation) and the urethra (demarcated by the indwelling catheter) changes its angle of inclination (urethral hypermobility). This patient did not show evidence of stress urinary incontinence, however.

posterior urethral valves in the infant male, and the postoperative urethra. In the female, it is a primary method of visualizing urethral diverticula.

3. For the evaluation of certain voiding dysfunctions (e.g., detrusor-external sphincter dyssynergia, neuropathic bladder), VCUG is sometimes combined with simultaneous pressure-flow recordings (videourodynamics).

4. For the evaluation of an ectopic ureter thought to insert into the urethra. Reflux into such ectopic ureters is fairly common.

C. Contraindications
1. There are no contraindications to VCUG except in the unusual instance of the patient who cannot be catheterized.

2. Occasionally, the examination cannot be satisfactorily performed because of the patient's voluntary or involuntary inability to void at the time.

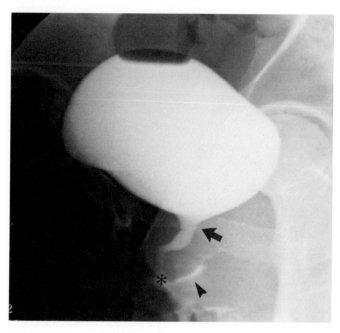

Figure 3-5 Normal female voiding cystourethrogram. Oblique projection of a normal bladder and female urethra during voiding. Note the smooth outline of the bladder, the widely funneled bladder neck (*arrow*), and the normal female urethra. An *asterisk* indicates the position of the urethral meatus. Some of the voided CM coats the perineum and refluxes into the distal vagina (*arrowhead*). A small amount of air was introduced into the bladder during catheterization. With the patient in the erect position, the air rises to the dome of the bladder and produces a black and white air–fluid level.

D. Technique

1. This procedure may be performed in males or females. It is best performed under fluoroscopic control.

2. The bladder is catheterized and filled with water-soluble CM (usually HOCM). When the patient has a strong desire to void, the catheter is withdrawn and the patient voids. Fluoroscopic images of micturition are obtained (Figs. 3-5 and 3-6). An estimate of the completeness of bladder emptying is made.

3. In patients who have undergone recent bladder neck or urethral surgery, voiding around an indwelling urethral catheter is initially performed to look for contrast ex-

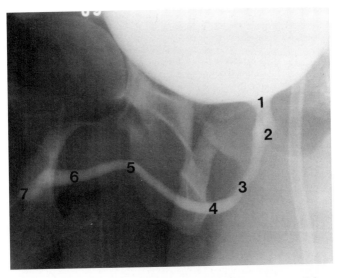

Figure 3-6 Normal male voiding cystourethrogram. A young adult male was being evaluated with videourodynamics for voiding dysfunction. A fluoroscopic image obtained during voiding shows a normal urethra as well as the lower half of the urinary bladder.
1, bladder neck; 2, verumontanum within prostatic urethra; 3, membraneous urethra (level of urogenital diaphragm); 4, bulbous urethra; 5, penoscrotal junction; 6, pendulous or penile urethra; 7, urethral meatus. A rectal catheter posterior to urethra is measuring intraabdominal pressure during the urodynamic study.

    travasation. If none is seen fluoroscopically, the urethral catheter may be removed and another void documented fluoroscopically.
4. Although the bladder is filled with the patient recumbent, voiding is usually performed with the patient standing.

E. Complications
These are essentially the same as those listed under cystography.

VII. RETROGRADE URETHROGRAPHY (RUG)
A. Purpose
To provide detailed visualization of the anterior urethra in the male. The procedure has little or no application in the female. Unlike a VCUG, the RUG incompletely visualizes the

posterior urethra because of the resistance to retrograde flow provided by the external urethral sphincter.

B. Indications

1. Detailed delineation of suspected or known urethral stricture (most common indication).
2. Suspected urethral trauma. RUG should be routinely performed before attempting passage of a urethral catheter.
3. Demonstration of urethral diverticula, fistulae, and neoplasms.

C. Contraindications

1. Acute urethritis, as discussed below.
2. Patients who are contrast-sensitive can manifest sensitivity if CM is absorbed during the procedure. LOCM should be employed in this situation.

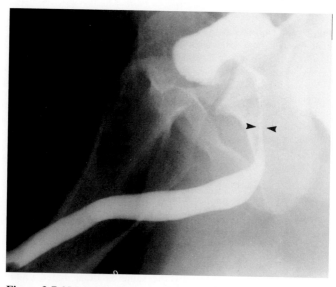

Figure 3-7 Normal retrograde urethrogram. The pendulous and bulbous portions of the urethra are maximally distended with the retrograde injection of CM through a catheter placed in the terminal portion of the urethra (fossa navicularis). *Arrowheads* show the location of the external urethral sphincter within the urogenital diaphragm. As most patients have some difficulty relaxing their external sphincter, only a small amount of CM is filling an underdistended prostatic urethra and entering the urinary bladder.

D. Technique

1. The most distal 1 to 2 cm of the urethra is occluded by means of a partially inflated Foley catheter balloon placed in the fossa navicularis. The remainder of the anterior urethra is filled with water-soluble CM.

2. Radiographic images of the urethra fully distended with CM are taken during injection (Fig. 3-7).

E. Complications

1. Reflux of CM from the urethra to the surrounding corpus spongiosum can occur during RUG. Such reflux is usually minimal and without clinical consequence except in the presence of urethritis when bacteria may be forced into the bloodstream. The procedure is relatively contraindicated in the face of infection. As mentioned above, LOCM is used for contrast-sensitive men.

2. Pulmonary embolism is a very real consideration if water-soluble CM are not used. For this reason, oily contrast agents are contraindicated for RUG.

VIII. LOOPOGRAPHY AND POUCHOGRAPHY

Anastomosis of the ureters to an isolated intact segment (loop) of ileum or transverse colon or to a detubularized large or small bowel segment (pouch) is the most common method of establishing permanent urinary diversion. The isolated but otherwise intact bowel loop serves as a conduit for urine propelling it outward toward the stoma in a continuous, rhythmic, isoperistaltic way. The detubularized pouch, on the other hand, lacks the contractility to propel urine to the outside, thus becoming a reservoir rather than a conduit. Therefore, detubularized pouches are continent of urine and require intermittent catheterization for emptying. The peristaltic loops do not. Be they loops or pouches, both types of urinary receptacles occasionally require radiologic evaluation. Radiologic examination of such bowel segments is referred to as loopography or pouchography.

A. Purpose and Indications

1. To evaluate the bowel conduit or reservoir for suspected intrinsic disease (e.g., filling defects, anastomotic or other leaks, loop stenosis), capacity, or peristaltic activity.

2. To visualize the upper urinary tracts by reflux. Reflux is normal with ileal conduits since the thin small-bowel wall precludes an antireflux ureteroileal anastomosis. Large-bowel receptacles, however, as well as detubularized segments, are often of an antirefluxing nature.

3. To evaluate patients with intact loop diversion whose upper urinary tracts show deterioration by serial IVUs or ultrasonograms (i.e., worsening hydronephrosis, renal calculi, renal scarring) or whose renal function is diminishing. In such patients the absence of reflux may indicate ureteroileal obstruction.

4. To localize the urinary diversion and probable site of ureteral implantation prior to interventional procedures on the diverted ureters.

B. Contraindications

1. There are no contraindications to the retrograde study of a urinary conduit or reservoir.

2. Patients with current or previous urinary tract infections should receive prophylactic antibiotics.

C. Technique

1. Following a KUB, the stoma of an ileal conduit is catheterized with a 14 or 16 French Foley catheter. By placing gentle traction on the catheter with its inflated balloon just below the anterior abdominal wall, CM is prevented from exiting the stoma. The conduit is filled with water-soluble CM by gentle hand injection until the ileum is well distended. Fluoroscopic images are obtained with particular attention given to the presence or absence of reflux. The catheter is then removed and the conduit and upper urinary tracts evaluated for emptying.

2. A continent urinary pouch or reservoir is also evaluated fluoroscopically. The stoma (for a cutaneous diversion) or urethra (for an orthotopic diversion) is catheterized and a Foley catheter placed into the reservoir. The reservoir is opacified with CM to capacity, which varies with time. At maturity, it should accomodate several hundred mL of fluid. Filling defects and leaks are documented, if present. Nonopaque mucus in the reservoir is an expected finding.

3. Although many pouches do not normally allow for ureteral reflux, reflux may be observed with a Studer pouch, in which the ureters are anastomosed to an isoperistaltic afferent loop of ileum, which drains into a detubularized ileal pouch. Although reflux does not occur in a normally functioning Studer pouch, the elevated intraluminal pressures generated during retrograde pouch opacification will fill the isoperistaltic afferent limb and diverted ureters (Fig. 3-8).

D. Complications

Pyelonephritis may accompany forceful reflux of infected urine.

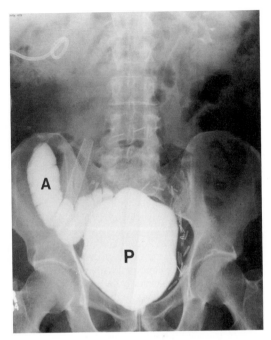

Figure 3-8 Normal pouchogram. The patient has undergone radical cystectomy for bladder cancer and surgical creation of an orthotopic continent urinary pouch of the Studer variety. A retrograde cystogram performed through a urethral Foley catheter fills the pouch (P) and isoperistaltic afferent limb (A). Although both components of the diversion are crafted from ileum, the detubularized pouch or reservoir no longer appears as a loop of bowel, whereas the afferent limb looks look a loop of ileum. There is faint contrast opacification of the left collecting system and proximal ureter secondary to reflux from the afferent limb, a normal finding. The right ureter is obstructed near its entry into the afferent limb and does not reflux, despite the present of an expandable metal stent (Wallstent) which was inserted percutaneously to maintain ureteral patency. Note the presence of a pigtail percutaneous nephrostomy catheter on the right.

IX. ANGIOGRAPHY
A. Basic Considerations
Angiography refers to the radiologic study of both the arterial and venous systems. There are various anatomic subdivisions. Those pertinent to the study of the urinary tract include:
1. Arterial: aortography, renal arteriography, adrenal arteriography

2. Venous: inferior venacavography, renal phlebography, adrenal phlebography, gonadal phlebography

B. Indications
1. Renal
   a. *Hypertension.* Angiography can be employed diagnostically both to image the arterial supply to the kidney and to sample renal vein blood for renin. Balloon angioplasty and metal stent deployment often complement angiographic demonstration of hemodynamically significant renal arterial stenoses.
   b. *Neoplasms.* Since the development of CT and MRI, angiography is infrequently employed in the diagnosis of renal masses. It is still used occasionally for the embolization (preoperative or otherwise) of certain renal neoplasms, including renal cell carcinoma and angiomyolipoma.
   c. *Renal trauma.* Most traumatic parenchymal and vascular lesions can be satisfactorily imaged by means of CT. Angiography is usually reserved to demonstrate an arterial bleeder or arteriovenous communication prior to ablation.
   d. *Evaluation.* For the evaluation (and potential ablation) of vascular abnormalities such as aneurysms and arteriovenous malformations.
   e. *Diagnostic.* In suspected embolism of the renal arterial tree, thrombosis of the renal artery or renal vein where the diagnosis is not clear by CT or MRI.
   f. *Preoperative.* To provide a preoperative arterial "road map" when intrarenal surgical dissection is contemplated. This is especially valuable when there is a high risk of anomalous vascular supply such as in a horseshoe kidney. In most of these cases, however, CT angiography or MR angiography has supplanted catheter angiography.
   g. *Donors.* In the preoperative evaluation of potential renal donors, CT angiography and MR angiography have supplanted catheter angiography in most institutions.
2. Adrenal gland
   a. Ablation of adrenal function by embolization or over-injection of the adrenal veins.
   b. For adrenal vein sampling of functioning adrenal tumors.
3. Other
   a. Gonadal phlebography is occasionally employed in the search for a nonpalpable undescended testis.
   b. Gonadal phlebography is also valuable in evaluating varicoceles and in treating them by means of venous

occlusion with balloons, coils, or sclerosing agents (Fig. 3-9).

C. Contraindications

1. Bleeding diathesis.
2. Hypercoagulation states such as polycythemia vera constitute a relative contraindication. Extremely small instruments should be used in these patients because of the risk of thrombosis.

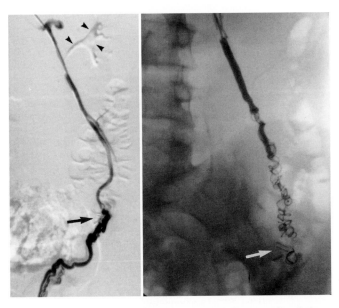

Figure 3-9 Left spermatic venogram. **A.** The left spermatic vein has been opacified by means of a catheter inserted from the femoral vein into the inferior vena cava, left renal vein, and left spermatic vein. Digital subtraction venogram shows a tortuous spermatic vein distal to three metallic clips (*arrow*) placed on that vein during a prior open surgical attempt to ligate the tortuous vein and relieve a symptomatic varicocele. The venogram shows venous recanalization and recurrent varicocele formation. Note the almost completely subtracted left pyelocalyceal system (*arrowheads*). **B.** Multiple metallic embolization coils have been inserted into the spermatic vein proximal to the metallic clips (*arrows*). Repeat spermatic venogram shows complete absence of contrast flow into the tortuous vein as previously demonstrated, a technically successful spermatic vein embolization procedure.

D. Technique for performing angiography

1. Percutaneous vascular catheterization (Seldinger technique)
   a. Arterial
   b. Venous
      By means of a percutaneous puncture usually into the femoral artery or femoral vein, a needle is inserted into the desired blood vessel and a guidewire is passed through it. The needle is removed and a catheter is passed over the guidewire until its tip is satisfactorily placed within the vascular system. CM is then injected.

2. Selective angiography
   a. Selective renal arteriography
      This is the most common method of performing renal arteriography. A catheter is inserted retrograde into the aorta as described and then manipulated until its tip comes to lie in the renal artery. A few mL of CM are injected and serial radiographs follow. Because of the rapid transit of the contrast through the vascular system, films must be exposed quite rapidly, often at the rate of several per second. Three phases of renal arteriography can be recognized: arterial, nephrographic, and venous.
   b. Selective renal phlebography
      The renal vein is selectively catheterized percutaneously and contrast material injected. Usually the renal artery needs to be temporarily occluded or constricted with epinephrine to slow blood flow and preclude the too rapid washout of contrast from the renal vein (Fig. 3-10).

3. Digital subtraction angiography
   With this technique, electronic subtraction and computerized image manipulation are carried out to provide visualization of the arterial tree after intravenous injection or after relatively small intra-arterial injections (Fig. 3-11).

E. Complications

Angiography is relatively safe when performed by trained personnel, however, there are certain well-recognized complications.

1. Vascular complications related to the puncture.
   a. Minor: transient spasm, small hematoma, pain.
   b. Major: bleeding, thrombosis, dissection, arteriovenous fistula, and pseudoaneurysm formation.

2. Physiologic complications secondary to the effect of CM injected directly into the kidney. These are transient and

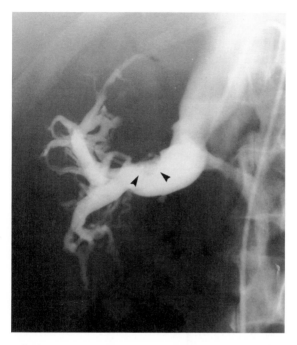

Figure 3-10 Right renal venogram. A catheter passed up the inferior vena cava has been inserted into the right renal vein and contrast material injected. Normal intrarenal venous arborization is demonstrated. There is small nonobstructing filling defect in the main renal vein (*arrowheads*) that represents a tumor thrombus from a renal cell carcinoma. To obtain this degree of intrarenal venous opacification, epinephrine is usually injected into the renal artery immediately prior to the venous injection. This slows arterial flow and maximizes retrograde venous opacification by minimizing the dilution of the injected contrast by inflowing unopacified arterial blood.

rarely lasting. Properly performed by currently recommended techniques, there is no permanent or lasting deleterious effect on renal function following the injection of CM into the renal artery.

3. Systemic effects of CM.

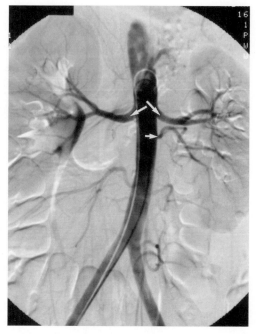

Figure 3-11 Normal digital subtraction angiogram (DSA). The patient is being evaluated as a potential renal donor. The aorta and proximal renal arteries are well opacified and appear normal. An image immediately prior to the contrast injection has been electronically subtracted from an image following the injection, thereby eliminating or "subtracting" all structures other than the vessels of interest. Minimal catheter movement during the injection accounts for the apparent presence of two pigtail catheters in the aorta, one white and the other black. Although most of the bowel and the opacified right pyelocalyceal system and ureter have been subtracted away, slight spatial misregistration accounts for their faint visualization. Note the presence of a single renal artery on the right and two arteries on the left (*arrows*).

X. RADIONUCLIDE IMAGING
A. Basic Principles
The flow of radioisotopes through the kidney and other GU structures can be monitored so that, in turn, vascular perfusion, parenchymal integrity, and, in the case of the kidney, outflow tract anatomy can be imaged. By means of radio-pharmaceuticals designed for specific physiologic functions, tissue isotopic distribution is imaged with a gamma cam-

era, which measures emitted gamma radiation as a function of time and spatial distribution. In this way, organ function can also be ascertained. Radiopharmaceuticals can be primarily morphologic agents or functional agents. Examples of some of the radiopharmaceuticals frequently employed for GU imaging are ^{131}I-ortho-iodohippurate, ^{99m}Tc-glucoheptonate, ^{99m}Tc-DTPA, ^{99m}Tc-DMSA, ^{99m}Tc-MAG$_3$, and [67]gallium citrate.

B. Indications

1. *Measurement of renal function.* Following a bolus injection of radionuclide, computer analysis of radioactivity versus time can analyze blood clearance rates to determine glomerular filtration rate, effective renal plasma flow, and fractionation of individual renal function. The ability to ascertain the function of one kidney has special significance when decisions regarding nephrectomy versus salvage operations must be made (Fig. 3-12). In cases of severe hydronephrosis, split renal functions before and after a period of nephrostomy drainage may show a surprising degree of renal functional improvement in the hitherto obstructed kidney.

2. *Hypertension.* Differential renal blood flow studies (performed before and after the administration of an angiotensin-converting enzyme inhibitor such as captopril) detect approximately 85 percent of cases of renal artery stenosis, but the study is complicated by an approximately 10 percent false-positive rate, mainly in patients with essential hypertension. Other difficulties with isotope screening in hypertension include problems in distinguishing unilateral renovascular lesions from unilateral renal parenchymal disease and problems recognizing bilateral vascular stenoses. The accuracy of the examination is decreased in the face of renal insufficiency.

3. *Renal functional impairment.* Radionuclide imaging is more sensitive than IVU in providing images of the kidney when renal function is diminished and is sometimes used in lieu of radiographic methods in evaluating patients with renal failure of unknown cause. However, anatomic detail is much less satisfactory than that provided by IVU. In cases of suspected obstructive uropathy, radionuclide studies are often not specific enough to compete with the other imaging modalities, specifically US, CT, or MRI.

4. *Contraindications to CM.* Although radionuclide methods are not as specific as radiographic studies, they represent an acceptable alternative in an attempt to gain some gross information about renal anatomy and differential

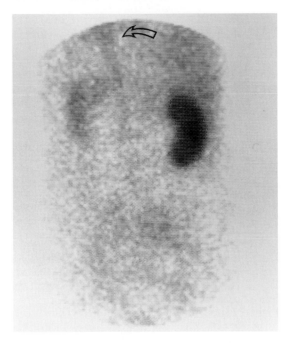

Figure 3-12 Renal scintigram in obstruction. **A.** Following intravenous injection of a bolus of ^{99m}Tc-MAG3, scintigraphic images show diminished perfusion of the left kidney when compared with the right. The proximal abdominal aorta is still evident (*arrow*).

function in those who cannot receive CM. Patients with renal failure and those with demonstrated unusually severe contrast sensitivity fall into this group.

5. *Evaluation of renal transplant failure.* Isotopic methods of imaging the kidney are very helpful in evaluating renal transplant complications including obstruction, extravasation, and stenosis of the arterial anastomosis. Differentiation between acute tubular necrosis and transplant rejection is a more difficult task.

6. *Questionable or intermittent obstruction.* The presence of intermittent obstruction, especially at the ureteropelvic junction, is often difficult to document. Using radionuclide methods, the rate of emptying of the collecting system after a diuretic challenge (washout or lasix renogram) can be evaluated and compared to standard emptying profiles.

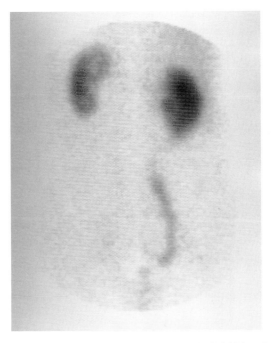

Figure 3-12 (*continued*)   **B.** Thirty min later, the left kidney has accumulated additional isotope but has not excreted it into the collecting system. Excretion occurred normally on the right, but there is persistent isotope in the distal right ureter indicating impaired emptying into the bladder. Computer analysis showed that 77 percent of the patient's overall renal function was being contributed by the right kidney and 23 percent by the left. The scintigrams give evidence of bilateral ureteral obstruction, much more severe on the left than the right. The patient had multifocal transitional cell carcinoma of the bladder with bilateral distal ureteral obstruction and azotemia. A percutaneous nephrostomy was performed on the better functioning right kidney. The kidneys are displayed as they are viewed by a nuclear camera positioned behind the patient.

       7. *Renal masses.* Occasionally, it is difficult or impossible to differentiate between a renal mass or pseudomass (pseudotumor) by IVU. In these cases, the use of radionuclides to provide a functional image of the renal parenchyma can be extremely important in showing whether there is a pathologic mass in the renal parenchyma. In the presence of an abnormality, there is

a photon deficient area in the kidney (cold spot). With pseudotumors no such defect is noticed. CT, US, and MRI can also distinguish between bona fide masses and pseudotumors and have supplanted isotopic techniques for this purpose in most institutions.

8. *Extravasation of urine.* Small urinary leaks can sometimes be undetectable with contrast studies. However, because small amounts of radionuclide can be detected readily with modern scanning techniques, small or early extravasations can be imaged much more readily with radionuclide studies than with conventional radiography.

9. *Vesicoureteral reflux.* Vesicoureteral reflux is usually demonstrated initially by VCUG. However, once demonstrated, it may be followed periodically by radionuclide cystourethrography, which is more sensitive than VCUG and imposes less of a radiation burden on the patient. Using agents such as ^{99m}Tc-DMSA, the renal scarring, which is often the consequence of reflux, can also be demonstrated.

10. *The "acute" scrotum.* When testicular torsion is suspected, a radionuclide flow study of the scrotum will demonstrate the viability of the testis and compare its perfusion to the opposite side. Increased nuclide perfusion favors epididymitis over torsion.

11. *Inflammatory lesions.* Inflammatory lesions of any organ result in abnormal uptake of ^{67}gallium citrate. Gallium scanning is useful in uncovering occult inflammatory foci in or around the kidneys or confirming the presence of a clinically atypical infection. Other agents such as ^{111}indium, which can be fixed to leukocytes, may also be used.

12. *Adrenal gland.* ^{131}iodine metaiodobenzylguanidine (MIBG), an adrenal medullary imaging agent, can readily and easily localize pheochromocytomas. Cholesterol analogues (Iodine-131 NP-59) have also been synthesized and have proved helpful in localizing hyper- and hypofunctioning adrenal lesions.

C. Contraindications

No contraindications to the use of radionuclides for diagnostic purposes exist although they should not be administered during pregnancy.

D. Technique

Techniques vary depending on the information desired. In general, a tracer dose of radioactive isotope bound to a specific pharmaceutical agent is administered and the patient is placed beneath a gamma camera where images (scans, scintigrams) are generated at intervals depending on the information sought. For flow studies, images are taken as frequently as every few seconds. For anatomic information, images are obtained by accumulating counts for several minutes. These images may be taken sequentially for as long as several hours, and under certain circumstances may even be delayed up to 24 or 48 hours. Recently, techniques for obtaining tomographic scintigraphy [single-photon emission computed tomography (SPECT)] have considerably improved the anatomic information provided by radionuclide images. When evaluating renal function, small radiation detectors or gamma cameras placed directly over the kidneys can be used to generate time–radioactivity curves. This is known as a renogram.

E. Complications
There are no complications of nuclear medicine diagnostic procedures. The radiation doses involved are minimal to modest and, in many cases, are less than those for comparable conventional radiographic studies or CT.

XI. ULTRASONOGRAPHY
A. Purpose
Ultrasound (US) can be used to image most parts of the GU system.
1. Advantages
   a. Noninvasive.
   b. Independent of organ function.
   c. CM not required, although newly developed ultrasound contrast agents often enhance the diagnostic yield of the examination.
   d. Characteristics of blood flow can be determined.
2. Disadvantages
   a. Inferior resolution compared to, for example, IVU or PYRG.
   b. Certain structures cannot be visualized, for example, the nondilated abdominal ureter.

B. Techniques
Two types of sonographic imaging can be employed in the urinary tract: Real-time gray-scale imaging and Doppler or flow imaging. The latter is frequently color coded and combined with real-time imaging. Real-time imaging allows consistent modification of transducer position to obtain optimal projections (Fig. 3-13).

C. Complications
None known.

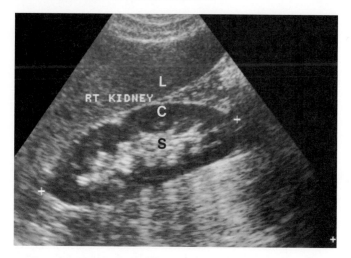

Figure 3-13 Normal nephrosonogram. Sagittal ultrasonogram of the right kidney shows normal renal cortex (C), slightly less echogenic than adjacent normal liver (L), the relatively sonolucent renal medullary pyramids (*arrowheads*), and the echogenic renal sinus (S). Electronic cursors have been placed at each renal pole to determine renal length.

D. Indications

1. Kidney
   a. *Renal masses.* US can detect fluid-filled renal masses with more than 98 percent accuracy. Solid mass lesions larger than 1 cm in diameter are also routinely identified. The sonographic patterns for cysts and solid masses are quite distinctive, although complex or complicated cysts may share certain imaging characteristics of solid lesions. The detection of neoplasms is aided by demonstrating flow within them by means of color-flow or power Doppler. This modality has value also in demonstrating intravenous and intracaval tumor extension with renal neoplasms. The ability to identify, characterize, and stage a renal mass lesion is dependent on the depth of the lesion beneath the skin and body habitus of the patient.
   b. *Impaired renal function.* The number, size, shape, and location of the kidneys, as well as the status of the renal pelvis, can be determined accurately. Dilated renal pelves and calyces usually indicate obstructive uropathy.
   c. *Unilateral nonvisualization at urography.* The cause for a nonvisualizing kidney can be frequently revealed

by US. In many cases, however, the study must be supplemented by other imaging modalities such as retrograde pyelography.

d. *To screen patients at risk for the presence of hydronephrosis.* US is extremely accurate in detecting volume changes in the upper urinary tract. False positives are not uncommon, but false negatives are rare.

e. *As a guide to biopsy and other interventional procedures.* US can outline the kidney (including renal transplants) and ascertain its depth below the skin, thus facilitating percutaneous renal biopsy with an aspiration biopsy needle guide. US is also very helpful in guiding needles into renal cysts or dilated renal collecting systems for antegrade pyelography preparatory to percutaneous nephrostomy.

f. *Renal pelvic filling defects.* These are most commonly caused by nonopaque calculi, urothelial neoplasms, and blood clots. Renal calculi are markedly echogenic, produce acoustic shadowing, and are readily detectable by US. Clots and tumors may also be demonstrated, but not necessarily differentiated.

g. *Evaluation of perinephric collections.* Fluid collections around the kidney consist of abscesses, urinomas, hematomas, or, in the case of a transplanted kidney, lymphoceles. Although these can all be recognized as echo-free masses in the perinephric space or around the kidney, differentiating one from the other is usually not possible by US alone. A complex fluid mass is more likely an abscess or hematoma than a lymphocele or urinoma.

h. *Renal surveillance.* Kidneys at risk for the development of specific diseases can be periodically monitored by US (for example, the contralateral kidney following nephrectomy for Wilms' tumor and evaluation of family members of patients with hereditary disorders such as polycystic disease and tuberous sclerosis). The status of existing diseases such as hydronephrosis can also be monitored to determine whether the process is static, improving, or worsening.

i. *Renovascular problems.* Utilizing color-flow Doppler sonography for the most part, arterial and venous lesions (e.g., occlusions, stenoses, aneurysms, fistulae, malformations) of the extra- and intrarenal arteries and veins can be demonstrated and flow velocities estimated. The technique allows for ready demonstration of bland and tumor thrombus in the renal vein and inferior vena cava.

j. *Renal transplant evaluation.* The transplanted kidney, because of its superficial position in the pelvis, is particularly well suited for US evaluation. The combination of Doppler and gray-scale sonography (duplex Doppler) makes it possible to trouble-shoot ailing renal allografts for such complications as rejection, renal artery stenosis, and arterial or venous thrombi, thereby helping to separate them from cyclosporine toxicity and acute tubular necrosis. Surgical complications such as hydronephrosis and lymphocele formation also lend themselves well to diagnosis by US.

k. *Fetal renal ultrasound.* In utero hydronephrosis can often be detected, although various etiologies cannot often be differentiated (posterior urethral valves, ureteropelvic junction obstruction, primary megaureter/megacalyces, multicystic kidney, vesicoureteral reflux, duplication anomaly, prune belly syndrome). The diagnosis of fetal hydronephrosis best serves to alert physicians to the need for additional urologic evaluation in the early neonatal period.

2. Ureter

   US has limited usefulness in most ureteral disorders, but is very successful in a few isolated circumstances. Dilated ureters may be seen, ureteroceles demonstrated within the bladder, and small calculi imaged, especially in the pelvic ureter. Color-flow demonstration of asymmetric jets of urine from the ureteral orifices into the bladder often indicate the presence of ureteral obstruction.

3. Bladder

   Uses of ultrasonography include the measurement of residual urine (when urethral instrumentation is not desired or is contraindicated), guidance for suprapubic aspiration, staging of bladder tumors, and evaluation of intravesical masses and diverticula.

4. Prostate and seminal vesicles

   a. US of the prostate can estimate prostatic size and sometimes distinguish benign from malignant enlargement. US staging of prostate cancer is limited. Intrarectal transducers may be used to scan the prostate and seminal vesicles (transrectal US or TRUS) through the rectal wall (Fig. 3-14). This is the most common method of localizing a suspicious prostate lesion for transrectal biopsy or a cystic lesion in a seminal vesicle for aspiration.

   b. TRUS should not be used as a routine screening modality in an asymptomatic population, but is helpful in the presence of a palpable nodule or elevated prostatic specific antigen level to identify suspicious

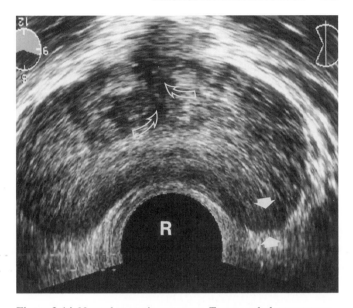

Figure 3-14 Normal prostatic sonogram. Transrectal ultrasonogram of the prostate gland (R, rectal ultrasound probe) displays fine low level echoes within the normal peripheral zone of the prostate (*arrowheads*). The central gland displays a brighter and coarser echo texture. The midline hypoechoic area on the anterior aspect of the prostate (*arrows*) represents the anterior fibromuscular stroma, a portion of the gland which normally impedes transmission of the ultrasound beam through the prostate. Prostate cancer often appears as discrete hypoechoic areas in the peripheral zone. BPH produces nodules and clusters of variable echogenicity in the central gland.

       lesions as well as to direct transrectal biopsies to suspicious foci (in addition to routine sextant biopsies).

5. Scrotum and external genitalia

  a. US can differentiate intratesticular from extratesticular masses as well as solid from cystic scrotal masses. US is helpful when inflammation or neoplasm of the testis or epididymis is associated with a secondary hydrocele that prevents adequate palpation of the underlying lesion. Color-flow Doppler is very helpful in the scrotum and external genitalia. Perfusion patterns often serve to differentiate inflammation from neoplasia and to substantiate a diagnosis of torsion or infarction.

  b. Undescended testicles can often be identified in the inguinal canal (but not within the abdomen) with US.

    c. In male sexual dysfunction, inadequacies of flow in the cavernosal arteries are readily identified, and this technique has become a standard part of the evaluation of the impotent patient. It can easily identified fibrous plaques (which may be calcified) in the tunica albuginea in Peyronie's disease. Retrograde filling of the urethra with saline during gray-scale scanning can identify strictures of the distal male urethra and assess the periurethral tissues for associated scarring. This technique was believed to allow for selection of the most appropriate treatment of urethral stricture, but it has not gained widespread acceptance.

    d. In the female, translabial or endoluminal (endourethral) US has been employed to identify simple and complex urethral diverticula, but is not favored by most urologists and radiologists over voiding cystourethrography and MRI.

6. Intraoperative US

This technique is often used to assist in partial nephrectomy in patients with one or more small renal tumors.

XII. COMPUTED TOMOGRAPHY
A. Basic Principles

A narrowly collimated x-ray beam is rotated about the patient and the amount of transmitted radiation is measured. Adjacent areas are compared. A computer processes the data and formats them as a digitized matrix of dots corresponding to an anatomic cross section of the body. The darkness of each dot is a function of the amount of radiation detected. A number of contiguous or slightly overlapping cross-sectional slices, each varying in thickness from 3 mm to 1 cm, are made through the anatomic areas of interest. Although many visceral structures can be recognized by their suggestive CT appearance, others have similar densities. To enhance structural differences, CM is frequently given. This is the same type as is used for urography and other urologic studies. Following administration of CM, multiple images are repeated. Many pathologic lesions can be recognized on the basis of their appearance before and after contrast administration (Fig. 3-15). The advantage of CT over ordinary radiography is not so much a difference in the type of information obtained or its spatial resolution, but rather the greater contrast resolution of CT, which is approximately 10 times that possible with conventional radiography. The useful display of tomographic cross-sectional anatomy in CT, relatively unaffected by surrounding high x-ray absorbing tissues such as bone, is another distinct advantage. Complex computer algorithms allow reconstruction of CT data into many forms, including different planes, such as coronal and sagittal.

B. Purpose

To visualize the urinary tract primarily in thin cross-sectional slices.

C. Techniques

1. Preparation is the same as for any procedure in which CM is to be administered except that a dilute mixture of barium or gastrografin is administered orally before the study to identify the small and large bowels and thereby avoid confusion of fluid-filled bowel with abdominal masses or lymph nodes. In those patients being studied specifically for high-density ureteral calculi, oral contrast material should be omitted.

2. After a series of preselected, noncontrast material enhanced CT scans through an area of interest, sections are repeated following contrast administration. CM allows better characterization and delineation of renal masses, permits evaluation of renal vein and caval patency in renal neoplasm, compares blood flow to each kidney, and helps differentiate vascular structures from solid masses, such as retroperitoneal lymphadenopathy. The contrast is usually administered as a rapid bolus using a power injector.

D. Complications

There are no complications specific to CT. The complications are limited to those described under contrast media. Contraindications are identical to those for IVU. Some unusually obese patients may not be candidates for CT because they cannot fit into the gantry or are too heavy for the table.

E. Indications

CT plays a major role in uroradiologic diagnosis. Indications have been broadening consistently as the efficacy of CT is fully appreciated. Some of its more important uses are:

1. Renal masses
   a. *Diagnosis.* CT is very accurate in detecting renal masses, identifying renal pseudotumors, and differentiating simple as well as complex cystic masses from solid lesions of the kidney. Because fresh blood is readily apparent on CT, hemorrhagic lesions and hematomas are easily recognizable. Renal parenchymal and urothelial neoplasms also have suggestive appearances on CT. In certain respects CT is competitive with US in evaluating renal masses, but in other respects, the two procedures are

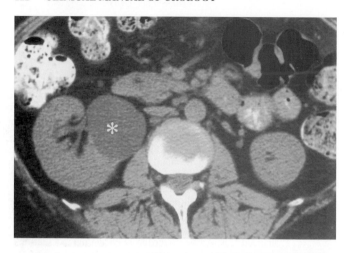

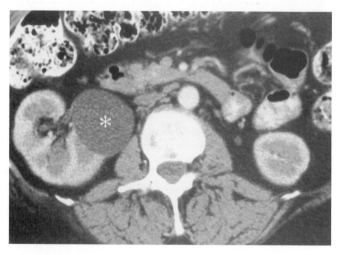

Figure 3-15 CT scan of a benign renal cyst. **A.** Unenhanced and CM-enhanced scans; **B.** 60 to 90 seconds after a bolus injection of CM, and **C.** 2 to 3 min after CM demonstrate a 5 cm in diameter benign renal cyst (*asterisk*) in the medial aspect of the interpolar portion of the right kidney. The well circumscribed and marginated water attenuation cyst does not enhance (increase in attenuation) following CM administration. Note that during **B,** the corticomedullary phase, the aorta and renal cortices have densely enhanced. The renal medullary pyramids have not yet received contrast-enhanced blood and have become well demarcated from brightly enhanced renal cortex.

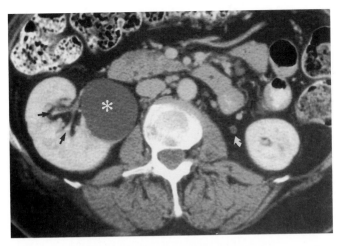

Figure 3-15 (*continued*)   **C.** A few minutes later, both cortex and medulla are opacified and are no longer distinguishable (similar to **A,** the unenhanced scan). A small amount of CM has begun to be excreted into calyces (*arrows*). Images of the left kidney show a normal lower renal pole and normal proximal ureter (*curved arrow*), not yet filled with CM. Neither the main renal arteries nor veins are seen at the level of these scans.

        complementary, especially if the mass is indeterminate on US.

  b. *Staging of renal neoplasms.* CT provides evidence of renal vein or IVC tumor thrombus, lymphadenopathy, and liver or adrenal metastases. It is very helpful in the preoperative evaluation of neoplasms.

  c. *Postoperative.* CT can detect local recurrence of neoplasm after partial or total nephrectomy for malignant disease.

2. Renal inflammatory disease
   CT is the most helpful imaging modality in identifying acute pyelonephritis, xanthogranulomatous or emphysematous pyelonephritis, and renal abscess and assessing inflammatory perinephric extension.

3. Hydronephrosis
   CT is superb for determining the level and etiology of hydronephrosis.

4. Perinephric effusions
   Perinephric abscess, urinoma, and hematoma can be readily recognized by CT and often differentiated by the CT attenuation or density values.

5. Trauma

CT is widely employed and very informative in assessing the extent of renal trauma and its possible complications, including extravasation, urinoma formation, and impaired renal viability.

6. Retroperitoneal masses

CT and MRI are the best methods of evaluating most retroperitoneal masses including neoplasms.

7. Retroperitoneal lymph nodes

CT and MRI are the most reliable methods currently available to evaluate enlarged retroperitoneal lymph nodes. This is an important part of the staging of many urologic tumors including those arising in the testis, bladder, and prostate.

8. Retroperitoneal fibrosis

In suspected cases of retroperitoneal fibrosis, CT can usually demonstrate the culpable fibrous plaque, and CT and MRI are the two most important diagnostic modalities in evaluating for the disease.

9. Renal pelvic filling defects

Many renal pelvic defects are attributable to nonopaque calculi. CT is exquisitely sensitive in detecting such calculi even though they are nonopaque on conventional radiography. In addition, some of the other causes for filling defects, including blood clots and neoplasms, can also be detected by CT. CT is also of some help in staging transitional cell carcinoma of the renal collecting systems.

10. Renal transplants

CT shares with MRI the ability to evaluate ailing renal transplants for hydronephrosis and perinephric fluid collections. Azotemia precludes the use of CM to evaluate vascular integrity.

Potential renal donors can be evaluated with cross-sectional and reconstructed CT images of renal parenchyma, vessels, collecting systems, and ureters (CT, CT angiography, and CT urography).

11. Urinary bladder

CT is valuable in staging tumors confined to the urinary bladder when the perivesical fat planes are preserved. However, perivesical stranding could be attributable to inflammation or tumor, thereby limiting the staging value of CT. Obvious lymphadenopathy can be detected. MRI surpasses CT as the dominant imaging study in staging bladder cancer. Both techniques are limited, however, by their inability to detect small or microscopic metastases in normal-sized lymph nodes and minimal or microscopic tumor invasion of peripelvic fat and contiguous surfaces.

12. Prostate and seminal vesicles
    With CT, congenital anomalies, cysts, and abscesses of the seminal vesicles can be well visualized and prostate abscesses detected. CT, however, has been replaced by MRI in assessing carcinoma of the prostate.
13. Adrenal gland
    For many years CT has been the study of choice for the evaluation of any patient with suspected adrenal pathology. It is quite useful in detecting pathology but is only helpful in precise diagnosis when an adrenal mass is of low attenuation (adrenal adenoma, myelolipoma, or uncomplicated cyst). Recently, adrenal CT has been replaced in many institutions by MRI for several purposes including the detection of pheochromocytoma and the differentiation of benign adenomas from adenocarcinomas or metastases.

XIII. MAGNETIC RESONANCE IMAGING
A. Basic Principles and Techniques

1. MRI is based on the interaction of externally applied radiofrequency (RF) pulses with the hydrogen nuclei (protons) of body tissues that have been aligned in a magnetic field. In response to such RF stimulation, the affected protons become temporarily realigned. When the pulse is removed, the nuclei begin to realign themselves in a matter of milliseconds. As they recover their original orientation, the protons emit RF signals of their own. The character of these RF waves, which are received by antennae (coils) in the MRI machine, are a function of the type of body tissue being examined and its location in space. Thus, when this information is digitized and computer-processed, anatomic images of slices of the body (much as in CT) are provided. Unlike CT, however, these images are multiplanar and capable of being tailored to reveal specific information (e.g., blood flow).

2. Blood-vessel imaging by means of MRI is known as magnetic resonance angiography (MRA). Images of the renal collecting system, ureter, and bladder can be obtained and reconstructed to simulate images from an IVU (magnetic resonance urography or MRU).

3. MRI machines can be classified on the basis of field strength. High field strength (1.5 T) and midfield strength (0.5 to 1.0 T) are generally used for most clinical work. No special preparation is necessary prior to undergoing MRI. The patient is placed in a gantry quite similar to that used for CT scanning. An initial series of images are made and studied by a radiologist. After this, contrast

agents such as gadolinium-DTPA may be administered and postcontrast images obtained. With imaging of the pelvis, an endorectal (or endovaginal) balloon-mounted surface coil is often utilized to obtain high resolution images.

B. Indications
1. Kidney
    a. *Renal masses.* MRI is very sensitive in differentiating cysts from malignant and benign (angiomyolipoma) neoplasms and pseudotumors from bona fide renal lesions (Figs. 3-16 and 3-17). As CT and US are also very reliable, MRI is usually reserved in these circumstances for patients with severe contrast allergy or renal dysfunction, or for those whose lesions are still indeterminate after other imaging studies have been performed (Fig. 3-18). The MR contrast agent, gadolinium, very rarely incites an allergic reaction and it does not have the same nephrotoxic potential as iodinated CM. There is no relationship between sensitivity to iodinated CM and to gadolinium.
    b. *Vascular lesions.* MRA depicts renal arterial and venous lesions with exquisite detail and is fast becoming the primary imaging study in patients with suspected renal aneurysms, arteriovenous communications, renal artery stenosis and infarction, and renal vein occlusion (Fig. 3-19). MRA is particularly useful in evaluating ailing renal transplants where extrarenal and intrarenal vascular problems occur not infrequently.
    c. *Renal donor evaluation.* As with CT, MR imaging of potential renal donors (a combination of MRI, MRA and MRU) can evaluate renal parenchymal, collecting system and ureteral morphology, and arterial and venous anatomy related to harvesting a donor kidney. Because MRI is limited in its ability to detect calcification, potential renal donors should also have a KUB to evaluate for the presence of renal calculi.
    d. *Staging renal neoplasms.* The excellent ability of MRI to visualize the renal vein, inferior vena cava, regional lymph nodes, liver, adrenal glands, and renal pelvis make it a logical choice for staging renal parenchymal and renal pelvic neoplasms. In many institutions, MRI is replacing CT for this purpose if a renal neoplasm is detected on IVU or US. MRI can also determine whether a small renal parenchymal neoplasm is amenable to partial nephrectomy.

e. *Miscellaneous.* MRI can be used to estimate overall and split renal function by means of evaluating dynamic enhancement and changes in perfusion, examine obstructed and inflamed kidneys, evaluate for the presence of blood in traumatized kidneys, and in many other situations that arise in clinical practice. It can often differentiate benign and malignant forms of retroperitoneal fibrosis, and radiation fibrosis from recurrent neoplasm.

2. Adrenal gland

As a result of improvements in tissue specificity with MRI, benign nonhyperfunctioning adrenal adenomas (often incidentally discovered during evaluation of patients with known or suspected malignancies) can usually be differentiated from adrenal metastases, and both myelolipomas and pheochromocytomas (adrenal and extraadrenal) readily identified. Because of its ability to image and display anatomy in multiple planes, the often difficult differentiation of adrenal neoplasms from upper pole renal neoplasms is simplified with MRI. Its multiplanar capabilities is also valuable in determining the origin of large abdominal masses whose sites of origin are not always obvious with other modalities. Such lesions often arise in the adrenal gland.

3. Bladder

MRI can more accurately stage bladder cancer than can CT because it can determine the depth of the tumor's penetration into the bladder wall in most cases and assess invasion of the perivesical fat. MRI is not more accurate than CT, however, in assessing adenopathy, since both modalities depend on changes in size as the criterion for positivity. As is well known from CT, nodes may be enlarged by hyperplastic changes and, conversely, small nodes may be infiltrated with tumor.

4. Prostate and seminal vesicles

a. *Carcinoma.* The primary role of MRI in the male pelvis is in staging carcinoma of the prostate. MRI surpasses all other modalities in this respect when an endorectal coil is utilized for imaging. With its associated increase in resolution and more favorable signal to noise ratio, MRI can usually detect gross extracapsular extension of tumor and seminal vesicle involvement, thereby preventing unnecessary surgery. Body-coil pelvic imaging is used to detect lymphadenopathy.

b. *Ejaculatory dysfunction.* MRI is also important in men with scanty or painful ejaculation, hematospermia, or unusual symptoms or signs pointing to

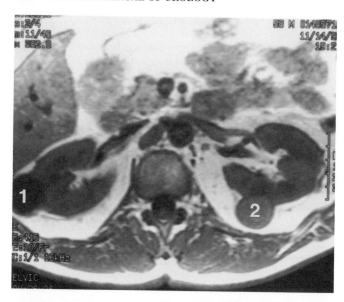

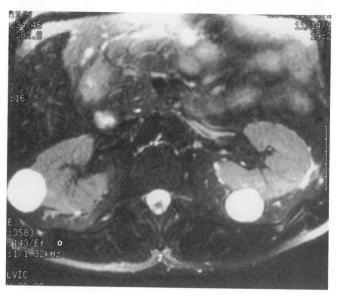

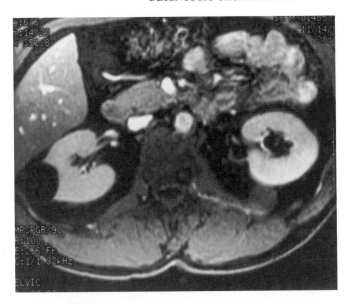

Figure 3-16 MRI of simple and complicated renal cysts. **A.** Axial
T1-weighted MR scan through the kidneys shows round masses
projecting from the lateral aspect of the right kidney (mass 1) and
posterior aspect of the left kidney (mass 2). The former is of lower
signal intensity (blacker) than normal renal parenchyma; the latter of
slightly higher signal intensity (grayer) than adjacent kidney. **B.** Axial
T2-weighted image at the same level as **A.** Both renal masses display
very high signal intensity (white). The kidneys are of medium signal
intensity (gray). **C.** Contrast-enhanced axial T1-weighted image again
demonstrates both renal masses. Neither appears different than on **A,**
before contrast was administered. Therefore, neither has peripheral
nor internal vascularity. The kidneys have become brightly enhanced
as have both the aorta and inferior vena cava. Mass 1 is a benign renal
cyst (dark on T1, bright on T2, no CM enhancement). Mass 2 is a
cyst filled with proteinaceous material or blood products (medium
gray on T1, bright white on T2, no enhancement). The simple renal
cyst requires no further investigation; the complicated cyst should be
imaged at least one more time, perhaps in 3 to 6 months, to assure
lesion stability and exclude an avascular renal neoplasm that has
undergone internal hemorrhage (an uncommon occurrence for an
avascular lesion).

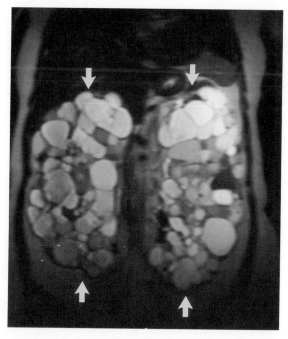

Figure 3-17 MRI of polycystic kidneys. Coronal T2-weighted image shows markedly enlarged kidneys (*arrows*) that contain innumerable round cysts. The "white" cysts contain simple cyst fluid, whereas the "gray" and "black" cysts contain blood products of varying age. The patient has autosomal dominant (adult) polycystic kidney disease with characteristic (and spectacular) MR findings.

        obstruction, stones, infection, and so forth, of the seminal tract or prostate gland.

  5. Testes

    a. *Testicular tumor.* Although MRI is not specific in differentiating the various types of gonadal neoplasms, it is helpful in distinguishing neoplasm from other conditions, such as infection, infarction, and hematoma, with which tumor may be confused.

    b. *Cryptorchidism.* Undescended testes located in the abdomen or inguinal canals can usually be visualized by MRI.

  6. Penis

    MRI can detect hematomas within the corporal bodies and disruptions of the tunica albuginea following trauma, as well as tunical plaques of Peyronie's disease.

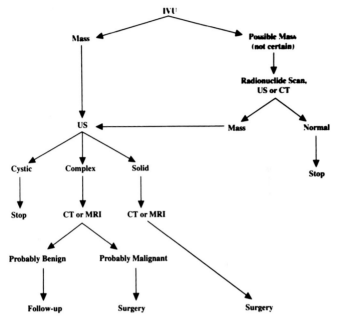

Figure 3-18 Workup for a renal mass.

7. Urethra

Using an endorectal or endovaginal coil, diverticula of the female urethra can easily be identified and their location with respect the bladder, size, and relationship to the urethra demonstrated. Occasionally, the neck of the diverticulum can be imaged. These factors considerably facilitate surgical correction. Carcinoma of the male and female urethras can also be easily staged with MRI.

C. Contraindications

1. Patients with pacemakers, implanted infusion pumps, cochlear implants, other implanted electronic devices, cerebral aneurysm surgical clips, and metallic ocular foreign bodies are not candidates for MRI. However, most surgical clips and prostheses used today are not ferromagnetic, and patients harboring them can be safely studied with MRI. When there is doubt about the nature of the metal, however, it is probably best to avoid the examination.

2. Claustrophobic patients usually respond well to tranquilizers, but those who do not will not easily tolerate MRI

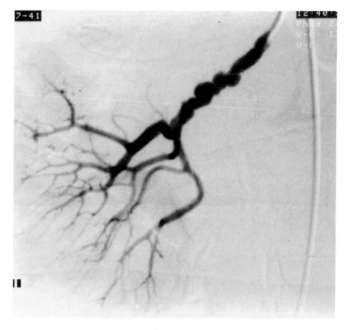

Figure 3-19 Fibromuscular dysplasia (FMD) of renal artery.
A. Selective digital subtraction angiogram (DSA) of right renal artery shows the characteristic beaded appearance of FMD. The distal renal arteries appear normal.

in a traditional "closed" magnet. Lower-field strength "open" magnets are now available, although images of the urinary tract obtained thereby are not as optimal as with higher-field strength magnets.

3. Very large or obese patients may be disqualified because of limitations in the diameter of the gantry opening or the weight limits of the examining table.

4. Although not yet shown to be deleterious, MR contrast agents should not be administered to pregnancy females. Pregnancy itself does not constitute a contraindication to MRI, as no ionizing radiation is involved.

D. Complications

No complications have been reported from exposure to magnetic fields. Some heat is generated within the body but it is of low magnitude. This varies with differing pulse sequences.

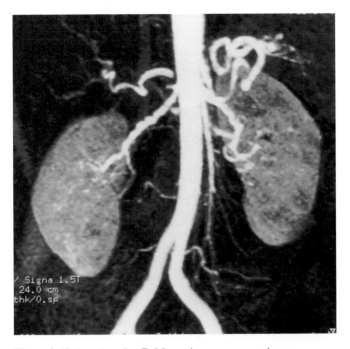

Figure 3-19 (*continued*)   **B.** Magnetic resonance angiogram (MRA) obtained after a bolus of gadolinium (but no catheter) shows the aorta and iliac arteries as well as many of the aortic branches. The changes of FMD are also well seen in the right renal artery. MRA does not image the intrarenal arterial tree but does simultaneously show the renal parenchyma, which the DSA does not.

BIBLIOGRAPHY

Davidson AJ, Hartman DS, Choyke PL, Wagner B: *Radiology of the Kidney and Genitourinary Tract.* Philadelphia: Saunders, 1999.

Dunnick NR, Sandler CM, Amis ES, Newhouse JH: *Textbook of Uroradiology.* Baltimore: Williams & Wilkins, 2000.

Pollack HM, McGlennan BL, Eds: *Clinical Urography.* Philadelphia: Saunders, 2000.

Resnick MI, Older RA: *Diagnosis of Genitourinary Disease.* New York: Thieme, 1997.

CHAPTER 4

Interventional Uroradiology

Marc P. Banner

I. **RENAL CYST ASPIRATION AND ABLATION**
   A. **Principles**
   1. To discriminate between simple and complex cystic lesions when imaging studies are inconclusive.
   2. To decompress and/or obliterate a symptomatic benign simple renal cyst.

   B. **Indications**
   1. Diagnostic aspiration with cytologic evaluation of the cyst fluid and radiographic evaluation of the interior of the cyst are performed when a definitive diagnosis of a benign simple cyst cannot be established with ultrasonography (US) or computed tomography (CT).
   2. Percutaneous ablation of a renal cyst is indicated if the lesion, by virtue of its size or location in the kidney, is producing pain, obstructive hydronephrosis, segmental compression of portions of the collecting system with stasis of urine resulting in stone formation, renin-dependent hypertension due to vascular compression and segmental ischemia, or pressure atrophy of adjacent renal parenchyma. Neither indication is encountered commonly in clinical practice.

   C. **Contraindications**
   1. An uncorrected bleeding diathesis.
   2. Small cysts, especially if hilar in location, that cannot be well imaged with US, CT, or fluoroscopy are best left undisturbed for fear of inadvertent injury to adjacent renal vessels. Follow-up imaging ensures that the lesion remains stable and benign in appearance.
   3. Aspiration of cysts in autosomal dominant polycystic kidney disease and of multilocular cysts, although not absolutely contraindicated, is rarely employed because of

the difficulty in localizing a specific cyst or locule and the unlikelihood of achieving complete decompression.

D. Technique

1. Renal cysts are aspirated with CT, fluoroscopic, or, most often, US guidance, using a 20-gauge needle.
2. If the procedure is being performed to establish the diagnosis of a benign cyst, one-half of the cyst volume is withdrawn for cytologic analysis and replaced with an equal volume mixture of water-soluble contrast material and air.
3. The mass is examined in multiple projections to outline the interior of the cyst with both positive and negative (air) contrast material.
4. If the cyst is being punctured to ascertain whether it is responsible for the patient's flank or back pain, as much fluid as possible is aspirated from the lesion.
5. If the cyst is to be ablated, a small catheter or sheath is initially placed in the lesion, the diagnostic study performed (if not previously done), the majority of the cyst fluid aspirated, a sclerosing agent instilled into the cyst for a variable length of time, and the catheter removed.
6. Many sclerosing agents can obliterate renal cysts. Absolute alcohol is most often used currently.

E. Results

1. Diagnostic renal cyst aspiration
    a. A typically benign renal cyst contains clear, amber to yellow fluid with no abnormal cells and exhibits a smooth cyst cavity.
    b. Hemorrhagic or infected cysts contain dark, cloudy, or bloody fluid, but also have a smooth lining and negative aspirate cytology.
    c. Positive cytology, an irregular cyst cavity, or an intracavitary fixed filling defect suggests a cystic neoplasm and usually dictates surgical exploration.
    d. Most renal cysts reaccumulate after diagnostic aspiration, even if the cyst is drained completely.
    e. The results of biochemical analysis of renal cyst fluid are generally nonspecific and unrewarding. Consequently, such studies are not routinely performed.
2. Therapeutic renal cyst ablation
    a. The majority of renal cysts can be permanently obliterated, thereby relieving the symptoms that prompted intervention (Fig. 4-1).

F. Complications

1. Complications of diagnostic cyst aspiration are infrequent.

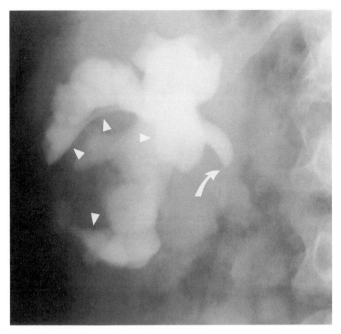

Figure 4-1 Renal cyst aspiration and ablation. **A.** Excretory urogram shows a large central renal mass that is splaying infundibula (*arrowheads*) and obstructing the UPJ (*arrow*) causing hydronephrosis. Ultrasonography showed the mass to be cystic in nature.

2. Improper needle placement may cause perinephric hemorrhage, inadvertent puncture of adjacent organs (e.g., lung, gastrointestinal tract), infection, arteriovenous fistula, and urinoma formation. Air embolism has not been reported.
3. Extravasation of water-soluble contrast into the perinephric tissues is innocuous; however, sclerosing agents, if extravasated, can cause fat necrosis, soft tissue fibrosis, or a febrile reaction.

II. PERCUTANEOUS NEPHROSTOMY (PCN)
A. Principles
1. PCN has become an important aspect of the diagnosis and management of a wide variety of urologic problems.
2. Its wide acceptance has stimulated the development of numerous additional techniques that, together with PCN, encompass the term interventional uroradiology.

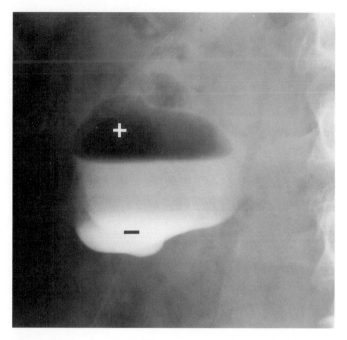

Figure 4-1 (*continued*)   **B.** Percutaneous renal cyst aspiration yielded clear amber fluid with negative cytology. A double-contrast renal cystogram shows that the cyst has a smooth inner wall as outlined by both positive (+) and negative (−) contrast material. A small plastic catheter has been left in the cyst for subsequent drainage and sclerosis.

B. Indications

1. Provide urgent renal drainage for relief of obstructive azotemia or anuria when retrograde drainage is not feasible, expedient, or possible. PCN is particularly beneficial when urosepsis accompanies obstruction. PCN preserves or improves renal function until the cause of obstruction can be relieved (with chemotherapy, radiotherapy, surgery, or simply time).

2. Provide access to the renal collecting system, ureter, or bladder for various therapeutic procedures, including ureteral stent placement; stone removal, disintegration, or dissolution; stricture dilation; biopsy of urothelial lesions; retrieval of foreign bodies; and nephroscopically directed surgical procedures (e.g., endopyelotomy, fulguration of urothelial tumors).

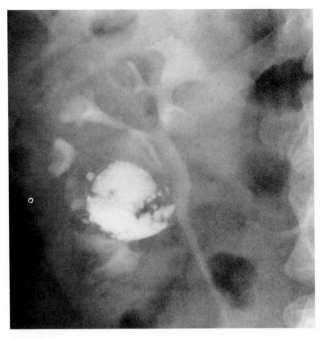

Figure 4-1 (*continued*)   **C.** Excretory urogram 6 months following cyst ablation shows residual opaque sclerosing agent in the renal cyst and resolution of obstructive hydronephrosis. The sclerosant will gradually resorb and disappear but will usually prevent cyst fluid reaccumulation.

      3. Provide urinary diversion in conjunction with ureteral stenting and/or obturation for ureteral fistulae or leaks or intractable vesicovaginal fistulae.

      4. Assess recoverable function of a chronically obstructed kidney, thereby helping to determine subsequent therapy.

C. Contraindications
    1. An uncorrected bleeding disorder.

D. Technique
    1. The renal collecting system is localized by means of renal excretion of contrast medium (if renal function is normal), antegrade pyelography, or US.
    2. The patient is placed prone and sedated. The flank is cleansed, and a subcostal skin entry site in the posterior axillary line is anesthetized.

3. A needle is advanced into the collecting system from the flank, urine aspirated, contrast material injected, and a guidewire inserted through the needle into the kidney. The procedure is monitored fluoroscopically.
4. The needle is removed and the nephrocutaneous track enlarged by passing fascial dilators over the guidewire.
5. A drainage catheter, usually an 8-French (F) "pigtail" catheter with a self-retaining mechanism, is passed over the guidewire and positioned in the renal pelvis. The guidewire is removed and the catheter is secured to the skin and attached to a closed gravity drainage bag (Fig 4-2).

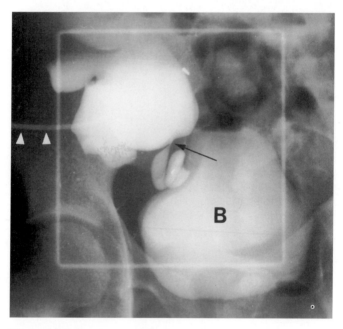

Figure 4-2 Percutaneous nephrostomy. Obstructive azotemia with anuria in a renal transplant recipient was relieved by percutaneous renal decompression. Following initial placement of the nephrostomy catheter (*arrowheads*), complete obstruction at the UPJ was present. With partial decompression of the renal pelvis, some contrast material passed through a stenotic UPJ (*arrow*), through a tortuous ureter and transplant ureteroneocystostomy, and into the urinary bladder (**B**). The patient subsequently had her native right ureter anastomosed to the transplant renal pelvis.

E. Results

1. Percutaneous renal drainage can be established in more than 98 percent of cases. Nondilated collecting systems and those filled with calculi are technical challenges and potential sources of failure of catheter placement, especially for those with relatively limited experience. In these cases, success rates of 85 to 90 percent can be expected.

2. PCN is well tolerated by the great majority of patients and those caring for them.

F. Complications

1. Serious complications related to PCN can be expected in approximately 4 percent of cases and minor complications in 15 percent. These include bleeding of varying severity (usually minor and transient but occasionally requiring transfusion or embolization), introduction of a new infection, exacerbation of existing sepsis, urine leak, penetration of adjacent viscera (e.g., pleura, bowel, gallbladder), and failure to establish drainage.

2. Catheter dislodgment and/or obstruction following PCN can be minimized by using self-retaining drainage catheters, routinely exchanged every few months.

III. URETERAL STENTING

A. Principles

1. Percutaneous ureteral stenting provides urinary diversion without the need for an external collection device when retrograde insertion of a ureteral stent is not possible or practical.

2. Most patients find a ureteral stent catheter more acceptable and convenient than a nephrostomy catheter.

B. Indications

1. Long-term stenting (months to years) is most frequently performed to bypass a ureteral obstruction.

2. Short-term stenting (weeks to months)
   a. Facilitates healing of postoperative or traumatic pyeloureteral leaks or ureteral fistulae by diverting the urinary stream.
   b. Prevents stricture formation as ureteral injuries or implantations (native or allograft ureters) heal by providing a mold around which ureteral epithelialization is facilitated.
   c. Maintains ureteral caliber following balloon dilation or incision of benign ureteral strictures.

3. Catheters percutaneously placed into the ureters facilitate intraoperative ureteral identification during difficult surgical dissections (e.g., revision of an obstructed ureteroileal diversion).

4. Ureteral stents are often used in conjunction with nonoperative treatment of renal and ureteral calculi. Prior to extracorporeal shock-wave lithotripsy (ESWL), stents are used.

   a. To manipulate mid or upper ureteral calculi into the kidney or, if this is not possible, bypass them.

   b. To prevent stones from migrating back into the ureter prior to therapy.

   c. To facilitate localization of renal and ureteral stones during ESWL.

   d. To allow for antegrade urinary drainage while stone fragments pass into the bladder. Stents are ideally inserted cystoscopically. Improperly positioned stents may require readjustment using fluoroscopy in the radiology department.

5. Antegrade insertion of ureteral stents prior to percutaneous therapy for renal calculi insure that stone fragments created during ultrasonic lithotripsy do not inadvertently migrate into the ureter.

C. Contraindications

1. The presence of active renal infection.

2. Markedly diseased, intolerant bladders (e.g., radiation cystitis, bladder invasion by adjacent neoplasm).

3. Bladder fistulae.

D. Technique

1. Following PCN, a guidewire and catheter are manipulated through the abnormal (often stenotic) ureteral segment and into the urinary bladder or a bowel conduit or urinary reservoir.

2. The catheter is replaced with a ureteral stent in which multiple side holes have been created where the stent will eventually be positioned in the renal pelvis. Kidney urine enters the stent through these side holes, travels through the catheter, and exits from its distal pigtail segment. Depending on ureteral caliber, urine may also flow around the stent. The proximal end of the stent protrudes from the skin and is obturated externally. This is an external ureteral stent catheter (Fig. 4-3).

3. An external ureteral stent can be periodically changed from the flank over a guidewire.

4. Urinary drainage can be totally internalized inserting an internal ureteral stent with a pigtail configuration at both

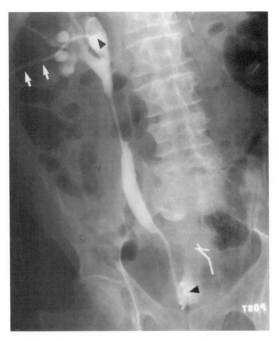

Figure 4-3 Percutaneous ureteral stenting. An elderly male with recurrent invasive transitional cell carcinoma of the bladder who has already undergone left nephroureterectomy (note surgical clips) now presents with azotemia and oliguria secondary to tumor obstructing the right ureteral orifice. A retrograde catheter could not be passed cystoscopically. A right percutaneous nephrostomy was performed, following which a nephroureteral stent could be passed into the bladder, bypassing the right distal ureteral obstruction. Loops in the catheter (arrowheads) in the kidney and bladder represent the proximal- and distal-most drainage portions of the stent. The portion of the catheter that protrudes from the flank (*arrows*) is only used to gain access to the stent for periodic replacement.

ends. The proximal pigtail is positioned in the renal pelvis and the distal pigtail in the bladder. Double pigtail stents must be periodically changed (at least every 6 months) cystoscopically (Fig. 4-4).

5. Patients who require ureteral stenting following ureteral diversion to a bowel conduit should have an external ureteral stent inserted in combined antegrade/retrograde fashion. A guidewire and catheter are first manipulated beyond the abnormal ureteral segment, through the bowel

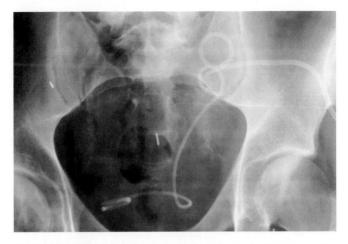

Figure 4-4 Percutaneous ureteral stenting. Ureteral obstruction with azotemia in a renal transplant necessitated percutaneous renal drainage. An internalized, so-called "double pigtail" ureteral stent has been passed in antegrade fashion through the distal ureteral obstruction (not shown) with the proximal pigtail positioned in the transplant renal pelvis and the distal pigtail in the bladder. A temporary pigtail nephrostomy catheter extends from the transplant to the skin. It is removed once satisfactory antegrade drainage through the stent has been demonstrated.

conduit, and out the stoma rather than into the bladder. The catheter is removed and a single pigtail drainage catheter passed retrograde into the renal pelvis. The distal end of this catheter protrudes through the stoma to drain into the urostomy collection bag. Internal ureteral stents should not be used in patients with ureteroenterostomies or continent urinary diversion reservoirs.

6. Catheters for intraoperative ureteral identification are percutaneously passed down the ureter to the point of ureteral obstruction. A PCN is also required to drain the kidney until surgical correction of the obstructed ureter has been accomplished.

7. Ureteral stents used as an adjunct to percutaneous nephrostolithotomy are passed into the pelvic ureter in conjunction with creation of a nephrocutaneous track through which endoscopes are inserted into the kidney.

8. Fluoroscopically guided retrograde perurethral catheter manipulations following unsuccessful retrograde endoscopic attempts to pass catheters beyond ureteral obstructions and fistulae can be accomplished in the radiology de-

partment. This approach employs standard interventional equipment (e.g., catheters, guidewires, sheaths) passed through or over partially inserted ureteral catheters.

E. Results
1. Both internal and external ureteral stents allow patients to lead as active a life as their underlying condition will permit.
2. Ureteral obstructions can often be negotiated in antegrade (percutaneous) fashion even if retrograde cystoscopic catheterization is not possible (e.g., neoplastic obstruction of a ureteral orifice, distal ureteral angulation secondary to prostatic enlargement, spread of prostatic malignancy, ureteral reimplantation, tight ureteral stenoses, or urethral stricture.
3. Approximately 85 to 90 percent of ureteral obstructions and fistulae can be stented percutaneously. Very tightly obstructed ureters and ureters that are both tortuous and encased by tumor or fibrosis are the most frequent causes of failure of antegrade stent placement.
4. Internal ureteral stents may not drain kidneys as well as a PCN, especially when ureteral obstruction is caused by extrinsic compression or if intravesical pressure is elevated at rest or during micturition.

F. Complications
1. Improperly positioned stents will not provide optimal urinary drainage. This problem can be rectified with percutaneous, cystoscopic, or ureteroscopic techniques.
2. Symptoms attributable to the intravesical coil of the stent (even when properly positioned) occur commonly, including microscopic hematuria, pyuria, lower abdominal pain, dysuria, urinary frequency, nocturia, and flank pain on voiding (due to renal reflux of bladder urine).
3. Fatigue fractures and encrustation of ureteral stents may occur if stents are not periodically replaced. This should be carried out at least every 6 months and more often in patients who form stones.

IV. PERCUTANEOUS URETERAL OCCLUSION
A. Principles
1. Patients with advanced and often incurable pelvic or retroperitoneal malignancies may develop fistulae from the ureters, bladder, or urethra to the skin, vagina, or bowel. These fistulae are often accompanied by dysuria, incontinence, and skin maceration.
2. Most of these patients have previously undergone many surgical procedures, chemotherapy, and/or radiotherapy

to palliate local cancer recurrence, are quite ill, and are usually not candidates for surgical urinary diversion.

3. Bladder drainage is usually either impractical or ineffective and often aggravates the clinical picture.

4. In the absence of complete ureteral obstruction, PCN alone does not satisfactorily divert urine, although it may decrease the amount of leakage at the fistula site.

5. Addition of external ureteral stents may further diminish leakage, but often aggravates bladder symptoms.

B. Indications

1. To terminate urinary leakage from ureteral, bladder, or urethral fistulae in patients as described above while, if possible, preserving renal function.

C. Techniques

1. A variety of techniques may occlude the ureter without the need for surgery, most of which require concomitant percutaneous renal drainage. They include the following.
   a. Ureteral obturation by percutaneously wedging a large catheter in the ureter proximal to a urinary leak.
   b. Other mechanical blocking devices, such as tissue adhesives, balloons, plugs, and coils.
   c. Percutaneous retroperitoneal ureteral clipping.
   d. Endoscopic ureteral fulguration.

2. Renal embolization can obliterate renal function on the side of a ureteral leak. PCN drainage is obviated.

D. Results

1. All of these approaches have been effective for variable periods of time, but, with the exception of embolization, require permanent PCN drainage, as these fistulae rarely heal.

2. These techniques do, however, improve the quality of life for patients with short life expectancies.

V. DILATION OF URETERAL STENOSES
A. Principles

1. Chronic ureteral stenting is not optimal therapy for benign postoperative ureteral strictures, although it may be appropriate for malignant ureteral obstructions.

2. Many benign ureteral strictures are amenable to balloon catheter dilation or endourologic incision.

3. These procedures, if successful, can spare patients the nuisance of chronic indwelling stents or the risks of additional surgery.

B. Indications

1. An attempt at balloon catheter dilation of all benign ureteral strictures should be made before relegating patients to additional surgery or to chronic PCN or indwelling ureteral stent drainage.

2. Endoscopic incision, employed alone or in combination with balloon dilation and ureteral stenting, can relieve certain ureteropelvic junction (UPJ) obstructions (both congenital and acquired) as well as postoperative ureteroenteral anastomotic strictures.

3. Balloon dilation of ureters encircled by sutures sometimes results in disruption of the offending ligature, thus saving the patient an operation.

4. Balloon dilation of vesicourethral anastomotic strictures that develop after radical prostatectomy is a nonoperative alternative to endoscopic incision and appears to be less likely to cause urinary incontinence.

C. Contraindications

1. Ureteral strictures caused by malignant disease, either primary or recurrent.

2. Inflammatory or traumatic urethral strictures appear to be more amenable to optical internal urethrotomy than to balloon dilation.

D. Technique

1. The strictured ureter is cannulated as described above.

2. Biopsies and/or other imaging studies are obtained to confirm that the stricture has a benign etiology.

3. A catheter with an inflatable balloon capable of withstanding 15 to 17 atmospheres of pressure is advanced across the stricture. The balloon is inflated with contrast material to approximately 30-F. A waist or narrowing in the balloon is evident at the stricture site upon initial inflation; this will disappear with continued or repeated inflations if a technically successful stricture divulsion has been accomplished (Fig. 4-5).

4. Balloons are left inflated for 5 to 10 min and then exchanged for ureteral stents, which remain in situ for 6 to 8 weeks to maintain luminal patency while ureteral musculature heals. Stenting is accomplished with the largest catheter that will be comfortably accommodated. This is generally 10-F if the stent traverses the intramural ureter, but may be larger if a ureteroenterostomy stricture is dilated and stented.

5. After 6 to 8 weeks, the stent is exchanged for a PCN and the efficacy of the dilation subsequently determined by

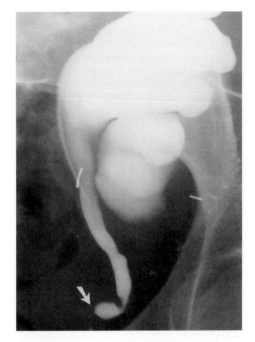

Figure 4-5 Catheter dilation of benign ureteral stricture.
A. Following percutaneous drainage of an obstructed renal transplant, a nephrostogram shows complete distal ureteral obstruction at the ureteroneocystostomy (*arrow*).

       means of nephrostograms and urodynamic studies prior to catheter removal.

6. Certain ureteral strictures in females can be dilated and stented in retrograde fashion per urethra with an internalized double pigtail catheter (usually 8-F).

7. Following removal of all catheters, an IVU should be obtained at 1, 6, and 12 months to insure that the ureter has remained patent.

8. Similar techniques have been adapted to treat congenital UPJ obstructions by endoscopic incision and stenting.

E. Results

1. Approximately 58 percent of all benign ureteral strictures can be successfully dilated with balloon catheters, usually with one session.

2. Some strictures that do not initially open up well following the first procedure will respond favorably to a second similar procedure.

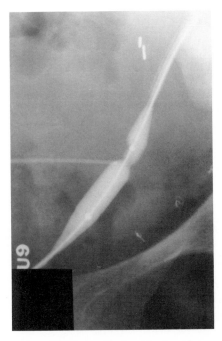

Figure 4-5 (*continued*)   **B.** The obstructed ureter has been percutaneously cannulated with a guidewire, and a balloon catheter has been inflated at the site of the ureteral obstruction. The residual narrowing or waist in the balloon represents the tightest and most resistant portion of the stricture.

3. The etiology and age of the stricture seem to influence the outcome of dilation therapy. Strictures not associated with ischemia or dense fibrosis may be successfully dilated (including those that occur in renal allograft recipients). Those associated with radiotherapy or surgical devascularization have a much lower rate of success.

4. Strictures that have been present for less than 3 months respond much better to dilation therapy than do those that are more chronic in nature.

5. Endoscopic incision followed by balloon dilation and ureteral stenting is more effective than balloon catheter dilation alone for ureteroenteral anastomotic and UPJ strictures.

6. Unsuccessful balloon dilation does not adversely affect other therapeutic options, including chronic indwelling ureteral stenting, surgical revision, or insertion of a metallic expandable ureteral stent (Wallstent or similar

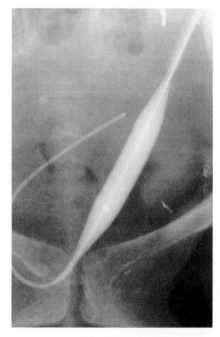

Figure 4-5 (*continued*)   **C.** With continued balloon inflation, the waist in the balloon eventually effaced, indicating successful divulsion of the ureteral stricture. The ureter was then stented for 6 weeks prior to catheter removal, with a favorable outcome.

device). Although often associated with favorable short-term results, the long-term efficacy of metallic stents has not yet been established.

F. Complications
1. No known permanent sequela have resulted from unsuccessful dilation therapy. Laceration of ureteral mucosa or wall may occur with balloon overdistention. These perforations heal uneventfully if the ureter is stented and probably do not affect the outcome of dilation therapy.

VI. PERCUTANEOUS PROCEDURES FOR UPPER URINARY TRACT CALCULI
A. Principles
1. Extracorporeal shock wave lithotripsy (ESWL) has become the preferred mode of therapy for most symptomatic renal and proximal ureteral calculi and, when used alone, effectively treats 70 to 80 percent of such cases.

2. When combined with endourologic and percutaneous procedures, ESWL can be used to treat over 90 percent of stone patients.

3. Distal ureteral calculi are managed by retrograde ureteroscopy or, in select cases, ESWL.

4. Percutaneous techniques for accessing and/or decompressing the kidney, as well as for extracting or disintegrating certain calculi, are still needed, both as primary therapy for patients with select stones, abnormal urinary tract morphology, or unusual clinical circumstances; and as secondary therapy when ESWL or ureteroscopy are ineffective or associated with complications.

B. Indications

Percutaneous techniques are important as an initial or additional procedure in the following circumstances.

1. Large stone volume (i.e., single calculus larger than 2.0 to 2.5 cm in diameter or multiple renal calculi with an aggregate diameter of 2.5 to 3.0 cm). The need for a PCN in place of, or prior to, ESWL also depends on the probable chemical composition of the stone (how easily it will disintegrate with ESWL) and whether a retrograde ureteral stent has been inserted prior to treatment. With a stent in place, stones that readily fragment with ESWL, but that are larger than those mentioned above, can be effectively treated with ESWL monotherapy.

2. Stones associated with compromised urinary drainage, such as anomalous or postoperative narrowings in the collecting system or ureter. In these cases, percutaneous stone therapy may be combined with endourologic treatment for the underlying obstructive process, such as endopyelotomy for UPJ stenosis, balloon dilation for infundibular or ureteral strictures.

3. Staghorn calculi, which are densely opaque and/or associated with a dilated renal collecting system, are best treated by initial PCN, percutaneous debulking of the stone with ultrasonic lithotripsy, and subsequent ESWL for residual stone fragments that remain after nephroscopy (Fig. 4-5). Those that are faintly opaque and only partially fill a nondilated collecting system may be effectively treated with a ureteral stent and ESWL.

4. Stones that do not adequately fragment with ESWL or ureteroscopy require a PCN for percutaneous ultrasonic lithotripsy and/or intrarenal irrigation with various solutions to dissolve residual stone fragments. Calculi that fall into this category are usually composed of cystine. Chemolysis is also used for residual fragments of uric acid and struvite calculi.

5. Patients in whom certain removal of a stone is important, as residual stone fragments persist in a significant percentage of patients following ESWL.

6. Patients with stones in calyceal diverticula or dilated calyces (especially in the lower renal poles) where there is an especially high likelihood of residual fragments after ESWL.

7. Stone-bearing patients whose body habitus (e.g., marked skeletal deformity) or renal location (e.g., certain anomalous, ectopic, and transplanted kidneys) renders them physically unsuitable for treatment with ESWL, especially with a water-bath lithotriptor.

8. When renal decompression is needed and endoscopic attempts have not been successful. This can either occur prior to or following lithotripsy, as in patients who develop an obstructing or otherwise symptomatic ureteral steinstrasse following ESWL of sizable upper tract calculi (see Chapter 9).

9. The percutaneous route is also well suited to the removal of foreign bodies (e.g., broken stent and guidewire fragments, internal ureteral stents, fungus balls) from the renal pelvis and/or ureter.

C. Contraindications

1. An uncorrected bleeding disorder.

2. An uninfected, stone-bearing but nonfunctioning (or very poorly functioning) kidney.

3. Active renal infection should be treated with antibiotics prior to elective percutaneous procedures. Emergency percutaneous decompression for an obstructing renal or ureteral calculus or steinstrasse with associated urosepsis is often the most effective treatment for the infection.

D. Technique

1. The technique of PCN is described above.

2. Puncture of the collecting system should be made through a posteriorly oriented, peripherally situated calyx, especially when the PCN track is to be dilated to accept a nephroscope for stone extraction or intracorporeal lithotripsy.

3. The percutaneous approach for staghorn calculi or other very large or unusually shaped calculi is made into that calyx that will allow for nephroscopic disintegration of the majority of the stone (also usually a posterior calyx).

4. Percutaneous therapy for calyceal or diverticular stones usually requires percutaneous access through the stone-bearing region.

5. A ureteral access catheter (5 or 6 F) is percutaneously passed into the ureter at the time of PCN. If renal

drainage is compromised (by calculi, anatomy, or the access catheter), an 8F PCN catheter is also placed into the collecting system.

6. The nephrocutaneous track is usually dilated in the operating room under anesthesia just prior to percutaneous nephrostolithotomy. This is accomplished by passing progressively larger fascial dilators or a large balloon catheter over a guidewire that has been inserted into the ureter through the previously placed ureteral access catheter.

7. Following percutaneous nephrostolithotomy, a 24-F Malecot catheter is inserted into the renal pelvis and placed to gravity drainage.

8. The number and location of residual stone fragments are documented with a subsequent nephrostogram and, if present, treated with ESWL, topical dissolution, or repeat nephroscopy (rigid or flexible) with stone extraction.

9. Dissolution therapy may require insertion of different or additional PCN or ureteral catheters to insure that the irrigating solution adequately bathes the stones and drains the kidney while maintaining normal intrarenal pressure (Fig. 4-6).

10. PCN with or without ureteral stenting may be needed for obstructing ureteral stone fragments that cannot be managed in retrograde endoscopic fashion.

11. If a guidewire cannot be passed through the stenotic infundibulum of a stone-bearing hydrocalyx or calyceal diverticulum, a small PCN catheter is coiled around the stone, the nephrocutaneous track allowed to mature, the track dilated to the stone (but not beyond), the stone extracted or disintegrated nephroscopically, and the stenotic infundibulum dilated with a balloon catheter or incised nephroscopically and then stented.

E. Results

1. PCN can be successfully performed in almost all cases. The procedure is technically challenging when calculi fill the collecting system and thwart attempted passage of guidewires and catheters. Distention of the collecting system by means of a previously inserted retrograde ureteral catheter may facilitate insertion of a PCN and/or a ureteral access catheter for drainage and/or subsequent ESWL, but is not routinely needed to accomplish these tasks.

F. Complications

1. Complications of PCN have been discussed previously.

2. Perforations of the collecting system or ureter occur occasionally when manipulating catheters and guidewires

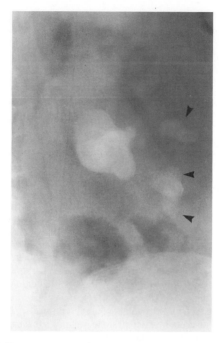

Figure 4-6 Percutaneous nephrostolithotomy. **A.** A middle-aged female with recurrent left flank pain has multiple left renal calculi, the largest a 3.2 × 2.8 cm stone in the renal pelvis. Smaller peripheral calculi are also present (*arrowheads*). The stone burden is too great to be safely treated with extracorporeal shock-wave lithotripsy. Therefore, percutaneous nephrostolithotomy is the treatment of choice.

around large renal or obstructing ureteral calculi or through stenotic urinary passages. These heal if nephrostomy drainage is adequate and, in cases of ureteral perforation, a ureteral stent is placed.
3. Complications related to topical stone dissolution include pain, fever, bacilluria, urothelial edema, and, if irrigating fluid is absorbed, electrolyte imbalance. Dissolution is temporarily halted until these problems are corrected.

VII. PERCUTANEOUS DRAINAGE OF RENAL AND RELATED RETROPERITONEAL FLUID COLLECTIONS
A. Principles
1. Percutaneous drainage of renal and related retroperitoneal abscesses is almost always clinically efficacious and usually obviates the need for surgical drainage.

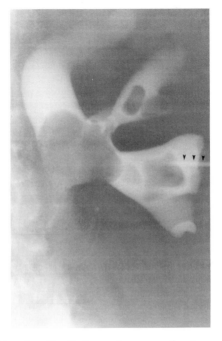

Figure 4-6 (*continued*)   **B.** A percutaneous nephrostomy needle (*arrowheads*) has been inserted into the lower pole of the stone-bearing left kidney. Injected contrast material opacifies the collecting system and shows the stones as filling defects. The large stone obstructs the renal pelvis. The nephrostomy track was subsequently dilated and the stones disintegrated under direct vision with a rigid nephroscope and ultrasonic lithotrite.

2. Percutaneous abscess drainage duplicates surgical management principles by providing decompression, evacuation, and continuous drainage without dissemination of infection. Standard retroperitoneal approaches for operative drainage are duplicated percutaneously by employing cross-sectional imaging for guidance.

B. Indications
1. A patient with a renal abscess or infected renal cyst who fails to improve with broad-spectrum antibiotics.
2. An infected renal or retroperitoneal fluid collection that requires drainage.

C. Contraindications
1. Absence of a safe percutaneous drainage route.

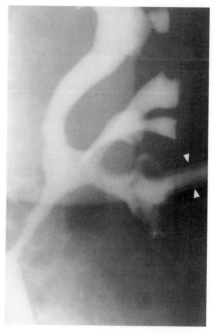

Figure 4-6 (*continued*)   **C.** A follow-up nephrostogram shows the collecting system to be free of stones. The apparent filling defect in the lower pole calyx represents one of the four wings of a large-bore Malecot nephrostomy catheter (*arrowheads* point to shaft of catheter). Injected contrast readily flows through the renal pelvis into the ureter. The catheter was then removed and the 1-cm flank incision healed rapidly.

    2. Small renal abscesses (less than 3 cm in diameter) can often be effectively treated with a course of intravenous antibiotics and may not require drainage.

    3. Abnormal coagulation parameters.

D. Technique

    1. The anatomic relationship of the fluid collection to its surrounding structures is assessed by cross-sectional imaging (CT or, less commonly, US). A safe, extraperitoneal route that avoids puncture of viscera, pleura, and major vessels or tracking pus across the peritoneum is planned for diagnostic needle aspiration and catheter placement.

2. Diagnostic aspiration with a 20- or 21-gauge needle along the planned drainage route confirms the diagnosis.

3. If diagnostic aspiration yields infected material, a catheter is introduced under fluoroscopic control, the abscess evacuated, and the catheter securely sutured in place to provide continuous drainage. Injection of contrast medium to evaluate the size and appearance of the abscess or whether it communicates with the collecting system is minimized at the time of the drainage to reduce the chances of inciting bacteremia or septic shock.

4. Septa within an abscess can usually be perforated with catheters and guidewires so that locules intercommunicate. Even so, multiloculated abscesses may require more than one catheter for complete drainage.

5. Multiple drainage catheters may be needed for renal abscesses that have spread retroperitoneally (one catheter for each component) or those that are associated with obstructive uropathy (PCN catheter and abscess drainage catheter).

6. Self-retaining pigtail or Malecot catheters, 10 to 14 F in diameter, placed to gravity drainage, effectively drain most urinary tract abscesses. Those with very viscous contents may be better drained with large sump catheters placed to suction drainage and periodically irrigated with saline. In general, abscesses related to the urinary tract are less viscous than are those that originate from the pancreas or gastrointestinal tract.

7. Following an initial favorable response to percutaneous therapy, patients with continued drainage can be changed from parenteral or oral antibiotics, discharged from the hospital with their drainage catheters in place, and followed as outpatients. Periodic follow-up catheter studies and CT scans are usually obtained at 1- to 2-week intervals (Fig. 4-7).

8. If a patient fails to improve on antibiotics and catheter drainage, a CT scan is obtained to detect undrained locules, enteric communications, or misplaced catheters.

9. Indications for catheter removal include the following.
   a. A satisfactory clinical response
   b. Defervescence
   c. Return of white blood cell count to normal
   d. Cessation of drainage
   e. Obliteration of the abscess cavity

10. Drainage catheters usually need to remain in place for an average of 2 to 4 weeks for most urinary abscesses. Renal abscesses usually resolve in less time than do those that have spread extrarenally. The track will close following catheter removal if all infected material has been evacuated.

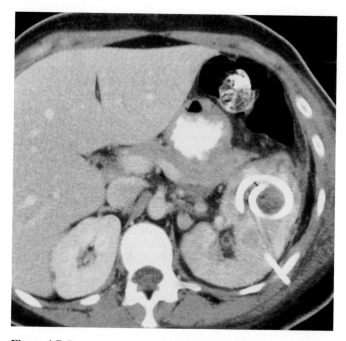

Figure 4-7 Percutaneous drainage of renal abscess. An abscess in the upper pole of the left kidney is being percutaneous drained with a pigtail catheter. The catheter is readily apparent on this contrast-enhanced CT, entering from the flank in a similar location as would a percutaneous nephrostomy catheter. The abscess is still present, expanding the anterior portion of the kidney and enhancing in heterogeneous fashion. With continued catheter drainage, the abscess resolved, obviating the need for surgical drainage.

E. **Results**

1. Percutaneous abscess drainage, by itself or in conjunction with other nonoperative or endourologic procedures, can be expected to cure approximately 72 percent of renal and related retroperitoneal abscesses, as determined by resolution of clinical signs and symptoms and CT scans.

2. These figures represent a significant improvement over cure and mortality rates from surgical drainage and reflect the abilities of cross-sectional imaging to diagnose abscesses earlier in their development, needle aspiration to confirm the nature of a fluid collection, and the efficacy of percutaneous drainage techniques.

3. In those patients not cured by percutaneous abscess drainage, the procedure will improve the patient's clini-

cal status in preparation for elective surgery to deal with underlying renal disease (e.g. nonfunctioning kidney, stone).

4. Percutaneous drainage will facilitate subsequent surgery (should it be needed) and decrease complications and patient morbidity.

F. Complications

1. Many patients develop transient bacteremia and febrile episodes following percutaneous abscess drainage. Some may develop septic shock.
2. These complications can be minimized by limiting catheter manipulation, lavage of the cavity, and/or contrast opacification of the abscess at the time of drainage.
3. A less than complete clinical response may result from only partial drainage of septated collections or premature catheter removal.
4. An infected, obstructed calyx or calyceal diverticulum may be mistaken for a renal parenchymal abscess and continue to drain urine after the infection has cleared. Specific measures must then be directed toward alleviating the calyceal obstruction by either dilating or occluding the neck of the diverticulum.

G. Percutaneous Drainage of Lymphoceles

1. Lymphoceles that occur after renal transplantation or pelvic surgery can be drained percutaneously, but may recur if drainage catheters are removed prematurely.
2. Sclerotherapy of the lymphocele cavity with tetracycline or povidone-iodine (Betadine) appears to be more effective in preventing fluid reaccumulation than simple catheter drainage alone (Fig. 4-8).
3. Needle aspiration alone of a lymphocele may be of temporary help but can lead to secondary infection of the closed space.

H. Percutaneous Drainage of Urinomas

1. Urinomas are chronic urine collections contained within a fibrous pseudocapsule that result from extravasation of urine due to obstruction of the renal collecting system, surgery, or trauma.
2. Urinomas may cause secondary ureteral obstruction.
3. Large urinomas can be aspirated or drained in conjunction with management of the cause of the urine leak (PCN and ureteral stenting).
4. Small (and occasionally large) urinomas will usually resorb spontaneously following relief of urinary obstruction or urinary diversion.

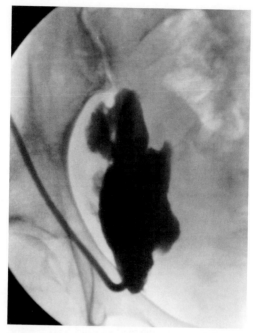

Figure 4-8 Percutaneous drainage of pelvic lymphocele. A lymphocele has formed following renal transplantation with resultant lower extremity edema. The fluid collection was percutaneously drained and a pigtail catheter inserted into the cavity. Subsequently, the lymphocele was percutaneously ablated with povidone-iodine (Betadine). Contrast opacification of the lymphocele 10 days following initiation of sclerotherapy shows a residual cavity in the right lower quadrant which was considerably smaller than it was at the time of initial drainage. The catheter was removed after 3 weeks of drainage and sclerotherapy.

VIII. URINARY TRACT BIOPSY TECHNIQUES
A. Principles

1. Soft tissue, visceral, and nodal lesions related to the urinary tract can readily be sampled for cytologic or histologic analysis when determination of the nature of the abnormality in question (benign or malignant) affects patient management. Prostate needle biopsy is considered elsewhere in this book.

2. Biopsies can be obtained with needles percutaneously placed into lesions or through catheters inserted percutaneously or endoscopically (transcatheter) into the urinary tract.

B. Indications

1. Primary diagnosis of upper urinary tract malignancy when imaging studies and cytology are not definitive.
2. Accurate staging of neoplastic disease by means of biopsy of radiologically visualized lesions.
3. Evaluation of the cause of ureteral obstruction in patients with a known current or past malignancy.
4. Evaluation of renal and adrenal masses in patients with a history of malignancy.

C. Contraindications

1. Contraindications to needle aspiration biopsy include the following.
   a. Hemorrhagic diathesis.
   b. Suspicion of an arteriovenous malformation in the area to be biopsied.
2. There are no contraindications to transcatheter brush biopsy.

D. Technique

1. Needle biopsy
   a. The biopsy site is localized by one of the following: fluoroscopy, excretory urography, retrograde pyelography, ileal loopography, US, CT, MRI, cystography, lymphangiography, or manual palpation. Most percutaneous biopsies are guided by CT or US, some by MRI, with operator preference, lesion size and location, and machine availability all determining factors.
   b. Biopsies performed with small (21 to 22 gauge), thin-walled needles yield samples for cytologic evaluation. Larger needles (14 to 20 gauge), often used in conjunction with automated, spring-loaded biopsy devices, yield specimens for histologic evaluation.
   c. Depth of needle insertion is ascertained by imaging the needle tip on CT, US (with an aspiration biopsy transducer), MRI, or, if employing fluoroscopy, by comparing the position of the needle tip with the biopsy site in various oblique fluoroscopic projections.
   d. The needle is placed directly into soft tissue or visceral abnormalities or immediately adjacent to an obstructed ureter at the point of narrowing or blockage. Most needle biopsies are obtained transperitoneally.
   e. Aspiration biopsies are obtained and evaluated immediately by a cytopathologist to ascertain the adequacy of tissue sampling. Additional biopsies are performed until diagnostic material is obtained.
   f. Large needles provide tissue cores of sufficient size for conventional histopathologic examination.

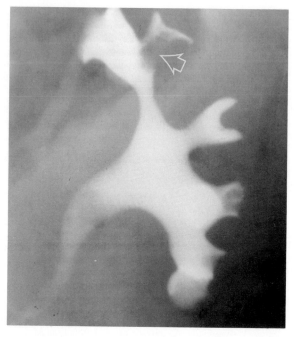

Figure 4-9 Transcatheter brush biopsy of transitional cell carcinoma.
A. An irregularly shaped filling defect (*arrow*) in an upper pole calyx is
seen in this patient with microscopic hematuria and a history of prior
bladder tumor. The remainder of the kidney and ureter are normal.

2. Transcatheter biopsy
   a. This approach is most frequently employed to obtain
      a brush biopsy of a pyelocalyceal or ureteral lesion
      suspicious for transitional cell carcinoma on noninva-
      sive imaging studies.
   b. An open-ended catheter is passed cytoscopically into
      the ureter or kidney. A guidewire on which is mounted
      a nylon brush is then passed through the catheter and
      the suspicious abnormality "brushed" under fluo-
      roscopy. Exfoliated cells retrieved by the brush are
      subjected to cytologic analysis (Fig. 4-9).
   c. A variety of brush configurations are available for ap-
      proaching lesions through the collecting system and
      ureter. Other biopsy instruments, including forceps
      and snares, can be passed through larger catheters or
      sheaths percutaneously or perurethrally inserted into
      the upper urinary tract.

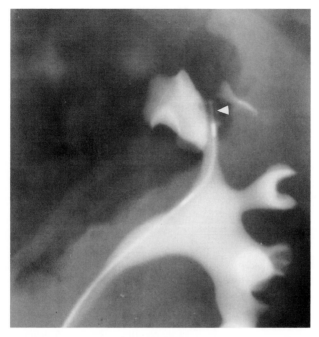

Figure 4-9 (*continued*)   **B.** Under fluoroscopic control, a nylon brush (*arrowhead*) attached to a guidewire is advanced beyond the end of a ureteral catheter (inserted cystoscopically) and "brushed" against the filling defect. Exfoliated cells were analyzed cytologically and shown to represent transitional cell carcinoma.

E. Results

1. Transcatheter and percutaneous brush biopsies yield true-positive results in over 90 percent of cases. False-positive results are very infrequent.
2. Cytologic demonstration of malignant cells generally alters patient management by obviating the need for more invasive diagnostic techniques (including ureteroscopy), surgical biopsy, or staging procedures.
3. Negative findings do not exclude the presence of malignancy, as they may represent sampling error.
4. Therefore, thin-needle aspiration or transcatheter brush biopsy is of value only when positive results are obtained.
5. Tissue core biopsies analyzed histologically will lessen false-negative results.
6. Biopsy of lymph nodes that exhibit filling defects on lymphography has a 70 percent correlation with surgical

lymphadenectomy results. However, positive aspirations may be obtained in as many as 15 percent of normal-appearing nodes.

F. Complications
1. Complications following aspiration biopsy are rare and include the following.
   a. Blood vessel injury with bleeding or arteriovenous fistula formation
   b. Peritonitis due to bowel leak
   c. Pneumothorax
   d. Seeding of the needle track with malignant cells. Only a handful of cases of spread of renal malignancy following aspiration biopsy have been reported. Nonetheless, because of the propensity for urothelial (but not parenchymal) tumors to spread along epithelial surfaces, they should not be biopsied percutaneously if it can be avoided.
2. Complications rarely accompany brush biopsy.
   a. Patient discomfort and hematuria relate to catheter manipulation and vigorous "brushing" of friable lesions.
   b. Collecting system or ureteral perforation with catheters or guidewires can occur but appears to be innocuous if adequate urinary drainage is maintained for a day or two after the procedure, usually with a retrograde ureteral catheter.
   c. Retroperitoneal seeding following perforation of a collecting system or ureter that harbored a urothelial neoplasm is a theoretical possibility.

IX. PERCUTANEOUS TRANSLUMINAL RENAL ANGIOPLASTY (PTRA)
A. Principles
1. PTRA is the most commonly employed nonoperative treatment alternative to surgical bypass grafting in patients with renovascular hypertension. Other vascular interventional techniques that also increase renal blood flow are intra-arterial thrombolysis, transcatheter thrombectomy, and arterial stents.

B. Indications
1. Indications for PTRA include the following.
   a. Correct proven renovascular hypertension.
   b. Correct the angiotensinogenic component in patients with essential hypertension plus superimposed renovascular hypertension.
   c. Facilitate medical management by permitting reduction or elimination of antihypertensive medications.

    d. Prevent renal failure due to impending renal artery occlusion.

    e. Reverse renal failure in patients with recent thrombosis of a stenotic renal artery.

2. The importance of PTRA depends on the etiology of the hypertension

    a. PTRA is the procedure of choice for fibromuscular renal artery disease; unilateral, short (less than 3 cm), nonostial atherosclerotic stenoses; and renal transplant arterial stenoses.

    b. PTRA will significantly improve patients with bilateral, nonostial atherosclerotic stenoses, postoperative vascular stenoses, and stenoses associated with worsening renal function and decreasing renal mass (serum creatinine less than 3.0 mg/dL).

    c. Lesser degrees of short- and long-term success with PTRA occur with ostial atherosclerotic stenoses, nonatheromatous lesions (e.g. neurofibromatosis, Takayasu's arteritis), stenoses associated with azotemia (creatinine greater than 3.0 mg/dL) for whom dialysis is imminent, and renal artery occlusions.

    d. PTRA plays a limited role in arterial stenoses associated with a renal artery aneurysm or in vessels arising from an aneurysm, or for those associated with severely diseased aortas, including abdominal coarctation (midaortic syndrome).

3. Intra-arterial streptokinase can lyse an occluding renal artery thrombus, following which PTRA can dilate an underlying stenosis.

4. Transcatheter thrombectomy can often immediately restore renal blood flow with minimal risk in patients with acute thrombotic or embolic renal artery occlusion. These patients not infrequently have underlying medical problems that increase the risk of surgical thrombectomy.

C. Contraindications

1. Contraindications are similar to those for surgical correction of a renal artery stenosis producing hypertension.

D. Technique

1. Antihypertensive drugs are reduced or eliminated to prevent hypotension after successful angioplasty.

2. PTRA is usually performed following diagnostic renal arteriography via the initial femoral puncture site. Occasionally, an axillary approach is required.

3. A catheter is selectively engaged in the renal artery and a guidewire used to cross the stenotic lesion.

4. The catheter is removed and replaced with a double lumen balloon catheter. The balloon is centered over the

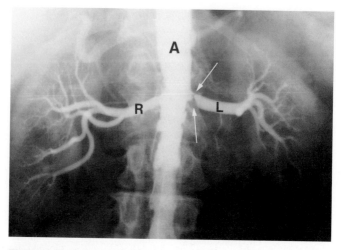

Figure 4-10 PTRA. **A.** Midstream aortogram in an elderly male with hypertension shows a tight stenosis at the origin of the left renal artery (*arrows*) and irregularity of the abdominal aorta, both attributable to atherosclerosis. A, aorta; L, left renal artery; R, right renal artery. PTRA with a balloon catheter was subsequently performed.

stenosis and inflated with contrast medium under fluoro-scopic control. The diameter of the balloon is matched to the normal portion of the renal artery adjacent to the stenosis, resulting in about 20 percent overdilation due to radiographic magnification.

5. Pressure measurements across the stenosis are obtained before and after angioplasty. Post-PTRA angiography assesses the anatomic success of the procedure.

6. Antispasmodics and vasodilators are often injected prior to crossing a stenosis to prevent or diminish the frequency or severity of renal artery spasm.

7. Intra-arterial administration of a fibrinolytic agent, such as streptokinase, may be used to lyse pre- or post-PTRA thrombotic occlusions.

8. Patients are anticoagulated prior to, during, and following PTRA.

E. Results

1. A technically successful PTRA (i.e., the procedure has resulted in either a cure or an improvement in the hypertension) occurs in 80 to 95 percent of cases, depending on the etiology of the stenosis (Fig. 4-10).

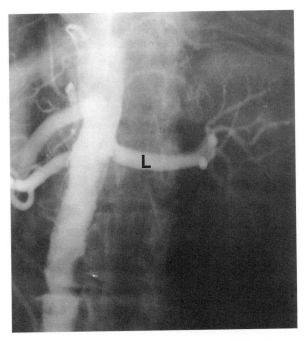

Figure 4-10 (*continued*)   **B.** Postangioplasty aortogram shows a widely patent left renal artery. The stenosis was successfully dilated and the patient's blood pressure reverted to normal. Resistant stenoses often benefit from transcatheter insertion of expandable metallic stents, similar in configuration to, though smaller than the one illustrated in Figure 3-8.

2. Recurrent stenoses occur in 10 to 20 percent of patients; they are most commonly seen when there is incomplete dilation of the lesion. Attempts at redilating a recurrent stenosis are generally good, but with a slightly decreased success rate.
3. The success and long-term patency rates of PTRA are greater in fibromuscular renal artery stenoses than in atherosclerotic lesions.
4. Technical failures occur most commonly when lesions are at a surgical anastomosis or at the origins of the renal arteries. Other failures are due to the inability to cross the lesion with a guidewire and/or catheter.
5. Advantages of PTRA over surgical treatment include:
   a. Decreased morbidity and mortality

     b. Shorter hospital stay with decreased recuperative period

     c. Restenoses following PTRA can be redilated percutaneously, stented, or corrected surgically

6. Experience with percutaneously placed self- or balloon-expandable, flexible, renal artery stents following unsuccessful PTRA has been that stents are an attractive and efficacious approach to improve renal blood flow. Their precise indications, true safety, and long-term efficacy is still being evaluated.

F. Complications

1. The complication rate of PTRA varies from 5 to 10 percent; most complications are minor.

2. Most procedure-related complications are easily managed and do not result in permanent deterioration of renal function or nephrectomy. Emergency surgical intervention is rarely needed.

3. Nonocclusive dissection of the renal artery usually requires nonemergent surgical bypass grafting.

4. Occlusive dissection of the renal artery requires surgical bypass.

5. Puncture site hematomas or thrombosis may or may not require surgery.

6. Renal artery rupture is an acute emergency that must be treated surgically.

7. Nonfilling of segmental intrarenal branches on the post-PTRA arteriogram is related to transient spasm or thrombosis, but does not usually produce lasting clinical sequela.

8. Idiosyncratic reactions to contrast media are rare. Transient contrast-induced renal insufficiency is a frequent problem, as many of these patients have preexisting azotemia, which is a primary risk factor for contrast nephropathy.

X. TRANSCATHETER EMBOLIZATION
A. Principles

1. Transcatheter techniques for vascular occlusion can be used to treat selected acute and nonacute clinical problems. Renal abnormalities and varicoceles account for most urinary tract embolizations.

2. A variety of embolic materials can be introduced through angiographic catheters. Particulate agents provide temporary vascular occlusion (hours to weeks). Mechanical, polymerizing, or sclerosing agents produce permanent occlusion.

B. Indications

1. Decrease blood flow through vascular renal or retroperitoneal tumors prior to surgical extirpation, facilitating surgical removal and perhaps enhancing an immune response and/or diminishing possible metastatic spread at the time of nephrectomy.
2. Control intractable bleeding from an incurable renal cell carcinoma, ameliorate tumor-related pain and paraneoplastic syndromes, and temporarily halt tumor growth (months to years).
3. Control renal hemorrhage secondary to traumatic aneurysms or arteriovenous malformation (AVMs).
4. Improve hypertension in patients with AVMs.
5. Ablate renal function by infarcting all renal tissue as an alternative to bilateral surgical nephrectomy in patients with the following.
   a. End-stage renal disease and nephrotic syndrome with severe renal protein loss, or uncontrollable hypertension.
   b. Ureterocutaneous fistulae usually secondary to irradiated pelvic malignancies.
6. Control posttraumatic pelvic hemorrhage.
7. Control intractable vesical hemorrhage associated with radiation cystitis when conservative urologic management is not effective or is contraindicated.
8. Occlude the internal spermatic vein in patients with testicular varicocele.
9. Diminish bleeding and/or symptomatology referable to uterine leiomyomata.

C. Contraindications

1. Lack of a valid indication for embolotherapy.
2. The presence of untreated renal infection.

D. Technique

1. An angiographic catheter is selectively introduced into the vessel(s) supplying the tumor, malformation, organ, or other area to be devascularized and one or more embolic agents are introduced. These include:
   a. Particulates [e.g., autologous clot, Gelfoam, polyvinyl alcohol (Ivalon), skeletal muscle]
   b. Mechanical agents (e.g., stainless steel coils, detachable balloons)
   c. Polymerizing fluids [e.g., isobutyl 2-cyano acrylate (bucrylate)]
   d. other agents (e.g., absolute alcohol, hot contrast material)

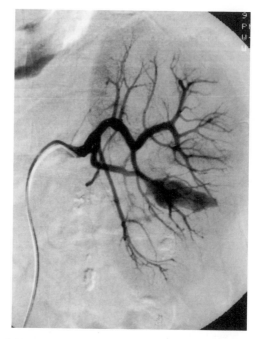

Figure 4-11 Renal embolization. **A.** Digital subtraction selective left renal arteriogram in a patient with persistent gross hematuria following percutaneous nephrostolithotomy shows a flame-shaped contrast collection in the lower renal pole representing a pseudoaneurysm that resulted from the prior percutaneous nephrostomy.

2. A renal artery occlusion balloon catheter helps prevent systemic reflux of embolic agents.
3. A postembolization arteriogram is obtained to assess the effectiveness of embolotherapy.
4. Therapeutic embolization should be deferred for at least 1 day after a diagnostic angiogram to decrease the contrast medium load to the remaining kidney.

E. Results
1. The efficacy of embolotherapy is apparent on the postembolization angiogram. Complete vascular occlusion may require the use of several embolic agents. For localized renal abnormalities (e.g., aneurysms, vascular malforma-

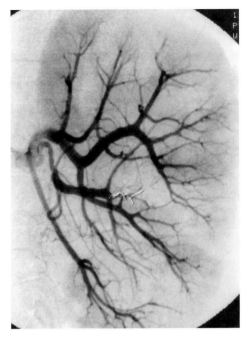

Figure 4-11 (*continued*)   **B.** The injured renal artery has been successfully occluded with several small metal coils. The remainder of the kidney remains well perfused.

tions), segmental vessel embolization maximizes preservation of functioning renal tissue (Fig. 4-11).
2. Internal spermatic veins supplying varicoceles may be occluded in 85 to 90 percent of cases. Sperm counts and motility subsequently increase in as many as 75 percent of infertile men.

F. Complications
1. *Postembolization syndrome.* Most patients experience pain in the area of the embolized vessel, nausea, vomiting, and/or fever lasting 24 to 48 hours. Some may develop an ileus. These symptoms are related to tissue ischemia and infarction.
2. *Reflux.* The most serious complication of renal artery embolotherapy is reflux of embolic material and undesired migration to other vessels (e.g., spinal cord and bowel

infarction, occlusion of the contralateral renal artery and peripheral vessels). Use of occlusion balloon catheters and slow injection of small quantities of embolic material help to prevent reflux. The rate of clinically significant reflux is generally 1 percent or less.

BIBLIOGRAPHY

Banner MP: *Radiologic Interventions: Uroradiology.* Baltimore: Williams & Wilkins, 1998.

CHAPTER 5
Lower Urinary Tract Infections in Women

Philip M. Hanno

I. INCIDENCE

Urinary tract infections (UTIs) account for more than 5 million office visits in the United States every year. About half of all adult women report that they have had a urinary tract infection at some time during their life. The prevalence of asymptomatic bacteriuria is about 1 to 2 percent in newborns. After the first year of life, infections are more common in females. During the ages 5 to 18 years, the prevalence is 1.2 percent in girls, fourfold the rate found in boys. The prevalence of bacteriuria in females rises about 1 percent per decade, up to almost 10 percent in elderly women. Approximately 20 percent of the women who develop a urinary tract infection will have frequent recurrences of infection (every 2 to 4 months) following the initial episode. The cost to the health care system for uncomplicated lower urinary tract infections has been estimated at $350 million annually. Thus, the problem of lower tract infection in women, while no longer considered to be a prelude to renal deterioration, continues to be a major one. The associated morbidity and lost time from work, cost of medications, and potential development of bacterial resistance are all drains on the health care budget, as well as quality of life.

II. DEFINITION AND CLASSIFICATION

The criteria for the presumptive diagnosis of urinary tract infection in a symptomatic patient include the following.

1. Symptoms of bladder irritation (dysuria, urgency or frequency of urination) or of infection of the kidney (flank pain, fever, costovertebral angle tenderness).
2. Urine sediment containing 8 to 10 or more white blood cells per high-powered field.
3. Quantitative urine culture revealing at least 100,000 microorganisms per milliliter of urine in a clean-voided specimen.

It is possible to have a bacterial urinary tract infection with a negative urinalysis and/or bacterial counts in the urine of less than

173

10^5. The entire clinical setting must be taken into account when making the diagnosis. Consistent sterile cultures can be used to rule out bacterial infection of the urinary tract as a cause of symptoms, and make one look to other diagnoses. The presence of 100,000 microorganisms per milliliter of urine in a patient without symptoms is termed "asymptomatic bacteriuria."

Urinary tract infections can be classified as to their site of origin. Cystitis refers to the nonspecific clinical syndrome of dysuria, urinary frequency, urgency, and suprapubic fullness. Vaginitis, urethritis, interstitial cystitis, and urethral syndrome can all present with similar symptoms. Fever, chills, and flank pain can indicate the presence of pyelonephritis, an interstitial inflammation caused by bacterial infection of the renal parenchyma. Based on symptoms, it is remarkably difficult to differentiate infection involving the upper tracts from bacteriuria confined to the bladder. Many patients with pure lower tract symptoms will have positive cultures of ureteral and renal pelvic urine. Similarly, some patients with flank pain will be found to have only cystitis on differential urine cultures. From a practical standpoint, it is not generally an important distinction, and localizing the site of infection in clinically uncomplicated infections is unnecessary.

Infections can be classified as uncomplicated (occurring in a normal urinary tract) or complicated (occurring in a patient with structural or anatomic impairments that decrease antibiotic efficacy). Perhaps the most useful classification of urinary tract infection is that devised by Stamey of Stanford. *First infections* refer to isolated or remotely occurring bacterial cystitis. These are the most common infections in women, occurring in 25 to 30 percent of women between the ages of 30 and 40 years. *Unresolved bacteriuria* occurs when the urine cannot be sterilized despite antibiotic treatment. Common causes include preexisting or acquired bacterial resistance, inadequate coverage of a second organism, rapid reinfection with a new organism during therapy, azotemia preventing access of the antibiotic to the urinary tract, and noncompliance with treatment. *Recurrent infection* is an infection diagnosed after successful treatment of an antecedent infection. This category represents 95 percent of recurrent UTIs in women. The other 5 percent may be caused by *bacterial persistence.* Sterilization of the urine is short-lived, and within weeks, a relapse with the identical organism occurs. Such infections indicate a site of persistent infection within the urinary tract that could represent a stone, enterovesical fistula, or infected anatomic anomaly such as a diverticulum in the urinary tract.

The most helpful laboratory guide for rapid diagnosis is careful microscopic examination of the urine. Documentation by urine culture can be helpful in diagnosing a first infection or evaluating patients with recurrent symptoms unresponsive to empirical therapy.

III. PATHOGENESIS

The bacteria responsible for urinary tract infections are normally present in the bowel. *Escherichia coli* is the most common, accounting for 85 percent of community-acquired infections and up to 50 percent of nosocomial infections. Other common organisms include *Proteus* sp., *Klebsiella* sp., *Enterococcus faecalis,* and *Staphylococcus saprophyticus.* The female urethra is short, and bacteria generally enter the bladder in an ascending fashion. Host-defense mechanisms can be more important than bacterial virulence or inoculum size in determining whether a clinical infection develops.

Vaginal mucosal introital colonization generally precedes infection, and is determined by bacterial adherence, the receptive characteristics of the epithelial surface, and the fluid that bathes both surfaces. Estrogens and pH affect attachment and colonization of the vaginal mucosa. Host-defense mechanisms include the antiadherence properties of the vaginal and bladder mucosa, the hydrokinetic clearance of bacteria through voiding, and changes in urine pH and composition that may inhibit bacterial growth. Women with recurrent urinary tract infections demonstrate increased adherence of bacteria in vitro to uroepithelial cells when compared to findings in women who have never had an infection. Studies suggest that this may be genetically determined.

Risk factors for UTI include sexual intercourse, use of a diaphragm or cervical cap, and spermacidal jelly, which can alter the normal vaginal flora. The ABO-blood group nonsecretor phenotype is at increased risk for vaginal colonization with uropathic bacteria. Urologic instrumentation, diabetes, and age-related changes in the elderly patient are also risk factors. Low estrogen levels allow vaginal pH to rise, resulting in a higher likelihood of vaginal colonization with *E. coli.* Personal hygiene habits are not related to recurrent UTI. The use of oral contraceptive agents is also unrelated.

IV. MANAGEMENT (Fig. 5-1)

A. Uncomplicated Isolated Cystitis

Urologic investigation in not routinely indicated in women with isolated episodes of acute urinary frequency, dysuria, and urgency suggestive of lower urinary tract infection. Diagnosis is often empiric, however, a urinalysis and/or culture can provide helpful documentation of the true diagnosis and causative organism. Examination of urine sediment after centrifugation will show microscopic bacteriuria in more than 90 percent of infections with 10^5 colony forming units (cfu)/mL. Pyuria will be seen in 80 to 95 percent of infections, and microhematuria in about 50 percent. It must be kept in mind that normal vaginal flora can appear to be gram-negative bacteria on

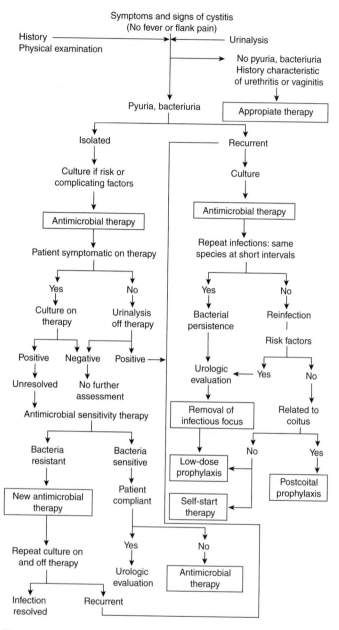

Figure 5-1 Management of acute cystitis. (*From Schaeffer AJ: Infections of the urinary tract. In: Walsh PC, Retic AB, Vaughan ED, Wein AJ, eds. Campbell's Urology, 7th ed.* Philadelphia: Saunders, 1998, p 589, with permission.)

urinalysis, and that pyuria may be noted in a variety of inflammatory conditions of the urinary tract. Alternatively, if the patient is drinking increased fluids and voiding frequently, the urine will be dilute, and signs of infection on urinalysis may be missing. If a urine culture is performed, it should be a carefully collected, midstream specimen to decrease the likelihood of any vaginal contamination. Approximately one third of women with acute symptomatic cystitis caused by *E. coli, S. saprophyticus,* or *Proteus* have colony counts of midstream urine specimens ranging from 10^2 to 10^4 cfu/mL. Thus, a pure culture in the presence of symptoms must be considered significant, regardless of colony count.

Clues in the history that may suggest an increased risk of complicated UTI include childhood infections, previous urologic surgery or instrumentation, urolithiasis, or the presence of diabetes. If hematuria is noted, the physician is obligated to be sure that it is no longer present after treatment of infection. If it is still present, a urologic imaging study and cystoscopy are necessary to rule out other urologic pathology. If a complicated UTI is suspected by history, a similar evaluation may be necessary after the infection has cleared.

Treatment of isolated cystitis is often empirical and not based on culture data. A drug should be chosen based on the following criteria: (1) the relative likelihood that it will be active against enteric bacteria that commonly produce UTIs; (2) its ability to achieve high concentrations in the urine; (3) its tendency not to alter the bowel or vaginal flora or to select for resistant bacteria; (4) its limited toxicity; and (5) its availability at reasonable cost to the patient. Because these organisms causing isolated UTI in the community are generally pansensitive to antibiotics, cost and convenience are major factors in drug selection. Urine levels of antimicrobial rather than serum levels are important for efficacy in eliminating bacteriuria. Care must be taken in interpreting antibiotic susceptibility tests, as they are often based on serum levels of drug. In the past, physicians prescribed treatment for 5 to 10 days. It is now apparent that 3 days of antibiotic will suffice to clear the vast majority of uncomplicated urinary tract infections. Single-dose therapy is slightly less efficacious.

B. Unresolved Bacteriuria

Persistent symptoms following treatment for UTI, necessitates repeat urine culture and sensitivity testing. Choice of antibiotic will depend on the results obtained, and a 7- to 10-day course would be reasonable. Repeat culture and bacterial identification (if positive) following treatment for unresolved bacteriuria is important in order to later differentiate the problem from recurrent infection from a site within the urinary tract.

C. Recurrent Bacterial Cystitis

A detailed culture history is critical in differentiating reinfection from a site outside the urinary tract as the cause of recurrent cystitis from reinfection from a site of bacterial persistence within the urinary tract. The former accounts for over 95 percent of cases of recurrent UTI, but the latter is important, as a full urologic evaluation is mandatory. Bacterial identification becomes important, as recurrent infections that occur after successful antimicrobial eradication (negative culture) and that are subsequently caused by varying strains of *Enterobacteriaceae* are pathognomonic for reinfection. The only confounding factor that might cause a similar scenario is reinfection from an enterovesical fistula with different organisms. In this unusual case, often the urine can never be sterilized, and infections may be with multiple rather than one organism, thus giving the suspicion of a fistula.

This author tends to be aggressive in evaluating patients with long histories of recurrent urinary tract infections in order not to miss a treatable etiology. A renal and bladder ultrasound will demonstrate normal anatomy, absence of infection stones, and low bladder urinary residual urine volume. Flexible office cystoscopy will rule out any urethral stenosis (very rare), urethral diverticulum, or local bladder pathology that might have been missed (herald patch representing a fistula, abnormal and chronically infected site of bladder mucosa, infected suture from previous surgery, etc.).

Once it is clear that the patient's problem represents recurrent cystitis from reinfection from a site outside the urinary tract, usually gram-negative introital colonization, one can discuss treatment strategies. The patient should be reassured that the problem is largely one of controlling the symptoms, and not a threat to her urologic health. It is a treatable nuisance that most patients can manage on their own without numerous visits to physicians offices. Years ago, many patients were treated with long-term, low-dose antibiotic therapy. This might have been 50 mg nitrofurantoin every evening for 6 months or half tablet of trimethoprim-sulfamethoxazole every other night for 6 months. At that point, treatment would stop in the hope that the introital colonization with uropathogenic gram-negative organisms had resolved, which tends to happen over time. Two or three episodes of UTI over the next 6 months would trigger another course of prophylaxis.

In an effort to decrease overall antibiotic usage, new and equally effective strategies have emerged. "Self-start" therapy relies on the patient to make the clinical diagnosis of UTI, not difficult in this unfortunately experienced group. Patients are given a prescription for an appropriate urinary antibiotic (nitrofurantoin, trimethoprim-sulfamethoxazole, cephalosporin), which they take for 3 days at the first sign of infection. Some physicians encourage dip-slide culture before and after medication. This author believes that if the symptoms respond quickly to 3 days of antibiotic treatment, culture is not necessary. Only if the symptoms do not respond or reoccur within a few days is a visit to the physician for appropriate culture and sensitivity testing required. Certainly, systemic symptoms such as fever and flank pain, or the presence of gross hematuria should trigger a visit to the physician. With appropriate patient education self-treatment seems to work very well in properly diagnosed recurrent UTI from reinfection.

Other options include single-dose therapy. Although this might clear the bacteria from the urinary tract, symptoms often persist for 48 hours, and the patient is left unsure as to whether more antibiotic or a different antibiotic is necessary. If infections seem to be exclusively related to intercourse, and frequency of intercourse is not too high, one can consider a prophylactic antibiotic just before sexual activity to prevent infection. Those having sex on a nightly basis might do better to treat symptomatic infections with short-term courses of antibiotics, thus limiting overall use of antibiotic.

V. CHOICE OF ANTIBIOTIC

There are many excellent, inexpensive, first-line antimicrobials to consider for the treatment of uncomplicated lower urinary tract infections in women (Table 5-1). Nitrofurantoin, while not effective against *Pseudomonas* and *Proteus* species, does cover the vast majority of pathogens encountered. It has high urine levels, a short half-life in the blood, and minimal effect on resident fecal and vaginal flora. It is associated with a low incidence of bacterial resistance. Trimethoprim with or without sulfamethoxazole (TMP-SMX) is another widely used and very effective treatment for UTI. Alone or in combination these drugs will not eradicate *Enterococcus* and *Pseudomonas* species. They are inexpensive and can clear the vaginal flora of gram-negative uropathogens, although the clinical significance of this is questionable. Skin rashes and gastrointestinal side effects prove the main drawbacks.

Cephalosporins, as a group, have poor activity against *Enterococcus*. First-generation drugs are reasonable to treat uncomplicated UTI, but the second- and third-generation members of this group would best be reserved for culture documented infections requiring their broader coverage. Ampicillin and amoxacillin, traditionally regarded as inexpensive first-line therapy, have generally fallen out of favor due to their interference with the fecal flora and the resultant emergence of resistant strains such that these drugs are now ineffective against as many as 30 percent of common urinary isolates.

Although the fluoroquinolones have a very broad spectrum of activity against most urinary pathogens including *Pseudomonas aeruginosa,* their routine use for treatment of uncomplicated UTI

Table 5-1 Reliable Coverage of Antimicrobials Used in the Treatment of Urinary Tract Infections of Commonly Encountered Pathogens.

ANTIMICROBIAL OR ANTIMICROBIAL CLASS	GRAM-POSITIVE PATHOGENS	GRAM-NEGATIVE PATHOGENS
Amoxicillin with ampicillin	*Streptococcus* Enterococci	*Escherichia coli* *Proteus mirabilis*
Amoxicillin with clavulanate	*Streptococcus*	*E. coli*
Ampicillin with sulbactam	*Staphylococcus* (not MRSA) Enterococci	*P. mirabilis* *Haemophilus influenzae, Klebsiella* spp.
Antistaphylococcal penicillins	*Streptococcus* *Staphylococcus* (not MRSA)	None
Antipseudomonal penicillins	*Streptococcus* Enterococci	Most including *Pseudomonas aeruginosa*
First-generation cephalosporins	*Streptococcus* *Staphylococcus* (not MRSA)	*E. coli* *P. mirabilis* *Klebsiella* spp.

Agent	Gram-positive	Gram-negative
Second-generation cephalosporins (cefamandole, cefuroxime, cefaclor)	*Streptococcus* *Staphylococcus* (not MRSA)	*E. coli, P. mirabilis* *H. influenzae, Klebsiella* spp.
Second-generation cephalosporins (cefoxitin, cefotetan)	*Streptococcus*	*E. coli, Proteus* spp. (incl. indole +) *H. influenzae, Klebsiella* spp.
Third-generation cephalosporins (ceftazidime, cefoperazone)	*Streptococcus*	Most, including *P. aeruginosa*
Aztreonam	None	Most, including *P. aeruginosa*
Aminoglycosides	*Staphylococcus* (urine)	Most, including *P. aeruginosa*
Fluoroquinolones	None	Most, including *P. aeruginosa*
Nitrofurantoin	*Staphylococcus* (not MRSA) Enterococci	Many Enterobacteriaceae (not *Providencia, Serratia, Acinetobacter*) *Klebsiella* spp.
Trimethoprim-sulfamethoxazole	*Streptococcus* *Staphylococcus*	Most Enterobacteriaceae (not *P. aeruginosa*)
Vancomycin	All including MRSA	None

MRSA, methicillin-resistant *Staphylococcus aureus*. (From Schaeffer AJ: *Infections of the urinary tract*. In: Walsh PC, Retic AB, Vaughan ED, Wein AJ, eds. *Campbell's Urology*, 7th ed. Philadelphia: Saunders, 1998, p 556, with permission.)

is controversial. Gram-positive activity is limited and efficacy against *Enterococcus* is poor. These are expensive, powerful oral agents. The fear that overuse may lead to the development of resistance and the fact that for most uncomplicated UTIs less expensive drugs are just as effective has tended to limit their use. They remain a valuable class of antibiotic, best restricted to complicated UTIs, pseudomonal infections, or treatment of resistant organisms.

VI. ASYMPTOMATIC BACTERIURIA OF PREGNANCY AND IN THE ELDERLY PATIENT

Pregnancy requires particular attention with regard to screening for bacteriuria and treatment of urinary infection. The prevalence of bacteriuria identified by screening is no higher in pregnant females than nonpregnant females of the same age. However, pregnancy results in physiologic changes that have important implications with regard to asymptomatic bacteriuria and progression of infection. With pregnancy, come increases in renal size, augmented renal function, hydroureteronephrosis, and anterosuperior displacement of the bladder. The frequency of acute pyelonephritis in pregnant women is significantly higher than in their nonpregnant counterparts. Studies suggest a 20 to 40 percent incidence of pyelonephritis if asymptomatic bacteriuria is untreated in this population. In addition, bacterial pyelonephritis in pregnancy has been associated with infant prematurity and perinatal mortality. These factors make it prudent to screen for asymptomatic bacteriuria in pregnancy, treat it aggressively, and obtain follow-up cultures. An initial negative screening urine culture need not be repeated, as these patients are unlikely to develop bacteriuria later in pregnancy.

The prevalence of bacteriuria in the elderly patient is surprisingly high. Up to 20 percent of women and 10 percent of men older than 65 years have bacteriuria. The figures are even higher for nursing home residents. The need for treatment of asymptomatic bacteriuria in the elderly is controversial. It is not uncommon for courses of antibiotics to be unsuccessful in long-term management of bacteriuria in this group of patients. Studies suggest that noncatheterized male and female residents of nursing homes with bacteriuria have no higher frequency of courses of antimicrobial treatment, infections, or hospitalizations than those without persistent bacteriuria. Clearly, symptomatic urinary tract infections in the elderly patient should be appropriately treated. In addition, it would seem prudent to treat any bacteriuria due to urea-splitting bacteria such as *Proteus mirabilis* to prevent stone formation. Otherwise, routine treatment of asymptomatic bacteriuria in the elderly patient appears unjustified.

BIBLIOGRAPHY

Engel JD, Schaeffer AJ: Evaluation of and antimicrobial therapy for recurrent urinary tract infections in women. *Urol Clin North Am* 25:681, 1998.

Faro S: New considerations in treatment of urinary tract infections in adults. *Urology* 39:1, 1992.

Hooton TM, Scholes D, Stapleton AE, et al: A prospective study of asymptomatic bacteriuria in sexually active young women. NEJM 343:992–997, 2000.

Kunin CM: Duration of treatment of urinary tract infections. *Am J Med* 71:849, 1981.

Kunin CM: *Urinary Tract Infections: Detection, Prevention, and Management,* 5th ed. Baltimore: Williams & Wilkins, 1997.

Nicolle LE: Asymptomatic bacteriuria—important or not? NEJM 343:1037–1039, 2000.

Schaeffer AJ, Stuppy, BA: Efficacy and safety of self-start therapy in women with recurrent urinary tract infections. *J Urol* 161:207, 1999.

SELF-ASSESSMENT QUESTIONS

1. The risk that a women who develops an initial urinary tract infection will have frequent recurrences is:
   a. 2%
   b. 10%
   c. 20%
   d. 50%
2. Lower urinary tract infection in women can best be considered:
   a. a prelude to renal deterioration.
   b. a symptomatic problem with no long-term sequelae.
   c. a sign of significant immunodeficiency.
   d. a major risk factor for urolithiasis.
3. The distinction between upper and lower tract bacteriuria:
   a. is clinically made on the basis of symptoms.
   b. determines the choice of antibiotic.
   c. is unnecessary from a practical standpoint.
   d. depends on serum antibody titers.
4. The most important determinant of bacterial urinary tract infection is:
   a. virulence of the bacteria.
   b. poor perineal hygiene.
   c. family history.
   d. a problem of the host-defense mechanism.
5. Which of the following does not require treatment?
   a. Asymptomatic bacteriuria of pregnancy
   b. Symptomatic urinary infection in a 75-year-old woman
   c. Asymptomatic bacteriuria in a 75-year-old woman
   d. Asymptomatic Proteus UTI in a 50-year-old woman

Answers

1. c
2. b
3. c
4. d
5. c

CHAPTER 6

Prostatitis and Lower Urinary Tract Infections in Men

Heather C. Selman
Michel Pontari

I. INCIDENCE AND RISK FACTORS

A. Urinary Tract Infections (UTIs)

UTIs are the most common nosocomial bacterial infections in the United States and account for more than 7 million visits to physicians annually. The majority of infections are in women, with 20 to 50 percent of women developing a UTI during their lifetime and an incidence of infection 30 times higher in adult women than adult men. However, UTIs are more common in male infants than female infants, perhaps due to the higher incidence of congenital genitourinary disorders in males, and uncircumcised infants have more UTIs than those who are circumcised. The incidence of UTIs is similar for men and women above the age of 50 years. The increased prevalence in men above this age is secondary to prostatic enlargement with resultant bladder outlet obstruction and residual urine, urinary tract instrumentation, immobility or decreased activity, and decreased prostatic secretions. Asymptomatic bacteriuria may range from 15 to 35 percent in institutionalized elderly men and is frequently polymicrobial.

B. Other Risk Factors

Other risk factors for UTIs include urethral stricture disease, neurogenic bladder, calculi, urethral catheters (5 percent per single catheterization and 5 percent increase per day of catheterization), external collecting devices, enteric fistulae, urachal cysts or sinuses, renal impairment, neutropenia, insertive anal intercourse, intercourse with an infected female partner, and lack of circumcision with inadequate meatal care. Diabetes mellitus can cause a neurogenic bladder with a large capacity and infrequent voiding. Elevated urinary glucose impairs phagocytosis.

II. PATHOGENESIS

A. Routes of Infection

The majority of uropathogens in men are introduced via the ascending route (through the urethra), as opposed to a hematogenous or lymphatic route, or direct extension.

B. Pathogens

Gram-negative enteric bacteria, particularly *Escherichia coli,* cause about 80 percent of UTIs in men. A smaller percentage are caused by *Klebsiella, Enterobacter,* and *Proteus.* About one-fifth of infections are caused by gram-positive organisms, such as enterococci and staphylococci. Two or more organisms may be the cause of infection in bacterial prostatitis, urinary fistulae, diabetes mellitus, or those resulting from foreign bodies or calculi.

C. Host Resistance

1. *Washout of bacteria during micturition.* A lower inoculum size is required when urine flow is obstructed.
2. *Bacterial antiadherence factors.* These include the mucopolysaccharide coating of the bladder epithelium and possibly urinary constituents including the normal flora of the urethra, Tamm-Horsfall mucoprotein, and immunoglublumins IgA and IgG.
3. *Prostatic antibacterial factor.* This is secreted by the prostate and has important antimicrobial activity. Spermine has some activity against gram-positive bacteria. Zinc is also felt to be antibacterial.
4. *Long male urethral length.* Long length inhibits retrograde ascent of bacteria. Furthermore, the male meatus, which is not located on the perineum, is less likely to come into contact with enteric bacteria compared to the female.

Table 6-1 Prevalence of Bacteriuria in Males

AGE GROUP	PERCENT
Infants	2
Young boys	0.1–0.5
Young adults	<0.01–0.03
Adults (30–65 years)	0.1
Elderly (> 65 years)	5–15

III. LOCALIZATION OF LOWER URINARY TRACT INFECTION—SEGMENTED BACTERIOLOGIC LOCALIZATION CULTURES

This four-glass urine test differentiates bacterial cystitis from chronic bacterial prostatitis.

A. **Technique (Fig. 6-1)**

The uncircumcised male must retract his foreskin prior to voiding and wipe glans with an alcohol swab. The first 10 mL of urine is collected in a sterile specimen container [voided bladder 1 (VB1)]. After voiding 200 mL, a midstream specimen is collected in a separate container (VB2). The patient then stops voiding and prostatic massage is performed. The expressed prostatic secretion (EPS) is gently milked by proximal to distal pressure on the bulbar urethra and is collected in a fresh container. The next 10 mL of voided urine is collected immediately following prostatic massage (VB3).

B. **Interpretation of Culture Results** (Fig. 6-2)

1. *VB1—identifies the urethral flora.* With urethral colonization or urethritis only, the VB1 is greatest.
2. *VB2—positive VB2 culture can result from bladder, prostatic, or urethral bacteria.* If the VB2 culture is positive, the patient should be treated with an antibiotic that will sterilize the bladder and urethra but will not diffuse into the prostate (e.g. nitrofurantoin for 3 days). After treatment, the localization cultures should be repeated.

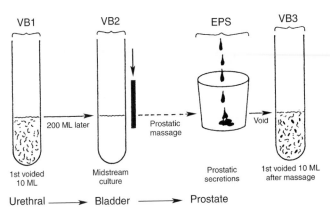

Figure 6-1 Bacterial localization procedure for male lower tract infection.

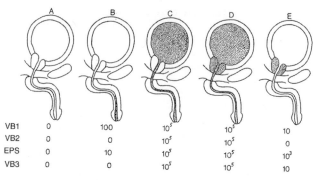

	A	B	C	D	E
VB1	0	100	10^5	10^5	10
VB2	0	0	10^5	10^5	0
EPS	0	10	10^5	10^5	10^3
VB3	0	0	10^5	10^5	10

Figure 6-2 Characteristic results of quantitative culture of VB1, VB2, EPS, and VB3 specimens (expressed as gram-negative bacilli per milliliter) in men with no urethral colonization by gram-negative bacilli **(A)**, urethral colonization only by gram-negative bacilli **(B)**, bacteriuria but no prostatic infection **(C)**, bacteriuria and coexisting prostatic infection **(D)**, and prostatic infection with suppression of bacterial growth in the urine with antimicrobial therapy **(E)**. *(Reproduced from Fowler JE Jr: Urinary Tract Infection and Inflammation. Chicago, Year Book Medical Publishers, 1989.)*

3. *EPS/VB3.* Cultures with substantially higher colony counts (tenfold) than VB1 indicate prostatic infection when VB2 culture is negative.

IV. BACTERIAL CYSTITIS
A. Signs and Symptoms
Urinary frequency, urgency, dysuria, nocturia, suprapubic discomfort, low back pain, and hematuria or terminally blood-tinged urine may be present. Systemic symptoms such as fever, chills, and rigors are absent. Elderly people may be asymptomatic or may have gastrointestinal symptoms, such as nausea and vomiting.

B. Diagnosis
1. *Urinalysis.* Positive leukocyte esterase and nitrite tests on dipstick suggest bacterial infection. On microscopic examination of a centrifuged specimen, greater than 10 WBC/HPF indicates pyuria. Red blood cells may be seen. Gram's stain is performed to look for bacteria. Casts are not seen.
2. *Urine culture.* Greater than or equal to 10^4 cfu per mL of urine indicates true bacterial infection in men as opposed to contamination from periurethral bacteria. (Higher

colony counts are required for the diagnosis in women due to the higher likelihood of contamination.) Polymicrobial growth without a predominant organism strongly suggests contamination.

3. *Diagnostic imaging and cystoscopy.* An intravenous urogram or renal ultrasound should be obtained after the first UTI to search for a possible urinary tract abnormality. Bladder ultrasound can evaluate the post-void residual urine volume. Cystoscopy should be performed after urine sterilization in men beyond middle age.

C. Treatment

1. *Bacterial cystitis.* Culture-appropriate antibiotics should be used for symptomatic men and asymptomatic men less than age 60 years for 7 to 10 days. Asymptomatic bacteriuria in elderly men need only be treated in the face of detrimental organisms (e.g. urea-splitting bacteria), abnormal urinary tracts, or urinary tract instrumentation. Men with UTIs can generally be managed as outpatients with trimethoprim-sulfamethoxazole (Bactrim, Septra), one double-strength tablet twice daily, or with a quinolone (ciprofloxacin 500 mg twice daily, ofloxacin 400 mg twice daily, or levofloxacin 250 mg once daily).

2. *Candidal cystitis.* This may be seen in catheterized patients or those with diabetes mellitus, immunosuppression, or on systemic antibiotics. The indwelling catheter should be removed, if possible, or changed. Any unnecessary steroid or antibiotic should be stopped. Continuous bladder irrigation with amphotericin B (50 mg/L sterile water every 24 hours) for 5 days may be used. Oral fluconazole 50 to 100 mg per day for 7 days is useful in treating *C. albicans.*

V. PROSTATITIS–CHRONIC PELVIC PAIN SYNDROME

A. Epidemiology

Prostatitis accounts for approximately one quarter of all male office visits for genitourinary tract symptoms. Half of all men will suffer from prostatitis symptoms sometime in their lives. Prostatitis accounts for approximately 2 million office visits to physicians in the United States annually.

B. Classification

Classification of the prostatitis syndromes is based on the presence of prostatic inflammation and bacterial infection. Only 10 percent of men with prostatitis syndromes have bacterial prostatitis. Classically, the four groups have been: acute bacterial prostatitis, chronic bacterial prostatitis, nonbacterial prostatitis, and prostatodynia. In 1995, the Chronic

Prostatitis Workshop of the National Institute of Diabetes, Digestive and Kidney Diseases reclassified the syndromes (Table 6-2). Acute bacterial prostatitis is class I. Chronic bacterial prostatitis is class II. Nonbacterial prostatitis and prostatodynia are class III, called chronic abacterial prostatitis–chronic pelvic pain syndrome (CPPS), and are subcategorized depending on the presence or absence of leukocytes in the EPS and/or semen. Class IV describes patients without symptoms but with the presence of inflammation in the EPS, semen, or prostate tissue on biopsy or resection. Class IV patients require no treatment as they are asymptomatic.

C. **Acute Bacterial Prostatitis**
   1. *Signs and Symptoms.* Possible prodrome of vague pelvic and systemic symptoms. Acute onset of dysuria, urgency, frequency, nocturia, perineal and low back pain, difficulty voiding, fever, chills, malaise. Prostate is enlarged, boggy, and tender on rectal examination although examination should be minimized to avoid bacteremia.
   2. *Laboratory results.* Elevated white blood count. Pyuria and bacteriuria on urinalysis. Urine culture most commonly grows *E. coli. Klebsiella, Proteus mirabilis, Enterobacter,* and *Staphylococcus aureus* are also common; *Salmonella* is rare. Granulomatous prostatitis may result from miliary tuberculosis or systemic mycosis.
   3. *Treatment.* Bed rest, antipyretics, analgesics, hydration, suprapubic cystotomy for urinary retention, stool softeners. Acutely ill patients may require hospitalization for hydration and broad-spectrum parenteral antibiotics (ampicillin and gentamicin) until culture and sensitivity results are available. These antibiotics are able to penetrate the generally impermeable prostatic epithelium due to alterations in the epithelial barrier during intense inflammation. Afebrile patients may be managed as outpatients with trimethoprim-sulfamethoxazole or a fluoro-

Table 6-2   National Institute of Diabetes, Digestive and Kidney Diseases Classifications of Prostatitis Syndromes

Class I	Acute bacterial prostatitis
Class II	Chronic bacterial prostatitis
Class III	Chronic abacterial prostatitis/
	chronic pelvic pain syndrome
	a. Inflammatory
	b. Noninflammatory
Class IV	Asymptomatic inflammatory prostatitis

quinolone for 3 to 4 weeks. Treatment is important to attempt to prevent the development of chronic prostatitis. *Salmonella* is treated with cotrimoxazole or chloramphenicol. Tuberculous and mycotic prostatitis are treated with antitubercular or antifungal therapies.

4. *Complications.* Prostatic abscess should be suspected in diabetic patients or in presence of continued spiking fevers despite adequate antibiotics and a fluctuant prostate. Computer tomography or transrectal ultrasound (TRUS) can diagnose a prostatic abscess. It can be drained by transurethral incision or TRUS-guided transperineal percutaneous drainage. Chronic prostatitis is a possible sequela of acute prostatitis.

D. Chronic Bacterial Prostatitis

1. *Signs and Symptoms.* Pelvic, perineal, or low back discomfort; dysuria and irritative voiding; clear discharge; recurrent UTI; pain during or after ejaculation. More insidious onset than acute prostatitis. Physical examination is normal.

2. *Laboratory results.* Bladder urine should first be sterilized with amoxicillin or nitrofurantoin. EPS and VB3 cultures show colony counts at least tenfold higher than VB2. Greater than 10 WBC/HPF in EPS. Culture documentation of prior bacteriuria. Recurrent bacteriuria between courses of antibiotics is common. *E. coli* in 80 percent of cases. *Klebsiella, Pseudomonas aeruginosa,* and *Proteus* less common. The role of gram-positive organisms, including *Staphylococcus epidermitis* and *Staphylococcus saprophyticus,* is debated as the anterior urethra is normally colonized by such organisms and contamination of the prostatitic secretions cannot be avoided. Localization studies for these organisms usually are not reproducible, do not produce an immune response in prostatic secretions, and do not lead to relapsing and recurrent UTI in untreated patients, as do gram-negative prostatic infections. Little evidence has been found that *Chlamydia trachomatis, Mycoplasma,* fungi, obligate anearobic bacteria, trichomonads, or viruses cause prostatitis. *Ureaplasma urealyticum* has been localized to the prostate in a small percentage of patients.

3. *Treatment.* Antibiotics are used either to eradicate the prostatic bacteria or to suppress bacteriuria and relieve symptoms. Curative antibiotics, such as trimethoprim-sulfamethoxazole (TMP-SMX) and the fluoroquinolones, are lipid soluble in order to penetrate the lipid membrane of the prostate and are concentrated within the prostate. TMP (160 mg) and SMX (800 mg)

twice daily or a fluoroquinolone in standard doses for 4 to 6 weeks are curative in 33 to 50 percent of patients. Treatment can be extended up to 12 weeks if cure is not obtained. A suppressive dose of one fluoroquinolone or TMP-SMX can be continued. Zinc and other vitamin supplements have not proven useful. Transurethral resection of the prostate should only be used in the presence of prostatic calculi or bladder outlet obstruction. Prostatic massage is of questionable benefit.

E. **Chronic Abacterial Prostatitis–Chronic Pelvic Pain Syndrome (CPPS)**
   1. *Signs and Symptoms.* The same as in chronic bacterial prostatitis. May be intermittent in nature.
   2. *Laboratory results.* WBC/HPF and lipid laden macrophages in EPS semen or VB_3 of patients with chronic abacterial prostatitis (class IIIa) or no WBC/HPF in EPS semen or VB_3 of patients with CPPS (class IIIb). No bacterial growth on urine or prostatic fluid cultures. Etiologic investigation is ongoing. Reflux of urine into prostatic ducts may be involved in chronic abacterial prostatitis. Pelvic floor tension myalgia and bladder neck/urethral spasms may play a role in CPPS. Patients with symptoms of bladder outlet obstruction should have a videourodynamic study to rule out bladder neck dysfunction. Patients with severe irritative voiding symptoms should have a urine cytology.
   3. *Treatment.* Nonsteroidal anti-inflammatory agents, hot sitz baths, tricyclic antidepressants for chronic pain, anticholinergics, repeated prostate massage, and 5 alpha-reductase inhibitors. Alpha-adrenergic blockers, muscle relaxants (diazepam), or even transurethral incision of the bladder neck or microwave thermotherapy can be used in patients with bladder neck/external sphincter spasms.

VI. **INFECTION OF THE SEMINAL VESICLES**
   This is rarely diagnosed in the absence of chronic bacterial prostatitis or epididymitis and may be suspected by the palpation of a hard, swollen mass above the prostate on rectal examination.

VII. **EPIDIDYMITIS**
   A. **Etiology**
      1. *Retrograde ascent* of urethral pathogen through the ejaculatory duct and vas deferens to the epididymis.
         a. Sexual transmission is responsible for most cases in men under age 35 years. *Chlamydia trachomatis* is most common, followed by *Neisseria gonorrhoeae.*

    b. Nonsexual transmission is responsible for most cases in men over age 35 years. The bacteria may be carried through the urethra by climbing an indwelling catheter as a scaffold.

2. *Antegrade descent* may occur when a bladder infection is present and is due to bladder outlet obstruction. May have recently undergone urinary tract instrumentation or operation (transurethral resection of prostate may lead to reflux of urine down vas deferens). A prostatic infection may rarely be the source of bacteria. An ectopic ureter emptying into a seminal vesicle is an uncommon cause of recurrent epididymitis.

3. *Hematogenous* spread of bacteria from a distant source may occur and can result in infection with organisms such as *Haemophilus influenza, Cryptococcus, Brucella,* or tuberculosis.

4. *Amiodarone* is selectively concentrated in the epididymis and can cause inflammation of the head of the epididymis. Dose reduction leads to resolution.

B. Signs and Symptoms

The epididymis may be swollen up to ten times its normal size. It is exquisitely tender. When the testicle is involved (epididymo-orchitis), the epididymis may not be palpable as a separate structure. A reactive hydrocele is common. Elevation of the testicle when the patient is recumbent may relieve the pain. Fever and symptoms of cystitis are frequent. Urethral discharge is occasionally present.

C. Laboratory Evaluation

Perform urinalysis and urine culture. Gram's stain of urethral specimen when sexually transmitted disease suspected.

D. Scrotal Ultrasound with Doppler Flow

Shows increased blood flow to the inflamed epididymis and helps differentiate from testicular torsion.

E. Differential Diagnosis

Testicular torsion, torsion of appendix testis, testicular abscess, testis tumor, mumps orchitis.

F. Treatment

Bed rest, scrotal elevation and support, ice packs, and pain relief with nonsteroidal anti-inflammatory agents. Men requiring urinary drainage should undergo placement of a suprapubic catheter. Surgical drainage of a scrotal abscess or testicular infarct may be necessary. Antibiotic therapy consists of treatment with a fluoroquinolone or trimethoprim-sulfamethoxazole for 10 days for an infection from a source in the bladder. If the infection is chlamydial, treat with doxycycline 200 mg initially, followed by 100 mg twice daily for 2 weeks. Ceftriaxone 250 mg intramuscularly, ciprofloxacin 500 mg orally, or ofloxacin 400 mg orally, in a single dose, will treat gonorrhea and should be administered when treating for *Chlamydia*.

VIII. URETHRITIS

Urethritis is one of the most common problems in ambulatory medicine and is commonly sexually transmitted. It is classified as gonococcal or nongonococcal (Table 6-3).

A. Gonococcal Urethritis

1. *Epidemiology.* Gonorrhea is second only to *Chlamydia trachomatis* as the most frequently reported infectious disease in the United States. The incidence has fallen in the last two decades. It accounts for approximately 35 percent of urethritis in men. A small proportion of men may be asymptomatic carriers. Human immunodeficiency virus (HIV) transmission may be facilitated by gonococcal infection.

2. *Etiology. Neisseria gonorrhoeae* is a gram-negative intracellular diplococcus. Incubation period is 1 to 14 days and is 2 to 5 days in 80 percent of cases.

3. *Signs and Symptoms.* Dysuria, itching, occasionally urinary frequency and urgency. A purulent urethral discharge is more common than a mucoid discharge. One to 3 percent of men are asymptomatic.

4. *Laboratory results.* Gram's stain has greater than 90 percent sensitivity and specificity and shows gram-negative diplococci within polymorphonuclear lymphocytes. Definitive diagnosis is made by culture of a urethral swab on Thayer-Martin and New York City media. The urethral specimen must be obtained at least 1 hour after voiding using a calcium alginate swab inserted 2 to 4 cm into the urethra and rotated gently; evaluation of the urethral discharge from the meatus alone is inadequate. Consider screening persons at high risk.

5. *Treatment.* Important are efficacy, minimizing noncompliance, and treatment of concurrent chlamydial infection. High resistance to penicillin and tetracycline exist in the United States. The following treatment regimens recommended by the Centers for Disease Control and Prevention have at least 95 percent efficacy.

    a. Ceftriaxone (Rocephin) 125 mg IM in a single dose.
    b. Cefixime (Suprax) 400 mg orally in a single dose.
    c. Ciprofloxacin (Cipro) 500 mg orally in a single dose.
    d. Ofloxacin (Floxin) 400 mg orally in a single dose.

Table 6-3 Classification of Urethritis

	GONOCOCCAL	NONGONOCOCCAL
Epidemiology	Lower socioeconomic group	Higher socioeconomic group
Pathogen	*N. gonorrhoeae*	*C. trachomatis, U. urealyticum, Trichomonas vaginalis,* herpes, condyloma, noninfectious
Incubation period	1–14 days (usually 2–5 days)	1–5 weeks
Discharge	Purulent, copious	Thin, mucoid, scant or absent
Gram's stain	Gram-negative intracellular diplococci	Inflammatory cells
Treatment	Ceftriaxone, cefixime, ciprofloxacin, ofloxacin	Doxycycline, azithromycin, tetracycline, erythromycin, metronidazole

e. Concurrent chlamydial infections occur in 15 to 45 percent of men. Presumptive treatment can be performed with doxycycline (Vibramycin) 100 mg orally twice daily for 7 days, azithromycin (Zithromax) 1 g orally in a single dose, or erythromycin base 500 mg orally four times daily for 7 days.

6. *Referral of sex partners.* Recent sex partners (last 30 days) should be referred for examination and treatment.

7. *Reporting.* Gonorrhea is reportable in all states.

8. *Counseling.* Offer screening for other sexually transmitted diseases, including *Chlamydia,* syphilis, hepatitis, and HIV. Review safe-sex options and methods of risk reduction.

B. Nongonococcal Urethritis

1. *Epidemiology.* Accounts for approximately 65 percent of urethritis in males. *Chlamydia* is the most frequently reported infectious disease in the United States.

2. *Etiology.* Urethral inflammation not caused by gonorrhea: *Chlamydia trachomatis* in 23 to 55 percent, *Ureaplasma urealyticum* in 20 to 40 percent, and *Trichomonas vaginalis* in 2 to 5 percent. Herpes simplex virus, human papillomavirus, and yeast have been implicated as well. Incubation period is usually 1 to 5 weeks. Noninfectious urethritis can result from foreign bodies, soaps, shampoos, vaginal douches, spermicidal agents, catheters, urethral instrumentation, and manual stimulation. May be seen with the systemic diseases Stevens–Johnson syndrome and Wegener's granulomatosis. Chronic urethritis may result from urethral strictures, urethral diverticula, meatal stenosis, periurethral abscesses, or bacteriuria. A cause cannot be found in up to 20 percent of cases.

3. *Signs and symptoms.* Dysuria, itching, meatal erythema, mucoid discharge. The discharge may only be evident before the first morning void as meatal crusting or staining of the underwear. Symptoms generally less severe than gonococcal urethritis.

4. *Laboratory results.* Gram's stain showing five or more polymorphonuclear leukocytes per oil immersion field of the urethral discharge, an intraurethral swab specimen, or VB_1, is diagnostic of urethritis. *Chlamydia* is an intracellular parasite of columnar epithelium and is best diagnosed by culture of an intraurethral swab taken 2 to 4 mm from the meatus. *Trichomonas* is diagnosed by wet mount of a urethral swab and by culture. *U. urealyticum* can be cultured on complex artificial media.

5. *Treatment.* The patient and sexual partners should be treated and should abstain from intercourse during treatment and until both are free of symptoms and signs.

   a. Doxycycline 100mg orally twice daily for 7 days.

   b. Azithromycin (Zithromax) 1 g orally in a single dose.

   c. Tetracycline 500 mg orally four times daily for 7 days. *U. urealyticum* is resistant in 6 to 10 percent of cases.

   d. Erythromycin base 500 mg orally four times daily for 7 days. Treatment of choice during pregnancy and lactation, and for tetracycline resistant ureaplasma.

   e. Ofloxacin (Floxin) 300 mg orally twice daily for 7 days.

   f. Metronidazole (Flagyl) 2 g orally in a single dose treats *Trichomonas.*

   g. Acyclovir treats herpes virus.

C. Postgonococcal Urethritis

Recurrent urethritis after effective treatment of gonorrhea, due to the inadequate treatment of concomitant infection with *Chlamydia* in 70 percent of cases.

D. Complications of Urethritis

1. *Epididymitis.* Develops in 1 to 2 percent of men with nongonococcal urethritis.

2. *Urethral stricture.* Approximately 20 years after gonococcal or nongonococcal urethritis.

3. *Disseminated gonococcal infection.* Occurs in 1 percent.

4. *Reiter's syndrome.* Occurs in 1 to 4 percent of cases of infectious nongonococcal urethritis. Associated with ankylosing spondylitis and HLA B-27. Arthritis, uveitis, and skin lesions occur 1 to 4 weeks after development of urethritis. Usually resolves spontaneously but may recur.

BIBLIOGRAPHY

Andriole VT, ed: *Infectious Disease Clinics of North America,* vol. 11, no. 3, 1997.

Centers for Disease Control and Prevention: 1998 Sexually transmitted diseases treatment guidelines. *MMWR 1998* 47, Jan 23, 1998 (No. RR-1).

Eykyn SJ: Urinary tract infections in the elderly. *Brit J Urol* 82(suppl 1):79, 1998.

Fowler JE Jr: *Urinary Tract Infection and Inflammation.* Chicago: Year Book Medical Publishers, 1989.

Krieger JN: Urethritis: Etiology, diagnosis, treatment and complications. In: Gillenwater JY, et al, eds: *Adult and Pediatric Urology.* St. Louis: Mosby, 1996, vol 2, chap 38, pp 1879–1915.

Krieger JN, Egan KJ: Comprehensive evaluation and treatment of 75 men referred to chronic prostatitis clinic. *Urology* 38:11, 1991.

Meares EM Jr, Stamey TA: Bacteriologic localization patterns in bacterial prostatitis and urethritis. *Invest Urol* 5:492, 1968.

Schaeffer AJ: Infections of the urinary tract. In: Walsh PJ, et al (eds): *Campbell's Urology.* Philadelphia: Saunders, 1998, vol. 1, pp 533–614.

Schmid GP, Fontanarosa PB: Evolving strategies for management of the nongonococcal urethritis syndrome. *JAMA* 274:577, 1995.

Wright ET, Chmiel JS, Grayhack JT, Schaeffer AJ: Prostatic fluid inflammation in prostatitis. *J Urol* 152:2300, 1994.

SELF-ASSESSMENT QUESTIONS

1. Which male age groups have the highest incidence of UTI? Why?
2. What are the most common organisms that cause lower urinary tract infections in men?
3. List three host-resistance factors.
4. When the VB2 culture is positive, what must be done to determine whether the patient has bacterial cystitis or bacterial prostatitis?
5. What does VB3 represent?
6. Under which circumstances should a positive urine culture from an elderly man (greater than 65 years) be treated?
7. What is the most common type of prostatitis? How is it treated?
8. When treating *Gonnorrhea,* what other organisms should always be treated?
9. What is the differential diagnosis of epididymitis?
10. What type of catheter should be placed in a patient with acute bacterial prostatitis or epididymitis when urinary drainage is required?

CHAPTER 7
Painful Bladder Syndromes

Philip Hanno

The two most common and least understood entities that are encompassed by the term *painful bladder* are urethral syndrome and interstitial cystitis (IC). The painful bladder disease complex includes a large group of urologic patients with pain in the bladder, irritative voiding symptoms (urgency, frequency, nocturia, dysuria), and sterile urine (Table 7-1). There are painful bladder diseases with well-known etiologies and pathogenesis. These include radiation cystitis, cyclophosphamide cystitis, carcinoma in situ, malacoplakia vesicae, and systemic diseases affecting the bladder. Cystitis and/or urethritis caused by organisms in low "insignificant" colony counts or by organisms like *Chlamydia,* which are not routinely cultured for, are common infectious processes causing symptoms that used to be ascribed to urethral syndrome. The differential diagnosis of pelvic pain also includes endometriosis in females and epididymitis, prostatodynia, and nonbacterial prostatitis (chronic pelvic pain syndrome) in males. In fact, symptoms attributed to prostatodynia in males are remarkably reminiscent of urethral syndrome in females.

Although the etiology of both urethral syndrome and IC remains in doubt, there is reason to believe that they may be varying manifestations of a single spectrum of disease, with the more self-limited forms and those with less in the way of clinical findings categorized as urethral syndrome. As current methods of investigation continue to shed light on this group of problems, we will likely see a continuation in the trend to diminish the use of the very nonspecific diagnosis of urethral syndrome.

I. URETHRAL SYNDROME

In 1945, the American physician Richard Cabot was quoted as having stated that "any pain within two feet of the female urethra for which one cannot find an adequate explanation should be suspected of coming from the female urethra." Urethral syndrome can be defined as a symptom complex consisting of urinary frequency, urgency, dysuria, and suprapubic discomfort without any objective findings of urologic pathology. Typically, these symptoms occur in

Table 7-1 Causes of Frequency and Urgency

Urinary tract infection
Upper motor neuron lesion habit
Large fluid intake
Pregnancy
Bladder calculus
Urethral caruncle
Radiation cystitis
Large postvoid residual
Genital condyloma
Diabetes mellitus
Cervicitis
Periurethral gland infection
Chemical irritants: contraceptive foams, douches, diaphragm, obsessive washing
Detrusor instability
Vulvar carcinoma
Diuretic therapy
Bladder cancer
Urethral diverticulum
Pelvic mass
Chemotherapy
Bacterial urethritis
Renal impairment
Diabetes insipidus
Atrophic urethral changes

From Hanno PM: Interstitial cystitis and related diseases. In: Walsh PC, Retic AB, Vaughan ED, Wein AJ, eds: *Campbell's Urology,* 7th ed. Philadelphia: Saunders, 1998, p 653, with permission.

women; however, there is no reason to assume that a similar entity does not occur in the male.

The diagnosis is one of exclusion. Urinalysis, cultures, cytologic studies, and cystoscopy—including cystoscopic examination under anesthesia if a diagnosis of IC is entertained—are all unremarkable. Nocturia is unusual.

Theories as to the etiology of urethral syndrome are varied. Hormonal imbalances, reactions to ingested or environmental chemicals, and allergic conditions have been proposed, with little supporting evidence, and are not widely accepted. Many authors have supported the idea of urethral stenosis and reported good results with urethral dilatation. However, diagnostic criteria are inconsistent, histologic studies claiming to document periurethral fibrosis are not reproducible, and a truly stenotic urethra in these patients is probably very rare.

Neurogenic and psychogenic causes of urethral syndrome have been explored, but the case for either of these is highly controversial. If the condition is strictly defined as occurring with sterile urine and negative urine cytology, evidence for an anatomic, infectious, inflammatory, or neurogenic cause is weak. One can then speculate that it might be psychogenic or that it may fall into the spectrum represented in its extreme by IC. It must be remembered that in few, if any, studies of urethral syndrome were patients clinically evaluated to exclude IC the way it is now defined.

Whereas infection often causes symptoms of urethral syndrome, by definition, bacterial urethritis, if diagnosed, would not be urethral syndrome. Stamm reported that many patients with urethral syndrome have pyuria, and a significant proportion of these patients actually have a chlamydial urethritis that can be treated successfully with appropriate antibiotics. Certainly, a trial of antibiotics can be justified, especially in patients with pyuria, even in the absence of positive cultures in symptomatic patients.

The same diagnostic techniques used in the evaluation of IC and detailed in the following section are useful in diagnosing urethral syndrome. Indeed, as both are essentially diagnoses of exclusion, the examiner must be sure that specific disease entities [nicely detailed in the National Institutes of Health (NIH) research definition of IC (below)] are indeed not responsible for the symptom complex. Although urine and urethral cultures are critical, urodynamics and cystoscopy under anesthesia with bladder distention can be postponed until symptoms have persisted 6 to 9 months, as many patients will experience spontaneous and long-lived remission of their symptoms. Urine cytology and imaging studies to rule out other conditions can also be withheld, assuming the symptoms resolve in a matter of weeks.

A course of antibiotics would seem to be the mainstay of treatment, even in the absence of positive cultures. Doxycycline, erythromycin, and metronidazole have been recommended to treat the fastidious organisms and anaerobes potentially missed on routine culture. When antibiotics fail, numerous other treatments have been recommended, including endoscopic and open surgical procedures designed to treat urethral stenosis, local fulguration or scarification of the urethra, and virtually the entire gamut of treatments used for IC and mentioned in the following section. The physician's time and reassurance may be the best medicine.

II. INTERSTITIAL CYSTITIS
A. Definition

IC remains a diagnosis of exclusion. With little certain about its etiology and little distinctive about its pathology, groups of basic scientists and clinicians working through the NIH have arbitrarily proposed a set of characteristics that have come to define the disease. Although originally meant to be criteria for entry into NIH-funded research projects on IC, for lack of anything better, they seem to have evolved into the de facto definition. Clearly, there are many patients with the syndrome who fall outside these guidelines.

The NIH diagnostic criteria for IC are as follows.

Criteria Required for Inclusion as Diagnostic of IC

A. One of the following two cystoscopic findings must be present.

1. *Glomerulations (pinpoint submucosal hemhorrages).* An examination for glomerulations should be undertaken after distention of the bladder with the patient under anesthesia and the fluid inflow pressure at 80 to 100 cm water for 1 to 2 min. The bladder may be distended up to two times before evaluation. The glomerulations must be diffuse—present in at least 3 quadrants of the bladder—and there must be at least 10 glomerulations per quadrant. The glomerulations must not lie along the path of the cystoscope (to eliminate artifacts due to instrumentation contact).

2. *A classic Hunner's ulcer.* A discrete bladder ulceration typically noted at the time of bladder distention and present in a distinct minority of patients.

B. One of the following two subjective symptoms must be present.

1. Pain associated with the bladder.
2. Urinary urgency.

The fulfillment of any of the following criteria *excludes* a diagnosis of IC.

1. A bladder capacity greater than 350 mL on cystometry carried out in a conscious patient using either a gas or liquid medium.

2. The absence of an intense urge to void in patients whose bladder has been filled to 100 mL of gas or 150 mL of water during cystometry at a fill rate of 30 to 100 mL/min.

3. The demonstration of phasic involuntary bladder contractions on cystometry using the fill rate described above.

4. A duration of symptoms of less than 9 months.

5. The absence of nocturia.

6. The occurrence of symptoms that are relieved by antimicrobials, urinary antiseptics, anticholinergics, or antispasmodics.

7. A frequency of urination during waking hours of less than eight times per day.

8. A diagnosis of bacterial cystitis or prostatitis within a 3-month period.

9. The presence of bladder or lower ureteral calculi.

10. A finding of active genital herpes.
11. The occurrence of uterine, cervical, vaginal, or urethral cancer.
12. A finding of a urethral diverticulum.
13. The presence of cyclophosphamide (or any type of chemical) cystitis.
14. The occurrence of tuberculous cystitis.
15. The demonstration of radiation cystitis.
16. The presence of benign or malignant bladder tumors.
17. A finding of vaginitis
18. An age of less than 18 years.

Certain of the exclusion criteria serve mainly to make an examiner wary of a diagnosis of IC, but should by no means be used for categoric exclusion of such a diagnosis. However, because of the ambiguity involved, these patients should probably be eliminated from research studies or separately categorized. Thus, the previous definition is best considered a "research definition" of IC. In particular, exclusion criteria 4–6, 8, 9, 11, 12, 17, and 18 are only relative. Specific pathologic findings represent a glaring omission from the criteria, as there is a lack of consensus as to which pathologic findings, if any, are required for a tissue diagnosis of IC.

Questions have arisen as to how specific the cardinal diagnostic finding of glomerulation really is. In a recent study, Waxman found 42 percent of women with symptoms consistent with IC and 45 percent of asymptomatic women subjected to bladder distention under anesthesia to have glomerulations. The National Institutes of Health Interstitial Cystitis Database Study found that more than 60 percent of patients regarded by researchers as definitely or likely to have IC would not meet the strict application of NIH guidelines. It would seem that the NIH guidelines are useful for selecting patients for research studies on IC, but too restrictive to be used by clinicians as the diagnostic definition of interstitial cystitis.

As a part of the painful bladder complex, IC is one of a group of diseases manifested by bladder pain, irritative voiding symptoms (urgency, frequency, nocturia, dysuria), and negative urine cultures. Diseases of known etiology include radiation cystitis, cyclophosphamide cystitis, cystitis caused by microorganisms that are not detected by routine culture methodologies, malacoplakia vesicae, and systemic diseases affecting the bladder. The Danish have characterized the painful bladder of unknown etiology into four subgroups: IC, detrusor myopathy, chronic unspecific cystitis, and eosinophilic cystitis.

There appear to be three groups of patients who show symptoms without an obvious cause. One group develops lower tract symptoms that resolve before any formal evaluation can be instituted. These are patients whom we would diagnose as suffering from urethral syndrome. A second group of patients has the symptom complex long enough to be referred to a urologist who elects to perform an evaluation including cystoscopy under anesthesia with hydrodistention of the bladder and biopsy. Those patients with glomerulations are considered to have IC. Those without these "typical findings of IC" are in a twilight zone, but are generally treated as if they have IC. The number of patients with urethral syndrome that would have findings of IC if they were evaluated with bladder distention under anesthesia is unknown.

The diagnosis of IC remains primarily a clinical diagnosis of exclusion. It is often based on the presence of unremitting symptoms of frequency, sensory urgency, and pain in the absence of other causes. Bladder biopsy would be helpful only to the extent that it is judged necessary to rule out other causes of the patient's symptoms. Bladder distention under anesthesia can help to make the diagnosis if glomerulations are found, can provide short-term relief from symptoms, and may change treatment decisions if clear bladder ulceration is noted or if capacity under anesthesia is less than 200 mL. Whether distention under anesthesia is necessary in all patients before initiating treatment for presumed IC is a hot topic of debate in the urologic community. This author believes that urodynamics are helpful in differentiating sensory urgency from motor urgency. A suggested diagnostic aliorithm is presented in Figure 7-1.

B. Epidemiology

The sole source of IC incidence and prevalence data until 1990 was Oravisto's regional population-based study. Studies of the metropolitan Helsinki, Finland area showed a prevalence of the disease in women of 18.1 in 10^5. The joint prevalence of both sexes was 10.6 in 10^5, and the annual incidence of new female cases was 1.2 in 10^5. Severe cases accounted for 10 percent of the total. Ten percent of cases were in men. The disease onset was commonly subacute rather than insidious, and full development of the classic symptom complex occurred in a short time. Generally, the disease did not progress continuously, but reached its final stage rapidly and then stabilized at that level. Subsequent major deterioration was the exception rather than the rule.

Many of the above findings were confirmed in 1989 in a major population-based study in the United States. Among a wealth of interesting data, the study revealed the following.

1. The prevalence of diagnosed IC in the United States approximates 43,500 cases, double the incidence found by Oravisto in Finland.
2. Late deterioration in symptoms is unusual (as per Oravisto).

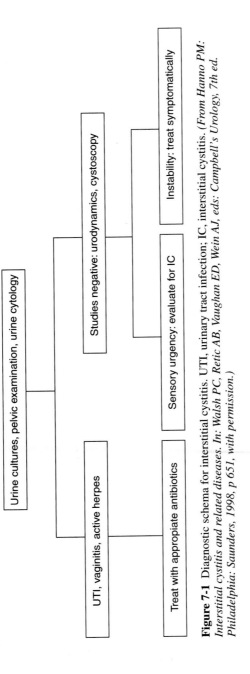

Figure 7-1 Diagnostic schema for interstitial cystitis. UTI, urinary tract infection; IC, interstitial cystitis. (*From Hanno PM: Interstitial cystitis and related diseases. In: Walsh PC, Retic AB, Vaughan ED, Wein AJ, eds: Campbell's Urology. 7th ed. Philadelphia: Saunders, 1998, p 651, with permission.*)

3. As many as 50 percent of patients experience spontaneous remissions with a duration ranging from 1 to 80 months (mean: 8 months).

4. IC patients are 10 to 12 times more likely than control subjects to report childhood bladder problems.

5. Patients with IC are twice as likely as controls to report a history of urinary tract infection; however, more than half of all IC patients report less than one such infection per year before the onset of IC.

6. The time from symptom onset to diagnosis varied from 24 months for patients most recently diagnosed to 51 months for members of the Interstitial Cystitis Association, a patient advocacy group.

7. Women who were diagnosed by the sampled urologists as actually having IC represented only 20 percent of the cases that presented with symptoms that were suggestive of this disease. The remaining cases were women who had been classified by a urologist as having painful bladder syndrome and sterile urine, but had not been diagnosed. Based on these data, it can be extrapolated that a possible half a million patients in the United States have this disease.

8. Household size, marital status, number of male sexual partners, and educational status did not seem to significantly differ in those patients diagnosed as having IC in comparison with the general adult female population.

9. Using well-developed quality of life indicators, which employed responses to subjective statements, IC females scored lower on nine such tests, compared with an identical set of tests given to a sample of U.S. females with chronic renal failure undergoing dialysis.

C. Etiology

Although there are no lack of theories, the etiology of IC remains obscure. This is not necessarily surprising in a disease as difficult to objectively categorize as this one is. Today, the general opinion is that the etiology is multifactorial and that it may be a syndrome rather than a specific disease.

Numerous studies have failed to find evidence of causative bacterial, fungal, and viral infection. Potential etiologies of IC tend to fall in and out of favor, and one of the most popular now concerns a possible deficiency in the bladder glycosaminoglycan (GAG) layer lining the luminal surface as a possible initiating event. A defective transitional epithelium may lead to molecular leaks of normal urine constituents into the bladder wall, setting up the symptom complex. While it is known experimentally that exogenous GAG is effective in providing an epithelial permeability barrier in bladders intentionally treated to remove this natural layer, it is not yet clear whether a defect in this layer is responsible for IC symptoms in the majority of patients, or whether such a defect might be a primary or secondary event in pathogenesis.

Many ultrastructural, biochemical, and functional studies of bladder GAG have failed to fully support this theory. Speculation about what might initiate a GAG abnormality is absent, and the possibility that if such an abnormality exists, it might be secondary to a primary unknown insult certainly is not unreasonable. In an effort to support the GAG theory, Parsons has shown that intravesical potassium instillation is more painful in a large percentage of IC patients than in normal subjects. Some patients do seem to respond to treatment with GAG (see below), and at least some cases of IC may be related to GAG abnormality.

Another intuitively enticing possibility is that the urine of IC patients is itself carrying a pathologic substance accounting for the disorder. Bladder pain developing years after substitution cystoplasty with bowel segments, and pouch pain occurring in IC patients with a continent diversion provide interesting clinical data for consideration. Although an intriguing theory, the toxic urine etiology remains to be proven.

Many studies have noted the presence of a mast cell infiltrate in the bladder wall in a subset of IC patients, suggesting a potential pathogenic role of the mast cell. The bladder mast cell contains many granules, each can secrete many vasoactive and nociceptive molecules. A number of conditions such as extreme cold, drugs, neuropeptides, stress, trauma, and toxins can trigger the mast cell to secrete some of its contents. In turn, these chemicals can sensitize sensory neurons, which can further activate mast cells by releasing neurotransmitters or neuropeptides. Additionally, the mast cell can directly cause vasodilatation and bladder mucosal damage while attracting inflammatory cells, thus causing many of the problems observed in IC.

The question then becomes why antihistamines have not been more effective in treatment. Although the evidence suggests that the mast cell may be related to the pathogenesis of the symptoms of IC in some patients, and, indeed, treatments such as amitriptyline and hydroxyzine have pharmacologic activity that is partly based on mast cell stabilization, the presence of mast cells is not necessary for a diagnosis of IC. Detrusor mastocytosis cannot be considered a marker for the disease. Researchers have found mast cell infiltration in the bladder to be a nonspecific finding, associated not only with IC, but also with other bladder pathology. With mast cell counts showing the highest elevations in patients with the ulcerative form of IC, the question as to whether these cells play a primary or secondary role in pathogenesis is unanswered.

For many years the autoimmune character of IC has been commented on. However, the lack of pathologic findings, the variable and usually poor response to immunosuppressants and anti-inflammatory agents, and the usual immediate relief upon diversion of the urinary stream speak against an autoimmune etiology. Although the immune mechanism may have at least a partial role in the pathophysiology of IC, many studies continue to cast doubt on this as a significant causative factor.

Through the work of T. Buffington at Ohio State University, a naturally occurring animal model of the disorder, now termed "feline interstitial cystitis," has been characterized and studied. These animals show nearly all of the characteristics of human IC including bladder glomerulations on hydrodistention, and most if not all of the symptoms as best as can be determined. Future work with this model may prove productive with regard to pathogenesis and treatment.

D. Treatment

The ultimate goal of therapy of any disease process is to neutralize the factor or factors responsible for the disease. As long as causative factors are unknown, treatments will be based on empiricism. Although the symptoms of IC can be controlled with one of a variety of treatments in the overwhelming majority of patients, there is little evidence that treatment accomplishes anything more than influencing the symptomatic expression of the disease rather than curing the condition.

Hydraulic distention under anesthesia is generally the initial therapeutic modality used in the treatment of IC, as it has been an initial part of the diagnostic process. Approximately 50 percent of patients experience some symptomatic relief following distention, although we have been impressed that an almost equal number experience some exacerbation of their symptoms. Both effects seem to be short lived.

Most physicians begin the treatment of diagnosed IC with symptomatic measures. Patients are instructed to avoid foods that they find aggravate their symptoms. Commonly, these include caffeinated beverages, highly acidic foods, and alcohol. Warm tub baths, mild analgesics, and stress reduction can be beneficial.

Oral drug therapy is generally indicated when conservative measures fail to significantly improve the quality of life. The tricyclic antidepressant amitriptyline has many actions that are theoretically beneficial to patients with IC. It is the most potent tricyclic antidepressant in terms of blocking H_1-histaminergic receptors, stabilizes mast cells in vitro, and has activity that might tend to stimulate predominantly beta-adrenergic receptors in the bladder-body smooth musculature, an action that would further facilitate urinary storage by decreasing the excitability of smooth muscle in that area. It has analgesic actions that are not clearly understood and sedative properties that can be potentially beneficial to IC sufferers. In a dosage gradually increasing to 75 mg at bedtime over 3 weeks, responses have been more than 50 percent with little tachyphylaxis.

Elmiron (sodium pentosanpolysulfate) is a synthetic GAG and a heparin analog partially excreted in the urine. When given orally in a double-blind, placebo-controlled trial, 38 percent of 74 patients treated for 3 months reported at least 50 percent improvement in pelvic pain compared to 18 percent in a placebo group. There was no significant improvement in frequency, urgency, or nocturia. Elmiron has been studied extensively in trials in the United States and Europe, and its value has been debated. It does appear that a subset of patients respond to it within 3 to 6 months at a dosage of 100 mg three times a day.

The antihistamine hydroxyzine is a third oral agent that has been reported to show benefit in small, uncontrolled studies for IC. In addition to its ability to inhibit bladder mast cell activation, it has potentially beneficial anticholinergic, anxiolytic, sedative, and analgesic properties.

Intravesical lavage with one of a variety of preparations remains the standard therapy for IC against which other treatments may be measured. Pool and Rives reported on 74 patients treated with intravesical silver nitrate. Excellent to good results were obtained in 89 percent of patients, with an average duration of response of 7.6 months. Burford and Burford also reported good results after using silver nitrate in conjunction with bladder fulgeration. O'Conor introduced the use of intravesical chlorpactin (WWCS-90) in treating IC. Messing and Stamey reported a 72 percent success rate and duration of response of 6 months.

One of the principal treatments for IC is the intravesical instillation of dimethyl sulfoxide (DMSO), a byproduct of the wood-pulp industry and a derivative of lignum. Its pharmacologic properties include membrane penetration, enhanced drug absorption, anti-inflammatory and analgesic effects, collagen dissolution, muscle relaxation, and mast cell histamine release. Stewart popularized the use of this agent in treating IC.

Intravesical BCG administered weekly for 6 weeks has been reported beneficial in 60 percent of patients with 89 percent demonstrating a long-term response of 24 to 33 months. This data will need to be confirmed in larger studies.

The rare patient with a discrete Hunner's ulcer can be treated with transurethral resection, fulgeration, or laser irradiation. Transcutaneous electrical nerve stimulation is effective in some patients.

Diagnosed IC/ Chronic urethral syndrome
Symptoms tolerable: self-help protocols, mild analgesics

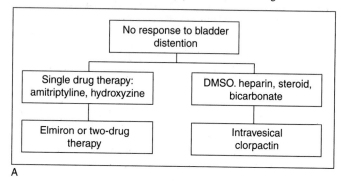

A

Failure of first-line therapy
Cross over to intravesical or oral Rx

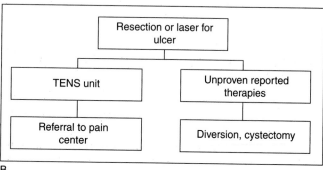

B

Figure 7-2 Treatment algorithm for interstitial cystitis. DMSO, dimethyl sulfoxide; TENS, transurethral electrical nerve stimulation. (*From Hanno PM: Interstitial cystitis and related diseases. In: Walsh PC, Retic AB, Vaughan ED, Wein AJ, eds: Campbell's Urology, 7th ed. Philadelphia: Saunders, 1998, p 652, with permission.*)

When standard treatments fail to relieve symptoms, referral of the patient to a pain clinic must be considered. The safe, controlled use of chronic opiate medication can be considered as an option.

It is certainly worthwhile to exhaust all reasonable conservative measures before proceeding to surgical therapy in a disease such as IC, which is chronic, not life-threatening, and subject to spontaneous remission of symptomatology. Augmentation cystoplasty with supratrigonal cystectomy can be considered in patients with a small capacity bladder measured under anesthesia. Patients with large capacity bladders and intractable symptoms may best be treated with diversion, with or without cystectomy. Success rates for major surgery are about 50 percent, and many patients will require the expertise of a physician trained in chronic pain management even after surgical management. Less than 5 percent of patients generally require any type of reconstructive or exenterative surgery.

Figure 7-2 provides a treatment algorithm. It is best to offer one treatment at a time, as the natural history of the disease with the tendency for spontaneous remission in symptom severity works in both the patient's and physician's favor.

BIBLIOGRAPHY

Hanno PM: Interstitial cystitis and related diseases. In: *Campbell's Urology, 7th ed.* Walsh PC, Retik AB, Stamey TA, Vaughn ED, Wein, AJ, eds. Philadelphia: Saunders, 1998, pp 631–662.

Hanno PM, ed: Interstitial cystitis. *Urol Clin North Am,* vol. 21, no. 1, 1994.

Hanno PM, Landis R, Matthews-Cook Y, et. al: The diagnosis of interstitial cystitis revisited: Lessons learned from the National Institutes of Health Interstitial Cystitis Database Study. *J Urol* 161: Feb, 1999.

Hanno PM, Staskin D, Wein AJ, Krane R, eds: *Interstitial Cystitis—Current Concepts.* London: Springer Verlag, 1990.

Parsons CL, Benson G, Childs SJ, et. al: A quantitatively controlled method to study prospectively interstitial cystitis and demonstrate the efficacy of pentosanpolysulfate. *J Urol* 150:845, 1993.

Peeker R, Aldenborg, F, Fall M: The treatment of interstitial cystitis with supratrigonal cystectomy and ileocystoplasty: Difference in outcome between classic and nonulcer disease. *J Urol* 159:1479, 1998.

Peters KM, Diokno AC, Steinert BW, Gonzalez JA: The efficacy of intravesical bacillus Calmette-Guerin in the treatment of interstitial cystitis: Long-term followup. *J Urol* 159:1483, 1998.

Waxman JA, Sulak PJ, Kuehl TJ: Cystoscopic findings consistent with interstitial cystitis in normal women undergoing tubal ligation. *J Urol* 160:1663, 1998.

SELF-ASSESSMENT QUESTIONS

1. Which of the following findings must be present to make a diagnosis of interstitial cystitis?
   a. Microhematuria
   b. Typical pathologic findings on bladder biopsy
   c. History of urgency incontinence
   d. Positive urinary culture
   e. Pelvic pain and/or urinary frequency
2. The NIH criteria for interstitial cystitis are best categorized as:
   a. criteria useful in treatment stratification.
   b. a clinical definition of IC.
   c. minimal criteria to make a diagnosis of IC.

    d. a summary of the pathologic findings necessary to make a diagnosis of IC by bladder biopsy.

    e. a research definition of IC.

3. The finding of glomerulations incidentally at cystoscopy in an asymptomatic patient suggests:

    a. urinary infection.

    b. undiagnosed interstitial cystitis.

    c. high likelihood of carcinoma in situ.

    d. no significant pathology.

    e. bladder instablility.

4. The presumed mechanism of action of pentosan polysulfate is:

    a. immunosuppression.

    b. bladder glycosaminoglycan replacement.

    c. antibacterial action.

    d. central analgesic effect.

    e. smooth muscle relaxation.

5. Surgical therapy for interstitial cystitis is best reserved for:

    a. early in the disease course.

    b. patients who fail oral therapy.

    c. patients who primarily have symptoms of frequency.

    d. a last resort after all conservative treatments have failed.

    e. patients who primarily have symptoms of pain.

Answers

1. e
2. e
3. d
4. b
5. d

CHAPTER 8
Pyelonephritis

Ira J. Kohn
Jeffrey P. Weiss

I. DEFINITION

Pyelonephritis is the term denoting infection of the upper urinary tract, that is, the kidney and renal pelvis. There are two forms: acute and chronic. Acute pyelonephritis is characterized by acute suppuration accompanied by fever, flank pain, bacteruria, and pyuria. Repeated attacks of acute pyelonephritis lead to chronic pyelonephritis characterized by progressive renal scarring, usually asymmetric and irregular, involving both the cortex and pelviocalyceal system.

II. DIAGNOSIS AND CLINICAL CHARACTERISTICS
A. Diagnosis

1. The diagnosis of acute pyelonephritis is usually made on clinical grounds. The definitive diagnostic method is catheterization of the ureters and renal pelvis for urinalysis (revealing pyuria and bacteruria) and culture. This is unnecessarily invasive, however.

2. Routine urinalysis reveals pyuria, bacteruria, and white cell casts.

3. Bacterial antibodies, if present, suggest upper tract infection. There is, however, a significant proportion of false positives using this criterion.

4. The Fairley bladder washout test obtains culture of ureteral urine without ureteral catheterization by culturing urine in the bladder after residual bladder urine is washed out.

5. Radiographic methods include: excretory urography (more useful in chronic than acute pyelonephritis in defining areas of cortical scarring); Tc-99m DMSA or glucoheptonate nuclear renal scans to detect areas of cortical scarring; and voiding cystourethrography (conventional radiographic or nuclear scanning techniques) to

document the presence of vesicoureteral reflux (VUR). The latter is a major etiologic factor in pyelonephritis. Because an intravenous urogram is often obtained, urologists should be familiar with excretory urography findings of acute pyelonephritis, including the following.

a. Generalized or focal renal enlargement probably secondary to inflammation and congestion.

b. Obstruction of renal tubules from surrounding parenchymal edema and vasoconstriction may impair contrast excretion resulting in diminished nephrograms or delayed calyceal imaging.

c. Dilation of the renal pelvis or ureter without obstruction secondary to impaired ureteral peristalsis caused by bacterial endotoxin.

For patients not responding to antibiotic therapy, febrile for 72 hours or longer, or with complicating factors such as diabetes or immunocompromised states, computed tomography (CT) has been found useful to rule out renal/perirenal abscess and other complicating factors. CT may specifically demonstrate renal enlargement, abnormal contour, perirenal inflammatory extension, abnormal nephrograms, and areas of impaired renal function. Localized pyelonephritis (lobar nephronia) or phlegmons may be particularly well diagnosed with CT, which is useful in both children and adults. Renal ultrasound is helpful where contrast studies are contraindicated, such as in cases of emphysematous pyelonephritis and lobar nephronia.

6. Renal biopsy with bacterial culture is mentioned only to be condemned not only because of excessive risk to the patient, but also because of the focal nature of renal infection, which may be easily missed by a random renal biopsy.

7. Because renal concentrating ability is impaired in pyelonephritis, it has been suggested that demonstration of an impaired renal concentrating mechanism in the presence of bacteriuria implies pyelonephritis as opposed to lower tract infection. However, this parameter is nonspecific due to statistical overlap in concentrating abilities between patients with upper and lower urinary tract infections.

8. Whereas acute pyelonephritis is usually diagnosed on clinical grounds, chronic pyelonephritis is diagnosed by radiologic and pathologic means showing scarred, contracted kidneys, either focally or diffusely, often with clubbing of underlying calyces. When unilateral, compensatory hypertrophy of the contralateral renal unit is often noted. For some of these patients, the urinary tract

infections resulting in renal scarring are so remote that bacteria cannot be cultured from the urine, resulting in the terms abacterial nephritis or interstitial nephritis. In many of these patients, however, bacterial antigens can be detected in renal tissue by immunofluorescent localization techniques.

B. Clinical Characteristics
1. In general, patients with pyelonephritis present with fever, flank pain, costovertebral angle (CVA) tenderness, and infected urine. Clinical presentation may vary from acute sepsis to cystitis with mild flank pain.
2. Additional acute symptoms usually include systemic malaise, nausea, and vomiting. Lower urinary tract symptoms of dysuria, increased urinary frequency, and urgency are often noted.
3. Approximately 75 percent of patients give a history of previous lower urinary tract infections.
4. Severe cases may cause sepsis, hypotension, and death in a compromised host.
5. Acute pyelonephritis can be self-limited. Multiple bouts can lead to progressive loss of tubules, thereby impairing renal concentrating ability. This is followed by glomerular damage late in the course (chronic pyelonephritis), producing azotemia and hypertension.
6. Some patients with chronic pyelonephritis present with a history of recurrent urinary tract infections. Many are totally asymptomatic, with the condition discovered incidentally either radiologically or secondary to complications of chronic azotemia (Fig. 8-1).

III. ETIOLOGY AND RISK FACTORS
A. Major Etiologic Factors in the Pathogenesis of Pyelonephritis
1. The first, and by far most the most common, factor is VUR of infected urine. Not all patients with reflux of infected urine into the renal pelvis will sustain renal damage. This leads to the concept of intrarenal reflux, or pyelotubular reflux via wide open papillary ducts, the absence of which is thought to be protective to the renal tubules and parenchyma.
2. Obstruction of the urinary tract from any cause contributes to pyelonephritis due to stasis and disabling of the washout mechanisms of urinary clearance of bacteria. Such obstruction can be congenital (e.g., ureteropelvic junction obstruction), acquired (e.g., stone disease), or associated with pregnancy (unilateral, usually right-sided, ureteral obstruction by the gravid uterus).

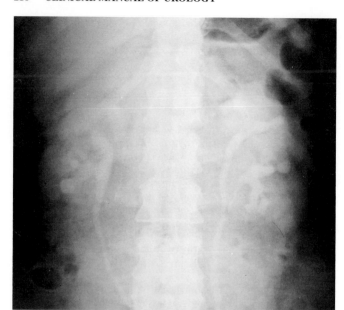

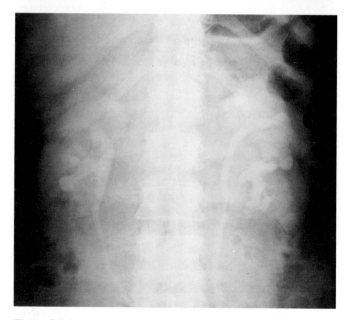

Figure 8-1 Intravenous pyelogram of a patient with chronic pyelonephritis caliectasis and renal scarring.

3. The third potential mechanism of bacterial invasion of the kidney is hematogenous; however, bacteria are unlikely to seat in the kidney in the absence of urinary obstruction. A fourth possible route of bacterial implantation in the kidney is via lymphatics, although this mechanism has been discounted.

B. **Risk Factors Increasing Vulnerability to Pyelonephritis**
   1. *Procedures.* Instrumentation of the genitourinary tract.
   2. *Diabetes mellitus.* Diabetic patients are more prone to pyelonephritis due to increased substrate availability in the kidney. Increased parenchymal destruction by gas-forming organisms leads to a rare complication of diabetes, emphysematous pyelonephritis, the treatment of which is usually nephrectomy (see below).
   3. *Neurogenic bladder.* This condition provides the urologist with a complex array of problems, among which are urinary retention, high-pressure VUR, hydronephrosis, and renal calculi.
   4. *Age.* In general, the frequency of bacteruria increases with age, with accelerated increases due to sexual activity in young women, and prostatic enlargement with urinary retention in elderly men. Acute pyelonephritis rarely causes renal scarring in most adults with normal urinary tracts. The growing kidneys of children with intrarenal reflux of infected urine appears to be the most vulnerable to scarring.
   5. *Gender.* Females are more likely to develop bacteria due to the short urethra in close proximity to the gastrointestinal (GI) tract and favorable milieu for bacterial proliferation compared with the male urethra.
   All of these especially promote the severity and persistence of infection in the kidneys of these patients.

IV. **BACTERIOLOGY**
   A. **Causative Agents**
      The origin of most bacteria causing pyelonephritis is in fecal flora. The majority (80 percent) of uncomplicated cases of pyelonephritis are caused by *E. coli.* Less common causative agents are:

      1. *Proteus*
      2. *Pseudomonas*
      3. *Enterobacter*
      4. *Klebsiella*
      5. *Serratia*
      6. *Citrobacter*
      7. *Enterococcus*
      8. *Staphylococcus*

Of interest is infection with *Proteus mirabilis* and some strains of *Klebsiella* that contain the enzyme urease, which is capable of splitting urea with the production of ammonia and an alkaline environment. The latter is favorable for precipitation of the salt struvite, or magnesium ammonium phosphate. Struvite tends to settle into branched calculi that harbor bacteria in their interstices; these calculi are extremely resistant to antibiotic therapy. Thus, eradication of infection in the presence of struvite calculi involves both antimicrobial therapy and complete removal of these "infected stones."

Pyelonephritis and secondary focal or diffuse renal abscess may occur in patients afflicted with AIDS due to opportunistic molds and fungi such as aspergillosis and mucormycosis.

B. Adherence

Because most bacteria contaminating the urinary tract are washed away before causing infection, it must be that those bacteria initiating infection somehow become adherent to the urothelium. Adherence is a property of bacteria afforded by fimbriated extensions of the cell wall (pili) that attach to uromucoid or glycolipid receptors of urothelial cells. It has been found that patients with chronic pyelonephritis and renal failure have a higher P-fimbriated receptor accessibility on uroepithelial cells than those with chronic pyelonephritis and normal renal function, a concept that may become useful for the detection of risk groups among patients with recurrent pyelonephritis. An additional property of bacteria enabling establishment of infection in the kidney is endotoxin, causing inhibition of ureteral mobility, with attendant stasis, ureteral dilatation, and enhancement of low-pressure intrarenal reflux at the level of the renal papilla. Thus, adhesiveness and endotoxins are major weapons of bacteria causing urothelial infection.

V. CONTRIBUTIONS OF IMMUNE AND INFLAMMATORY RESPONSE

If adhesiveness and endotoxins promote bacterial infection in the urinary tract, the immune response stems the tide against cellular damage, with some caveats.

A. Antibody Response

Bacterial invasion of the kidney brings forth primarily a humoral (antibody) response as opposed to cell-mediated immunity.

B. Inflammatory Response

1. Activation of the complement cascade attracts polymorphonuclear leukocytes (chemotaxis) that phagocytize bacteria while at the same time causing release of

metabolites [known as superoxide radicals (O_2^-) that damage not only bacteria, but also surrounding normal host tissue (e.g., renal tubules)].

2. Experimental studies of renal venous blood after renal infection reveal rapid activation of serum complement indicating a triggering of the ongoing inflammatory reaction, as well as rapid rise in venous renin levels. This is suggestive of an important renovascular occlusive phenomenon resulting from renal parenchymal infection, which may result in ischemic tissue damage.

Thus, renal tissue becomes an "innocent bystander" in this subcellular biochemical skirmish, the basis of renal injury in pyelonephritis. There is evidence that suppression of superoxide radicals by the administration of superoxide dismutase and a xanthine oxidase inhibitor (allopurinol) may reduce the inflammatory response and its attendant tissue destruction. A summary of the pathogenesis of pyelonephritis is offered in Figure 8-2.

VI. SPECIAL CASE: XANTHOGRANULOMATOUS PYELONEPHRITIS (XGP)

A. Definition
XGP is an unusual inflammatory lesion of the kidney associated with obstructing stones and chronic renal infection (Fig. 8-3).

B. Symptoms and Signs
Aside from the usual symptoms of pyelonephritis, XGP frequently causes nonfunction of the affected kidney and the process is invariably unilateral. Radiologic imaging often reveals renal calculi and a renal mass. Perirenal fat may be involved with adjacent subcapsular inflammatory response.

C. Bacteriology
Proteus and *E. coli* are the primary microbes associated with XGP.

D. Pathology
Grossly, these kidneys consist of yellow-white nodules, pyonephrosis, and hemmorrhage. Histopathologic examination reveals a granulomatous type of chronic inflammation with lipid-laden macrophages known as xanthoma cells.

E. Treatment
The major difficulty with this entity is its distinction from a malignant lesion, notably renal cell carcinoma; radiologic studies may be ambiguous and xanthoma cells may resemble clear cell adenocarcinoma on frozen section pathology.

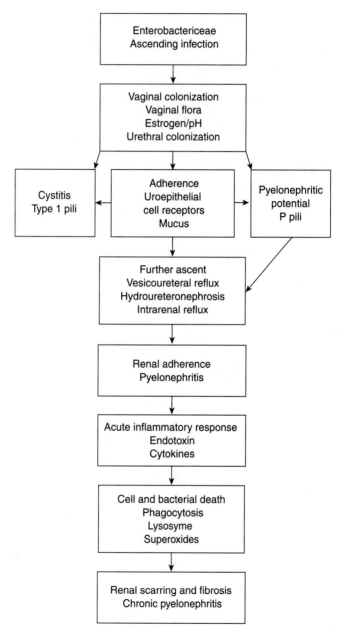

Figure 8-2 Pathogenesis of pyelonephritis.

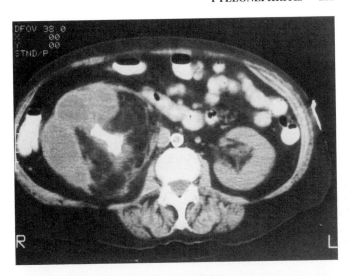

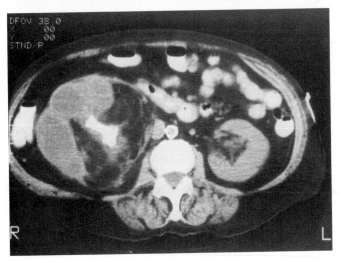

Figure 8-3 Computed tomography scan without intravenous contrast. The image reveals a large, right renal stone and mixed density of the renal parenchyma suggestive of a mass, with marked stranding of fat in the renal sinus in a 74-year-old woman who presented floridly septic. Pathology from right radical nephrectomy revealed xanthogranulomatous pyelonephritis.

One tipoff to the diagnosis is the presence of large, often branched calculi in the presence of a renal mass associated with either focal or global renal nonfunction. However, XGP is usually treated with nephrectomy.

VII. PATHOLOGY
A. Histopathologic Characteristics
Acute pyelonephritis is characterized by the presence of acute inflammation and focal bacterial abscess formation in random areas of the kidney.

B. Pathogenesis
1. *Acute pyelonephritis.* Infection begins in the interstitium and spreads to destroy tubules, giving rise to white cell casts seen on urinalysis. Glomeruli are characteristically resistant to acute infection. As the cortex is more vascular than the medulla, greater inflammation is present both cortically and in the subcapsular area despite the fact that bacterial invasion may begin in the medulla. A collection of purulent exudate extending out of the capsular area gives rise to perinephric abscess.
2. *Chronic pyelonephritis.* As these abscesses in and about the kidney heal, they become replaced with contracted scar tissue infiltrated by chronic inflammatory cells (lymphocytes, plasma cells). These form the basis of the distorted cortical and pyelocalyceal anatomy seen in chronic pyelonephritis. Although glomeruli may be spared or fibrotic, periglomerular fibrosis is common in conjunction with atrophied tubules.
3. *Thyroidization.* A particular pattern of tubular damage consisting of dilated tubules filled with hyalin and leukocyte casts, resembling the thyroid colloid, is called thyroidization.
4. Collectively, the scarring process of chronic pyelonephritis produces the familiar small, irregularly shaped kidney in its end stage.

VIII. COMPLICATIONS
A. Renal Insufficiency
Acute renal failure is an exceedingly rare complication of acute bacterial pyelonephritis, although case reports exist in both adults and children. The small kidney resulting from chronic repeated attacks of pyelonephritis contributes to progressive azotemia and chronic renal failure. In particular, 13 percent of patients with end-stage renal disease have chronic pyelonephritis as a primary etiologic factor.

B. Hypertension

One half to three quarters of patients with chronic pyelonephritis are hypertensive. The mechanism of hypertension in this disease is probably due to fibrosis of the renal parenchyma with resulting ischemia and secondary activation of the renin-angiotensin system. Although hypertension can accelerate progressive renal failure, the fact that nephrectomy cures hypertension in selected patients demonstrated to have elevated ipsilateral renal vein renin levels suggests that the renal disease caused the hypertension in these patients and not vice versa.

C. Renal Abscess

Renal abscess may follow insufficient treatment of focal bacterial nephritis (lobar nephronia). CT, ultrasound, and needle aspiration will make the diagnosis; treatment is percutaneous aspiration and prolonged antimicrobial therapy or definitive surgical drainage (Fig. 8-4).

D. Perinephric Abscess

Most cases arise from preexisting renal factors such as renal calculi, ureteral calculi, hydronephrosis, renal cystic disease, or infected carcinoma. Diagnosis and treatment are similar to those for renal abscess.

E. Emphysematous Pyelonephritis

This condition is characterized by an acute necrotizing parenchymal and perirenal infection caused by gas-forming uropathogens. Although the exact etiology remains unknown, diabetic patients seem to be at increased risk. This is probably due to impaired host immune response and high tissue levels of glucose serving as substrate for the production of carbon dioxide via fermentation by responsible microorganisms. Complicating factors can include urinary tract obstruction secondary to calculi or sloughed necrotic papillae. Women are affected more commonly than men, and almost all cases have been reported in adults, with minimal risk for juvenile diabetic patients. Intrarenal parenchymal gas defined by plain x-ray, CT scan, or ultrasound is pathognomonic and establishes the diagnosis (Fig. 8-5). The process may be bilateral in 10 percent of affected patients. Immediate nephrectomy in combination with appropriate antibiotics has lowered the mortality from 75 percent to 25 percent. Aggressive percutaneous renal and perirenal drainage has been reported to yield success in nonsurgical and selected cases. Most cases of emphysematous pyelonephritis are caused by *E. coli,* with cases secondary to *Klebsiella, Proteus,* and *Candida albicans* reported as well.

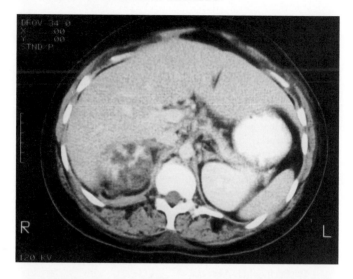

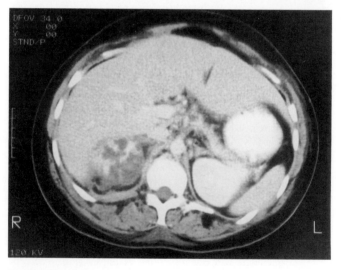

Figure 8-4 Computed tomography scan of renal abscess at upper pole of right kidney.

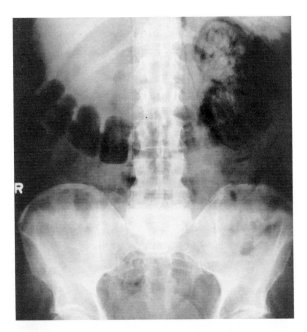

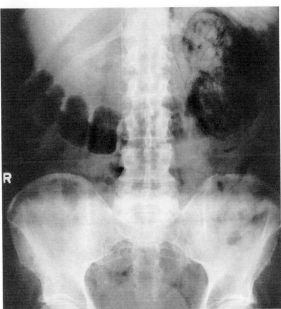

Figure 8-5 Scout radiograph of abdomen revealing left pneumopyelogram consistent with emphysematous pyelonephritis.

225

IX. TREATMENT (FIG. 8-6)

A. Acute

1. Acute *uncomplicated* pyelonephritis can potentially be managed on an outpatient basis with a 2-week course of appropriate oral antibiotics, such as trimethoprim-sulfamethoxasole or fluoroquinolones. For patients who are vomiting and dehydrated, septic, or with *complicated* pyelonephritis, treatment is initiated with intravenous hydration and antibiotic therapy (usually a penicillin and an aminoglycoside, substituting vancomycin in penicillin-allergic patients). Initiation of therapy with cephalosporins is recommended for pregnant patients presenting with pyelonephritis. Once clinically stable, patients are converted to appropriate oral antibiotics based on the antimicrobial sensitivities of blood and urine cultures at presentation. Duration of antibiotic treatment for complicated pyelonephritis is 3 weeks. Experimental studies have shown that early antibiotic treatment is rewarded with diminished tendency toward renal scarring.

2. Control of pain and nausea with narcotic analgesics, nonsteroidal antiinflammatory drugs, and antiemetics.

3. Most patients will have persistent fevers, which should trend downward during the first 72 hours following initiation of antibiotics. For patients febrile beyond 72 hours or not otherwise clinically responding to treatment, CT scanning or ultrasonography is recommended to check for complicating factors, such as renal abscess or urinary obstruction.

3. Patients promptly responding to therapy should undergo subsequent evaluation for urinary obstruction, calculi, or other factors, with intravenous urography and/or ultrasonography.

4. The pediatric patient should be studied with voiding cystourethrography and nuclear renal scanning to evaluate for vesicoureteral reflux and renal scarring/dysfunction, respectively.

5. Ten to 30 percent of patients with acute pyelonephritis relapse following a 2-week course of antibiotics, the majority being cured by a second 2-week course of antibiotics.

B. Chronic

In chronic pyelonephritis, the physician must search for predisposing risk factors such as obstructive uropathy, reflux, or struvite calculi. These factors should be treated surgically, occasionally in conjunction with the use of chronic suppression with appropriate urinary antiseptics such as penicillin, nitrofurantoin, or trimethoprim-sulfamethoxisole. Urease inhibitors, such as acetohydroxaminic acid, may be useful to

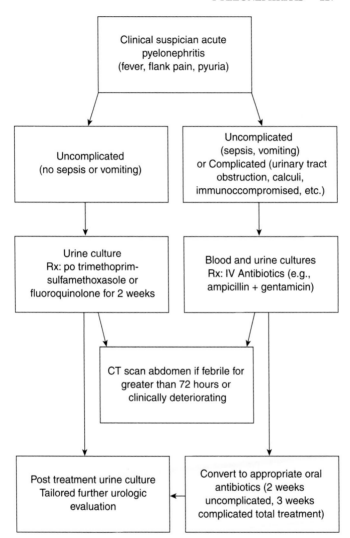

Figure 8-6 Management of acute pyelonephritis.

mitigate growth and development of struvite calculi. Patients with a unilaterally scarred, contracted kidney in addition to hypertension may be candidates for nephrectomy to protect the normal kidney from nephrosclerosis, exacerbation of the hypertension, and progressive renal disease.

X. SUMMARY

The salient features of this discussion of pyelonephritis include distinction of acute from chronic forms; methods of diagnosis and treatment; and identification of risk factors, causative agents, and underlying mechanisms of tissue damage found in this disease. Pyelonephritis is a clinical diagnosis that may be supported by several laboratory tests. Excretory urography and voiding cystourethrography remain the mainstay of adjunctive diagnostic methods. Treatment should be aimed at the acute form, with the intent of reducing the incidence of its chronic form and attendant complications. Although the bacteriology and corresponding antimicrobial therapies are straightforward, the discussion of more recent advances in the understanding of immunologic and biochemical mechanisms at work in pyelonephritis holds promise for greater success in treatment directed at halting the transformation of acute into chronic pyelonephritis.

BIBLIOGRAPHY

Bailey RR, Lynn KL, Robson RA, Smith AH, Maling TM, Turner JG: DMSA renal scans in adults with acute pyelonephritis. *Clin Nephrol* 46:99, 1996.

Bergeron MG: Treatment of pyelonephritis in adults. *Med Clin North Am* 79:619, 1995.

Blanco M, Blanco JE, Alonso MP, Blanco J: Virulence factors and O groups of Escherichia coli isolates from patients with acute pyelonephritis, cystitis, and asymptomatic bacteruria. *Eur J Epidemiol* 12:191, 1996.

Chen MT, Huang CN, Chou YH, Huang CH, Chiang CP, Liu GC: Percutaneous drainage in the treatment of emphysematous pyelonephritis: 10-year experience. *J of Urol* 157:1569, 1997.

Eastham J, Ahlering T, Skinner E: Xanthogranulomatous pyelonephritis: Clinical findings and surgical considerations. *Urology* 43:295, 1994.

Figueroa AJ, Stein JP, Cunningham JA, Ginsberg DA, Skinnner DG: Xanthogranulomatous pyelonephritis in a pregnant woman: A case report and review of the literature. *Urology* 48:294, 1996.

Fridovich I: Superoxide radical: An endogenous toxicant. *Annu Rev Pharmacol Toxicol* 23:239, 1983.

Greenfield SP, Montgomery P: Computed tomography and acute pyelonephritis in children. *Urology* 29:137, 1987.

Hudson MA, Weyman PJ, et al: Emphysematous pyelonephritis: Successful management by percutaneous drainage. *J Urol* 136:884, 1986.

Jacobson SH, Kallenius G, et al: P-fimbriae receptors in patients with chronic pyelonephritis. *J Urol* 139:900, 1978.

Janson KL, Roberts JA, et al: Noninvasive localization of urinary tract infections: Clinical investigations and experience. *J Urol* 130:488, 1983.

Johnson JR, Ireton RC, Lipsky BA: Emphysematous pyelonephritis caused by *Candida albicans*. *J Urol* 136:80, 1986.

Kaack MB, Dowling KJ, et al: Immunology of pyelonephritis. VIII. *E. coli* causes granulocytic aggregation and renal ischemia. *J Urol* 136:1117, 1986.

Kanel KT, Kroboth FJ, et al: The intravenous pyelogram in acute pyelonephritis. *Arch Intern Med* 148:2144, 1988.

Koh KB, Lam HS, Lee SH: Emphysematous pyelonephritis: Drainage or nephrectomy? *Br J Urol* 71:609, 1993.

Lavocat MP, Granjon D, Allard D, Gay C, Freycon MT, Dubois F: Imaging in pyelonephritis. *Pediatr Radiol* 27:159, 1997.

Lorentz WB, Iskander S, et al: Acute renal failure due to pyelonephritis. *Nephron* 54:256, 1990.

Malek RS, Elder, JS: Xanthogranulomatous pyelonephritis: A critical analysis of 26 cases and of the literature. *J Urol* 119:589, 1978.

Meyrier A: Long-term risks of acute pyelonephritis. *Nephron* 54:197, 1990.

Millar LK, Wing DA, Paul RH, Grimes, DA: Outpatient treatment of pyelonephritis in pregnancy: A randomized controlled trial. *Obstet Gynecol* 86:560, 1995.

Roberts JA: Pathogenesis of pyelonephritis. *AUA Update Series,* vol. 2, lesson 8, 1983.

Roberts JA: Pathogenesis of pyelonephritis. *J Urol* 129: 1102, 1983.

Roberts JA: Pyelonephritis, cortical abscess, and perinephric abscess. *Urol Clin North Am* 13:637, 1986.

Roberts JA, Kaack MB, Baskin G: Treatment of experimental pyelonephritis in the monkey. *J Urol* 143:150, 1990.

Senn E, Zaunbauer W, et al: Computed tomography in acute pyelonephritis. *Br J Urol* 59:118, 1987.

Shokeir AA, El-Azab M, Moshen T, El-Diasty T: Emphysematous pyelonephritis: A 15-year experience. *Urology* 49:343, 1997.

Stamey TA, Pfau A: Some functional, pathologic, bacteriologic, and chemotherapeutic characteristics of unilateral pyelonephritis in man. *Invest Urol* 1:134, 1963.

Stamey TA: *Pathogenesis and Treatment of Urinary Tract Infections.* Baltimore: Williams & Wilkins, 1980.

Stein JP, Spitz A, Elmajian DA, et al: Bilateral emphysematous pyelonephritis: A case report and review of the literature. *Urology* 47:129, 1996.

Tsugaya M, Hirao N, et al: Computerized tomography in acute pyelonephritis: The clinical correlations. *J Urol* 144:611, 1990.

Walsh PC, Retik AB, Vaughan ED, Wein AJ eds: *Campbell's Urology.* 7th ed. Philadelphia: Saunders, 1998.

Wan YL, Lo SK, Bullard MJ, Chang PL, Lee TY: Predictors of outcome in emphysematous pyelonephritis. *J Urol* 59:369, 1998.

CHAPTER 9
Nephrolithiasis

John J. Pahira
Amir A. Razack

I. EPIDEMIOLOGY

1. The annual incidence of nephrolithiasis in the United States is 16 to 24 cases per 10,000 persons.
2. The prevalence of nephrolithiasis in the United States is 7 percent in males and 3 percent in females.
3. Nephrolithiasis accounts for 7 to 10 of every 1000 hospital admissions.
4. Males have three- to fourfold increased risk of developing stones over females (high urinary citrate concentrations in women) with peak age at onset of 20 to 40 years.
5. With no treatment, 10 percent of all first time stone formers will have recurrent disease within 1 year, and 50% within 10 years.
6. Uric acid and calcium stones are more frequent in males, whereas infectious stones are more common in females.
7. The incidence of kidney stones has increased in industrialized countries due to high dietary protein intake. Bladder stones are more common in underdeveloped countries.

II. COMPOSITION OF RENAL STONES

1. *Calcium oxalate.* 36 to 70 percent.
2. *Calcium phosphate (hydroxyapatite).* 6 to 20 percent.
3. *Mixed calcium oxalate and calcium phosphate.* 11 to 31 percent.
4. *Magnesium ammonium phosphate (struvite).* 6 to 20 percent.
5. *Uric acid.* 6 to 17 percent.
6. *Cystine.* 0.5 to 3 percent.
7. *Miscellaneous.* Xanthine, silicates, and drug metabolites. 1 to 4 percent.

III. PATHOGENESIS AND PHYSIOCHEMICAL PROPERTIES

A. Factors Influencing Stone Formation

1. Genetics
   a. Idiopathic hypercalciuria inherited as an autosomal dominant trait.

      b. Cystinuria inherited as an autosomal recessive defect on chromosome 2.

      c. Primary hyperoxaluria, type 1 and 2, are inherited as an autosomal recessive.

      d. Lesch-Nyhan syndrome is an X-linked disease causing hyperuricemia.

      e. Familial renal tubular acidosis (RTA), Ehlers-Danlos syndrome, Marfan's syndrome, Wilson's disease.

  2. Environmental

      a. Dietary factors:

         i. High protein and sodium intake increase risk of calcium stones.

        ii. High purine diets lower urinary pH and cause hyperuricosuria.

       iii. Vitamin B_6 (pyridoxine) deficiency results in increased formation and excretion of oxalate.

       iv. Dehydration, inadequate fluid intake, vitamin C excess, calcium supplements, calcium-containing antacids.

      b. Geographical factors:

         i. Higher during summer months.

        ii. Higher in Southeast United States and lower in Mid-Atlantic and Northwest regions.

B. Physical and Biochemical Parameters

  1. Supersaturation not dependent solely on the solute concentration but also on ionic strength, complexion, urine volume, and urine pH. Ionic strength is determined by the presence of monovalent ions in the urine. Its increase will allow more crystals to be in solution without supersaturation. The presence of certain substances in the urine, such as citrate and phosphate, that naturally complex with any potential solute reduces the free ion activity.

  2. Urinary organic (e.g., glycosaminoglycans, nephrocalcin, Tamm-Horsfall protein, uropontin) and inorganic inhibitors (e.g. citrate, pyrophosphate) inhibit various phases of stone formation.

  3. Epitaxy is overgrowth of one type of crystal on the surface of a preexisting one that is of different type. This process of heterogeneous nucleation is seen with amorphous calcium phosphate and uric acid facilitating the crystallization of calcium oxalate salt.

  4. Crystal retention can occur due to the interaction between renal epithelial cells and salt crystal, which results in their internalization and submucosal plaque formation (Randall's plaques). These crystals aggregate and erode toward the papillary surface to form a nidus for further stone growth. Reduced urine output and stasis due to

anatomic abnormalities of the genitourinary tract can facilitate stone formation. A horseshoe kidney, calyx or bladder diverticula, obstructive disorders, and medullary sponge kidney can all predispose to increase crystal retention.

C. Etiological Factors of Specific Stone Types

1. Calcium stones

   Calcium oxalate develops in acidic urine (pH less than 6.0). Calcium phosphate develops in alkaline urine (pH higher than 7.5). With calcium phosphate stones, rule out urinary tract infection, Renal Tubular Acidosis (RTA), and hyperparathyroidism. Promoters of calcium stones include: hypercalciuria, hypocitrauria, hyperuricosuria, hyperoxaluria, dietary factors, and absence of inhibitors (Table 9-1).

   a. *Hypercalciuria.* Normocalcemic hypercalciuria (idiopathic hypercalciuria) occurs in 30 to 60 percent of calcium oxalate stone formers. Also in 5 to 10 percent of nonstone formers. Absorptive hypercalciuria (AH) is characterized by intestinal hyperabsorption of calcium possibly due to increased serum calcitrol (1,25 dihydroxy vitamin D) and increased sensitivity of vitamin D receptors. Hyperabsorption occurs in the jejunum. Suppression of parathyroid hormone (PTH) function increases filtered load of calcium with decreased renal tubular reabsorption of calcium leading to excess urinary calcium loss. Serum calcium is normal. Stones are of three distinctive types (Table 9-2).

   Renal hypercalciuria (Renal leak) is characterized by impaired proximal tubular reabsorption of calcium and increased serum PTH, with subsequent increase in the synthesis of $1,25(OH)_2D$ maintaining serum calcium homeostasis. Hypercalciuria occurs even during fasting state.

   Resorptive hypercalciuria (subtle hyperparathyroidism) is characterized by increased bone resorption

Table 9-1 Normal Values of Urinary Excretion of Substances Affecting Stone Formation

SUBSTANCE	MEN (Mg/d)	WOMEN (Mg/d)
Urinary calcium	< 300	< 250
Urinary uric acid	< 800	< 750
Urinary citrate	450–600	650–800
Urinary oxalate	< 45	< 45

Table 9-2 Summary of Laboratory Findings

	PHPT	AH-I	AH-II	AH-III	RH	HUCN
Serum Ca	↑	N	N	N	N	N
Serum Po	↓/N	N	N	↓	N	N
Serum PTH	↑	N/↓	N/↓	N/↓	↑	N
Urine Ca	↑/N	↑	↑	↑/N	↑	N
Urinary Ca (fasting)	↑/N	N	N	N	↑	N
Urinary Ca (1 g Ca load)	↑/N	↑	↑	↑	↑/N	N
Urine uric acid	N/↑	N/↑	N/↑	N	N/↑	↑
Bone density	N/↓	N	N	N	N/↓	N

PHPT, Primary hyperparathyroidism; AH-I, absorptive hypercalciuria, type I; AH-II, absorptive hypercaliuria, type II; AH-III, absorptive hypercalciuria, type III; RH, renal hypercalciuria; HUCN, hyperuricosuric calcium oxalate nephrolithiasis.

due to underlying primary hyperparathyroidism with excessive PTH. Hyperparathyroidism indirectly enhances intestinal calcium absorption by stimulating calcitrol production. Increased urinary calcium exceeds the tubular absorption capability.

Hypercalcemic hypercalciuric states are seen in the following.

1. Primary hyperparathyroidism is the second most common cause of calcium stones (1 to 5 percent). Caused by adenoma in 85 percent and diffuse multigland hyperplasia in 15 percent of patients. Stones are primar-ily calcium phosphate. Fasting urinary calcium is elevated.

2. There is an increased production of 1,25(OH)$_2$D by the macrophage within the sarcoid granuloma in sarcoidosis. Stones are primarily calcium oxalate. PTH levels are low or immeasurable.

3. Other etiologies include hypervitaminosis D, milk–alkali syndrome, immobilization, Paget's disease, multiple myeloma, and other malignancies (lung, breast, renal cell, head and neck cancers).

b. *Hypocitrauria.* Seen as a sole abnormality in 5 percent of patients with stones, and in 50 percent of patients who have other associated metabolic disturbances. Citrate forms a soluble salt with calcium and inhibits the formation of calcium oxalate or calcium phosphate crystals. Acidosis is the most important etiologic factor. It reduces urinary citrate by enhancing tubular citrate reabsorption and metabolism to bicarbonate. Causes of hypocitraturic calcium stones include:

1. Chronic diarrheal syndrome associated with enteric hyperoxaluria
2. Distal renal tubular acidosis (type I RTA)
3. Idiopathic
4. High salt and animal protein containing diet
5. Hypokalemia
6. Thiazide induced hypokalemia and intracellular acidosis
7. Urinary tract infection (UTI) with bacteria degrading citrate

c. *Hyperuricosuria.* Ten to 20 percent of patients with hyperuricosuria have calcium oxalate stones. Uric acid crystals may act as a nidus facilitating the nucleation of calcium oxalate crystal and may also decrease the activities of some urinary inhibitors. At a urinary pH of less than 5.5, the dissociated form of uric acid predominates and the urine will be saturated with monosodium urate, which can induce heterogeneous nucleation of calcium oxalate. It can also enhance calcium oxalate crystallization by complexing with urinary inhibitors. Causes of hyperuricosuria include:

1. Chronic diarrheal diseases (regional enteritis, short gut syndrome, and inflammatory bowel diseases).
2. High dietary purine intake.
3. Increased endogenous uric acid production as in patients with myeloproliferative disorders, acute tumor lysis syndrome after a radiation or chemotherapy.

d. *Hyperoxaluria.* Oxalate forms insoluble complexes with calcium in the gastrointestinal tract and in the urine. The activity of stone disease correlates better with the urinary oxalate level rather than urinary calcium.

   i. *Dietary hyperoxaluria.* High dietary content of oxalates or vitamin C may increase urinary oxalate to 50 to 60 mg/d. A low calcium diet (under 500 mg/d) increases urinary oxalate excretion. Reducing oxalate in diet helps treat this condition.

   ii. *Enteric hyperoxaluria.* Seen in small bowel malabsorption of variable etiology, this includes, inflammatory bowel disease, bowel resection, and jejunoileal bypass. There is an increase of intestinal bile salts and fatty acids, which bind to calcium salt and form calcium soaps. As there is less calcium available to bind with luminal oxalate, there is increased oxalate available for absorption. Colonic mucosal permeability to free oxalate is also increased. Both factors contribute to significant gut absorption of oxalate. These patients tend to have low urinary citrate and magnesium as a result of chronic metabolic acidosis and hypokalemia due to ongoing diarrhea. Treatments include lowering dietary oxalate and fat, combined with oral calcium, citrate, and magnesium supplements. Cholestyramine helps to bind fatty acids and bile salts in the gut.

iii. *Primary hyperoxaluria (PH).* PH Type I is an autosomal recessive trait in which the conversion of glyxoalate to glycine is diminished due to a defect in the enzyme alanine-glyoxylate aminotransferase activity. This results in increased conversion of glyoxalate to oxalate. There is increased oxalate production and excretion early in childhood. These patients present with early stone formation, nephrocalcinosis, tubulointerstitial nephritis, and subsequent renal failure. PH Type II is a rare deficiency of D-glycerate dehydrogenase and glyoxalate reductase. Only 21 cases have been reported.

2. Uric acid stones

a. Uric acid is an end product of purine metabolism of endogenous or exogenous sources. It is a weak acid with pK of 5.35 at physiologic pH. At a urine pH of less than 5.5, the majority of uric acid exists in its insoluble undissociated form, which is the major constituent of uric acid stone. As the urine pH increases to higher than 5.5, more soluble dissociated monosodium urate crystals are formed, favoring calcium oxalate and calcium phosphate stone formation. Stones are usually round, smooth, yellow-orange, and radiolucent. The main risk factor for crystallization of uric acid is the high concentration of urate, which is attributable either to a high excretion of urate or to a low urine volume and a low urinary pH. Although most patients with uric acid nephrolithiasis excrete more than 750 mg/d of uric acid, idiopathic uric acid stone disease can occur without hyperuricosuria. The latter is an autosomal dominant disorder in which patients have acid urine with low ammonium excretion. Between 80 to 90 percent of patients with hyperuricosuric nephrolithiasis are men.

b. Struvite stones (triple phosphate, infected stone) True struvite stones are composed of a combination of magnesium ammonium phosphate ($MgNH_4PO_4 \cdot {}_6H_2O$) and carbonate apatite ($Ca_{10}(PO_4)_6 \cdot CO_3$). Fifty percent of struvite stones may contain a nidus of another stone composition. A urine pH equal to or higher than 7.2 and the presence of ammonia in the urine are essential for the crystallization of ammonia in the urine. Struvite stones form only when urease producing organisms split urea into ammonia, bicarbonate, and carbonate ion. The most common organism associated with struvite calculi is *Proteus mirabilis.* Others include, *Hemophilus influenzae, Staphylococcus au-reus,* and *Yersinia enterocolitica,* and to a lesser extent *Ureaplasma urealyticum, Klebsiella pneumoniae, Pseudomonas* species, and enterococci with the exception of *E. coli.* Because of increased susceptibility of women to urinary tract infection, struvite stones are more common in females than men with a ratio of 2:1. However, struvite stones formed in the bladder are more frequent in men. Factors that predispose to urinary tract infections increase the likelihood of struvite stone formation. These include congenital or acquired anatomic abnormalities, neurologic disorders, and indwelling foreign bodies. In patients with spinal cord lesions, 8 percent will form renal calculi, with 98 percent of the stones composed of struvite.

3. Cystine stones
   An autosomal recessive disorder due to the mutation in the SLC3A1 amino acid transporter gene on chromosome 2. This causes an impaired transtubular reabsorption of filtered dibasic amino acids (cystine, ornithine, arginine, and lysine) and results in excessive urinary excretion. Cystine precipitates in hexagonal plates due to its low solubility to form the major constituent of cystine stones. Heterozygotes (asymptomatic) excrete more than 400 mg of cystine per day, whereas homozygote stone formers excrete more than 600 mg/day. Positive urine cyanide-nitroprusside colorimetric reaction is a qualitative screen.

IV. CLINICAL MANIFESTATIONS OF NEPHROLITHIASIS

1. Asymptomatic nephrolithiasis may be discovered during the course of radiographic studies undertaken for unrelated reasons.

2. Pain is the most common symptom, varies from mild ache to severe intense pain requiring hospitalization and parenteral analgesic medications. Renal colic occurs when stones produce obstruction. Typically, it begins suddenly in the early morning hours and intensifies over a period of 15 to 30 min into a steady pain that causes nausea and vomiting. The pain develops in paroxysms that are related to movement of stone in the ureter and associated ureteral spasm. Paroxysms usually last 20 to 60 min. Obstruction occurs at one of four sites along the course of the ureter: the ureteropelvic junction, midureter at the level of iliac vessels, the posterior part of the pelvis in women, and the ureterovesical junction. The site of obstruction determines the location of pain. An upper ureteral or renal pelvic obstruction lead to flank pain, with costovertebral angle tenderness that may radiate laterally around the flank and into the abdomen. On the other hand,

lower ureteral obstruction causes pain that can radiate to the groin and the ipsilateral testicle or labia. Renal colic can be due to the passage of blood clots or sloughed papillae.

3. Microscopic or gross hematuria occurs in 95 percent of patients. Hematuria may be absent if the stone is causing complete obstruction.

4. Nausea and vomiting are frequently associated with renal colic.

5. Frequency, urgency, and dysuria can result from stone impaction at the ureterovesical junction and/or associated urinary tract infection.

6. Another symptom can be low-grade fever without associated infection.

7. Staghorn calculi do not produce symptoms unless small pieces break off and pass into the ureter. They can cause chronic renal failure over years if present bilaterally.

V. EVALUATION OF PATIENTS WITH NEPHROLITHIASIS

The National Institutes of Health (NIH) consensus conference on prevention and treatment of kidney stones suggested that all patients, even those with a single stone, should have a basic work up to rule out systemic causes of nephrolithiasis. More comprehensive evaluation needs to be done in certain groups of patients including:

1. All children.

2. Patients in the demographic group in which stones are not expected (e.g., black women).

3. Patients with growing or recurrent stone (metabolically active disease).

4. Patients with a strong family history of stones.

5. Patients with systemic diseases or underlying metabolic disorders that predispose to stone formation.

6. When the recovered stone is not composed predominantly of calcium oxalate.

7. Solitary kidney.

A detailed evaluation should be undertaken 3 to 4 weeks after the last episode of renal colic, and as the patients resume their normal fluid and dietary intakes.

A. Medical History

The following questions should be considered to identify specific risk factors.

1. Chronology of stone events: age at first stone passage, number and size of stones passed, the particular kidney involved with each event, spontaneous passage versus

need for active intervention, and the symptoms noted with each episode.

2. The presence of systemic diseases or underlying metabolic disorders that enhance stone formation (e.g., Crohn's disease, colectomy, sarcoidosis, hyperparathyroidism, hyperthyroidism, RTA, and gout).

3. The presence of a family history of stones.

4. Intake of medication that can increase the risk of stone formation (e.g., acetazolamide, ascorbic acid, salicylic acid, calcium containing antacids, triamterine, acyclovir, and indinavir).

5. Occupation and life style, as professionals have a greater tendency to stone formation than manual laborers. High protein and sodium dietary intake increases risk of stone formation. Habitual tea drinking may lead to oxaluria.

6. The analysis of previous stones.

B. Physical Examination

May provide clues to underlying systemic causes (tophi secondary to gout, enterocutaneous fistulas with Crohn's disease, metastatic breast cancer as a cause of hypercalcemia).

C. Laboratory Tests

1. *Urinalysis.* High specific gravity can indicate inadequate hydration. Low urine pH (less than 5.5) is seen with uric acid stones, whereas high urine pH (at or about 7.2) is seen in patients with RTA and struvite stones. Microscopic or gross hematuria. The presence of white blood cells in the urine may be seen in the absence of infection. Crystalluria can help in defining stone type (hexagonal cystine crystal, coffin lid phosphate crystal, rhomboidal uric acid crystal). Bacteriuria must be further evaluated with urine culture.

2. *Urine culture.* Early detection of urinary tract infections is important. Determine the presence of urease-producing bacteria.

3. *Cystine screening.* Addition of sodium nitroprusside to urine with cystine concentration higher than 75 mg/L alters the urine color to purple-red.

4. *Blood tests.* CBC may show mild peripheral leukocytosis. WBC higher than $15,000/mm^3$ may suggest an active infection. Serum chemistry includes serum calcium, phosphate, uric acid, sodium, potassium, chloride, bicarbonate, albumin, and serum creatinine. If serum calcium level is elevated, an intact PTH should be checked.

5. *Twenty-four hour urine collection.* Done as a part of the comprehensive workup. Urine is collected in a container with boric acid as preservative, which may falsely lower

urinary pH. Collection is done to determine total urine volume, pH, calcium, citrate, magnesium, oxalate, phosphate, sodium uric acid (cystine, if screening test is positive), and creatinine.

6. *Stone analysis.* Analysis with x-ray crystallgraphy or infrared spectrography.

7. *Urinary acidification test.* With oral ammonium chloride load (0.1 gm/kg body weight) given over 30 min for the diagnosis of distal type I RTA. Urine pH fails to drop below 5.3.

D. Radiologic Evaluation

1. *Plain film of the kidneys, ureter, and the bladder (KUB).* This is 90 percent sensitive in detecting urinary calculi. Determining the size, number, and location of the stones provide a rational planning of stone removal. Most of the stones (92 percent), with the exception of pure uric acid, cystine, and xanthine stones, are at least partially radiopaque and can be detected by a KUB. KUB has the advantage of being quick, inexpensive, easily obtainable, and provides accurate measures of stone size. Its limitations include the inability to detect nonopaque calculi and those that are less than 2 mm in size. It is difficult to differentiate renal from extrarenal calculi on supine film. The study can not be used in pregnant patients.

2. *Intravenous pyelogram (IVP).* The diagnostic procedure of choice. High sensitivity and specificity for determining stones location and the degree of obstruction. IVP can detect radiolucent stones and define anatomic abnormality contributing to stone formation. Patients are requested to strain their urine if they have to void during the procedure in response to intravenous contrast that induces diuresis.

3. *Ultrasonography (US).* Procedure of choice in patients known to have allergy to contrast and pregnant females. Sensitivity of ultrasonography to renal calculi is less than radiography. False-negatives occur in the presence of small renal calculi or in obese patients. Calculi in the ureter between the level of the iliac crest and the uretrovesical junction cannot be evaluated satisfactorily. Detect radiolucent calculi and urinary tract obstruction if present. Used to follow size of existing stones and the formation of new ones. Used to rule out other etiology in patient presenting with acute flank pain.

4. *CT scans.* A noncontrast-enhanced CT scan is the most rapid and cost effective method for rapidly diagnosing nephrolithiasis and obstruction in patients with acute flank pain. It has a sensitivity of 97 percent and specificity of 96 percent. More sensitive than radiography,

sonography, or both combined in detecting all type of stones. Helical or spiral CT scanning is superior to non-helical CT, as it requires less cooperation from patient.

VI. MANAGEMENT OF NEPHROLITHIASIS
A. Treating Patients with Acute Renal Colic
1. Aggressive intravenous fluid hydration is usually not necessary unless the patient is dehydrated and unable to take fluid orally. It may actually aggravate the degree of obstruction and increase patient discomfort.
2. Parenteral analgesic
   a. Parenteral use of analgesic may be needed if pain is severe and associated nausea and vomiting render patients unable to use medication via the oral route.
   b. The newer parenteral nonsteroidal anti-inflammatory drugs (NSAIDs)(Ketorolac-Toradol), when compared to the standard narcotic analgesics (Mepridine-demerol), were as effective, if not more, in alleviating renal colic.
   c. The risk of NSAID-related renal dysfunction due to their hemodynamic effects or direct tubulointerstitial diseases can be increased in states of dehydration or the concomitant administration of radiocontrast materials.
   d. NSAIDs (Ketorolac) should be avoided in older patients, patients with renal failure, volume depletion, or bilateral ureteral obstruction, and in the pregnant patients.
   e. NSAIDs are appropriate for patients with renal colic who have a known addiction to narcotics, or in those who need to immediately return to a setting where they can not be under the influence of narcotics.
   f. Epidural analgesia can be used for a pregnant patient with a symptomatic calculi.
3. There is no benefit from using smooth muscle relaxants such as nifedipine.
4. Referral to the urologist should be made if the following occur:
   a. Persistent pain.
   b. Patient unable to pass the stone due to size (larger than 8 mm).
   c. Urinary extravasation detected on IVP study.
   d. High-grade obstruction with a large stone.
   e. Patient with a solitary kidney.
   f. Failure of outpatient conservative measures to induce the passage of stone.
   g. The presence of urinary infection, especially when there is obstruction.
   h. Early referral of pregnant patients.

B. Medical Treatment of Nephrolithiasis

1. General conservative measures
   a. Nonpharmacological intervention may reduce the 5-year incidence of stone recurrence by approximately 60 percent.
   b. High fluid intake of at least 8 to 10 (10 oz) glasses per day, to keep urine volume more than 2 L/d. Patients are instructed to drink to keep their urine clear.
   c. Relatively low animal protein diet (0.8 to 1.0 g/kg/d) helps to reduce stone formation. Patients are instructed to eat 8 oz of meat, chicken, or fish per day, and to have a vegetarian day per week.
   d. A low-sodium diet (2 to 3 g/d or 80 to 100 mEq/d) is effective in reducing calcium excretion in hypercalciuric patients. Patients are instructed to avoid salty food and the salt shaker.
   e. The role of dietary calcium restrictions is controversial because extreme dietary calcium restriction can reduce bone density and cause a negative calcium balance. In recent studies, high calcium intake did actually reduce the incidence of oxalate stones, presumably by increasing intestinal binding of calcium to oxalate. We advise patients to have one serving of dairy with each meal and to avoid dietary calcium at night.
   f. Avoid stone provoking drugs (e.g., Calcitrol, calcium supplements, loop diuretics, Probenicid).

2. Specific medical therapy of different stone types
   1. Calcium stones
      a. *Absorptive hypercalciuria type I.* Thiazide diuretics decrease urinary calcium by as much as 150 mg/d, both by inducing mild volume depletion, which results in compensatory rise in the proximal tubular reabsorption of sodium and calcium, and directly by enhancing distal tubular calcium reabsorption. Chlorthalidone 25 to 50 mg daily or Indapamide 2.5 to 5 mg/d, hydrochlorothiazide (HCTZ) 25 to 50 mg twice a day, or trichloromethiazide (Naqua) 2 to 4 mg/d can be used. Continued sodium restriction is stressed (evaluated by 24-hour urinary sodium of less than 100 mEq/d).

      Hypokalemia secondary to diuretic use may reduce citrate excretion, thus, supplementation with potassium citrate (Urocit-K tablet, Polycitra-K crystals, Polycitra syrup) 30 to 100 mEq a day is required.

      A potassium-sparing diuretic such as amiloride can be added at a dose of 5 to 10 mg/d. Potassium supplements should not be given with amiloride, since the combination can lead to severe hyperkalemia. Avoid triamterine because of its propensity to stone formation.

Sodium cellulose phosphate is a nonabsorbable calcium and magnesium binding resin. As it binds to intestinal calcium, more oxalate is unbound and available for absorption. Thus, dietary oxalate should be restricted. Dosage is 2.5 to 5.0g given with each meal. Long-term use can induce negative calcium balance and mandate monitoring bone density. Magnesium supplement may be necessary.

b. *Absorptive hypercalcemia type II.* Dietary calcium restrictions include a moderate restriction of 600 mg/d or one to two servings of dairy with meals. Dietary sodium restriction is essential to decrease hypercalciuria. Thiazide and potassium citrate supplements are offered when the above conservative measures are not effective.

c. *Absorptive hypercalciuria type III.* Orthophosphate (Neutra-Phos-K) reduces serum 1,25(OH)2 D levels and increases urinary inhibitory activity. Recommended dosage is 250 to 500 mg three to four times daily.

d. *Renal hypercalciuria.* Thiazide enhances tubular calcium reabsorption. This normalizes serum calcium and suppress PTH. HCTZ 50 mg twice daily or trichloromethiazide (Naqua) 4 mg/d can be given. Dietary sodium is restricted to 2 g/d, and keep urinary sodium less than 100 mEq.

Potassium citrate supplementation includes:
1. Polycitra K syrup 15 to 30 mL twice daily.
2. Polycitra K crystals 1 packet twice daily.
3. Urocit K 10 to 20 mEq twice daily.

e. *Hyperuricosuric calcium oxalate nephrolithiasis.* Increase fluid intake. Decrease dietary purine intake, especially red meat, fish, and poultry. Urinary alkalization with potassium citrate to keep urinary pH higher than 6.5. Urinary alkalization, with pH higher than 7.5 may facilitate precipitation of calcium phosphate crystals.

Xanthine oxidase inhibitor (Allopurinol) (recommended dose 100 to 300 mg/d) may reduce stone formation by 80 percent. It is given when serum uric acid is higher than 8 mg/dL or urinary uric acid is greater than 800 mg/24 hours.

f. *Hypocitrauria.* Potassium citrate increases intracellular pH, and hence citrate production. Urocit K

10 to 20 mEq two or three times daily can be used. The goal is to keep urinary citrate above 400 mg.

Ingestion of 4 ozs of lemon juice a day mixed with water as lemonade for a total volume of 2 L may increase urinary citrate by twofold.

  g. *Enteric hyperoxaluria.*

    i. Phase I

      1. Treat underlying disease (regional enteritis, blind loop syndrome, biliary tract disease, etc.).

      2. Increase fluid intake.

      3. Low dietary fat (50 g/d) and oxalate.

      4. Calcium supplementation, 2 to 3 tablets (500 mg each) with each meal. Use calcium citrate, better than calcium carbonate.

      5. Cholestyramine, 1 to 4 g four times a day after meals and at bed time.

    ii. Phase II

      1. Added to phase I after it has been unsuccessful.

      2. Potassium citrate (Urocit-K), 10 to 20 mEq, two or three times daily.

      3. Magnesium supplement with magnesium gluconate, 0.5 to 1 g three times daily.

      4. Allopurinol as 300 mg daily should be added if the stones contain uric acid.

      5. Pyridoxine (Vitamin B_6) 25 to 50 mg twice to four times daily.

  h. *Primary hyperoxaluria.* Pyridoxine (vitamin B_6) can decrease endogenous production of oxalate. It is given as 100 to 800 mg/d. Oral orthophosphate (2 g of elemental phosphorus per day) can be given in four divided doses. Others include oral magnesium and citrate supplements. Increase fluid intake. A combined liver/kidney transplant may be necessary in pyridoxine-resistant patients.

2. Uric acid stones

  a. Increase fluid intake especially at night to increase urine volume to 3 L per day.

  b. Decrease dietary animal protein to decrease sulfur content.

  c. Decrease dietary purine to decrease uric acid contents.

  d. Urinary alkalinization with potassium citrate to keep urine pH above 6.5. Patient to check his or her urine pH using nitrazine papers and adjust the dose accordingly. If urine pH remain at or below 6.0, check patient compliance to low protein diet and medication intake.

  e. Acetazolamide (Diamox) is given at a dosage of 250 to 500 mg at bedtime to maintain urine pH acceptable at night.

f. Allopurinol is given if urinary uric acid remains at or above 1 g/d despite good dietary compliance and a urine pH equal to or above 6.5. The recommended dose is 100 to 300 mg/d.

3. Cystine stones

a. If urine cystine is below 500 mg/L increase fluid intake to maintain urine output more than 3 L a day. Urinary alkalinization with potassium citrate is used to keep urine pH 7.0 to 7.5. This increases cystine solubility by threefold. Decrease dietary purines and sodium intake.

b. If urine cystine is above 500 mg/L or the above measures are ineffective, D-penicillamine is used. It forms a soluble disulfide with cysteine, thereby decreasing the availability of free cysteine to form cystine. Each 250 mg dose, decreases cystine concentration by 75 to 100/d. Therapy has many side effects and should be discontinued once stone dissolution occurs. Tiopronin (Thiola, mercaptopropionylglycine) has been shown to be as effective as D-Penicillamine, but with a better safety profile. Thiolia is now used more widely than D-Penicillamine. Captopril contains sulfhydryl groups, which bind to cysteine and by this decreases urinary cystine excretion. It is better tolerated than other medications and a good choice when thiols are not tolerated.

C. Nonmedical management of nephrolithiasis

1. General

a. On presentation, 66 to 75 percent of stones are located in the ureter, 80 percent of which are in the distal ureter.

b. On presentation, 10 to 15 percent of stones are bilateral.

c. Seventy-five to 80 percent of stones pass spontaneously.

d. Indications for nonmedical interventions includes persistent renal colic refractory to oral pain medications, the presence of obstructive uropathy secondary to stones, refractory hematuria, infected struvite stone, and the size and stone location (stones larger than 10 mm lodged at the renal pelvis).

e. Therapeutic modalities:

1. Extracorporeal shock wave lithotripsy (ESWL)
2. Percutaneous nephrostolithotomy (PCNL)
3. Rigid and flexible ureteroscopy (URS)
4. Combination treatment
5. Open surgical approaches

f. Factors influencing therapeutic choice are the following.

i. *Stone burden (size and number).* ESWL treatment of large stones (larger than 2 cm) creates a large quantity of fragments called "steinstrasse" (street of stone), which may accumulate in the ureter and cause obstruction. Stones larger than 2 cm in diameter are best treated with PCNL due to higher stone-free rates and lower retreatment rates. Multiple smaller stones may be easily targeted by ESWL. Most complete staghorn calculi are best managed initially by percutaneous debulking followed by ESWL of residual fragments.

ii. *Stone location.* Renal and upper ureteral stones are best managed with ESWL (75 percent) or PCNL. Lower ureteral stones are best managed with ureteroscopy using basket extraction or in situ lithotripsy with Holmium laser or electrohydrolic lithotripsy. A free-floating stone in the renal pelvis is most likely to be broken by ESWL. Lower pole calyceal stones are more accessible with PCNL than those in the upper pole. Narrowed calyceal infundibulum or ureteropelvic junction decreases the stone free rate after ESWL and stones are best managed percutaneously.

iii. *Stone composition.* If stone analysis is not available, composition is suggested by history and radiographic appearance. Pure calcium phosphate and calcium oxalate monohydrate stones may be refractory to ESWL. Calcium oxalate dihydrate stones fragment easily with ESWL. Cystine calculi are resistant to fragmentation with ESWL but may be degraded by ultrasonic energy. Uric acid calculi are easily fragmented by ESWL.

iv. *Extraurinary factors.* The presence of retroperitoneal masses, bony abnormalities such as scoliosis, coagulation abnormalities, pregnancy, cardiac pacemakers, and extra-renal vascular calcifications may influence the choice of therapy.

2. Shock wave lithotripsy
   a. The first application of ESWL was in Munich, West Germany, in February 1980.
   b. First commercially available kidney stone lithotripter, the Dornier Human Model 3 (HM3), was introduced in 1983.
   c. The first patient treated in the United States with ESWL was at the Methodist Hospital of Indiana in February 1984.
   d. Principle: focused high-pressure shock waves would release energy when passing through two different mediums of different acoustic impedance. This energy results in fragmentation of stones.
   e. Lithotripsy devices share four main features.

    1. Energy source (electrohydraulic, piezoelectric, electromagnetic).

    2. Coupling mechanism (water bath or water cushion and gel).

    3. Focusing device (ellipsoid, spherical disc, acoustic lens).

    4. Stone localization (fluoroscopy, ultrasound).

f. The HM3 device is the most common lithotriptor in use. An ellipsoid reflector and fluoroscopy guidance is used to localize the stone. One third of the energy is unreflected and unfocused leaving the ellipsoid slightly ahead of the focused waves. These unfocused waves, called *precursorial shock waves,* are painful when it strikes the skin. Newer devices now eliminate the water bath of the HM3 and deliver shock wave energy across a soft membrane that couples to the patient with gel.

g. Contraindications of ESWL:

    1. Absolute: pregnancy, bleeding diathesis, and obstruction below the level of the stone.

    2. Relative: calcified arteries and/or aneurysms and cardiac pacemaker (pacemaker should be reprogrammed).

h. Complications of ESWL:

    i. Complications related to stone fragments include renal colic due to the passage of stone fragments or obstruction, steinstrasse (most are passed with minimal symptoms but 7 percent requires intervention), and incomplete fragmentation.

    ii. Complications related to shock waves include skin bruising, subcapsular and perinephric hemorrhage, pancreatitis, hearing loss, and urosepsis.

i. *Efficacy of ESWL.* Success rate for renal stones less than 2 cm is 78 to 91 percent with an 80 percent success rate for upper and middle pole calyceal calculi versus 60 percent with lower pole calyceal calculi. A 62 to 90 percent success rate is found for nonimpacted upper ureteric calculi, especially when the stone has been present for less than 8 weeks. There is only a 54 to 80 percent success rate for mid-ureteral stones due to the difficult localization of the stone with the shock wave machine and manipulation up to the renal pelvis. Newer generation lithotripters improve localization of ureteral calculi. The original Dornier HM3 lithotriptor, with its large focal zone, delivers more energy into the patient during lithotripsy causing more localized pain which requires the administration of anesthesia. The newer second- and third-generation lithotriptor produce low pressure shock waves, wider entry sites through the skin, and smaller focal spot size, which result not only in decreased in local pain but also in a decrease in fragmentation efficiency.

j. *Adjunctive modalities.* Stents are used with stone burdens greater than 1.5 cm to decrease the risks of obstruction and sepsis. Stents are used to increase the treatment success with upper or mid-ureteral calculi by pushing the stone into the renal pelvis or simply by passing the stone.

k. *Combined therapy.* Large stone burdens or staghorn calculi often require initial debulking with percutaneous procedures followed by ESWL for residual stones.

3. Percutaneous nephrolithotomy

   a. Indications

      i. *Staghorn calculi.* The American Urological Association (AUA), in 1994, published recommendations targeting the treatment of staghorn calculi. Their guidelines recommended PCNL as first line treatment followed by ESWL or repeat PCNL as needed.

      ii. *Large renal stone burden.* Primary PCNL for calculi greater than 3 cm carries a success rate approaching 100 percent, with a lower rate of ancillary procedures (8 percent).

      iii. *Large lower pole renal calculi.* Have much lower success rate with ESWL due to the impedance of gravity-assisted drainage. PCNL is more cost effective than ESWL for lower pole calculi greater than 2 cm.

      iv. *Cystine calculi.* Although cystine calculi are ductile (firm) and resistant to ESWL, they are actually softer than other calculi types in terms of microhardness. This feature makes them suitable for ultrasonic lithotripsy.

      v. *Abnormalities of renal and upper tract anatomy.* Percutaneous approach is favorable in patients with ureteropelvic junction obstruction, caliceal diverticula and obstructed infundibula (hydrocalyx), ureteral obstruction, malformed kidneys (e.g., horseshoe and pelvic), and obstructive or large adjacent renal cysts.

      vi. *Abnormalities of patient anatomy.* Occasionally, obesity or musculoskeletal deformity may prevent the use of ESWL. In contrast, the effectiveness of PCNL is not affected by obesity, although modification of the technique is necessary.

    vii. *Shock wave lithotripsy and ureteroscopy failures.*

    viii. *Nephrolithiasis in transplanted kidneys.* With the kidney located superficially in the iliac fossa, ultrasound can localize the site of the calculi with precision then appropriate access for PCNL is obtained.

  b. Contraindications of PCNL include uncontrolled bleeding diathesis, untreated urinary tract infection, and inability to obtain optimal access for PCNL due to obesity, splenomegaly, or interposition of colon.

  c. Technique is to establish an access at lower pole calyx, dilation of tract with balloon dilator or Amplatz dilators under fluoroscopy and stone removal with graspers or its fragmentation using electrohydaulic, ultrasonic, or laser lithotripsy. A council catheter is left as a nephrostomy drainage with ureteral stenting if necessary. Antegrade nephrostogram is performed in 24 to 48 hours to ensure adequate drainage.

  d. Complications of PCNL include hemorrhage (5 to 12 percent), perforation and extravasation (5.4 to 26 percent), damage to adjacent organs (1 percent), ureteral obstruction (1.7 to 4.9 percent), and infection and urosepsis (3 percent).

  e. PCNL has success rates of 98 percent for renal stones and 90 percent for ureteral stones.

4. Ureteroscopy

  a. Remains the gold standard for the treatment of middle and distal ureteral calculi.

  b. Rigid ureteroscopes are easier for stone manipulation because of better flow and visibility.

  c. Flexible ureteroscopes are available for diagnostic and therapeutic uses. Because of their deflection capabilities, they can access the entire upper urinary tract.

  d. The stones are removed using the stone basket or graspers. On the other hand, endoscopic lithotripsy devices are used for stone fragmentation (electrohydaulic, ultrasonic, or laser lithotripsy).

  e. Efficacy of URS includes success rates of 98 to 99 percent for distal ureteral calculi, 51 to 97 percent for mid-ureteral calculi, and 58 to 88 percent for upper ureteral calculi.

  f. Complications of URS include failure to retrieve the stone, mucosal abrasions, false passages, and ureteral perforation; complete ureteral avulsion; ureteral stricture (3 to 11 percent); and urosepsis.

5. Open surgery
    a. Since era of ESWL, advanced PCNL, and ureteroscopy techniques, its role has diminished to less than 1%.
    b. It is still indicated for large complete staghorn calculi and large stone burdens in conjunction with UPJ obstruction.

BIBLIOGRAPHY

Barcelo P, Wuhl O, Servitge E, et al: Randomized double-blind study of potassium citrate in idiopathic hypocitraruric calcium nephrolithiasis. *J Urol* 150:1761–1764, 1993.

Begun FP, Foley D, Peterson A, White B: Patient evaluation, laboratory and imaging studies. *Urol Clin North Am* 24:97–116, 1997.

Breslau NA, Brinkley L, Hill KD, Pak CY: Relationship of animal protein-rich diet to kidney stone formation and calcium metabolism. *J Clin Endocrinol Metab* 66:140, 1988.

Bushinsky DA: Nephrolithiasis. *J Am Soc Nephrol* 9:917–924, 1998.

Coe FL, Parks JH, Asplin JR: the pathogenesis and treatment of kidney stones. *N Eng J Med* 327:1411, 1992.

Curhan GC, Rimm EB, Willett WC, Stamfer MJ: Regional variation in nephrolithiasis incidence and prevalence among United States men. *J Urol* 151:838, 1994.

Curhan GC, Willett WC, Speizer FE, Stampfer MJ: A prospective study of the intake of vitamin C and B_6, and the risk of kidney stones in men. *J Urol* 155:1847; 1996.

Dretler SP: The physiologic approach to the medical management of stone disease. *Uro Clin North Am* 25:613–623, 1998.

Ehreth JT, Drach GW, Arnett MI, et al: Extracorporeal shock-wave lithotripsy: Multicenter study of kidney and upper ureter versus middle and lower ureter treatments. *J Urol* 152;1379, 1994.

Evan AP, Willis LR, Conners B, et al: Shock wave lithotripsy-induced renal injury. *Am J Kidney Dis* 17:445, 1991.

Fine JK, Pak CY, Preminger GM: Effect of medical management and residual fragments on recurrent stone formation following shock wave lithotripsy. *J Urol* 153:27, 1995.

Goldfarb S: Diet and nephrolithiasis. *Annu Rev Med* 45:235–243, 1994.

Hess B, Hasler-Strum U, Ackermann D, Jaeger P: Metabolic evaluation of patients with recurrent idiopathic calcium nephrolithiasis. *Nephrol Dial Transplant* 12:1362, 1997.

Labrecque M, Dostaler L, Rousselle R, Nguyen T, Poirier S. A meta-analysis: Efficacy of nonsteroidal anti-inflammatory drugs in the treatment of acute renal colic. *Arch Intern Med* 154:1381–1387, 1994.

Lingeman JE: Lithotripsy and surgery. *Semin Nephrol* 16: 487–498, 1996.

Lingeman JE, Woods JR, Toth PD: Blood pressure changes following extracorporeal shock wave lithotripsy and other forms of treatment for nephrolithiasis. *JAMA* 263:1789, 1990.

Low RK, Stoller ML: Uric acid-related nephrolithiasis. *Urol Clin North Am* 24: 135–148, 1997.

Monk RD. Kidney stones: Clinical approach to adults. *Semin Nephrol* 16:375–388, 1996.

Pak CY, Resnick MI, Preminger GM: Ethnic and geographic diversity of stone disease. *Urology* 50:504–507, 1997.

Parivar F, Low RK, Stoller ML: Influence of diet on urinary stone disease. *J Urol* 155:432, 1996.

Riese RJ, Sakhaee K: Uric acid nephrolithiasis, pathogensis and treatment. *J Urol* 148:765, 1992.

Saklayen MG: Medical management of nephrolithiasis. *Med Clin North Am* 81:785, 1997.

Segura JW: Surgical management of urinary calculi. *Semin Nephrol* 10:53–63, 1990.

Segura JW, Preminger GM, Assimos DG, et al: Ureteral Stones Clinical Guidelines Panel summary report on the management of ureteral calculi. *J Urol* 158:1915, 1997.

Smith LH: The pathophysiology and medical treatment of urolithiasis. *Semin Nephrol* 10:31–52, 1990.

Smith LH, Drach G, Hall P, et al: National High Blood Pressure Education Program (NHBPEP) review paper on complications of shock wave lithotripsy for urinary calculi. *Am J Med* 91:635, 1991.

Smith RC, Rosenfield AT, Choe KA, et al. Acute flank pain: Comparison of noncontrast-enhanced CT and intravenous urogram. *Radiology* 194:789, 1995.

Stoller ML, Litt L, Salazar RG: Severe hemorrhage after extracorporeal shock-wave lithotripsy. *Ann Intern Med* 111:612, 1989.

Tiselius H: Investigation of single and recurrent stone formers. *Miner Electrolyte Metab* 20:321–327, 1994.

Wang LP, Wong HY, Griffith DP: Treatment options in struvite stones. *Urol Clin North Am* 24:149–171, 1997.

Wolf S, Clayman RV. Percutaneous nephrostolithotomy: What is its role in 1997? *Urol Clin North Am* 24:43–57, 1997.

SELF-ASSESSMENT QUESTIONS

1. In patients with hypercalciuria caused by "renal leak" of calcium, the best test to distinguish this condition from "absorptive hypercalciuria" is:
   a. hypocitraturia.
   b. 24-hour urinary calcium level.
   c. increased serum PTH.
   d. serum calcium.

2. Which diagnosis in not in the differential for pure calcium phosphate stone composition.
   a. hyperparathyroidism
   b. urinary tract infection
   c. hypocitraturia
   d. renal tubular acidosis

3. The most common laboratory findings in patients with uric acid nephrolithiasis are low 24-hour urine volume and elevated serum uric acid. True or false?

4. Which statement regarding the use of sodium cellulose phosphate is not true?
   a. It needs to be taken with each meal.
   b. Long-term use may induce negative calcium balance.
   c. It is important for patients to restrict dietary oxalate.
   d. It will help reduce intestinal hyperabsorption of calcium secondary to increased PTH in "renal leak" hypercalciuria.
   e. Patients often need magnesium supplementation while using sodium cellulose phosphate.

5. For patients who initially respond to thiazaides for treatment of "renal leak" hypercalciuria but on later follow up have recurrent hypercalciuria, the most likely cause is that:
    a. they can no longer store excess calcium and have increased filtered load.
    b. PTH levels are elevated secondary long-term thiazide use.
    c. excessive sodium intake reduces effectiveness of the thiazide.
    d. long-term thiazide use decreases potassium level.

6. For patients with "absorptive hypercalciuria" type III which statement is false?
    a. Urinary 1-25 hydroxy vitamin D levels are elevated.
    b. Urinary phosphate is high and serum phosphate level is low.
    c. Urinary citrate is low.
    d. This condition is best treated with orthophosphate.

7. Which statement is not true?
    a. In cystinuria four amino acids are elevated in the urine, but only cystine causes stones.
    b. Only homozygotes will excrete large enough cystine levels to form stones.
    c. Hydration and urinary alkalinization are the first line of medical treatment.
    d. Cystine stones respond well to ESWL treatment.

8. Which condition is unlikely to respond to potassium citrate therapy?
    a. uric acid nephrolithiasis
    b. cystine nephrolithiasis
    c. renal tubular acidosis
    d. renal leak hypercalciuria being treated long term with thiazide
    e. type III hypercalciuria

9. In the evaluation of patients with uric acid nephrolithiasis you often do not find elevated 24-hour uric acid levels because in the acid environment of the 24-hour urine the uric acid will precipitate out of solution and is not measured. True or false?

10. Which statement is not true?
    a. Cystine staghorn calculi are best managed with percutaneous debulking.
    b. Ureteroscopy is most effective for stones in the distal ureter.
    c. Uric acid renal calculi are not suitable for ESWL because they cannot be localized on fluoroscopy.
    d. Struvite staghorn calculi are best managed with a combination of percutaneous debulking and chemolysis or secondary ESWL.

Answers

1. c
2. c
3. False
4. d
5. c
6. c
7. d
8. e
9. True
10. c

CHAPTER 10

Emergency Room Urology

Rajesh Shinghal
Christopher K. Payne

This chapter outlines the typical problems the urologist is called upon to evaluate in the emergency department (ED). Through application of basic urologic principles and simple diagnostic procedures, most of these problems can be expediently triaged and often definitively treated in the ED. Some of the most common reasons for emergency urologic consultation—trauma, urolithiasis, urinary tract infections, sexually transmitted diseases—are covered in greater detail elsewhere in the book and the reader is encouraged to cross-reference these chapters.

I. PAIN IN THE URINARY TRACT
A. General Concepts
1. *Local pain.* Felt in or near the involved organs.
2. *Referred pain.* Originates in a diseased organ but is felt at a distance from that organ, due to common innervation of the site of the pathology and the location of perceived pain.
3. Because of common innervation, urologic pain is frequently referred to other sites in the body; therefore the consultant must always consider the many gastrointestinal and gynecologic conditions with similar symptoms. Many of these may represent surgical emergencies (Table 10-1).
4. Pain is usually caused by distention (bladder in retention, ureter and/or renal pelvis with passing stone).
5. Severity of pain is related to the time of onset of the distention. Chronic obstruction can lead to severe, yet painless dilation, whereas acute, mild dilation can be dramatically painful.
6. Other causes of pain include renal capsular distention, ischemia, inflammation, and infection.

B. Flank Pain and Renal Colic
1. Differential diagnosis
   The challenge is in distinguishing between the patient with a calculus and the patient with pyelonephritis, while

Table 10-1 Differential Diagnoses for Common Sites of Urologic Pain

SITE OF PAIN	ETIOLOGIES (A PARTIAL LIST)
Flank	Renal colic (calculi), pyelonephritis, renal trauma, renal vein thrombosis, cholecystitis
Right lower quadrant (RLQ)	Renal colic (calculi), appendicitis, PID, Meckel's diverticulum, perforated ulcer
Left lower quadrant (LLQ)	Renal colic (calculi), diverticulitis, PID, IBD
Suprapubic	Cystitis, urinary retention, constipation
Inguinal	Renal colic (calculi), inguinal or femoral hernia, torsion of undescended testis
Scrotal	Testicular torsion, epididymitis, referred pain from renal colic (calculi), inguinal hernia

PID, Pelvic Inflammatory Disease; IBD, Inflammatory Bowel Disease
Note the multiple manifestations of renal colic. Consider endometriosis as a source of abdominal and pelvic pain in any premenopausal woman.

keeping in mind other, less common entities. The examiner must always consider the possibilities of clot colic, renal vein thrombosis (history of arrhythmias, prosthetic heart valves, or hypercoaguable states), and renal ischemia (suspect after deceleration injury), as well as the variety of intra-abdominal emergencies that can be confused with urologic problems (appendicitis, bowel obstruction, diverticulitis, ovarian torsion, ectopic pregnancy).

2. History
   a. *Renal colic.* Renal colic classically is of sudden onset. It is characterized by waves of pain that are caused by intermittent ureteral contractions and result in increased intrarenal pressure. Associated nausea and vomiting are common. Patients are often writhing but find no relief with change of position. Pain can be referred to the groin, scrotum, or testicle in men and to the groin or vulva in women, depending on the level of obstruction.

b. *Pyelonephritis.* Flank pain from pyelonephritis is more typically subacute in onset, constant and unrelenting in nature, and exacerbated by movement. A prodrome of cystitis symptoms is a helpful clue. There will usually be a high, spiking fever that is much less common with urinary calculi.

c. Ask about previous history of urolithiasis, UTIs, and urologic surgery.

3. Diagnostic studies

a. *Urinalysis.* Often helps to confirm the clinical diagnosis; with a patient having an uncomplicated stone, examination typically reveals red cells with few white cells or bacteria. Infected urine has red cells, white cells, and bacteria; white cell casts are diagnostic of pyelonephritis. A normal urinalysis does not rule out urologic pathology but should alert the clinician to the possibility of other disease processes. Crystals may help to identify the composition of calculi. When possible, the consultant should examine the urine him/herself.

b. *Non-contrast CT scan (NCCT).* This imaging modality is being used with increasing frequency by most ED physicians in evaluating flank pain. Virtually all calculi, with the exception of Indavir stones, can be visualized and the degree of hydronephrosis, if any, can be assessed rapidly. Although the positive predictive value of NCCT is high for detecting calculi, there are no specific signs for pyelonephritis unless IV contrast is given. NCCT may also reveal other abdominal pathology that account for the patient's symptoms.

c. *Plain radiograph [kidneys, ureters, and bladder film (KUB)].* Approximately 85 percent of stones are radiopaque and can be identified on a plain film. Care must be taken not to miss stones overlying the sacrum or lateral spinal processes and not to misinterpret pelvic phleboliths.

d. *White count and serum creatinine.* Although not truly diagnostic studies, they are useful in triaging the ED patient and should generally be obtained when evaluating patients with flank pain.

e. *Urine culture.* Although not immediately helpful, a properly obtained culture must be collected in the ED from all patients with flank pain.

Principle: When the patient's history, physical findings, urinalysis, and radiologic studies are all in accord with the diagnosis of a urinary calculus, the patient can usually be diagnosed and triaged from the ED without further evaluation (i.e., admitted or treated and discharged with follow-up). When these data are contradictory, further studies must be obtained so that an accurate diagnosis can be made and appropriate therapy instituted.

    f. *Intravenous urogram (IVU or IVP).* A key study in the diagnosis and planning of treatment of urolithiasis, the urogram is optimally performed after the patient has been properly prepared so that the films will be of the highest quality. Always inquire about previous contrast reactions and check the serum creatinine before administering intravenous contrast.

    g. *Other studies.* Ultrasound, contrast-enhanced computed tomography (CT), or nuclear renal scans may occasionally be obtained in the ED to triage the patient.

4. Indications for admission for renal calculi

    Many of these patients may require ureteral stenting or percutaneous nephrostomy tube placement.

    a. Obstructing stone in a patient with a solitary kidney.

    b. Fever and infection associated with an obstructing stone.

    c. Inability to maintain oral hydration.

    d. Pain refractory to oral analgesics.

    e. High-grade obstruction from a stone that is too large (more than 1 cm) to pass spontaneously (a relative indication).

Principle: A patient discharged with a diagnosis of a stone should be instructed to maintain aggressive oral hydration and strain his or her urine. A clear plan for urologic follow-up should be in place.

5. Pyelonephritis

    Although some clinicians prefer to admit all patients with pyelonephritis, selected cases can be successfully managed on an outpatient basis. Young, healthy patients with no underlying urologic disorder or immunodeficiency can be given a trial of outpatient therapy if they are moderately ill. A 14-day course of oral antibiotics such as fluoroquinolones are first-line therapy for outpatients. Again, a clear plan for follow-up with a primary care physician or urologist is essential.

C. Suprapubic Pain

1. *Differential diagnosis.* Urinary retention, cystitis, bladder stones, interstitial cystitis, various gastrointestinal and gynecologic problems. From a urologic standpoint, retention and cystitis must be diagnosed and treated in the ED, other entities can be evaluated on an outpatient basis.

2. *History and physical examination.* Obtain a history about voiding function prior to onset of pain. Inquire about gross hematuria or a history of urinary retention. Attempt to palpate the bladder during the abdominal examination. A pelvic examination in women is often critical. For the unusual patient with a continent reconstruction or bladder augmentation, maintain a high degree of suspicion for pouch rupture.

3. *Laboratory evaluation.* Collect a voided urine for urinalysis and a catheterized postvoid residual urine to rule out retention and send for culture (retention discussed in detail below). Consider general surgical or gynecologic consultation in patients with significant pain if the above studies are negative.

D. Acute Scrotum

Principle: Testicular evaluations can be quite challenging. Do not underestimate the acute scrotum!

1. Differential diagnosis
   Includes a number of conditions of widely varying immediacy, several of which are discussed elsewhere. The usual dilemma is differentiating torsion and epididymitis (Table 10-2).
   a. Testicular torsion
   b. Epididymitis

Table 10-2 Diagnosis of Testicular Torsion Versus Epididymitis

	TORSION	EPIDIDYMITIS
Age	Puberty to 4th decade, most commonly; occasionally neonates	Puberty to 8th decade
Onset	Acute	Gradual/subacute
Nausea	Common	Unusual
Pain	Severe	Moderate to severe
Pyrexia	Absent	May be present
Urinalysis	Normal	Pyuria common
Manual scrotal elevation	Pain constant	Pain diminished
Testicular position	Elevated/ abnormal lie	Normal

    c. Torsion of appendix testis/appendix epididymis

    d. Trauma (with intratesticular bleed or testicular rupture)

    e. Incarcerated hernia

    f. Testicular tumor (with acute bleed)

    g. Idiopathic scrotal edema

    h. Acute hydrocele

    i. Henoch-Schönlein purpura

2. Testicular torsion

    a. *Symptom complex.* Classically, the sudden onset of severe testicular pain that is constant and progressive, often associated with nausea, but not with fever, urethral discharge, or cystitis symptoms. Usually pubertal and teenage boys.

    b. *Physical examination and laboratory studies.* The testicle is high in scrotum, with a horizontal lie, absent cremasteric reflex, and no relief with elevation of the testis. The urinalysis is normal.

    c. *Radiology studies.* Color Doppler ultrasound has become a useful adjunct to the history and physical examination. Some clinicians consider it an essential part of the acute scrotum evaluation, if obtained in an expedient manner. False-positive and false-negative results have been reported. Nuclear scanning, while very accurate, is more difficult to obtain emergently.

    d. *Manual detorsion.* An attempt can be made to manually detorse the testicle. Manual detorsion is performed by rotating the testicle in a medial to lateral direction. If the consultant is at the patient's feet looking up, the left testicle would be turned clockwise and the right testicle turned counterclockwise. More than one complete turn may be necessary. Although manual detorsion can be performed in the ED by a urologist, emergent surgery is still required to assure complete detorsion and perform contralateral orchiopexy.

    e. *Surgery.* All patients should undergo immediate exploration to detorse and fix the testicle in the scrotum and for fixation of the contralateral testicle, as the bell-clapper anomaly is often bilateral. Necrotic or marginally viable gonads should be removed to reduce the risk of infection and decrease the risk of immune-mediated damage to the remaining gonad

    f. *Extravaginal torsion.* A rare form occurring in utero and in neonates. The spermatic cord rotates above the testis because the gubernacular attachments to the scrotal wall have not yet developed. There will be a hard, scrotal mass that does not transilluminate and is nontender. These testicles can occasionally be saved, but the value of operation and contralateral fixation versus the risk of surgery in a newborn remains controversial.

3. Torsion of testicular appendages

   a. *Origin.* The appendix testis and appendix epididymis, embryologic remnants of the müllerian system, may undergo torsion that can clinically simulate testicular torsion.

   b. *Symptoms.* Most often seen in prepubertal boys. Pain is more gradual in onset and mild in severity compared to testicular torsion.

   c. *Physical examination.* Classic physical findings are point tenderness and the "blue-dot sign" over the superior–posterior portion of the testicle. A reactive hydrocele may be found.

   d. *Treatment.* When the diagnosis is certain, the vast majority of cases will respond to analgesics such as NSAIDs alone. Inform the patient that the pain and scrotal swelling may worsen in the subsequent 48 to 72 hours after diagnosis.

   e. *Surgery.* Surgical exploration and excision of the torsed appendix are required in all questionable cases.

Principle: The etiology of an acute scrotum can usually be ascertained using the history, physical examination, and urinalysis. In most cases, color Doppler ultrasound can provide additional helpful information. Do NOT delay surgical exploration to obtain these studies if the history and physical are diagnostic of testicular torsion. When in doubt, it is always most prudent to take the patient to the operating room for exploration.

II. GROSS HEMATURIA
A. Etiology

1. *Common causes.* Infections, stones, malignancies (bladder, kidney), benign prostatic hyperplasia (BPH), trauma, postoperative.

2. *Less common causes.* Radiation or chemical (cyclophosphamide) cystitis, sickle cell disease/trait, glomerulonephritis, coagulopathy, vascular infarction/thrombosis, gastrointestinal or gynecologic pathology.

B. History and Evaluation

An algorithm for evaluating and initially treating the patient with gross hematuria is presented in Figure 10-1. Two key points should be emphasized: (1) determine if the hematuria is due to a UTI, if so, most patients do not need further workup; (2) determine if the patient is emptying his or her bladder well. If these questions can be answered, the patient may

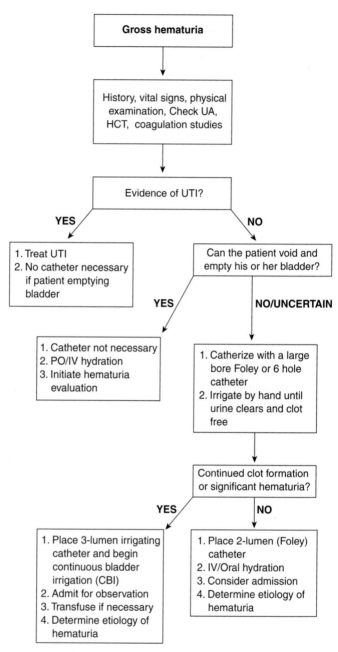

Figure 10-1 Gross hematuria evaluation and treatment algorithm.

be triaged and treated efficiently. When feasible, cystoscopy during an episode of gross hematuria can be valuable. This is particularly helpful in cases of intermittent bleeding from the upper tracts.

Principle: All patients presenting to the ED with gross hematuria must have urologic follow-up, even if the bleeding spontaneously resolves. Bladder tumors classically bleed intermittently and diagnosis can be delayed if patients are not appropriately counseled.

III. URINARY RETENTION

A. History

Age, general health, premorbid voiding symptoms, history of urethral strictures, previous episodes of retention, prior urologic manipulation or surgery (e.g., radical prostatectomy, TURP), medications (sympathomimetics, anticholinergics), and incontinence (sign of overflow retention).

B. Etiology

1. Anatomic obstruction
   a. BPH (most common)
   b. Urethral stricture
   c. Bladder neck contracture
   d. Prostate cancer (uncommon)
2. Functional obstruction
   a. Neurologic disease (CNS or peripheral)
   b. Medication side effect
   c. Pain (nociceptive retention), for example, postoperative or posttrauma
   d. Psychogenic

C. Management

The following outline is a standard management schema. However, prior to instrumenting the patient, a urologic history and a physical examination concentrating on the abdomen and perineum should be obtained. In most cases, a rectal examination should be performed. This information may significantly change the approach to the patient (i.e., the patient with acute prostatitis may be better served by a suprapubic tube initially; a patient with recurrent urethral strictures should be approached with a small catheter).

1. Attempt to pass an average-size Foley catheter (18 French). Consider instilling 10 to 20 mL of lubricating jelly into the urethra at this point, particularly if others have attempted catheterization and failed. The urologist will often be called upon to place a catheter in an otherwise healthy individual with no risk factors for anatomic

obstruction. Adequate lubrication of the catheter and urethra is perhaps the single most helpful intervention.

2. If this fails, try to determine the site of obstruction (urethra from stricture, prostate, bladder neck) and choose an appropriate catheter. For obstruction at the prostate secondary to BPH, attempt to pass a large, coudé-tipped Foley catheter (20 or 22 French) after instilling lubricating jelly into the urethra. The larger catheter will push aside the lateral prostatic lobes and the coudé tip will ride up over the median lobe when BPH is the cause of obstruction. For urethral strictures or bladder neck contractures, use a smaller catheter (12 or 14 French); however, most strictures significant enough to cause retention will not be bypassed with a smaller catheter.

3. If the previous is unsuccessful, the patient should be evaluated by a urologist. There are a number of options at this point that should be tailored to each situation.

   a. *Flexible cystoscopy.* Serves as a diagnostic and therapeutic modality and increasingly available at many hospitals with bedside cystoscopy carts. For strictures and bladder neck contractures, a guidewire can be passed under direct vision and a Council tip catheter can be passed over the wire. If a guidewire is not available, place a filiform under direct vision alongside the cystoscope and then dilate.

   b. *Filiforms and followers.* Useful in those with a history of prior urethral surgery, TURP, or RRP. Carefully pass a filiform into the bladder then thread a follower for drainage and dilation. Filiforms and followers carry an increased risk of iatrogenic trauma compared to cystoscopy.

4. When blind attempts at transurethral drainage are fruitless or inadvisable, the urology consultant will commonly elect to place a percutaneous suprapubic tube (SPT) with one of many commercially available kits designed for use under local anesthesia.

5. No patient in retention should be instrumented, drained, and then discharged from the ED without a clear plan for urologic follow-up.

D. Potential Complications after Relief of Obstruction

1. Post-obstructive diuresis (urine output more than 200 mL/h for 2 h)

   a. Caused by a combination of tubular damage and osmotic load and a transient impairment in the nephron's ability to concentrate urine.

   b. May result in hyponatremia, hypokalemia, hypovolemia, hypomagnesimia.

    c. Risk factors for post-obstructive diuriesis—hypertension, long-standing obstruction, signs of volume overload, renal failure, solitary kidney.

    d. Most patients do not exhibit a post-obstructive diuresis.

    e. Those patients that do develop a post-obstructive diuresis will often require admission for IV hydration and electrolyte monitoring.

2. *Hypotension.* Can be secondary to vasovagal response to relief of distention or relief of pelvic venous compression following bladder drainage.

3. *Hemorrhage ex vacuo.* An uncommon and rarely reported complication. Hematuria caused by bladder mucosal disruption following relief of long-standing obstruction. Hematuria resolves spontaneously in most cases.

IV. OLIGURIA AND ANURIA
A. Definition
Anuria is defined as urine output of less than 50 mL/24 h.

B. Differential Diagnosis
The causes of anuria are myriad; a careful history and physical examination will usually narrow the list of possibilities to a handful of causes, which can then be pursued through appropriate laboratory and radiographic tests.

Principle: The urologist is called upon to treat or exclude all types of obstructive uropathy in the anuric patient. Although it is not always possible or even appropriate to do so in the ED, the workup should be done promptly.

C. Evaluation and Treatment
1. Physical examination and urethral catheterization
Even when the patient is not in urinary retention, an indwelling Foley catheter will usually be necessary to monitor response to therapy.

2. Ultrasonography

    a. *Bilateral hydronephrosis.* Cystoscopy with bilateral retrograde pyelograms and double-J ureteral stent placement or bilateral percutaneous nephrostomy tube placement are diagnostic and therapeutic maneuvers. Alternatively, noncontrast CT or MRI of the abdomen can be obtained for diagnostic purposes in the patient with normal renal function, volume status, and electrolyte balance. In general, relief of obstruction is first and foremost.

    b. *No hydronephrosis.* Obstructive uropathy is unlikely in this setting, although false negative may be seen in dehydration, at the acute onset of obstruction, in retroperitoneal fibrosis, and in patients with an intrarenal collecting system. A nuclear renal scan is essential to complete the evaluation if the cause is unknown. Arteriography is needed only if the nuclear scan shows absent perfusion and other causes of prerenal azotemia have been ruled out.

c. *Unilateral hydronephrosis.* Either the dilated side is not truly obstructed or the nondilated side functions minimally. In either case, cystoscopy with retrograde catheterization of the dilated side will clarify the situation and treat the patient who is obstructed.

V. PRIAPISM

A. Definition

Priapism is the pathologic prolongation of penile erection, accompanied by pain and tenderness, but not by sexual excitement, and not relieved by orgasm.

B. Classification

1. Low-flow or ischemic
   a. Idiopathic
   b. Oral or injectable therapy for impotence
   c. Prescription drug—trazadone, chlorpromazine, others
   d. Recreational drug—alcohol, cocaine
   e. Sickle cell disease
   f. Neoplasm—leukemia, genitourinary neoplasm
2. High-flow or nonischemic
   a. Trauma (the vast majority of cases)
   b. Idiopathic

Principle: It is critical to diagnose high-flow priapism to avoid potentially traumatic interventions that are uniformly ineffective (e.g., shunting). Observation is appropriate if the diagnosis is established.

C. Pathophysiology

Great advances have been made in recent years in the understanding of the physiology of penile erection and priapism (Broderick and Lue). Priapism is a result of impairment of detumescence resulting in an abnormal steady state of penile blood flow and drainage. This can be either a high- or low-flow state depending on the inciting event, with the latter being much more common.

D. Evaluation

1. History and physical examination
   Identify risk factors and obtain medication and drug history. Penis is fully firm and 60 to 100 percent erect except

for the glans, which will be flaccid. Tenderness to palpation increases with time in ischemic priapism. Inspect for any evidence of perineal trauma.

2. Corporal aspiration, penile blood gas determination, and CBC
   Useful in differentiating between low- and high-flow priapism. In the former, the aspirate is dark, whereas in high-flow priapism, bright red arterial blood is seen. CBC diagnoses cases of malignant priapism due to leukemia. See Figure 10-2 for penile blood gas ranges.

E. Treatment

1. *Low-flow priapism.* A treatment algorithm for most causes of low-flow priapism is outlined in Figure 10-2 with corporal aspiration, irrigation, injection of alpha-agonists, and surgical shunting employed sequentially. Recommended doses of therapeutics are listed as follows.
   a. Epinephrine: 10 to 20 μg in normal saline per dose.
   b. Phenylephrine: 100 to 200 μg in normal saline per dose.
   c. Both of these medications have significant hemodynamic side effects. Blood pressure and pulse monitoring is mandatory in high-risk patients such as the elderly and patients with a history of hypertension or coronary artery disease.

2. *Sickle cell priapism.* More common in pediatric patients and African Americans. A result of red blood cell sludging impairing venous outflow.
   a. Initial management should include intravenous hydration and oxygenation. If no response, hypertransfusion has been effective in some cases.
   b. If conservative measures fail, proceed to corporal irrigation and shunting procedures.

3. *High-flow priapism.* Almost always posttraumatic where a fistula between the corporal tissue and a cavernosal artery has been created.
   a. Cavernosal blood gas determination is diagnostic (Fig. 10-2).
   b. Radiologic evaluation with angiography is the most useful initial study. Embolization at the time of angiography is considered first-line therapy. Color Doppler ultrasound can be a useful initial diagnostic study if angiography is not available. High-flow priapism may be observed as this is not an ischemic state.

4. Nonspecific therapies such as enemas, prostatic massage, pressure dressings, estrogens, antispasmodics, ice packs, anticoagulants, and anesthesia are outmoded. Sedation and analgesics may be appropriate but are not substitutes for effective, standard therapy as outlined previously.

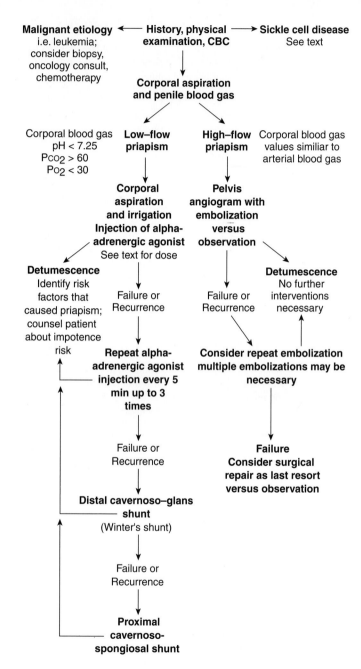

Figure 10-2 Priapism management algorithm.

F. Sequelae

Vascular thrombosis and fibrosis of the erectile tissues leading to impotence is reported in 50 percent of patients, regardless of treatment, by historical data. The patient should be so informed at the outset. There is evidence that early intervention improves outcome but even prompt, appropriate therapy may not prevent ultimate damage.

VI. FORESKIN EMERGENCIES

A. Phimosis

The uncircumcised foreskin cannot be retracted over the glans. This rarely requires emergency treatment as the patient can usually be catheterized with a coudé tip catheter if necessary. Nasal speculums can provide exposure to the meatus. In unusually severe cases, a dorsal slit may be required to allow catheterization. A dorsal slit is the initial treatment of choice for the patient with severe balanitis associated with phimosis. The initial incision is made at the 12 o'clock position after an adequate penile anesthetic block has been established.

B. Paraphimosis

The uncircumcised foreskin has been left in the retracted position resulting in obstruction to venous and lymphatic drainage and progressive edema. Treatment is immediate manual reduction. The consultant's fingers are placed behind the foreskin and steady pressure is applied to the glans (Fig. 10-3). Dorsal slit may also be used if manual reduction is not successful.

C. Zipper Injuries

A common source of genital lacerations, initial management involves adequate analgesia and disassembly of the zipper. Using a wire cutter or bone cutter, the median bar of the zipper is completely cut, allowing the teeth of the zipper to fall apart (Fig. 10-4).

D. Foreign Bodies

1. *External rings.* Often used as sexual aids, these constricting bands can cause edema, urethral fistula, or necrosis if left in place chronically. Most can be acutely managed with standard ring cutters. Likewise, pierced objects can become a nidus of infection. Immediate removal of the object and debridement if necessary constitute the initial management.
2. Intraurethral foreign bodies
   a. Evaluate radiographically.

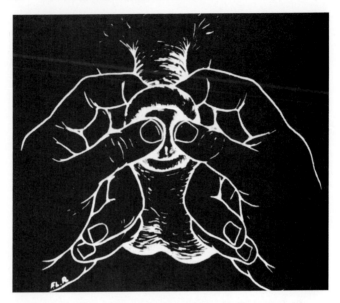

Figure 10-3 Manual reduction of paraphimosis. *(Reproduced from Lawrence PF: Essentials of Surgical Subspecialties. Baltimore, Williams & Wilkins, 1993 with permission.)*

    b. Do not catheterize the patient. Place a suprapubic tube if in retention.

    c. If distal to the external sphincter, the object will be palpable and can often be removed endoscopically.

    d. If proximal to the sphincter, open extraction is usually required.

E. Post-Circumcision Complications

    1. *Hematoma.* Most common problem. Can usually be drained by removing a stitch or two and evacuating the clot. Replace dressing.

    2. Bleeding

       a. Apply steady pressure for 10 to 15 min. If not effective, soak gauze in lidocaine containing 1:100,000 epinephrine and apply pressure with gauze for an additional 10 to 15 min.

       b. Skin edges may be cauterized with silver nitrate sticks.

       c. Significant bleeding may require suture placement under penile block with lidocaine.

    3. *Disruption of incision.* If small, no treatment; if major, place a few interrupted sutures under penile block.

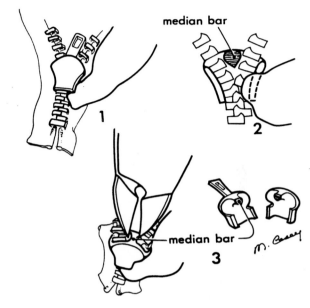

Figure 10-4 Technique for zipper disassembly in penile avulsion injuries. *(Reproduced from Flowerdrew R, et al. Management of the penile zipper injury. J Urol 117: 671, 1977, with permission.)*

4. *Infection.* Uncommon and usually minor; can almost always be treated with oral cephalosporins.

BIBLIOGRAPHY

Broderick GA, Lue TF: Priapism and the physiology of erection. American Urological Association Office of Education Baltimore, MD *AUA Update Series,* vol. 7, lesson 29, 1988.

Flowerdrew R, Fishman IJ, Churchill BM: Management of the penile zipper injury. *J Urol* 117:671, 1977.

Gulmi F, Felsen D, Vaughan ED: Pathophysiology of urinary tract obstruction. In: Walsh P, Retik AB, Vaughan ED, Wein AJ, eds: *Campbell's Urology,* 7th ed. Philadelphia: Saunders, 1998, p 375.

Somers WJ, Badalament RA, York JP, et al: Urology: Diseases of the genitourinary system. In: Lawrence PF, Bell RM, Dayton MT, eds: *Essentials of Surgical Subspecialties.* Baltimore: Williams & Wilkins, 1993, p 381.

CHAPTER 11
Urologic Trauma

Steven B. Brandes
Michael Yu

Traumatic injuries to the genitourinary system are commonly divided into injuries to the external genitalia, urethra, bladder, ureter, and kidney. The primary goal in the management of such traumatic injuries is to preserve the maximal amount of functional tissue while minimizing the complications. Complications can occur because of missed urologic injury at the time of initial presentation, the nature and severity of the injury itself, and/or inadequate or inappropriate initial management. Minimizing delayed complication occurrence can be achieved by appropriately staging the injuries, followed by the proper selection of surgery or expectant therapy.

I. TRAUMATIC RENAL INJURIES
A. Introduction
1. At major urban trauma centers, the kidneys are injured in 1.1 to 5 percent of all trauma cases. Renal trauma comprises about half of all GU trauma. Both kidneys are at equal disposition for injury.
2. Depending on the trauma center, renal injuries commonly result from blunt trauma (80 to 90 percent) and from penetrating trauma (10 to 20 percent). The percent of penetrating renal injuries are highest (up 30 percent) at inner-city trauma centers.
3. Blunt trauma includes falls from height, motor vehicle and cycle accidents, and direct blows to the abdomen, flank, and back.
4. Children (less than 16 years-old) are more prone to renal injury due to the relative large size of the kidney, scant perirenal fat, underdeveloped Gerota's fascia, and incomplete ossification of the lower ribs.
5. Penetrating renal injuries are the result of gunshots and stab wounds. Of penetrating abdominal wounds, only 7 to 10 percent involve the kidney. Conversely, associated

injuries occur in 77 to 100 percent of penetrating renal trauma.
6. The majority of renal injuries are grade 1. Such injuries heal spontaneously without adverse sequelae and require no imaging or active treatment.
7. Of traumatic renal injuries, only 4 percent of blunt trauma and 67 percent of penetrating trauma are significant renal injuries (grade 2 to 5).
8. Proper radiographic staging of renal injuries (grade 2 to 5) enables the potential management in a nonoperative/conservative fashion.

B. Initial Evaluation

1. Hematuria is the hallmark of renal injury. The degree of hematuria, however, does not correlate well with the extent of injury. The first voided or catheterized urine is analyzed for blood. Dipstick is adequate for the detection of microscopic hematuria. A small percentage of renal injuries, including 19 to 40 percent of renal pedicle injuries, will not present with hematuria.
2. Blunt trauma
   a. A history is gathered to quantify the forces involved in the renal injury, such as the speed of the vehicle and the height of the fall.
   b. Falls from a height or high-speed motor vehicle accidents imply deceleration injury and the need to rule out renal pedicle and ureteropelvic junction (UPJ) injury.
   c. All patients with severe multiple trauma to the flank, abdomen, or lower chest should be suspected of having a renal injury, regardless of the presence or absence of hematuria.
   d. Seemingly minor trauma that results in a significant renal injury usually occurs in a congenitally abnormal kidney (e.g., UPJ).
   e. Physical examination can detect clinical indicators of blunt renal injury, such as flank ecchymosis, lower rib fractures, and transverse process fractures.
3. Penetrating trauma
   a. Information on the type of firearm used and the caliber of the bullet is helpful to differentiate between high and low velocity missiles. The entrance and exit wound sites should also be noted. High velocity missiles (faster than 2200 ft/sec) cause both entrance and exit wounds, extensive soft tissue injury, and often delayed tissue necrosis due to a "blast" effect. Low velocity missiles generally do not cause severe renal injuries, unless the missiles passes through the renal hilum or collecting system.

    b. Site of the stab wound (SW) in relation to the anterior axillary line (AAL) is important. Entrance wounds anterior to the AAL and below the nipple line are often associated with intra-abdominal injuries. Wounds posterior to the AAL are less likely to have associated intraperitoneal organ injury, and thus these renal injuries can usually be managed conservatively. It is also important to note the length of the knife blade, so as to help predict the degree or depth of the injury.

C. Indications for Renal Imaging

1. Blunt trauma and gross hematuria. Hematuria is the hallmark of renal injury. However, hematuria does not correlate and cannot predict the degree or extent of renal injury. Hematuria is absent in up to 40 percent of renal vascular injuries. Hematuria is not a sensitive or specific test to differentiate minor from major renal injuries

2. Blunt trauma, microscopic hematuria, and shock. Significant microscopic hematuria is more than 5 RBC/HPF in the first voided or catheterized specimen. Shock is considered as systolic blood pressure less than 90 mm Hg during transport or on arrival in the emergency room.

3. Major acceleration or deceleration injury (e.g., fall from height, high-speed auto accident).

4. Microscopic or gross hematuria after penetrating flank, back, or abdominal trauma; or when the missile path, as evidence by entrance and exit sites, are in line with the kidney.

5. Pediatric (younger than 16 years) trauma patient with any degree of significant hematuria.

6. Associated injuries and physical signs suggesting underlying renal injury (e.g., flank ecchymosis/tenderness, lumbar spine fractures, 11th or 12th posterior rib fractures).

D. Imaging Studies

1. Intravenous urogram (IVU)

    a. In stable patients, abdominal computed tomography (CT) has generally replaced the IVU in the trauma setting. Prior to the advent of CT, IVU with nephrotomography were first-line studies employed to outline cortical borders and thus demonstrate more clearly any cortical lacerations, intrarenal hematomas, and/or areas of poor vascular perfusion. Such imaging can accurately stage the renal injury in 85 to 90 percent of cases.

    b. In unstable patients who require immediate laparotomy, a one-shot IVU should be performed prior to any renal exploration. Two mL per kg of body weight of standard 60 percent intravenous contrast is given, followed by a single abdominal radiograph 10 min later. No scout film is necessary. In children, 2 to 3 mL/kg of nonionic contrast is preferred.

c. The one-shot IVU determines the function of the contralateral kidney, the presence and extent of any urinary extravasation, and in penetrating injuries, the likely course of the missile. The nephrogram of the injured kidney is often poorly opacified and worsened by any hemodynamic instability. IVP performed during hypotension usually results in a faint nephrogram and delayed excretion simulating a pedicle injury.

d. Failure to visualize an enhancing kidney, persistence of the renal nephrogram, or enhancement of only a segment of the kidney, suggest significant renal parenchymal or pedicle injury.

e. Significant perirenal hematoma is suggested by an obscured renal outline, loss of the ipsilateral psoas margin, and/or displacement of the bowel or ureter. Abnormal or equivocal studies generally warrant further imaging or surgical exploration.

2. Computed tomography

a. CT is the imaging study of choice for evaluating the hemodynamically stable trauma patient. It is both sensitive and specific for demonstrating contusions, hematomas, renal parenchymal lacerations, and urinary extravasations; delineating segmental parenchymal infarcts; and for determining the size and location of the retroperitoneal hematoma and/or associated intra-abdominal organ injuries.

b. CT can also accurately define the extent of renal parenchymal vascular perfusion and evaluate any injuries to the hilum and great vessels. Renal vein injuries, however, are often difficult to detect, but are inferred by the presence of hematoma medial to the kidney that displaces the renal vasculature.

c. Renal artery occlusion and renal infarct are noted by lack of parenchymal enhancement or by a persistent "cortical rim sign." The rim sign, however, is usually not seen until 8 hours or more after injury.

d. Helical CT imaging is very quick and thus may understage many traumatic renal injuries. To detect renal parenchymal and venous injuries, later imaging into the nephrogram phase (longer than 80 sec) is often needed to detect renal parenchymal and venous injuries. To select urine and blood extravasation, delayed images (2 to 10 min) are also often needed.

3. Ultrasonography

a. Primarily used in Europe for evaluating renal trauma. Accurate and reliable in experienced hands.

   b. Useful for demonstrating perirenal fluid collections. Limitations, however, include an inability to distinguish fresh blood from extravasated urine and to identify vascular pedicle injuries or segmental infarcts.
   c. Visualization is poor when associated injuries are present, such as rib fractures, bandages, ileus, open wounds, and immobility. Pulsed Doppler, furthermore, is needed to diagnose a vascular injury.
4. Arteriography
   a. Presently, rarely used to evaluate renal injury since the advent of CT. More time-consuming, requires more technical expertise, more invasive, and provides little extra information over CT.
   b. Arteriography and superselective embolization, however, have important roles in the evaluation and treatment of posttraumatic delayed renal bleeding or arteriovenous fistulas. In recent anecdotal reports, arteriography and endoluminal stent placement have also been successful in managing renal artery intimal tears from blunt trauma.

E. Injury Scaling

The Organ Injury Scaling Committee of the American Association for the Surgery of Trauma has classified five grades of traumatic renal injuries (Table 11-1), ranging from least to most severe (I to V). Grades I and II renal injuries are considered minor and are commonly managed expectantly. Grade III are those with deep parenchymal lacerations that do not involve the collecting system. Grade IV injuries have deep parenchymal lacerations, urinary extravasation, heavy bleeding, and/or vascular injury. Grade IV also includes confined renal arterial and venous injuries. Only life-threatening injuries are graded V, namely pedicle avulsion or totally shattered kidney.

F. Indications for Renal Exploration

To select a nonoperative management strategy, the renal injury needs to be imaged and accurately staged. An incompletely staged renal injury requires surgical exploration. Not all penetrating renal injuries require surgical exploration. Roughly three of four renal gunshot wounds, one of two renal stab wounds, and only 2 percent of blunt renal injuries demand exploration.

1. *Blunt trauma.* The overall evaluation and management of adult renal injuries is detailed in Figure 11-1.
2. *Absolute indications.* Persistent and potentially life-threatening renal bleeding.

Table 11-1 AAST Classification of Traumatic Renal Injuries

GRADE	INJURY	INJURY DESCRIPTION
I	Contusion	Micro or gross hematuria with no renal injury on radiographic studies.
	Hematoma	Subcapsular hematoma, nonexpanding and without parenchymal laceration.
II	Hematoma	Perirenal hematoma, nonexpanding and well contained.
	Laceration	Renal cortex laceration <1cm in depth and without urinary extravasation.
III	Laceration	Renal cortex laceration >1cm in depth and no urinary extravasation.
IV	Laceration	Renal cortex laceration extending into the collecting system (as noted by contrast extravasation on imaging).
	Vascular	Renal artery or vein injury with a contained hematoma. Segmental renal artery or vein injury (noted by a segmental parenchymal infarct). Thrombosis of the main renal artery.
V	Laceration	Completely shattered kidney.
	Vascular	Avulsion of the renal hilum with kidney devascularization.

After Moore EE, Shackford SR, Pachter HL, et al: Organ injury scaling: Spleen, liver, and kidney. *J Trauma* 29:1664, 1989.

   a. Signs of continued renal bleeding are the presence of a pulsatile, expanding or unconfined retroperitoneal hematoma. Such retroperitoneal hematomas should be explored.
   b. Stable retroperitoneal hematomas can be safely observed, as long as proper preoperative or intraoperative radiographic studies document a renal injury that can be observed safely.
   c. Grade V injuries involve avulsion of the main renal artery or vein or a shattered kidney with massive tissue destruction. By definition, these injuries are life-threatening, and thus demand surgical exploration to prevent potential exsanguination.
3. *Relative indications.* Devitalized parenchyma.
   a. A major devitalized renal segment (more than 25 percent) is a relative indication.
   b. When associated with intra-abdominal injuries (e.g., colon, pancreas), urinary extravasation, extensive re-

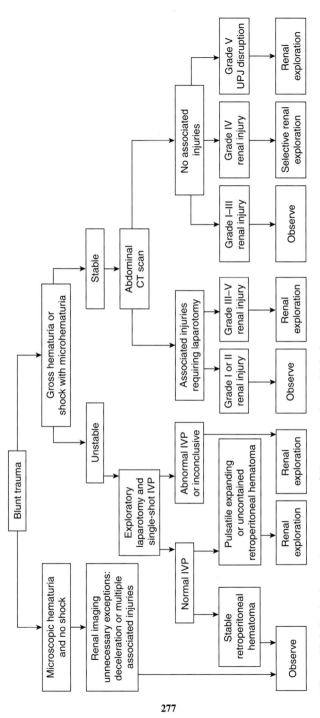

Figure 11-1 Evaluation and management of blunt traumatic renal injuries.

277

nal injury, and a large retroperitoneal hematoma, renal exploration should be particularly considered.

4. *Relative indications.* Urinary extravasation.
   a. In itself, does not demand surgical exploration. The majority (more than 75 percent) resolve spontaneously (usually within 72 hours).
   b. Contemporary series support the safety and efficacy of the nonoperative management of most blunt renal injuries with urinary extravasation.
   c. Complications (e.g., delayed urinomas or persistent urinary leaks), however, occur slightly more frequently. Yet, when they do occur, they can be successfully managed percutaneously or endoscopically, and do not decrease the renal salvage rate.
   d. UPJ avulsion injuries do not heal spontaneously and are best managed by prompt surgical repair. In all blunt renal injuries it is also important that delayed images visualize contrast distal to the UPJ to rule out a complete disruption. Medial extravasation of contrast is suggestive of UPJ injury.

5. *Relative indications.* Incomplete staging.
   a. Complete definition of the renal injury by appropriate imaging studies permits the selection of nonoperative management.
   b. Incomplete staging demands either further imaging or renal exploration.

6. *Relative indications.* Arterial thrombosis.
   a. Renal artery occlusion usually occurs from a major deceleration injury where the main renal artery is stretched and the less elastic intima is torn, leading to vessel thrombosis and kidney infarction.
   b. Renal salvage is remote after 12 hours of ischemia.
   c. If the contralateral kidney is normal and diagnosis prompt, it is controversial to attempt revascularization because overall, preservation of renal function is poor. In only 20 to 56 percent of such cases is more than 17 percent of differential function preserved.
   d. Patients with isolated renal artery thrombosis not associated with extensive bleeding or urinary extravasation are best managed conservatively, particularly when renal ischemia exceeds 12 hours. Blood pressures should also be periodically monitored for the development of renal induced hypertension. Revascularization should be reserved only for bilateral renal artery occlusion or unilateral occlusion in a solitary kidney, regardless of the ischemic time.

7. *Relative indications.* Celiotomy for associated injuries. When the abdomen is explored for an associated intra-abdominal injury (in particular, colon and pancreas), it is reasonable to also repair all preoperatively staged grade III and IV renal injuries. Although somewhat controversial, repair of radiographically staged grade III to IV renal injuries at the time of celiotomy is safe and effective and helps reduce potential urologic complications, such as urinoma, abscess, fistula, hydronephrosis, and stone formation.

G. Penetrating Trauma

Overall evaluation and management of adult penetrating renal trauma is detailed in Figure 11-2.

1. *Absolute indications.* The absolute indications for exploration are the same as for blunt renal injuries, namely persistent or potentially life-threatening renal bleeding.

2. *Relative indications*
   a. Theoretically, grade for grade, renal injuries should be managed the same way whether the mechanism is penetrating or blunt. This is true for grade I and II renal injuries, which can be managed conservatively.
   b. Penetrating grade III and IV renal injuries, however, particularly stab wounds, generally should be managed surgically due to a high rate of delayed bleeds (24 percent). This discrepancy may be due to a delayed gunshot blast injury, which is not seen on initial imaging, and to arteriovenous fistula formation, which more commonly occurs after a stab wound.
   c. Since all gunshot wounds (GSWs) that penetrate the peritoneal cavity undergo celiotomy, unexpected retroperitoneal hematomas are often encountered. All retroperitoneal hematomas demand exploration unless preoperative CT staging shows the renal injury to be grade I or II. One-shot IVP is often not sensitive enough for such staging.
   d. Stab wounds to the kidney posterior to the anterior axillary line are less likely to have associated visceral injuries, and thus more likely to undergo successful conservative management of their renal injury.

H. Management

1. Surgical methods of renal exploration and reconstruction
   a. The injured kidney is best exposed through a standard midline transperitoneal incision from the xiphoid process to the symphysis pubis.
   b. In the stable trauma patient, associated intra-abdominal injuries should be systematically examined and

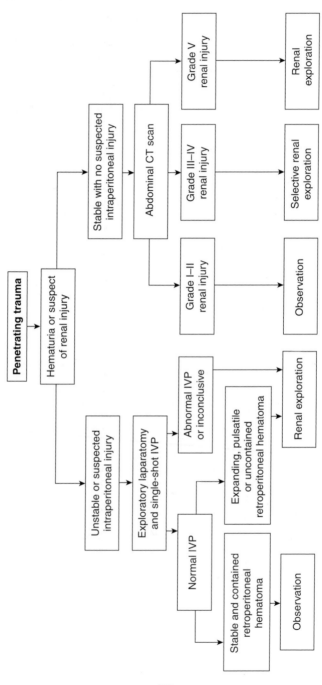

Figure 11-2 Evaluation and management of penetrating trauma to the kidney.

repaired prior to the kidney injury. When renal bleeding is massive or persistent (as in a renal hilar injury), however, the kidney should be explored first.

c. Classic teaching dictates that vascular control take place before renal exploration. The efficacy of consistent proximal vascular control of the renal pedicle prior to opening Gerota's fascia is demonstrated by a reduction in the overall nephrectomy rate, from the usual 31 to 56 percent, to a low of 11 to 15 percent.

d. Temporary occlusion of the renal artery is uncommon (11 to 17 percent) and usually needed in patients with renal vascular injuries, those in shock, and those with large or expanding retroperitoneal hematomas. Bleeding from the cut edge of the injured kidney usually can be easily controlled by digital compression, with no need for arterial occlusion.

e. Nephrectomy should be reserved for irreparable vascular or parenchymal injuries or for persistent hemodynamic instability, and thus as a life-saving maneuver.

f. In the absence of persistent hemodynamic instability or coagulopathy, renal reconstruction is safe and effective.

g. The method of kidney reconstruction is dictated by the degree and location of the injury, and not by the associated intra-abdominal injuries. Even a concomitant pancreatic or a colonic injury with frank fecal contamination are not contraindications to renal reconstruction. Furthermore, the resulting complication rates are only slightly increased.

h. The following are reconstructive principles for renal injures.

1. Broad exposure of the kidney and injured area.
2. Temporary vascular occlusion for brisk renal bleeding, when not well controlled by manual compression of the parenchyma.
3. Sharp excision of all nonviable parenchyma.
4. Meticulous hemostasis.
5. Watertight closure of the collecting system.
6. Parenchymal defect closure by approximation of the capsular edges over a Gelfoam bolster or coverage with omentum, perinephric fat, peritoneum, or polyglycolic acid mesh.
7. Interposition of a omental pedicle flap between the vascular, colonic, or pancreatic injury and the injured kidney.
8. Ureteral stent placement for a renal pelvis or ureteral injury.
9. Retroperitoneal drain.

2. *Nonoperative and conservative.* Properly staged and selected renal injuries can be successfully managed conservatively with the following steps.
   a. Strict bed rest until the urine visibly clears.
   b. Close monitoring of vital signs.
   c. Hematocrit, blood drawn every 6 hours until stable.
   d. Broad-spectrum antibiotics.
   e. Transfusions to keep the hematocrit stable. The confined spaces of the retroperitoneum and Gerota's envelope can tamponade and limit bleeding. Transfusion requirements of more than 4 to 6 units in 24 hours demand repeat imaging and possible arteriography and embolization or surgical exploration.
   f. For grade IV renal injuries, consider re-imaging the kidney 3 to 5 days after initial injury for persistent urinary leakage.

I. Complications after Renal Trauma

1. Complications are dependent on the grade of the initial renal injury and the method of management, and usually occur within 1 month of injury.
2. Early complications
   a. Prolonged urinary extravasation is the most common complication after renal trauma. Urinomas occur in less than 1 percent of renal trauma cases. Small, uninfected, and stable collections do not require intervention. Larger collections are prone to abscess formation and sepsis, and can commonly be easily managed by percutaneous catheter drainage.
   b. Shock from massive blood loss.
   c. Renal infarction.
   d. Abscess formation.
3. Late complications
   a. Other complications include delayed bleeding, arteriovenous fistula, abscess, urinary fistula, and hydronephrosis. In general, complications are usually of minimal long-term morbidity, can be successfully managed noninvasively, and do not significantly prolong the length of stay.
   b. Renal vascular hypertension after renal trauma is commonly transient. Sustained or delayed hypertension, such as by a Page or Goldblatt kidney are renin mediated and rare events (less than 1 percent). Careful monitoring of blood pressure for several months after injury should still be employed.
   c. Perinephric fibrosis that involves the UPJ, as usually seen after a lower pole kidney injury, can result in hydronephrosis. To prevent such occurrences, interposi-

tion of perirenal fat or omentum between the kidney and the ureter is effective.

d. At 3 to 6 months after a renal injury, follow-up imaging (IVU or CT) should be obtained to evaluate for delayed hydronephrosis, vascular compromise, or renal atrophy.

II. URETERAL AND RENAL PELVIS INJURIES

A. Mechanisms of Injury

1. External trauma

   a. Penetrating ureteral injuries are rare, with only 2.5 percent of all abdominal GSWs involving the ureter. Overall, ureteral injuries are 95 percent due to penetrating and 5 percent to a blunt mechanism (such as rapid acceleration or deceleration, as in falls from a height or motor vehicle accidents).

   b. High velocity missiles cause more surrounding and delayed tissue injury than low velocity bullets. GSWs near the ureter can result in severe ureteral contusion due to a blast effect.

   c. After a deceleration injury the kidney is often dislocated, and tears can occur at its fixation points, namely the UPJ and hilar vasculature. Another mechanism for injury is hyperextension of the back, where the ureter is avulsed by being stretched by the lumbar and lower thoracic vertebral bodies. This classically occurs in children because they are very limber.

2. Surgical trauma

   a. Ureteral injuries usually occur during difficult and/or bloody pelvic operations. Overall, the ureter is injured in only 0.5 to 1.0 percent of pelvic operations.

   b. Iatrogenic injuries commonly occur during the course of the following surgeries. Urology: ureteroscopy, vesicourethral suspension, or radical prostatectomy; gynecology: hysterectomy, salpingo-oophorectomy, or cystocele repair; colorectal surgery: abdominoperineal resection; and vascular surgery: aortic and iliac graft surgery.

   c. Of all surgeries, iatrogenic ureteral injury most commonly occurs during hysterectomy. Sites of common injury are at the uterine vessels and the cardinal and uterosacral ligaments.

B. Diagnosis of Ureteral Injury

Successful surgical management of collecting system injuries requires a high index of suspicion, early diagnosis (and thus a low threshold for urinary tract imaging), and an intimate knowledge of ureteral anatomy and blood supply.

1. Preoperative diagnosis
   a. Hematuria (gross or microscopic) is not a reliable sign and is absent in 23 to 45 percent of penetrating ureteral injuries and absent in 31 to 67 percent of blunt UPJ injuries. In the absence of hematuria, a high index of suspicion is required to diagnose ureteral injuries reliably. Furthermore, injuries can be missed due to multisystem life-threatening injuries that preclude radiographic evaluation
2. Missed ureteral injury diagnosis
   a. Ureteral injuries are morbid and potentially lethal when they are unrecognized and present in a delayed fashion.
   b. Clinical signs of a missed injury usually do not become obvious for days. Early physical signs are usually nonspecific and include: prolonged ileus, elevated BUN (blood urea nitrogen), persistent flank or abdominal pain, palpable abdominal mass, prolonged drainage from drain sites, urinary obstruction, sepsis, abscess, or peritonitis.
3. Imaging
   a. *IVU.* Intravenous urography is the primary imaging study employed to evaluate ureteral integrity. Accuracy in diagnosing a ureteral injury is very variable and thus considered unreliable. IVP findings suggestive of ureteral injury are incomplete visualization of the entire ureter, ureteral deviation or dilatation, urinary extravasation, hydronephrosis, and delayed or nonvisualization of the injured renal unit. Retrograde pyelography (RPG), although accurate in demonstrating the site presence and location of extravasation, it is both time consuming and cumbersome. RPG thus has little role in the acute trauma setting.
   b. *CT.* CT has been used with increasing frequency to evaluate ureteral trauma. Medial perirenal extravasation of contrast is the most common finding of renal pelvic/ureteral injury. The use of quick imaging spiral CT scanners or the presence of hypotension or significant renal injury can make opacification of the collecting system poor and thus decrease overall imaging sensitivity. On CT or IVU, avulsion of the UPJ can be inferred by the presence of medial perirenal contrast extravasation and no filling of the ipsilateral ureter. Lacerations of the UPJ also have medial contrast extravasation; however, contrast is seen in the ipsilateral ureter distal to the UPJ.
4. Intraoperative diagnosis
   a. The majority of penetrating ureteral injuries are diagnosed intraoperatively.

    b. Direct exploration is the most accurate method for diagnosis.

    c. Ureteral peristalsis is not a reliable indication of viability or of adequate vascularity.

    d. The most reliable way to determine ureteral viability is by incision and monitoring for a bleeding edge.

    e. Intravenous indigo carmine is also helpful in identifying ureteral injury by extravasation of blue dye from the injury site. Cystotomy and retrograde injection of indigo carmine by pediatric feeding tube is another method to test ureteral integrity.

C. Classification

1. Location of the ureteral injury.
2. Mechanism and manner of injury: avulsion (UPJ), contusion, transection, devascularization, crush, ligation, resection, fulguration.
3. AAST Injury Scale.

D. Associated Injuries

1. Patients with penetrating ureteral injuries are usually multiorgan system injured. Over 90 percent have concomitant bowel, iliac vessel, liver, and vena caval injury.
2. Patients with blunt ureteral trauma also commonly suffer from associated injuries (77 percent), such as the liver, long bones, head, and diaphragm.

E. Management

1. General considerations. The patient's overall physical condition, presence of associated injuries, any delay in diagnosis, and the level and full extent of ureteral injury.

    a. Promptly diagnosed ureteral injuries should be explored and reconstructed through a midline transperitoneal incision.

    b. Lack of bleeding from the cut edge suggests ischemia and warrants ureteral debridement until viable tissue appears.

    c. Ureteral contusions or bruising due to potential proximity blast injury should be, at a minimum, stented and a retroperitoneal drain placed. With severe contusions, the ureter should be segmentally resected, debrided and reanastomosed over a stent. If the blast injured ureter is not resected, then a double-J stent and retroperitoneal drain adjacent to the area of concern should be placed.

    d. Major iatrogenic ureteral crush injuries should have the segment excised. Formal reconstruction is dependent on the location of the injury (see below). Minor crush injuries should have a stent placed either endo-scopically or through a cystotomy.

e. The surgical principles for successful ureteral repair are:

1. Careful ureteral mobilization preserving the adventitia.
2. Debridement of nonviable tissue to a bleeding edge.
3. Mucosa-to-mucosa, spatulated, tension-free, and water-tight anastomosis.
4. Ureteral stenting/urinary diversion.
5. Isolation of repair from associated injuries (e.g., omental interposition for associated bowel, vascular, or pancreatic injuries).
6. Retroperitoneal drain.

2. Distal ureteral injuries (below the iliac vessels)

a. *Ureteroneocystostomy.* After the proximal end of the ureter is debrided to viable tissue and spatulated, a re-fluxing ureteral reimplantation into a fixed (floor/trigone) rather then mobile area of the bladder (dome) is preferred. A tunneled nonrefluxing reimplant is generally unnecessary and slightly increases the chance for ureteral stenosis. Ureteral stenting is for 4 to 6 weeks.

b. *Vesico-psoas hitch.* With greater distal ureteral loss, a psoas hitch to the ipsilateral psoas minor tendon usually bridges the gap. The contralateral superior vesical pedicle is divided to improve bladder mobilization. Care is taken not to entrap the genitofemoral nerve. The ureter is then reimplanted over a ureteral stent, and a suprapubic tube placed.

c. *Transureteroureterostomy.* A transureteroureterostomy (TUU) is particularly useful when there are associated rectal, major pelvic vascular, or extensive bladder injuries. Relative contraindications to a TUU are a prior history of urothelial cancer, genitourinary tuberculosis, nephrolithiasis, pelvic irradiation or infection, retroperitoneal fibrosis, or chronic pyelonephritis. The injured ureter is brought across the midline through a window in the colonic/sigmoid mesentery, usually cephalad to the inferior mesenteric artery, so as not to kink the ureter. The end-to-side ureteral anastomosis is stented and drained.

d. *Other procedures.* Ileal interposition, Boari flap, renal displacement, or autotransplantation are best reserved for delayed and controlled reconstructive settings.

3. Midureteral injuries

a. *Ureteroureterostomy.* The majority of complete transections, regardless of mechanism, can be repaired by primary ureteroureterostomy. Both ureteral segments are spatulated and a watertight, tension-free anastomosis performed over a double-J ureteral stent. In select cases, TUU may also be an option.

4. Upper ureteral injuries
   a. *Ureteroureterostomy.* Injuries to the upper third of the ureter are best repaired by primary ureteroureterostomy.
   b. *UPJ injuries.* UPJ injuries are usually avulsions after blunt trauma. Avulsion of the UPJ is the most common blunt ureteral injury seen, and occurs primarily in children (less than 16 years). Incomplete UPJ lacerations can often be successfully managed expectantly. Complete UPJ tears (avulsion) will not resolve spontaneously and demand primary surgical repair, ureteral stenting, and a retroperitoneal drain.

5. The unstable patient
   a. When the patient is too unstable to undergo lengthy ureteral reconstruction, a "damage control" approach of temporary cutaneous ureterostomy over a single "J" ureteral stent should be performed. An alternative method of last resort is ureteral ligation proximal to the injury, followed by a percutaneous nephrostomy tube when stable. Intraoperative placement of a nephrostomy tube should be avoided.
   b. Definitive reconstruction is delayed (up to 2 weeks) until the patient has stabilized from other injuries.

F. Management of Complications and Delayed Diagnosis

1. Delayed recognition of ureteral injuries is common, occurring in 8 to 57 percent of cases. Significant morbidity, including sepsis, abscess formation, hydronephrosis, and loss of renal function occurs in up to 50 percent of such patients. Other complications include ureteral stricture and fistula, urinary extravasation and urinoma formation, infection, and loss of renal function.

2. Ureteral injuries that are diagnosed within 2 weeks of initial trauma and have no significant infection should be surgically explored and repaired. If iatrogenic ligation of the ureter is found, the suture should be removed and the ureter stented.

3. Injuries that are diagnosed after 10 to 14 days should undergo proximal urinary diversion by percutaneous nephrostomy tube, percutaneous drainage of any urinoma or abscess, and when possible, antegrade stent placement across the injured ureter. Definitive ureteral reconstruction is usually delayed for 3 months.

III. BLADDER TRAUMA
A. Introduction

1. The majority (86 percent) of bladder injuries are due to blunt abdominal trauma from motor vehicle accidents, falls from height, and crush injuries.

2. Roughly 90 percent are associated with pelvic fractures, whereas 9 to 16 percent of all pelvic fractures have a ruptured bladder. The minority (14 percent) are due to penetrating trauma, namely GSWs and stab wounds.

3. Bladder ruptures are roughly 60 percent extraperitoneal, 30 percent intraperitoneal, and the remaining 10 to 12 percent are combined injuries.

4. Most bladder injuries in children are intraperitoneal. This is due to the child's bladder being an intra-abdominal organ and thus vulnerable to external trauma.

B. Mechanisms of Injury

1. Intraperitoneal
   a. Intraperitoneal bladder rupture occurs by severe blunt lower abdominal or pelvic trauma to a distended or full bladder.
   b. Elevated bladder pressures are transmitted into bladder rupture at the dome, its weakest and most mobile point. Ruptures are commonly several centimeters in length. Empty bladders are seldom injured.
   c. High mortality is due to associated injuries.

2. Extraperitoneal
   a. Nearly always associated with pelvic fracture.
   b. Injuries are commonly anterolateral and near the bladder base, and primarily due to shearing forces and to a lesser degree, to perforation by bony spicules.
   c. Extravasated urine is confined to the pelvis when the urogenital diaphragm is intact. When the superior fascia of the urogenital diaphragm (which is contiguous with Dartos, Colles', and Scarpa's fasciae) is ruptured, urine can infiltrate the scrotum, perineum, and abdominal wall. When the inferior fascia is disrupted, urine can also infiltrate the penis or thigh.

C. Signs and Symptoms

1. Nearly all bladder ruptures present with hematuria. Blunt injuries have 95 to 100 percent gross hematuria, and the remaining under 5 percent microhematuria. Penetrating bladder injuries have roughly 50 percent microscopic and 50 percent gross hematuria.

2. Patients commonly complain of pelvic or lower abdominal pain and inability to urinate. Signs of bladder rupture are suprapubic tenderness, low urine output, and gross

hematuria. On rectal examination, landmarks are commonly indistinct due to a large pelvic hematoma.

3. Intraperitoneal bladder ruptures that are diagnosed late often present with azotemia, hyperchloremic metabolic acidosis, hypernatremia, hyperkalemia, as well as elevation in serum levels of BUN.

4. Women with bladder rupture need a careful pelvic examination for possible vaginal or urethral tears.

D. Associated Injuries

1. Bladder injuries are rarely isolated, with 94 to 97 percent with associated injuries, mainly pelvic and long bone fractures and head and spinal and visceral injuries.

2. Mortality rates are high (16 to 53 percent) primarily due to severe pelvic fracture and pelvic hemorrhage and late multisystem organ failure.

3. In 10 percent and less than 2 percent of bladder ruptures, male urethral and renal injuries occur, respectively. Most urethral injuries are type III posterior injuries.

4. In women with a bladder injury or pelvic fracture, a thorough pelvic examination is important to determine any concomitant vaginal or urethral laceration.

E. Imaging

Definitive diagnosis is by a formal retrograde filling imaging study. Antegrade filling cystograms by Foley catheter clamping are unreliable due to inadequate bladder distention.

1. Cystography

Gravity filling of bladder with dilute contrast, via a Foley, to at least 300 mL or until extravasation. Films in at least two projections are preferred, but are often not possible due to a pelvic fracture. Post drainage films are essential so as not to miss 10 to 15 percent of injuries. Extent of injury commonly does not correspond to the degree of extravasation.

2. Cystography findings by injury type

a. *Bladder contusion.* Bladder mucosal or muscle wall injury without loss of wall continuity. Bladder outline commonly distorted, but no extravasation. Diagnosis of exclusion, with a normal abdominal CT (or IVP) and normal retrograde urogram (RUG).

b. *Interstitial rupture.* Non-full-thickness tear of the bladder wall. Bladder outline commonly distorted, but no extravasation.

c. *Intraperitoneal rupture.* Contrast outlines loops of bowel, fills cul-de-sac, and eventually paracolic gutters. Usually all above the superior margin of the acetabulum.

    d. *Extraperitoneal rupture.* Flame-like or star-burst contrast extravasation. Usually all below the superior margin of the acetabular line.

    e. *Large pelvic hematoma.* Bladder is "tear-drop" shaped due to pelvic hematoma compression of the bladder on both sides. In addition to being elongated, the bladder is lifted out of the pelvis. The degree of bladder distortion often corresponds to the severity of the pelvic hemorrhage.

3. *CT cystography.* As accurate as conventional cystography, as long as the bladder is retrograde filled to at least 300 mL or until extravasation. No post drainage images are needed.

F. Management

The overall evaluation and management of lower urinary tract trauma is detailed in Figure 11-3.

1. Intraperitoneal injuries and all penetrating bladder injuries

    a. The size and number of intraperitoneal ruptures can only be reliably assessed by surgical exploration, and not by cystography.

    b. For penetrating injuries, each missile tract is explored, all debris removed, all devitalized tissue debrided, and then the injury is closed.

    c. In iatrogenic penetrating injuries the entire bladder should be thoroughly inspected for more then one injury.

    d. After formal bladder repair, the urine is diverted by Foley and/or SP tube. Large-bore catheters are used to facilitate bloody drainage. The Foley is removed once the urine is clear. After 10 to 14 days, the SP tube is commonly removed.

2. Blunt extraperitoneal bladder injuries or interstitial ruptures

    a. Isolated injuries can be successfully managed by Foley catheter drainage. By 10 days, 87 percent are healed. The remaining 13 percent will heal by prolonging urinary diversion up to 1 month.

    b. When the abdomen is explored for associated injuries, all extraperitoneal bladder ruptures also should be repaired at the same time. The bladder should be exposed through a midline abdominal incision and the bladder opened at the dome to avoid the lateral pelvic hematomas. Opening the pelvic hematoma may cause bacterial contamination and release the tamponade effect. Bladder lacerations are closed from an intraperitoneal approach. The bladder neck and ureteral orifices need inspection for possible injury. Gently cannulate the ureter or give intravenous indigo carmine to assess ureteral integrity. Urinary drainage is by large bore SP tube and Foley catheter. No drain is placed.

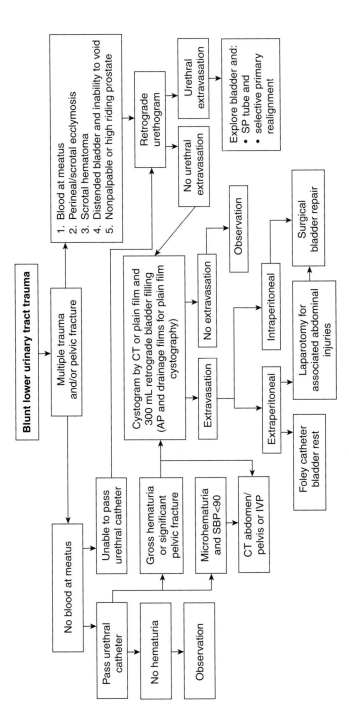

Figure 11-3 Algorithm for the evaluation and management of blunt trauma to the bladder and/or urethra.

3. *Bladder neck.* All bladder lacerations that extend into the bladder neck demand formal and prompt repair.
4. *Complications.* After appropriate treatment, complications are rare and are mostly infectious, such as urinary tract infection, peritonitis, pelvis abscess, and pelvic hematoma infection.

IV. URETHRA

A. Introduction

Urethral injuries are relatively uncommon, and are usually divided into anterior or posterior injuries. The vast majority are due to blunt trauma. Posterior urethral injuries are due to pelvic fracture and anterior urethral injuries to straddle-type injury. Penetrating injuries also occur, and are usually due to a gunshot wound to the anterior urethra. The management goal for urethral injuries is to minimize the chances for the debilitating complications of incontinence, impotence, and urethral stricture.

B. Anatomy

Fascial anatomy is important to defining and understanding urethral injuries. The male urethra can be divided into the anterior urethra (the bulbous and pendulous) and into the posterior urethra (the prostatic and membranous). From a surgical perspective, the urethra is divided into five divisions. The prostatic urethra extends from the prostatic base to apex. The membranous urethra lies within the GU diaphragm, contains the external striated urethral sphincter, and lies between the prostatic apex and bulbar urethra. The bulbar urethra is the urethral segment covered by the bulbospongiosus (ischiocavernosus) muscle. The pendulous urethra is the longest segment and starts at the distal margin/end of the bulbospongiosus muscle. The fossa navicularis is the last and most distal division.

C. Posterior Urethral Injuries

The posterior urethra is injured in 1.6 to 9.9 percent of pelvic fractures. Urethral injury is complete in 73 percent and partial in 27 percent.

1. Mechanism
   a. The posterior urethra is fixed in place at two locations, the membranous urethra to the ischiopubic rami by the urogenital diaphragm, and at the prostatic urethra to the symphysis by the puboprostatic ligaments. Urethral injuries are thus the result of the following.
      1. Shearing forces between a fixed prostate and a mobile bladder, resulting in bladder neck injury.
      2. Shearing forces between a fixed membranous urethra and a mobile bulbar urethra; resulting in membranous urethral (external sphincter) injury.

      3. Direct laceration by pelvic bone fragments (rare).

      4. Distraction caused by pelvic fracture between the symphysis and pubic rami.

  b. Urethral injury in women is rare due to short length, mobility, and lack of attachments to the pubic symphysis. When it does occur, it is commonly a partial, anterior, and longitudinal laceration. In extreme cases, varying degrees of complete avulsion can also occur, as well as associated vaginal laceration and pelvic fracture. In contrast to men, injuries to the female urethra and bladder neck are usually due to sharp edges of bony fragments that also concomitantly injure the vaginal vault. A pelvic examination is important for all women with a pelvic fracture.

2. Classification

  a. Two urethral injury scales are commonly employed. In both scales, fascial anatomy, as well as the degree and location of the urethral injury are important to injury classification. Grades of injury are determined by retrograde urethrography as detailed in Table 11-2.

  b. The urogenital diaphragm separates the pelvis from the perineum and is the most important fascial landmark in posterior urethral injuries.

3. Signs and symptoms

  a. When a urethral injury is suspected, catheterization should be avoided. Attempted catheter passage can convert a partial urethral injury into a complete one and/or potentially infect the pelvic hematoma.

  b. In the young, conscious patient, inability to pass a catheter is often due to a contracted external sphincter and not a urethral injury.

  c. Ability to void does not rule out a partial urethral tear.

  d. With prostatomembranous disruption, the prostate usually feels cranially and posteriorly displaced or not palpable. To the inexperienced examiner, a normal positioned prostate is often mistakenly labeled as "high riding." Furthermore, a tense pelvic hematoma can feel like a prostate on palpation, or blur the planes and make palpation difficult.

  e. Signs of urethral injury (physical findings are more apparent more than 1 hour after injury) include:

      1. Blood at the meatus (98 percent sensitive, due to spasm of the bulbospongiosus muscle); the amount of urethral bleeding correlates little with the severity of injury.

      2. Gross hematuria.

      3. Perineal ecchymosis or hematoma (GU diaphragm is disrupted).

4. Scrotal or penile hematoma.
5. Difficulty passing a Foley catheter.
6. Distended bladder and inability to void.
7. Nonpalpable prostate.
8. Classic triad: blood at meatus, inability to void, and distended bladder.
9. Female urethral injury is suspect when a pelvic fracture presents with vaginal bleeding and laceration, urethrorrhagia, and/or hematuria, labial swelling, or inability to void.

4. Imaging studies
   a. *KUB/pelvic films.* On pelvic film, urethral injury is suggested by pelvic ring disruption, and often associated with anterior and bilateral pubic ramus fractures, significant widening of the sacroiliac joint, or open book fracture with pubic diastasis.
   b. *RUG.* Retrograde urethrography (RUG) is the procedure of choice to evaluate for urethral injury. Contrast medium instilled in a small volume (20 to 30 mL), ideally under fluoroscopy. Large volumes of contrast will only obscure the full extent of urethral injury. Extent of urethral injury is graded radiographically (see Table 11-2).

5. Associated injuries
   a. Injury of the posterior urethra results from severe force and is associated with multiple injuries. From the associated injuries and subsequent complications, mortality rates are as high as one-third.
   b. Associated intra-abdominal injuries are bladder (10 to 20 percent), spleen (8 to 21 percent), followed by liver and bowel. At the time of SP tube placement, a cystogram or direct inspection should be performed. On physical examination, attention to the perineum, penis, and scrotum is also essential.
   c. All blunt posterior urethral injuries are associated with a pelvic fracture, and usually involve the anterior pelvic ring (e.g., pubic ramus and symphysis). Overall, urethral injury occurs in 3.5 to 15 percent of pelvic fractures.
   d. In female urethral injuries, associated vaginal lacerations are common, as is a increased incidence of vesicovaginal fistula.

6. General management
   a. Management goals for urethral injuries are preserving continence and potency, and avoiding the pelvic hematoma infection.
   b. Despite previous controversy, it is generally felt that the complications of impotence and incontinence re-

Table 11-2 Classifications of Urethral Injuries

URETHRAL INJURY SCALE

GRADE	DESCRIPTION OF INJURY
Type I	Urethra stretched. No evidence of extravasation on retrograde urethrogram (RUG).
Type II	Partial or complete disruption of the prostatomembranous junction, but the urogenital diaphragm remains intact. Contrast extravasation remains above the GU diaphragm on RUG. This is an uncommon injury.
Type III	Both the prostatomembranous urethra and the urogenital diaphragm are disrupted, with damage to the proximal bulbar urethra. Contrast extravasates above and below the GU diaphragm (often into the perineum). This is the most common type of posterior urethral injury (66–85%).
Type IV	Urethral injury with extension into the bladder neck and prostatic urethra.

AAST URETHRAL INJURY SCALE

GRADE	INJURY	DESCRIPTION OF INJURY
I	Contusion	Blood at meatus with normal RUG.
II	Stretch injury	Urethral elongation and no extravasation on RUG
III	Partial disruption	Extravasation at injury site, and contrast able to enter bladder on RUG.
IV	Complete disruption	Extravasation at injury site and no contrast enters bladder; urethral separation < 2 cm.
V	Complete disruption	Complete transection with urethral separation > 2cm or extension into the prostate, bladder neck, or vagina.

From Moore EE, Cogbill TH, Malagoni MA, et al: Organ injury scaling. *Surg Clin North Am* 75:293, 1995

sult from the initial injury itself and not the management method chosen.

c. Primary surgical dissection and urethral reconstruction, however, have much higher complication rates. Primary open surgical repair results in a high risk of uncontrolled venous pelvic bleeding by opening the pelvic hematoma, higher rates of postoperative impotence and incontinence, excessive urethral debridement and subsequent stricture, and is technically difficult.

d. Impotence after pelvic fracture or blunt perineal trauma is primarily vascular (80 percent). This is due to direct corporal cavernosal or internal pudendal artery injury that leads to corporeal veno-occlusive dysfunction and to cavernous arterial insufficiency. Only secondarily is impotence neurogenic [(resulting from prostatic plexus and/or cavernous nerve injury, and from nervi erigentes (S2–S4) injury)].

D. Complete Urethral Disruption

1. The ideal method of management is still controversial. The most accepted method is the most conservative one, namely suprapubic tube urinary diversion followed by delayed urethrotomy or urethroplasty.

2. Generally, it is the injury itself and not the method of repair that effects complications. Primary suturing of the urethral ends is the exception, where high rates of impotence and incontinence occur, as well as potentially, releasing the tamponade effect and convert an incomplete to a complete injury.

3. Presently, primary realignment has become a popular management option. Contemporary primary realignment is not the cumbersome interlocking "railroading" of sounds of yesteryear, but rather endoscopy with flexible cystoscopes from above and below, guidewires, and Seldinger technique catheter placement, all under fluoroscopic guidance. Others have used magnetic tipped catheters and fluoroscopy to stent the urethra. Timing of the realignment in the stable patient is at the time of injury. In the unstable patient, it is delayed a few days until the patient is stable (e.g., usually concomitantly with early repair of the associated orthopedic injuries). Traction should not be applied to the catheter. The Foley is maintained for 4 to 6 weeks, and acts as a guide for the prostate back into its normal position. Present series are small, but rates of incontinence and impotence appear as good, and slightly better as to stricture, than a delayed approach.

4. For the urologist who sees these injuries only occasionally, the best and easiest approach is open cystotomy and SP tube placement. Clear urine on opening suggests no major bladder injury. Care should be taken to avoid the prevesical/retropubic fascial planes and not to disrupt the pelvic hematoma. Concomitant bladder injuries are

closed from within the bladder. Prevesical drains are not used since they increase the potential for pelvic hematoma infection. Over the next 3 to 6 months, the hematoma slowly reabsorbs and allows the prostate to descend into a more normal position. For complete urethral disruptions, a delayed approach assumes an inevitable urethral stricture, which eventually necessitates a staged open urethroplasty. Management and evaluation of posterior urethral strictures is detailed in the chapter on urethral strictures.

E. Partial Urethral Disruption

1. Incomplete lacerations usually heal spontaneously. Primary management is urinary diversion by suprapubic tube. If gross hematuria is noted on tube placement, the bladder should be formally explored. If no gross hematuria is noted, a cystogram should be done.

2. A voiding cystourethrogram (VCUG) is performed after 2 to 3 weeks of urinary diversion. Subsequent urethral scarring is usually minimal. When strictures do occur, they are usually short and can often be successfully managed by urethrotomy.

F. Bladder Neck Injury

1. Early repair of a bladder neck (BN) injury is important to avoid incontinence, infection, and fistula formation.

2. Diagnosis of injury can be made by cystogram or by palpation at the time of bladder exploration.

3. For simple lacerations, urinary drainage is by prolonged urethral catheter and SP tube. For complete disruption or avulsion, repair is demanded, yet often technically difficult. To minimize scarring and bladder neck entrapment, some advocate omental pedicle flap placement.

4. Male children are typically more susceptible than adults to bladder neck injury and thus posttraumatic incontinence. This is primarily due to an immature prostate that is so small that injury extends trans-prostatically and into the bladder neck.

G. Blunt Anterior Urethral Injuries

1. Introduction

   a. In contrast to posterior urethral injuries, blunt anterior urethral injuries are caused by direct injury to the penis and urethra, have few associated injuries, and relatively low morbidity rates. Such injuries are classically the result of a "straddle" injury to the perineum, where the bulbar urethra is crushed against the pubic bone when the patient falls astride an object.

2. Anatomy
   a. The urethra and corpus spongiosum is surrounded by a fascial tunica albuginea, which is further enveloped by Buck's fascia, which also surrounds each corpora cavernosa of the penis and inserts into the GU diaphragm.
   b. When Buck's fascia remains intact, blood and urine from the injured urethra remain contained within the penis. A "sleeve-like" penile ecchymosis and swelling results.
   c. When Buck's fascia is disrupted, blood and urine from the injured urethra can spread to the scrotum, abdominal wall, perineum, and thigh, as contained by the Dartos, Scarpa's, and Colles' fasciae. These superficial fascial planes are all contiguous, and thus fluid or infection spread is limited by the fascial attachment sites, namely the clavicles, the urogenital diaphragm, and the fascia lata of the medial thigh, respectively. Extravasation extension into the perineum results in the classic "butterfly sign" hematoma (as limited by insertions at the fascia lata).

3. Signs and symptoms
   a. Patients with suspected urethral injury should not be allowed to void or have a Foley catheter passed until the urethra is evaluated by RUG.
   b. Signs of potential anterior urethral injury include:
      1. History of direct perineal trauma or straddle injury.
      2. Blood at the meatus (the most important predictor).
      3. Perineal and/or scrotal swelling and ecchymosis or tenderness (e.g., butterfly sign hematoma).
      4. Penile hematoma.
      5. Inability to void.

4. Classification and Management of Injuries
   a. *Contusions.* Such injuries typically occur when a Foley catheter with an inflated balloon is traumatically removed or the balloon inflated in the anterior urethra. Blood at the meatus or initial or terminal hematuria is present here, but no extravasation of contrast noted on retrograde urethrography. If the patient can void easily and the urine relatively clear, no Foley catheter or additional treatment is necessary.
   b. *Lacerations.* Based on retrograde urethrography, lacerations are considered complete or incomplete, with the later having contrast proximal to the injury extravasation site and into the bladder. Incomplete lacerations usually heal rapidly and with a low stricture rate. Treatment is usually proximal urinary diversion by suprapubic tube for 14 to 21 days. Urethral catheterization is discouraged because it risks convert-

ing an incomplete tear into a complete one. Complete lacerations, on the other hand, have a high stricture rate, which usually require a delayed (months later) open surgical repair. Patients who develop complete occlusion of the urethra should have SP drainage for 3 to 6 months before definite repair. Patients who delay presentation and have extensive extravasation also require placement of a perineal subcutaneous drain and debridement of all devitalized or infected tissue. Drains may also need to be placed in the scrotum and penis.

5. Complications
   a. Delay in diagnosis or treatment predisposes the genitalia to infection of the extravasated urine and blood, with possible development of abscess formation, sepsis, and fasciitis.
   b. The major long-term complications after initial management are urethral stricture, penile curvature, penile foreshortening, erectile dysfunction, and urinary incontinence.

H. Penetrating Anterior Urethral Injuries

GSWs to the urethra are uncommon. They occur in 2 to 7 percent of all civilian GU GSWs. An associated urethral injury is present in 18 to 57 percent of GSWs to the penis. Half of perineal GSWs also involve the urethra.

1. Signs and symptoms
   a. The amount of contrast extravasation on RUG usually does not correlate with the severity of the injury. If hemodynamic conditions allow, a RUG should be performed for the following.
      1. All penetrating wounds to the penis or perineum (in particular, GSWs).
      2. Blood at the penile meatus.
      3. Gross hematuria (microscopic hematuria is not predictive of injury).
      4. A suspected urethral injury.

2. Management
   a. A primary repair approach is generally employed for stab wounds and for low velocity GSWs. Strictures rates approach 80 percent for urinary diversion and stenting compared to 10 to 12 percent for primary repair.
   b. Surgical management generally is conservative debridement and primary end-to-end anastomosis over a silastic Foley catheter. Due to a rich blood supply, all contused corpora spongiosum should be debrided very conservatively, so as to avoid cordee, stricture, and fistula formation.

  c. When the urethral injury defect is so extensive (as with high velocity GSWs or shotgun blasts) that primary mobilization cannot approximate the urethral edges, the urethra should be marsupialized and a suprapubic tube placed. After 3 to 6 months, a delayed second-stage urethroplasty can be performed.

VI. EXTERNAL GENITALIA
A. Introduction
The etiology of traumatic injuries to the external genitalia are roughly one-half penetrating, one-half blunt, and the remaining 10 percent burns and industrial accidents. Extensive genital injuries are often complex problems of diagnosis, management, and reconstruction. In addition to cosmetic and functional disfigurement, such injuries can have devastating psychological and emotional effects.

B. Penetrating Injuries
Although relatively uncommon, at urban trauma centers 28 to 68 percent of all penetrating urologic injuries are to the external genitalia.

 1. *Associated injuries.* In the military experience of high velocity gunshots and land mine fragments, genital GSWs are rarely isolated, and are associated with major injuries to the lower extremities, abdomen, and chest. Mortality rates are up to 25 percent. In the civilian experience of mostly low velocity gunshots, genital injuries are commonly isolated or associated with soft tissue injuries (60 percent) and no mortalies. Other less common injuries are vascular, bowel, skeletal, and other intra-abdominal.

 2. *Management.* General surgical principles for managing GSWs elsewhere in the body apply to external genitalia trauma. Wounds of the corpora cavernosum and spongiosum, however, should be treated more like vasculature, with limited debridement and a good hemostatic closure. In general, management consists of meticulous hemostasis, vigorous saline lavage, removal of foreign bodies, hematoma evacuation, conservative debridement of devitalized tissue, repair of associated injuries, and primary wound closure.

 3. Scrotal injuries

  a. All penetrating scrotal GSWs, deep to Dartos fascia or with marked scrotal swelling, demand prompt surgical exploration. Even if the tunica albuginea is intact on exploration, draining the hematocele often shortens the disability course and prevents hematocele infection and testis atrophy. With highly selected cases of scrotal GSWs, testis evaluation by ultrasound and subsequent conservative management has been advocated.

b. The goal of scrotal exploration is testis preservation, in order to maintain androgen production and cosmesis. Fertility is not commonly preserved.

c. The injured testis is salvaged by debriding all extruded and devitalized seminiferous tubules, followed by primary tunica albuginea closure. A dependent Penrose drain is also placed. Despite efforts for preservation, GSWs to the testis result in orchiectomy in 25 to 71 percent of cases, or on average, 50 percent. After military-type, high velocity missile injuries, the orchiectomy rate approaches 90 percent.

4. Penile injuries

a. All GSWs to the penis demand a retrograde urethrogram. This is because 14 to 57 percent have an associated urethral injury.

b. Gunshot wounds to the penis that penetrate deep to Buck's fascia demand surgical exploration. Corporal injuries that are not repaired early can result in erectile dysfunction, penile scarring, curvature, pain, and infection.

c. Penile injuries are commonly explored by degloving the penis by a subcoronal circumferential incision. Surgical exposure can also be achieved through a curvilinear incision made at the base of the penis. Upon exposing the penile fascia, defects in the Buck's fascia and tunica albuginea are closed primarily.

d. The main goal of treatment is to prevent penile deformity or erectile dysfunction. Return to sexual activity is 4 to 6 weeks after repair. Potency is maintained in 87 to 100 percent of patients after surgical repair.

e. Penile injuries from high velocity missiles are often more extensive, requiring complex staged repairs, and occasionally, penectomy.

C. Blunt Genital Injuries: Testis Rupture

The most common causes for blunt testis rupture are motorcycle and auto accidents, followed by sporting activities.

1. *Signs and symptoms.* Testis is painful on palpation and nausea and vomiting are commonly present. The degree of scrotal swelling and ecchymosis present varies greatly. When marked scrotal swelling is present, it is difficult by physical examination to determine testis integrity and/or to distinguish it from a hematocele or hematoma of the cord or epididymis.

2. *Diagnostic procedures.* The most reliable test for tunica albuginea integrity is surgical exploration. When physical

examination of the testis is equivocal due to scrotal swelling, ultrasound of the scrotum has been widely used to help evaluate testis integrity. Inhomogeneous and irregular echo patterns are the most reliable sonographic predictors of seminiferous tubule extrusion and hemorrhage. A break in the echodense pattern of a linear tunica albuginea also suggests injury, but is much less reliable.

3. *Management.* Despite a hematocele, testis injury with an intact tunica can be successfully managed conservatively. Close follow-up is mandatory to assess for persistent bleeding or signs of infection. All blunt scrotal trauma with testis rupture demands early surgery. Early exploration offers the patient his best chance for testis salvage. When the bluntly traumatized testis is repaired promptly, salvage rates are 91 to 95 percent. When the scrotum is explored in a delayed fashion (days later), the salvage rate drops to 55 percent, and time to recovery is prolonged. The methods of testis exploration and repair are the same as for penetrating injuries, where all necrotic and extruded tubules are debrided and the tunica closed primarily.

D. Blunt Genital Injuries: Penile Fracture

1. The most common etiology is a direct blow to the erect penis during intercourse or masturbation.

2. Fracture is a tear in the tunica albuginea of the penis. Erection thins out the tunica and makes it more susceptible to injury.

3. Common presentation is a patient who reports a "cracking or popping" sound, immediate pain, rapid detumescence, penile swelling, and penile deviation away from the injury.

4. Associated urethral injury occurs in 15 to 22 percent of fractures. Unless blood is at the meatus, hematuria is present, or voiding is difficult, routine urethrography is not required.

5. Location of the fracture can often be identified on physical examination by a palpable defect in the tunica, focal tenderness, or overlying hematoma with contralateral penile deflection.

6. Ultrasonography has a limited role as negative results do not exclude a rupture.

7. Cavernosography can accurately diagnose and localize the rupture site. However, it is rarely indicated because it is an invasive, time-consuming, and difficult to interpret test.

8. Management is prompt exploration, hematoma evacuation, and primary repair of the tunica albuginea with absorbable suture. Tears in the tunica are commonly transverse and mid-shaft. Surgical repair results are relatively

complication free. Conservative management, however, is often complicated by penile fibrosis and by pain and angulation with erection.

E. Penile Amputation

Amputation of the penis is usually an act of self-emasculation by an acutely psychotic and young patient. On a less common basis, penis loss is the result of assault or accident (motorcycle accident, severe burn, or industrial machinery).

1. *Management.* All patients who present to the hospital with amputated genitals should be considered candidates for repair, regardless of late presentation or active psychosis. Transsexuals are also candidates for penis reattachment. Of patients who amputate their penis, roughly 95 percent undergo successful psychological rehabilitation and do not repeat self-emasculation or castration. On arrival at the hospital, the patient should be evaluated by a team approach of a urologist, a surgeon experienced in microvascular surgery, and a psychiatrist. The amputated penis, after being cleaned of blood and debris, should be promptly cooled to 4°C to minimize ischemic damage. Successful replantation of the penis is most dependent on limiting warm ischemic time. When warm ischemic time exceeds 12 hours, reimplantation is more likely to fail. Proper and prompt cooling, however, can prolong successful replantation up to 24 hours.

2. *Goals.* The goals of penile reconstruction are both cosmetic and functional (normal erectile function and a patent urethra). The corpora cavernosa is first reapproximated, then the urethra/corpus spongiosum over a Foley catheter, followed by a microvascular repair of the dorsal vein, artery, and nerves, when technically possible. When the amputated penis cannot be located or is damaged beyond repair, the penile stump is closed in standard partial penectomy fashion.

3. *Post replantation complications.* The most common are necrosis of the skin covering the amputated penis and glans skin slough. Other complications are penile numbness and poor sensation, followed by urethral stricture at the anastomotic site.

F. Testis Amputation

1. Self-castration is commonly accompanied with emasculation, and is seen mainly in transsexual and psychotic patients.

2. Unlike the penis, the testes can not tolerate prolonged periods of warm ischemia. The upper limit for attempting testicular replantation is less than 4 to 6 hours.

3. Testis replantation is technically demanding and time-consuming microvascular surgery. Attempts are made when both testes or a single testis with an atrophic or absent contralateral testis are amputated.

G. Genital Skin Avulsion Injuries

1. *Introduction.* In the past, the main cause of genital skin loss was farm or other rotary machinery, where the machine tore off entangled clothing, carrying with it the genital skin. The incidence has been largely reduced by improved safety measures. Presently, the main cause for genital skin avulsion is deceleration injuries while riding a motorcycle or bicycle. Typically, when genital skin is avulsed, it separates from the underlying tissue loose areolar tissue along avascular fascial planes. On the penile shaft, skin loss is superficial to Buck's fascia, whereas on the scrotum, skin loss is superficial to the external spermatic fascia. The underlying cord, testes, penile corpora, and urethra remain uninjured.

2. Management
   a. *Scrotal skin.* Since the scrotal skin is totally dependent on the terminal branches of the pudendal arteries, completely amputated scrotal skin cannot be replanted. The scrotum has an excellent blood supply and is greatly elastic and compliant. Scrotal skin loss of less than 60 percent can be closed primarily. More extensive scrotal skin loss (more than 60 percent) cannot be closed primarily. For such injuries where there are no major associated injuries and the scrotal wound clean and fresh, the most appropriate management is immediate skin grafting and scrotal reconstruction. When the wounds are contaminated or potentially infected, or the patient unstable, it is preferable to leave the testes and cords exposed and in the perioperative period manage them with frequent dressing changes. After about 5 days of dressing changes, the testes are placed in subcutaneous thigh pouches. Thigh pouches ease subsequent scrotal reconstruction, reduce the size of any perineal skin defect, do not require labor-intensive dressing changes, and well protect and cover the testes. Furthermore, in elderly or disabled patients where fertility and cosmesis are not of concern, leaving the testes in thigh pouches is a viable long-term option. Total scrotal reconstruction can be performed with autologous meshed skin grafts, mobilization of thigh flaps, or the use of tissue expanders.
   b. *Penile skin.* Penile skin avulsion usually demands immediate reconstruction. When penile shaft skin injury

or loss is circumferential, any skin that remains on the penis distal to the skin avulsion needs to be excised up to the coronal sulcus. In so doing, potential disfiguring chronic lymphedema is avoided. The goals for reconstruction are to create a cosmetically acceptable penis that can functionally have erections and carry urine. If the remaining skin is insufficient for primary closure, then a non-meshed thick split thickness skin graft is applied to the denuded penis. Meshed skin grafts should be used only for the impotent patient because meshed graft contracture can restrict erections. For the elderly and impotent patient, another option is to bury the denuded penis in a sub-Dartos tunnel in the scrotum.

H. Genital and Perineal Burns

1. Thermal burns to the genitalia are usually the result of fire (flame) and, to a lesser degree, boiling water or grease (scald).

2. Most burns of the scrotum or perineum are first- and second-degree burns and thus can heal with only local topical antimicrobial care (usually 1% silver sulfadiazine) and seldom require debridement.

3. Penile shaft skin is very thin and thus more prone to full thickness burns.

4. By definition, genital and perineal burns demand intensive care unit or burn center admission.

5. Burns to the genitalia and perineum commonly occur in association with extensive burns that usually exceed 40 percent of total body surface area. Isolated burns to the penis are rare and are usually the result of assault or child abuse.

6. Initial evaluation includes complete physical examination, laboratory evaluation (including urinalysis), tetanus prophylaxis, intravenous antibiotics, and estimate of the overall extent and depth of the burn. Initial management consists of aggressive fluid and electrolyte resuscitation.

7. A Foley catheter or suprapubic tube should be placed early to prevent urinary retention and to monitor urine output. Foley catheters are usually appropriate and relatively free of complications. Foley catheters, however, are not appropriate in patients with full thickness (third-degree) burns of the glans penis or ventral penis. To avoid pressure necrosis of the anterior urethra, suprapubic urinary diversion is best is such patients.

8. For third-degree genital burns, especially where the demarcation between viable and devitalized tissue is obvious, prompt skin debridement and immediate reconstruction by skin grafting is recommended. Prompt surgical

intervention reduces infection rates, shortens recovery time and hospital stay, and prevents delayed scar contracture.

9. Burns to the glans penis should not be debrided and grafted unless obviously necrotic. Overzealous debridement and grafting creates a poor cosmetic result. After initial eschar formation, the burned glans usually heals spontaneously.

BIBLIOGRAPHY

Kidney

Brandes SB, McAninch JW: Reconstructive surgery of the injured upper urinary tract. *Urol Clin North Am* 26:183, 1999.

Carroll PR, Klosterman P, McAninch JW: Early vascular control for renal trauma: A critical review. *J Urol* 141:826, 1989.

Carroll PR, McAninch JW, Klosterman P, Greenblatt M: Renovascular trauma: Risk assessment, surgical management, and outcome. *J Trauma* 30:547, 1990.

Cass AS: Ureteral contusion with gunshot wounds. *J Trauma* 24:59, 1984.

Eastman JA, Wilson TG, Ahlering TE: Urological evaluation and management of renal-proximity stab wounds. *J Urol* 150:1771, 1993.

Haaas CA, Dinchman KH, Nasrallah PF, Spirnak JP: Traumatic renal artery occlusion: A 15-year review. *J Trauma* 45:557, 1998.

Holcroft JW, Trunkey DD, Minagi H, et al: Renal trauma and retroperitoneal hematomas-indications for exploration. *J Trauma* 15:1045, 1975.

Husmann DA, Gilling PJ, Perry MO, et al: Major renal lacerations with a devitalized fragment following blunt abdominal trauma: A comparison between nonoperative (expectant) versus surgical management. *J Urol* 150:1774, 1993.

Kantos A, Sclafani SJA, Scalea T et al: The role of interventional radiology in the management of genitourinary trauma. *Urol Clin North Am* 16:255, 1989.

Mathews LA, Smith EM, Spirnak JP: Nonoperative treatment of major blunt renal lacerations with urinary extravasation. *J Urol* 157:2956, 1997.

Rosen MA, McAninch JW: Management of combined renal and pancreatic trauma. *J Urol* 152:22, 1994.

Scott RF Jr, Selzman HM: Complications of nephrectomy: Review of 450 patients and a description of a modification of the transperitoneal approach. *J Urol* 95:307, 1966.

Wessells H, Deirmenjian J, McAninch JW: Preservation of renal function after reconstruction for trauma: Quantitative assessment with radionuclide scintigraphy. *J Urol* 157:1583, 1997.

Wessells H, McAninch JW: Effect of colon injury on the management of simultaneous renal trauma. *J Urol* 155:1852, 1996.

Wessells H, McAninch JW, Meyer A, Bruce JE: Criteria for nonoperative treatment of significant penetrating renal lacerations. *J Urol* 157:24, 1996.

Ureter

Boone TB, Gilling PJ, Husman DA: Ureteropelvic junction disruption following blunt abdominal trauma. *J Urol* 150:33, 1993.

Brandes SB, Chelsky MJ, Buckman RF, Hanno PM: Ureteral injuries from penetrating trauma. *J Trauma* 36:766, 1994.

McGinty DM, Mendez R: Traumatic ureteral injuries with delayed recognition. *Urology* 10:115, 1977.

Presti JC, Carroll PR, McAninch JW: Ureteral and renal pelvic injuries from external trauma: Diagnosis and management. *J Trauma* 29:370, 1989.

Bladder

Carroll PR, McAninch JW: Bladder trauma: Mechanisms of injury and a unifiedmethod of diagnosis and repair. *J Urol* 132:254, 1984.

Merchant WC, Gibbons MD, Gonzales ET: Trauma to the bladder neck, trigone,and vagina in children. *J Urol* 131:747, 1984.

Corriere JN Jr, Sandler CM: Management of the ruptured bladder: 7 years experience with 111 cases. *J Trauma* 26:830, 1986.

Urethra

Colapinto V, McCollum RW: Injury to the male posterior urethra in fractured pelvis: A new classification. *J Urol* 118:575,1977.

Dixon CM, Hricak H, McAninch JW: Magnetic resonance imaging of traumatic posterior urethral defects and pelvic crush injuries. *J Urol* 148:1232,1992.

Husmann DA, Boone TB, Wilson WT: Management of low velocity gunshot wounds to the anterior urethra: The role of primary repair versus urinary diversion alone. *J Urol* 150:70, 1993.

Webster GD, Mathes GL, Selli C: Prostatomembranous urethral injuries: A review of the literature and a rational approach to their management. *J Urol* 130:898,1983.

External Genitalia

Bhanganada K, Chayavatana T, Pongnumkul: Surgical management of an epidemic of penile amputations in siam. *Am J Surg* 146:376, 1983.

Brandes SB, Buckman RF, Chelsky MJ, et al: External genitalia gunshot wounds: A ten-year experience with fifty-six cases. *J Trauma* 39:266, 1995.

Carroll PR, Lue TF, Schmidt RA et al: Penile replantation: Current concepts. *J Urol* 133:281, 1985.

Jordan GH, Gilbert DA: Management of amputation injuries of the male genitalia. *Urol Clin North Am* 16:359, 1989.

McAninch JW. Management of genital skin loss. *Urol Clin North Am* 16:387, 1989.

McAninch JW, Kahn RI, Jeffrey RB, et al. Major traumatic and septic genital injuries. *J Trauma* 24:291, 1984.

McDougal WS, Peterson HD, Pruitt BA Jr: The thermally injured perineum. *J Urol* 121:320, 1979.

Waguespack RL, Thompson IM, McManus WF, Pruitt BA: Genital and perineal burns. *AUA Update Series* 15:30, 1995.

SELF-ASSESSMENT QUESTIONS

1. All of the following require radiographic imaging of the upper urinary tracts after a blunt trauma, except:
   a. a 12-year-old with microscopic hematuria (> 5 RBC/HPF) and systolic blood pressure over 90 mm Hg.
   b. gross hematuria.
   c. penetrating abdominal trauma and microscopic hematuria.

     d. a fall from a two-story building and normal urinalysis.

     e. a 42-year-old with microscopic hematuria and normal blood pressure.

2. A high-speed motor cycle accident victim with abdominal pain was taken to the operating room for an emergent laparotomy, where a large, contained, stable and nonpulsatile right retroperitoneal hematoma was noted. One-shot IVU shows a barely discernible nephrogram on the right and prompt uptake and excretion the left. The next step is to:

     a. perform a nephrectomy.

     b. perform an on table arteriogram.

     c. isolate the proximal renal vessels, open Gerota's fascia, and explore the kidney.

     d. perform a retrograde urogram.

     e. close and obtain a postoperative abdominal CT scan.

3. A 12-year-old boy is stuck by a car from behind, throwing him backward and onto the hood of the car. He undergoes a noncontrast CT scan that shows no parenchymal renal injury. Associated injuries are orthopedic. He is observed and after 5 days develops fever and chills. On ultrasound, a medial perinephric fluid collection is noted. The most likely urologic injury is:

     a. renal artery avulsion.

     b. UPJ disruption.

     c. adrenal hemorrhage.

     d. renal vein injury.

     e. none of the above.

4. A 20-year-old gunshot wound victim underwent a celiotomy and repair of small bowel injuries. He recovered quickly from his injuries, but represented 3 weeks later with fever, chills, and abdominal pain. CT scan with intravenous contrast noted a 10 cm urinoma and continued extravasation of contrast from the mid-ureter into it. The best management for this patient is?

     a. Immediate laparotomy and repair of the collecting system

     b. Percutaneous nephrostomy tube placement and percutaneous drainage of the collection

     c. Intravenous antibiotics and observation.

     d. Retrograde urogram and placement of a ureteral stent

     e. Percutaneous urinoma drainage only

5. Which of the following bladder injuries demand prompt surgical intervention?

     a. Extraperitoneal bladder rupture and associated grade 3 urethral disruption

     b. Extraperitoneal bladder rupture, as well as a bladder neck injury

     c. Intraperitoneal bladder rupture

     d. Extraperitoneal bladder rupture and celiotomy performed for associated intra-abdominal injuries

     e. All of the above

6. A small rural hospital receives a 32-year-old multi-injured trauma patient after an auto accident. ER retrograde urethrography extravasation of contrast from the proximal bulbar urethra with no contrast entering the bladder. The local trauma surgeon calls you for advice on managing this patient. What would you recommend?

     a. Bladder exploration and primary realignment

     b. Primary suturing of ends of the disrupted urethra

     c. Attempt a gentle Foley catheter placement

     d. Suprapubic tube placement and prevesical drain

     e. Suprapubic tube, bladder exploration and no prevesical drain

7. An acutely psychotic 35-year-old male patient presents to the emergency room 6 hours after amputating his penis. The organ is located and properly cleaned and cooled. The best management for this patient is?
   a. Close the penis as for a partial penectomy
   b. Perineal urethrostomy and close the penis as for a partial penectomy
   c. Attempt a microvascular re-implant of the penis.
   d. Perform a total penectomy and perform a perineal urethrostomy
   e. Refer to plastic surgeon for transgender operation

8. An 18-year-old male sustained a blow to the perineum while playing on a trampoline. Retrograde urethrography notes a partial bulbar urethral injury and on physical examination there is penile and scrotal ecchymosis. Which of the following is true?
   a. Buck's fascia is intact
   b. Buck's fascia is ruptured
   c. Colle's fascia is ruptured
   d. Scarpa's fascia is ruptured
   e. None of the above

9. A 22-year old, healthy and potent male was in a motorcycle accident and suffered a degloving injury of the penile skin. On physical examination, the penile skin is nearly all gone, except for a 2-cm circumferential band of sub-coronal skin. What is the best management?
   a. Non-meshed split thickness skin graft
   b. Meshed split thickness skin graft
   c. Bury penis in a sub-Dartos pouch
   d. Remove residual skin up to the coronal sulcus, followed by a non-meshed skin graft.
   e. Dermal graft

10. Which of the following are suggestive of blunt urethral injury associated with pelvic fracture?
   a. Blood at the urethral meatus
   b. Malgaigne and pubic rami pelvic fractures
   c. Perineal ecchymosis
   d. Inability to void
   e. All of the above

Answers

1. e	6. e
2. c	7. c
3. b	8. b
4. b	9. d
5. e	10. e

CHAPTER 12
Urethral Stricture Disease

Steven B. Brandes

I. GENERAL

An anterior urethral stricture is a scar of the urethral epithelium. Commonly, it extends into the underlying corpus spongiosum. The scar (stricture) is composed of dense collagen and fibroblasts and thus contracts in all directions, shortening urethral length and narrowing luminal size. Strictures are usually asymptomatic until a lumen size below 16 French (F).

A. Anatomy

1. The relative location of the urethra within the spongiosum changes along the divisions of the urethra. In the pendulous and glandular urethra, the lumen lies in the center of the spongiosum. In the bulbar urethra, the lumen lies progressively dorsal. The anatomic location of the lumen in relation to the spongiosum is critical for selecting the sites for internal urethrotomy.

2. The blood supply to the corpus spongiosum is dual, with a proximal and distal blood supply. The main arterial supply is the common penile artery, a branch off the internal pudendal. The bulbar artery is the proximal urethral blood supply. The distal blood supply comes from the dorsal arteries of the penis and the multiple circumflex and perforators to the spongiosum from the corpora cavernosum.

3. The blood supply to the penile skin is the external pudendal artery, a medial branch of the femoral artery. The scrotal skin is supplied anteriorly, mainly by branches of the external pudendal, while posteriorly, the main supply is the scrotal artery, a branch of the internal pudendal. These distinct blood supplies allow for mobilization of different skin flaps for urethral reconstruction.

II. ANTERIOR URETHRAL STRICTURES

A. Etiology

1. Most urethral strictures are the result of occult blunt perineal trauma (e.g., straddle injury) or instrumentation

(e.g., traumatic catheter placement or removal or chronic indwelling Foley catheter)

2. Inflammatory strictures, such as secondary to gonococcal or chlamydial urethritis, are relatively uncommon today. At the turn of the century or in contemporary impoverished countries, over 90 percent of strictures are inflammatory, and commonly involve the bulbar and pendulous urethra. In Western countries, the most common cause for inflammatory strictures is balanitis xerotica obliterans (BXO), a form of lichen sclerosus et atrophicus, where whitish atrophic plaques commonly affect the glans, meatus, and preputial skin. It is a common cause of phimosis, and thus is often temporally apparent after circumcision. BXO starts off as inflammation of the glans that can extend into the meatus and fossa, and result in severe meatal stenosis, high pressure voiding, and eventually, inflammation of the periurethral (Littre) glands. Potentially, panurethral stricture disease can occur in this manner.

B. Physical Examination Signs and Symptoms

1. As the urethral lumen gradually strictures down, obstructive voiding symptoms worsen in an insidious pattern. Symptoms include weak urinary stream, straining to void, sprayed stream, hesitancy, incomplete emptying, urinary retention, and post-void dribbling. Urinary frequency and dysuria are also common initial complaints.
2. Meatal stricture have a deviated or splayed urinary stream.
3. Palpation of the urethra can often reveal firm areas consistent with spongiofibrosis/ periurethral scarring. A tender mass along the urethra is usually a periurethral abscess.
4. Urinary peak flow rate less than 10 mL/sec indicates significant stricture.
5. Urinalysis to assess for urinary tract infection.

C. Differential Diagnosis

1. Bladder outlet obstruction from an enlarged prostate (BPH).
2. Bladder neck contracture after transurethral surgery or prostatectomy.
3. Urethral carcinoma—biopsy needed for diagnosis.
4. Urethral polyp.

D. Stricture Evaluation

1. *Retrograde urethrography (RUG) and voiding cystourethrography (VCUG).* Dynamic contrast imaging is the best approach despite the advent of newer imaging modalities. Both studies are commonly needed to fully

assess stricture length, location, and caliber and the functional significance of the stricture. Although accurate for determining pendulous urethral stricture length, they will often underestimate the actual bulbar urethral length, often up to 50 percent.

2. *Ultrasonography.* Particularly useful for bulbar urethral stricture evaluation, sonography of bulbar strictures accurately corresponds to the true intraoperative length. When the bulbar stricture length as noted on RUG/VCUG is 11 to 25 mm, sonography can help with treatment decision making. Strictures or sonogram found to be shorter than 25 mm can be treated by an end-to-end urethroplasty, whereas those longer then 25 mm require a graft or flap for reconstruction. The advantage of using sonography then, is that true stricture length can be determined preoperatively, and thus graft or flap mobilization can be performed first, in the supine position. In so doing, patient time in lithotomy and positioning complications are limited.

3. *Endoscopy.* With the use of a pediatric cystoscope or flexible ureteroscope, the degree of urethral lumen elasticity and inflammation can be assessed. In general, the worse the spongiofibrosis, the worse the distensibility. Endoscopy is useful for confirming or clarifying urethrography and the examiner can visually assess urethral mucosa and associated scarring.

4. Calibration (bougie-à-boule)

E. Complications of Urethral Strictures

1. Complications of stricture disease are:
   a. Urethral discharge
   b. Urinary tract infection (UTI)
   c. Cystitis
   d. Chronic prostatitis or epididymitis
   e. Periurethral abscess
   f. Urethral diverticulum and calculus
   g. Urethrocutaneous fistula
   h. Urethral cancer (one third to one half of males with urethral cancer have a history of stricture disease)
   i. Bladder stones (due to chronic urinary stasis and infection)

F. Treatment Options

1. Management of urethral strictures should not be considered a reconstructive ladder. The practice of repeat dilatations and urethrotomies before considering urethroplasty should be abandoned. The goal of stricture management is cure and not just temporary management. Open surgical urethroplasty has a long-term success rate of roughly 90 to

95 percent and should be considered the gold standard by which all other methods should be judged.
2. Stricture management techniques are:
    a. Urethral dilatation
    b. Internal urethrotomy
    c. Excision an primary anastomosis
    d. Free graft (skin, buccal mucosa, bladder epithelium)
    e. Penile or preputial island flap
    f. Scrotal island flap
    g. Combined tissue transfer

G. Urethral Dilatation

1. By and large, dilatation is only a management tool and not a cure. It is usually reserved for patients who are not candidates for more aggressive surgical intervention.
2. Classically, dilatation has employed Van Buren urethral sounds or filiform and followers to 22 F. The least traumatic and safest methods, however, are serial catheter dilatation over several weeks or balloon dilatation.
3. Dilatation is potentially curative only for pure epithelial strictures with minimal to no spongiofibrosis.
4. To be effective, the scar needs to be stretched without causing more scarring. The best chance for doing so is to stretch the scar without causing bleeding. Bleeding from the urethra means that the scar was torn and the stricture will soon recur and result in worsened stricture length and density.
5. Overall, long-term success is poor and recurrence rates high. Once interval dilatation is discontinued, the stricture will recur.

H. Internal Urethrotomy

1. Internal urethrotomy encompasses all methods of transurethral incision or ablation to open a stricture.
2. The goal of cutting a stricture is to have epithelial regrowth before scar reapproximation. At best, the result of urethrotomy is to create a larger caliber stricture that offers no obstruction to voiding.
3. Urethrotomy is potentially curative for short strictures (smaller than 1 cm) that have minimal spongiofibrosis.
4. After each successive urethrotomy, there is a period of fleeting good urinary flow, followed by worsened degree of spongiofibrosis and a lingering stricture. There are also reports of lumen obliteration, as well as hemorrhage, sepsis, incontinence, local veno-occlusive erectile dysfunction, glans numbness, and priapism (particularly true for deep cuts made at 12 o'clock).
5. In the short term (less than 6 months), success rates are 70 to 80 percent. After 1 year, however, recurrence rates approach

50 to 60 percent, and by 5 years, 74 to 86 percent (depending on stricture length and degree of spongiofibrosis).

6. Direct visual urethrotomy by cold knife in Sasche fashion, with a deep cut at 12 o'clock (generally to 22 F) is the traditional method. Due to the location of the lumen in the spongiosum, in the bulbar urethra, cuts are better at 2 and 10 o'clock, whereas in the pendulous urethra, at 12 o'clock. Others prefer multiple circumferential radial incisions to open up the urethra.

7. Attempts to improve the mediocre long-term results of internal urethrotomy have been made with laser urethrotomy. Contact mode Nd:Yag lasers have been used to "chisel" out the scar. Results, however, are not superior to standard techniques.

I. Urethroplasty

Urethroplasty is scar revision surgery. Prior to any urethroplasty the scar should be stable and no longer contracting. Thus, it is preferred that the urethra not be instrumented for 3 months prior to planned surgery. If the stricture patient goes into urinary retention, a suprapubic tube should be placed. General guidelines for management are detailed in Figure 12-1.

1. Excision and Primary Anastomosis (EPA)
   a. Excision of the complete scar and primary anastomosis (EPA) is the optimal stricture repair.
   b. The technique of EPA involves circumferential mobilization of the strictured urethra from the penoscrotal junction to proximal bulb, complete excision of the scarred tissue, urethral spatulation, and reapproximation of the two urethral ends in two layers (urethral mucosa and spongiosal adventitia). The distal urethral segment relies on a good distal blood supply for survival, which may be impaired in patients with prior hypospadias.
   c. EPA is appropriate for bulbar urethral strictures under 2.5 cm in length. Reapproximation of longer strictures can result in ventral curvature, pain, and tension on the anastomosis. Overall, long-term success approaches 95 to 100 percent.
   d. Recurrence after EPA is due to inadequate excision of the fibrosis and inadequate urethral mobilization (where excess anastomotic tension results in ischemia). For strictures longer then 2.5 cm, the dorsal urethral plate can be anastomosed and an onlay graft of skin or buccal mucosa placed ventrally.

2. Grafts
   a. A graft is a tissue transfer that is dependent on the host blood supply for survival. The process is called a graft

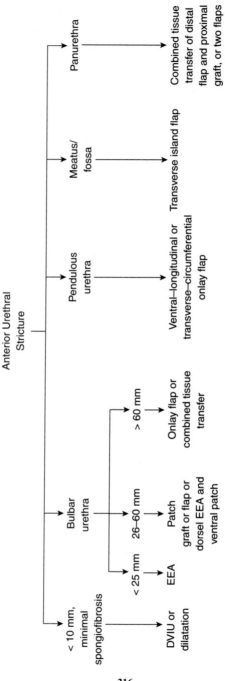

Figure 12-1 Algorithm for the management of anterior urethral stricture reconstruction. DVIU, direct visual internal urethrotomy; EEA, end-to-end anastomosis.

"take" and occurs in two stages, imbibition and inosculation.

b. Imbibition is nutrient absorption from the host bed in the first 48 hours.

c. The second phase is inosculation, which take place from 48 to 96 hours after grafting. Inosculation is graft revascularization by blood vessels and lymph joining from the host bed to the graft.

d. Conditions for graft success are well-vascularized host bed, rapid onset of imbibition, good apposition and immobilization of graft, and rapid onset of inosculation.

e. Skin grafts

　　1. Split thickness skin graft comprises the epidermis and superficial section of the papillary dermis.

　　2. Dermal graft comprises the deep papillary and the reticular dermis.

　　3. Full thickness skin graft involves all layers, the epidermis, papillary dermis, and the reticular dermis.

f. Free-graft urethroplasty

The primary grafts used are penile skin, buccal mucosa or bladder epithelium. Grafts are highly successful in the bulbar urethra as an onlay or patch technique, and where a spongioplasty to cover the graft can be performed. Buccal mucosa is easy and quick to harvest, minimally morbid, and has excellent take (up to 86 percent), mostly due to a thin lamina propria and thick epithelium. Urethrotomy is traditionally directed ventral. Dorsal urethrotomy (Barbagli) and grafting has gained recent popular use. Full-thickness skin grafts are used in urethral reconstruction because of their high "take," and contacts little (15 to 25 percent). Split-thickness grafts are not be used in one-stage urethroplasty because in unsupported tissue they can contact as much as 100 percent. Penile skin should be avoided when the penile skin is not abundant or also affected by BXO. Grafts are particularly useful in the obese patient with a bulbar stricture, where time in lithotomy needs to be minimized.

g. Meshed graft two-stage urethroplasty

　　i. Usually reserved for patients who have undergone failed urethroplasties or where the urethra and local skin are severely scarred, two-stage reconstruction is also indicated when stricture is associated with a fistula or abscess or lack of sufficient well-vascularized local skin for a one-stage reconstruction.

　　ii. The technique by Schreiter is a modification of the original two-stage urethroplasty by Johanson. After ventral urethrotomy to marsupialize the urethra, a meshed skin graft (4 to 5 cm in width) is tacked to the Dartos and urethral edges. After 6 months of graft maturation, the urethra is created by tubularizing the tissue in standard Thiersch-Duplay fashion.

3. Flaps

A flap is a tissue transfer where the donor blood supply is left intact. The success of a flap is described as "survival" and has better overall success than grafts.

a. *Penile and preputial island flaps.* Penile flaps are the mainstay of urethral reconstruction. Penile skin flaps rely on the rich vascular collaterals within the tunica Dartos for its blood supply. The anterior lamella of Buck's fascia is elevated to ensure taking the entire Dartos. Elevation is basically along avascular planes and thus bloodless. Island flaps are versatile and can be mobilized to all areas of the anterior urethra. Success rates of 85 to 90 percent are with onlay flaps where the urethral plate remains intact. Completely tubularized flaps have a near 50 percent failure rate. Depending on the location and the length of the stricture, flaps can be ventral–longitudinal (Orandi, for pendulous urethra), ventral–transverse (Jordan/Devine, for fossa strictures), or transverse–circumferential (Quartey, McAninch, or Q-type, for anterior urethra) and rotated to reach the defect. Proper mobilization will not put the flap on tension or cause penile torsion. The advantages of transverse–circumferential flaps is that they are always hairless, can be mobilized to any area of the anterior urethra, and are long (10 to 15 cm). Ventral flaps require less mobilization but hair is often present at the proximal aspect and limited in use to the pendulous urethra.

b. *Scrotal skin island flaps.* Indicated for bulbar strictures where time in lithotomy needs to be minimized or where other tissues are not available. When mobilizing a scrotal flap of skin, care should be taken to choose a non-hair bearing area. Otherwise, a hairy urethra can result, which is complicated by recurrent infection, sprayed urinary stream, and stone formation. A hairless patch of skin can often be found in the midline and the posterior scrotum. If the scrotum is hairy, the skin island can be expanded by epilation. After the initial epilation, the patient is reassessed 6 weeks later for a second treatment. The scrotal blood supply is dependent on the superficial external pudendal and the scrotal arteries. A scrotal flap is based on the Dartos for its blood supply, and is used as a patch onto an intact urethral plate. The disadvantages of scrotal skin over penile skin are it is more difficult to work with, tends to contract (and from redundancy, more prone to sacculation), and has a unilateral blood supply.

c. *Combined tissue transfer.* Occasionally, stricture length is so long that flap length is insufficient. In these cases, a combination of distal flap and proximal graft are used. Two island flaps can also be used. In so doing, panurethral strictures can be reconstructed in a single stage.

III. POSTERIOR URETHRAL STRICTURES
A. Urethral Distraction Injury Strictures

1. Urethral distraction injuries occur in up to 10 percent of pelvic fractures and are mainly due to high-speed motor vehicle accidents and occupational related injuries.

2. Urethral strictures develop in nearly all patients after a complete urethral disruption. Initial management by primary realignment appears to decrease overall stricture incidence.

3. Three to 6 months after initial injury, the prostate and bladder descend as the pelvic hematoma is reabsorbed and organized.

4. The eventual stricture length is commonly only 1 to 2 cm. Such relatively short strictures can be easily bridged by a one-stage urethroplasty.

5. The stricture involves, to varying degrees, spongiofibrosis of the distal bulb and membranous urethra. The other potential segments of "stricture" are not true strictures of the urethra, but rather scar tissue in the intervening space between the dislocated prostate and the pelvic diaphragm.

6. Less then 10 percent of urethral strictures are complex, that is with long urethral defects (longer than 6 cm) or associated with anterior urethral strictures, rectal or bladder neck injury, fistulas (urethrocutaneous or recto-urethral), or chronic periurethral cavities.

B. Stricture Evaluation

1. Although newer modalities, including ultrasound and magnetic resonance imaging (MRI) have been employed, dynamic fluoroscopic imaging with a simultaneous VCUG and retrograde urethrogram (RUG) remain the gold standard. When fluoroscopic images are confusing, MRI is helpful in surgical planning.

2. Before presenting for urethral reconstruction, the patient also must have:

a. No evidence of pelvic abscess or infection.

b. A competent bladder neck. Because the external/membranous urethra is damaged, a competent bladder neck is essential to assure continence after reconstruction. A static cystogram followed by voiding can assess bladder neck function.

c. No urethral instrumentation in the last 3 months (the scar must be stable).

C. Urethroplasty

1. One-stage open urethroplasty is the gold standard for correcting posterior urethral strictures. Long-term success rates approach 90 to 95 percent. Such surgery, however, is technically demanding and time consuming.

2. Multiple minimally invasive techniques have been reported, most being some modification of the "cut to the light" procedure. Long-term results have been poor and such techniques should be considered temporizing measures and not methods for cure.

3. Posterior urethroplasty is essentially a urethral flap detached from its proximal vascular supply and dependent on distal retrograde blood flow from the dorsal and circumflex arteries of the penis.

4. Patients with anterior urethral strictures, hypospadias, or traumatic bilateral pudendal artery occlusion, therefore, have a compromised retrograde/collateral urethral blood supply. One-stage posterior urethroplasty is relatively contraindicated in such patients.

5. Urethroplasty failure is commonly due to tension on the anastomosis, compromised retrograde urethral vascularity, and/or inadequate apical resection of scar.

6. Surgical methods to achieve a tension-free, mucosa to mucosa anastomosis of bulb to prostate are:

   a. Urethral mobilization from the penoscrotal junction to perineal membrane and judicious resection of apical scar (for strictures less than 3 cm in length).

   b. Separation of the corpora cavernosal bodies in the midline (for strictures 3 to 5 cm).

   c. Inferior pubectomy (for strictures longer than 5 cm or distorted pelvic anatomy).

   d. Rerouting the urethra under the crus of the corpora (for strictures longer than 6 cm).

   e. Combined transpubic/retropubic approach (employed for defects more than 6 cm or orthopedic deformity that precludes adequate perineal access).

   f. Urethral substitution with tubularized flap or two-stage graft urethroplasty (reserved for very long strictures, associated anterior urethral stricture/hypospadias, or as salvage for failed one-stage urethroplasty).

D. Post-Prostate Surgery Strictures

1. Membranous urethral strictures occur after up to 6 percent of transurethral resection of the prostate (TURP) procedures. Etiology is trauma of using too large a resectoscope or catheter or from over aggressive distal prostate resection. After radical prostatectomy, membranous urethral strictures are also rare, and are the result of poor mucosa–mucosa apposition.

2. TURP, simple prostatectomy, and radical prostatectomy all damage the internal urethral sphincter and thus continence is subsequently dependent on the external striated sphincter.

3. Strictures involving the external sphincter are best managed by urethral dilatation. Urethrotomy or other surgical repair can often result in incontinence.

BIBLIOGRAPHY

Dixon CM, Hricak H, McAninch JW: Magnetic resonance imaging of traumatic posterior urethral defects and pelvic crush injuries. *J Urol* 148:1162, 1992.

Morey AF, McAninch JW: Reconstruction of posterior urethral disruption injuries: Outcome analysis in 82 patients. *J Urol* 157:506, 1997.

Orandi A: One-stage urethroplasty. *Br J Urol* 40:717, 1968.

Pansadoro V, Emiliozzi P: Internal urethrotomy in the management of anterior urethral strictures: Long-term follow-up. *J Urol* 156:73, 1996.

Quartey JKM: One-stage penile/preputial island flap urethroplasty for urethral stricture. *J Urol* 134:474, 1985.

Schreiter F, Noll F: Mesh graft urethroplasty using a split-thickness skin graft of foreskin. *J Urol* 142:1223, 1989

Waterhouse K, Abrahms JI, Gruber H, et al: The transpubic approach to the lower urinary tract. *J Urol* 109:486, 1973.

Webster GD: Management of complex posterior urethral strictures. Problems Urol 1:226,1987.

Webster GD, Koefoot RB, Sihelnik SA: Urethroplasty management in 200 cases of urethral stricture: A rationale for procedure selection. *J Urol* 134:892, 1985.

SELF-ASSESSMENT QUESTIONS

1. A 25-year-old man with a 3.5 cm bulbar urethral stricture is best managed by:
   a. internal urethrotomy.
   b. urethral dilatation.
   c. end–end urethroplasty.
   d. buccal mucosal graft patch urethroplasty.
   e. laser urethrotomy.

2. The arterial blood supply to the penile skin is the:
   a. superficial inferior epigastric.
   b. external pudendal.
   c. penile artery.
   d. internal pudendal.
   e. gonadal.

3. A 16-year-old adolescent with a history of penoscrotal hypospadias presents with a 8 cm pendulous urethral stricture. Over the years, he has undergone nine operations on his urethra. The best management is:
   a. circular fasciocutaneous onlay flap urethroplasty.
   b. perineal urethrostomy.

   c. meshed graft, two-stage urethroplasty.

   d. buccal mucosa onlay graft urethroplasty.

   e. ventral–longitudinal onlay flap urethroplasty.

4. 34-year-old with a 2 cm pendulous, mid-penile urethral stricture. The best long-term treatment is:

   a. buccal mucosal onlay graft.

   b. internal urethrotomy.

   c. fasciocutaneous onlay flap urethroplasty.

   d. meshed graft, two stage urethroplasty.

   e. urethrotomy and periurethral triamcinolone injection.

5. Two-stage meshed graft urethroplasty is usually reserved for patients with:

   a. multiple failed urethroplasties.

   b. severely scarred local skin.

   c. hypospadias "cripple."

   d. severe stricture associated with fistula or abscess.

   e. all of the above.

6. Which of the conditions are key for graft success (take)?

   a. Rapid onset of imbibition

   b. Well-vascularized host bed

   c. Immobilization of the graft

   d. Rapid onset of inosculation

   e. All of the above

7. When using a combined tissue transfer techniques of a buccal mucosal graft and a fasciocutaneous flap for a bulbar pendulous stricture, the best to place the graft is:

   a. the meatus.

   b. the fossa.

   c. the pendulous urethra.

   d. the bulb.

   e. all of the above.

8. Which of the following are relative contraindications to performing a posterior urethroplasty?

   a. Open bladder neck noted on cystogram

   b. Pelvis abscess

   c. Pelvic infection

   d. Failed "cut to the light" procedure 3 weeks ago

   e. All of the above

9. During an end–end urethroplasty, what is the primary blood supply to the distal urethra?

   a. Dorsal artery of the penis

   b. Central cavernosal artery

   c. Superficial external pudendal artery

   d. Urethral artery

   e. Inferior epigastric artery

10. A 67-year-old man with no prior voiding dysfunction now presents with a 0.3 cm bulbar urethral stricture after open heart surgery. The initial best management is:

   a. end–end urethroplasty.

   b. buccal mucosal graft.

   c. fasciocutaneous flap.

   d. internal urethrotomy.

   e. dorsal patch graft.

Answers   1. d, 2. b, 3. c, 4. c, 5. d, 6. e, 7. d, 8. e, 9. a, 10. d

CHAPTER 13
Urinary Fistulae

Eric S. Rovner

A fistula represents a nonanatomic epithelialized connection between two or more body spaces. Although most fistulae are iatrogenic, they can also occur as a result of congenital anomalities, neoplastic or inflammatory processes, radiation therapy, trauma, and parturition.

I. VESICOVAGINAL FISTULA
A. General Considerations
Vesicovaginal fistulae (VVF) are the most common acquired fistula of the urinary tract.

1. Because fistulas result in considerable patient discomfort, are invariably unexpected, and finally, may be acquired as a result of surgical treatment of an unrelated problem, considerable emotional distress often accompanies the diagnosis and subsequent treatment.

2. VVF have been known about since ancient times, however, it was not until 1663 that Hendrik von Roonhuyse first described surgical repair. In 1852, James Marion Sims published his now famous surgical series describing a method of surgical treatment of VVF using silver wire in a transvaginal approach. Of note, it was not until the thirtieth attempt at closure of VVF that he achieved success.

B. Etiology
The most common cause of VVF differs in various parts of world. In the industrialized world, the most common cause (75 percent) is injury to the bladder at the time of gynecologic surgery; usually abdominal hysterectomy, whereas the remainder are due to vaginal hysterectomy or anti-incontinence surgery such as anterior colporrhaphy. Obstetric trauma accounts for very few VVF in the United States and other industrialized nations.

In the developing world, where routine perinatal obstetrical care may be limited, VVF most commonly occur as a result of prolonged labor with resulting pressure necrosis to the anterior vaginal wall and underlying trigone of the bladder from the baby's head. In some instances, VVF can result from the use of forceps or other instrumentation during delivery. Obstetric fistulas tend to be larger, located distally in the vagina, and may involve the proximal urethra.

1. Other causes of VVF include urologic or gynecologic instrumentation, pelvic malignancy (cervical cancer, etc.), inflammatory diseases, radiation therapy, and trauma.

2. Post-hysterectomy VVF are thought to result from an unrecognized incidental cystotomy near the vaginal cuff or as a result of tissue necrosis from a suture placed through both the bladder and vaginal wall during closure of the vaginal cuff.

C. Presentation

1. The most common complaint is constant urinary drainage per vagina although small fistulas can present with intermittent wetness that is positional in nature.

   a. VVF must be distinguished from urinary incontinence due to other causes including stress (urethral) incontinence, urge (bladder) incontinence, and overflow incontinence.

   b. Patients may also complain of recurrent cystitis, perineal skin irritation due to constant wetness, vaginal fungal infections, or rarely, pelvic pain. When a large VVF is present, patients may not void at all and simply have continuous leakage of urine into the vagina.

   c. VVF following hysterectomy or other surgical procedures may present upon removal of the urethral catheter or 1 to 3 weeks later with urinary drainage per vagina.

      i. VVF resulting from hysterectomy are usually located high in the vagina at the level of the vaginal cuff (Fig. 13-1).

   d. VVF resulting from radiation therapy may not present for months to years following completion of radiation. These tend to represent some of the most challenging reconstructive cases due to the size, complexity, and the associated voiding dysfunction due to the radiation effects on the urinary bladder. The endarteritis as a result of the radiation therapy can involve the surrounding tissues, limiting reconstructive options.

D. Evaluation

1. History

2. Physical examination

   a. A pelvic examination with a speculum should always be performed in an attempt to locate the fistula and assess the size and number of fistulae.

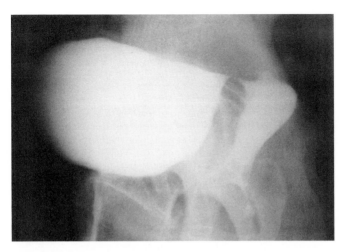

Figure 13-1 VCUG demonstrating a VVF high at the level of the vaginal cuff in a patient following hysterectomy. The vagina and fistula tract are well specified. VCUG, voiding cystourethrogram; VVF, vesicovaginal fistula.

    b. Palpate for masses or other pelvic pathology that may need to be addressed at the time of fistula repair.

    c. An assessment of inflammation surrounding the fistula is necessary as it can affect timing of the repair.

    d. The presence of a VVF can be confirmed by instilling a vital blue dye or sterile milk into the bladder per urethra and observing for discolored vaginal drainage.

       i. A double dye test can confirm the diagnosis of urinary fistula as well as suggest the possibility of an associated ureterovaginal or urethrovaginal fistula. A tampon is placed per vagina. Oral phenazopyridine is administered and vital blue dye is instilled into the bladder. If the tampon is discolored yellow-orange at the top, it is suggestive of a ureterovaginal fistula. Blue discoloration in the midportion of the tampon suggests VVF, whereas blue staining at the bottom suggests a urethrovaginal fistula.

3. Urine culture and urine analysis

4. Cystoscopy and possible biopsy of the fistula tract is performed if malignancy is suspected.

    a. Note the location of fistula relative to ureters; repair of the fistula may require reimplantation of ureters if the fistula involves the ureteral orifice.

5. Voiding cystourethrography
   a. Some small fistulas may not be seen radiographically unless the bladder is filled to capacity and a detrusor contraction is provoked during filling.
      i. Assesses for vesicoureteral reflux.
      ii. Examines for multiple fistulae including urethrovaginal fistula.
      iii. Assesses size and location of fistula.
6. Intravenous urography and/or retrograde pyeloureterography
   a. Assesses for concomitant ureteral injury and/or ureterovaginal fistula, which has been reported to occur in up to 12 percent of patients.
7. Cross-sectional pelvic imaging (MRI/CT) if malignancy is suspected.

E. Therapy

1. Nonsurgical management
   a. Catheter drainage is the initial treatment in most cases when the VVF is recognized early in the clinical course. Antibiotics and topical estrogen creams are adjuvant measures to prevent infection and promote healing.
   b. Fulguration of the fistula followed by catheter drainage has been shown to have some efficacy in small (less than 5 mm), uncomplicated fistulae.
   c. Adjuvant measures (such fibrin glue, etc.) have been used by some clinicians in conjunction with fulguration and catheter drainage as a "plug" in the fistula as well as a "scaffolding" to allow the ingrowth of healthy tissue.
2. Surgical management
   a. Success rates approach 90 to 98 percent regardless of surgical approach.
   b. Adherence to basic surgical principles are essential to achieve success in the repair of all urinary fistula (Table 13-1).
   c. Choice of the optimal surgical approach to VVF is controversial and there are numerous factors to consider (Table 13-2). No single approach is applicable to all VVF.
      i. *Transabdominal approach.* Generally performed as described by O'Conor. Through a midline infraumbilical incision, the bladder is exposed and opened in the sagittal plane down to the level of the fistula. The bladder is separated off the vagina beyond the level of the fistula. The fistulous tract

Table 13-1 Principles of Vesicovaginal Fistula Repair

Successful fistula repair requires the adherence to certain basic surgical principles:

1. Good hemostasis.
2. Judicious use of cautery.
3. Adequate exposure of the fistula tract.
4. Watertight closure of each layer.
5. Well-vascularized, healthy tissue for repair. The use of topical estrogens can be helpful to improve vaginal tissue quality preoperatively.
6. Multiple layer closure.
7. Tension-free, nonoverlapping suture lines.
8. Adequate urinary drainage after repair.
9. Prevention of infection (use of pre-, post-, and intraoperative antibiotics).
10. Adequate preoperative nutritional repletion.

---

is debrided back to healthy tissue from both bladder and vaginal sides. The bladder and vagina are closed separately. Often, well-vascularized tissue such as omentum is interposed between the vagina and bladder as an additional layer to promote healing and prevent recurrence.

ii. *Transvaginal approach.* Many approaches have been described including Sims, Latzko, and Raz. Through a vaginal approach, the vaginal wall is mobilized circumferentially about the fistula tract. Either the fistula tract is excised, with edges of the debrided tract forming the first layer of closure, or the tract is left in-situ, with fistula edges rolled over forming the primary layer of closure. The perivesical fascia on either side of the first layer of closure is then imbricated over the primary suture line forming the second layer. A labial fat pad (i.e., Martius flap), peritoneal flap, or gracilis muscle flap may be placed over the suture lines as a well-vascularized flap similar to the omental flap in the transabdominal approach. Finally, a flap of vaginal wall is advanced over the repair forming the final layer of closure.

3. Regardless of approach, maximal urinary drainage (urethral and suprapubic catheters) is maintained postoperatively. A cystogram is usually obtained 2 to 3 weeks following repair to confirm successful closure.

Table 13-2 Abdominal versus Transvaginal Repair of Vesicovaginal Fistula

Vesicovaginal fistula may be repaired through a transvaginal or transabdominal (transvesical) approach. There is no preferred approach for all fistulas; the "best" approach depends on the particular characteristics of the fistula and surgeon's experience.

	ABDOMINAL	TRANSVAGINAL
Length of hospitalization	4–7 days	1–2 days
Timing of repair	Usually delayed 2–6 months from the time of initial injury	May be done immediately in the absence of infection
Location of ureters relative to fistula tract	Fistula located near ureteral orifice may necessitate reimplantation	Reimplantation may not be necessary even if fistula tract is located near ureteral orifice
Sexual function	No change in vaginal depth	Potential risk of vaginal shortening or stenosis
Location of fistula tract/depth of vagina	Fistula located low on the trigone or near the bladder neck may be difficult to expose	Fistula located high at the vaginal cuff may be difficult to expose and repair transvaginally
Use of adjunctive flaps	Omentum, peritoneal flap, intestine	Labial fat pad (Martius fat pad); peritoneal flap; gracilis muscle; labial myocutaneous flap
Relative indications	Large fistulas; located high in a deep vagina; radiation fistulas; failed transvaginal approach; small capacity bladder requiring augmentation; need for ureteral reimplantation; inability to place patient in the lithotomy position	Uncomplicated fistulas, low fistulas, vaginal exposure may be difficult some nulliparous patients.

II. URETEROVAGINAL FISTULA

A. Etiology

Most ureterovaginal fistula are secondary to unrecognized distal ureteral injuries sustained during gynecologic procedures including: abdominal or vaginal hysterectomy, cesarean section, anti-incontinence surgery, and so forth. Occasionally, they may be secondary to endoscopic instrumentation, radiation therapy, pelvic malignancy, penetrating pelvic trauma, or other pelvic surgery (vascular, enteric, etc.).

1. Risk factors for ureteral injuries include a prior history of pelvic surgery, endometriosis, radiation therapy, and pelvic inflammatory disease.
2. Up to 12 percent of vesicovaginal fistulae may have an associated ureterovaginal fistula.

B. Presentation

May present with clear drainage per vagina or unilateral hydroureteronephrosis and flank pain secondary to partial ureteral obstruction. Flank pain, nausea, fever, and clear vaginal drainage following pelvic surgery is very suggestive of ureteral injury. Patients will almost invariably have a normal voiding pattern due to a normal contralateral upper unit.

C. Evaluation

1. *Intravenous urography.* A urogram may demonstrate partial obstruction, hydroureteronephrosis, and drainage into the vagina.
2. *Cystoscopy and retrograde pyelography.* These are performed to evaluate for bladder injury and to visualize the distal ureteral segment if not well seen on the urogram. An attempt at retrograde stenting is reasonable if the pyeloureterogram demonstrates ureteral continuity. Prolonged internal diversion with ureteral stenting may result in resolution of the fistula.
3. *CT/MRI.* Cross-sectional imaging can be useful to evaluate for pelvic malignancy when indicated or evaluate for a urinoma in patients with persistent fevers.
4. *Cystogram or cystometrogram.* In cases where a long segment of distal ureter is involved and a Boari flap is being considered for reconstruction, a cystogram or cystometrogram can be useful to evaluate the bladder capacity. In addition, a cystogram should evaluate for vesicoureteral reflux.

D. Therapy

1. *Percutaneous drainage and possible antegrade stenting.* If high-grade partial obstruction exists in the setting of sepsis, percutaneous drainage and a course of antibiotic therapy is indicated prior to definitive repair (Fig. 13-2). If retrograde stenting is unsuccessful but the pyeloureterogram shows continuity of the ureteral lumen, then an attempt at antegrade stenting can be made.

2. Ureteral stenting (see above).

3. *Surgery.* When stenting is unsuccessful, ureteral reimplantation (with or without psoas hitch) is performed. It is not necessary to excise the distal ureteral segment or even close the fistula unless vesicoureteral reflux is present.

4. Fistulas resulting from advanced pelvic malignancy may best be treated by urinary diversion.

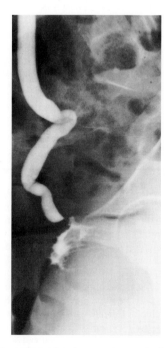

Figure 13-2 Antegrade nephrostogram demonstrating ureteral dilation and drainage into the vagina following abdominal hysterectomy. No contrast enters the urinary bladder consistent with complete ureteral obstruction and ureterovaginal fistula.

III. URETHROVAGINAL FISTULA

A. Etiology

Usually postsurgical (urethral diverticulectomy, anti-incontinence surgery, etc.), although they can occur as a result of trauma, instrumentation (catheterization), radiation, and child birth.

B. Presentation

Urethovaginal fistulae are often asymptomatic if located in the distal third of the urethra (beyond the continence mechanism), otherwise the presentation is similar to VVF. Occasionally, these patients may present with symptoms suggestive of stress or urgency incontinence and cystourethrography will be necessary to make the diagnosis. Dyspareunia or recurrent urinary tract infections (UTIs) are sometimes seen.

C. Evaluation

1. Voiding cystourethrography *VCUG*. Voiding images must be obtained in patients with a competent bladder neck and proximal sphincteric mechanism or the fistula will not be demonstrated.
2. *Cystoscopy*. Useful to evaluate for concurrent abnormalities of the bladder and urethra.

D. Therapy

1. Catheter drainage can be useful in a limited number of cases if the fistula is noted promptly.
2. Transvaginal surgical excision with urethral reconstruction, multiple layer closure using periurethral fascia, a labial fat pad (Martius flap), and vaginal wall flaps is usually highly successful.

IV. ENTEROVESICAL FISTULA

A. General Considerations

Enterovesical fistulas can form between any segment of bowel in the pelvis (colon, ileum, etc.) and the bladder.

B. Etiology

The most common cause of enterovesical fistula is diverticular disease of the colon (50 to 70 percent). Other common causes include neoplastic disease (colon cancer), inflammatory bowel disease (Crohn's disease), radiation therapy, and trauma.

C. Presentation

1. Enterovesical fistula may present with recurrent UTIs, fecaluria, pneumaturia, and hematuria.

2. Presentation with sepsis or GI symptoms is rare.
3. Gouverneur's syndrome (suprapubic pain, urinary frequency, dysuria, and tenesmus) is the hallmark of enterovesical fistula.

D. Evaluation
1. *Charcoal test.* The oral administration of activated charcoal can confirm the diagnosis of enterovesical fistula. Several hours after ingestion, flecks of charcoal can be noted in the urine.
2. *Cystoscopy and possible biopsy.* Endoscopic visualization has the highest yield for the identification of enterovesical fistula.
   i. Eighty to 100 percent of cases demonstrate bullous edema, erythema, or exudation of feculent material from the fistula site.
   ii. Generally, colonic fistulas occur on the left side and dome of the bladder, whereas small bowel fistulas occur on the dome and right side of the bladder.
   iii. Biopsy of the fistula is indicated in cases where malignancy is suspected.
3. *Colonscopy and barium enema.* Although less common than diverticular disease, it is important to exclude primary intestinal malignancy as the cause for the fistula.
4. *CT or MRI of the pelvis.* Air in the bladder, as seen on cross-sectional imaging, in the absence of prior lower urinary instrumentation (cystoscopy, catheterization, etc.) is highly suggestive of an enterovesical fistula. CT scan with contrast is generally considered to have the best diagnostic yield.
5. VCUG may demonstrate the fistulous connection. In some cases, however, the fistula can act as a "flap valve" and contrast will not be seen entering the bowel.

E. Therapy
1. *Bowel rest and hyperalimentation.* Total parental nutrition may allow the spontaneous closure of some enterovesical fistulae.
2. *Medical therapy.* This is most applicable in enterovesical fistula secondary to Crohn's disease. Appropriate use of corticosteroids, sulfasalazine, and antibiotics may promote spontaneous resolution.
3. Surgery. The application of surgery may involve either one-stage or a multistage approach depending on the presence or absence of inflammation, malignancy, and adjacent organ involvement. In those cases managed with staged procedures, a temporary fecal diversion is performed at the time of fistula repair.

i. The surgery involves laparotomy, separation of the bladder from the bowel, excision of the fistula tract, and primary closure of the involved viscera.

ii. In some cases, partial cystectomy and/or bowel resection may be necessary.

iii. Interposition of well-vascularized tissue such as omentum between the bowel and bladder may promote healing and prevent recurrence.

V. RECTOURETHRAL FISTULA

A. Etiology

May occur following radical prostatectomy, external beam radiotherapy for pelvic malignancy, pelvic brachytherapy, inflammatory diseases of the pelvis (prostatic abscess), or following penetrating pelvic trauma. During radical prostatectomy, the anterior rectal wall injury can be injured during dissection of the apical portion of the prostate. A postoperative rectourethral fistula can form from the reconstructed vesicourethral anastomosis to the injured portion of the rectum.

B. Presentation

May present with recurrent UTI's, fecaluria, pneumaturia, or, rarely, urine per rectum. A defect may be palpable at the level of the vesicourethral anastomosis. If a Foley catheter is indwelling it can be palpable on rectal examination.

C. Evaluation

1. Voiding cystourethrography will demonstrate a fistula between the rectum and urethra.

2. Intravenous urography may be used if there is concern for ureteral injury.

3. Barium enema can be helpful to rule out concurrent colonic malignancy.

4. Cystoscopy and/or colonoscopy.

5. CT or MRI of the pelvis can be utilized to evaluate for inflammatory collections or other pelvic masses (e.g., malignancy).

D. Therapy

Many approaches have been advocated for repair of this complex problem. Often, however, despite successful repair of the fistula and reconstitution of the GI and GU tracts, the patient may have severe problems with urinary and fecal incontinence postoperatively and should be counseled regarding this possibility prior to attempted repair. Both staged repairs and one-stage repairs have been advocated, although most clinicians would agree that fecal diversion should be performed as an initial measure. In staged repairs, the GI tract is reconstituted only after the fistula has been repaired. Surgical options include:

1. *Colostomy and urethral catheter drainage.* An attempt at fecal diversion and urethral drainage is a reasonable option in most patients. With prolonged fecal diversion, the fistula may close over the urethral catheter.

2. *Colostomy followed by a combined abdominal and/or perineal approach.* The rectum is separated off the urethra and both are closed primarily. Well-vascularized tissue such as omentum is interposed between the layers.

3. *Colostomy followed by a transrectal approach (York-Mason or transphincteric approach).* The fistula is exposed using either anal dilation and a speculum, or by transecting the anal sphincters. The fistula is then repaired in multiple layers by advancement and rotation of rectal wall flaps.

VI. OTHER URINARY FISTULA

A. Urovascular Fistula

Most commonly, these fistulae occur between the ureter and surrounding blood vessels such as the iliacs. Vigorous hematuria in the setting of indwelling stents in a previously irradiated patient or a patient with a history of vascular surgery should alert the physician to the possibility of this type of fistula. If the patient is in extremis (exsanguinating, etc.), immediate surgical intervention is indicated. If the patient is stable, imaging studies including CT, MRI, or angiography may be indicated. In some cases, surgery can be avoided with the use of interventional radiological techniques.

B. Vesicouterine Fistula

These rare fistulae most commonly occur following low segment cesarean section. They may present with Youssef's syndrome: menouria, apparent amenorrhea, patent cervix, and urinary continence. Treatment is usually surgical and involves either hysterectomy and closure of the bladder (if the patient has completed child-bearing) or excision of the fistula tract and separate closure of the bladder and uterus with interposition of omentum. Occasionally, successful treatment has been seen with hormonal induction of amenorrhea and catheter drainage.

BIBLIOGRAPHY

Gerber, Glenn S, Schoenberg HW: Female urinary tract fistulas. *J Urol* 149:229–236, 1993.

Goodwin WE, Scardino PT: Vesicovaginal and ureterovaginal fistulas: A summary of 25 years of experience. *J Urol* 123:370–4, 1980.

Leach GE: Urethrovaginal fistula repair with Martius labial fat pad. *Urol Clin North Am* 18:409–413, 1991.

Raz S, Bregg KJ, Nitti WVW, Sussman E: Transvaginal repair of vesicovaginal fistula using a peritoneal flap. *J Urol* 150:56–59, 1993.

Stothers L, Chopra A, Raz S: Vesicovaginal fistula. In: Raz S, ed. *Female Urology,* 2nd ed. Philadelphia, Saunders, 1997, pp. 490–506.

Stovsky MD, Ignatoff JM, Blum MD, Nanninga JB, O'Conor VJ, Kursh ED: Use of electrocoagulation in the treatment of vesicovaginal fistulas. *J Urol* 152:1443–1444, 1994.

Velagapudi SRC, Pollack HM, Weiss JP: *Acquired Fistula of the Urinary Tract.* Houston, vol. 12, AUA Update Series, AUA Office of Education, 1993, pp. 138–143.

Zimmern PE, Hadley HR, Staskin, DR, Raz S: Genitourinary fistulae: Vaginal approach for repair of vesicovaginal fistulae. *Urol Clin North Am* 12:361–367, 1985.

SELF-ASSESSMENT QUESTIONS

1. All of the following are true regarding vesicovaginal fistula (VVF) except:
   a. The most common cause of VVF in the United States is obstetrical trauma.
   b. VVF resulting from radiation therapy may not present for several months following completion of the radiation.
   c. VVF can be repaired through a transabdominal or transvaginal approach with similar success rates.
   d. Stress urinary incontinence can co-exist with VVF.
   e. Repair of a VVF using a transvaginal approach can be associated with postoperative dyspareunia.

2. A 45-year-old female presents with continuous urinary leakage following successful treatment of cervical cancer with radical hysterectomy and external beam radiotherapy several years prior. A vesicovaginal fistula is suspected. Which of the following is not usually indicated as part of the initial evaluation?
   a. Cystography (VCUG)
   b. Gas cystometrogram
   c. Cystoscopy and possible biopsy
   d. Intravenous urography
   e. Double dye test

3. A 58-year-old female with recurrent UTIs, grade III cystocele, and stress urinary incontinence undergoes a Raz bladder neck suspension and anterior colporrhaphy for treatment of the stress incontinence and prolapse. Intraoperatively, a urethral diverticulum is encountered and excised. Two weeks following surgery, the patient complains of recurrent debilitating incontinence. Post-void residual is minimal. Potential etiologies for the incontinence include all of the following except:
   a. urethrovaginal fistula.
   b. recurrent urethral diverticulum.
   c. de novo urgency incontinence.
   d. intrinsic sphincter deficiency.
   e. vesicovaginal fistula.

4. Rectourethral fistula can result from all of the following except:
   a. radical perineal prostatectomy.
   b. radical retropubic prostatectomy.
   c. abdominoperineal resection.

    d. stab wound to the scrotum.

    e. radiation therapy to the pelvis.

5. A 72-year-old female with a history of colon cancer presents with urinary frequency, recurrent UTIs, and hematuria. Gross inspection of the urine reveals particulate matter. Office cystoscopy reveals bullous edema and erythema adjacent to the dome of the bladder. Appropriate initial evaluation would include all of the following except:

    a. bladder biopsy.

    b. intravenous urography.

    c. CT of the pelvis.

    d. double dye test.

    e. urine culture.

Answers

1. a
2. b
3. b
4. c
5. d

CHAPTER 14

Voiding Function and Dysfunction

Alan J. Wein
Eric S. Rovner

The lower urinary tract (LUT) functions as a group of interrelated structures with a joint function in the adult to bring about efficient and low pressure bladder filling, low pressure urine storage with perfect continence, and periodic complete voluntary urinary expulsion, again at low pressure. Because in the adult the LUT is normally under voluntary neural control, it is clearly different from other visceral organs which are regulated solely by involuntary mechanisms. For description and teaching, the micturition cycle is best divided into two relatively discrete phases: bladder filling and urine storage and bladder emptying and voiding. The micturition cycle normally displays these two modes of operation in a simple on–off fashion. The cycle involves switching from inhibition of the voiding reflex and activation of storage reflexes to inhibition of the storage reflexes and activation of the voiding reflex—and back again. First some relevant facts regarding the anatomy, neuroanatomy, physiology and pharmacology of the lower urinary tract are summarized. We then answer certain important functional questions related to the filling and storage phase and the emptying and voiding phase of micturition. Certain "rules" are formulated that must be satisfied for the lower urinary tract to function normally. By extrapolation, these rules are used as a basis for a very simple functional classification of voiding dysfunction and as a framework to understand urodynamic evaluation and the rationale for all types of treatment. The neurourologic evaluation, classification schemes for voiding dysfunction, and the more common types of neurogenic and non-neurogenic voiding dysfunction are considered; followed by a synopsis and summation of pertinent points relative to all types of treatment for filling and storage and for emptying and voiding disorders. Benign prostatic hyperplasia (BPH) is discussed in Chapter 15.

I. RELEVANT LOWER URINARY TRACT ANATOMY AND TERMINOLOGY, PHYSIOLOGY, AND PHARMACOLOGY

A. Bladder, Urethra, Smooth and Striated Sphincter

1. The designation lower urinary tract (LUT) includes the bladder, urethra, and periurethral striated muscle. Anatomically and embryologically, the bladder traditionally has been divided into detrusor and trigone regions. The terms bladder *body* and bladder *base* refer to a functional rather than anatomic division of bladder smooth muscle. This is based on distinct differences in neuromorphology and neuropharmacology between the smooth muscle lying circumferentially above (body) and below (base) the level of the ureterovesical junction. The *smooth sphincter* refers to the smooth muscle of the bladder neck and proximal urethra. This sphincter is not anatomic but physiologic. Others refer to this area as the internal sphincter, the proximal sphincter, and simply, the bladder neck sphincter. Although most would accept the facts that the proximal urethra is that portion of the lower urinary tract between the bladder neck and "urogenital diaphragm" in both genders and that it contains smooth muscle capable of affecting urethral resistance, there is virtually no physiologic, pharmacologic, or pathologic change that affects the smooth muscle of the most proximal urethra without also affecting the smooth muscle of the bladder neck. Normally, resistance increases in the area of the smooth sphincter during bladder filling and urine storage and decreases during an emptying bladder contraction. In the human *proximal urethra* there is a thick, primarily longitudinal smooth muscle layer and a thinner outer circular layer. The longitudinal layer is felt by many clinicians, but not all, to be continuous with the musculature of the bladder base. Teleologically, this arrangement is consistent with a tonic role of the circular layer in maintaining closure during filling and storage and a phasic role for the longitudinal layer in contributing to the opening of the urethra during voiding. The bladder body does not contain discrete unidirectional layers of smooth muscle as suggested by some older texts. In the bladder base, there is a more or less layered-like arrangement of smooth muscle, loosely organized into inner and outer longitudinal and middle circular layers. The superficial and deep layers of the trigone musculature lie on the posterior bladder base smooth muscle.

2. The classic view of the *external urethral sphincter,* or *external sphincter,* is that of a striated muscle within the leaves of a "urogenital diaphragm" that extends horizon-

tally across the pelvis. It is responsible for stopping the urinary stream when the command "stop voiding" is obeyed. The *striated sphincter* concept expands this definition to include intramural and extramural portions. The *extramural* portion corresponds roughly to the "classic" external urethral sphincter, although there is no unbroken sheet of muscle that extends across the pelvis in either male or female and, thus, there is no true urogenital diaphragm. The *intramural* portion denotes skeletal muscle that is intimately associated with part of the urethra in both sexes above the maximal condensation of extramural striated muscle and which is continuous from that level for a variable distance to the bladder neck in the female and at least to the apex of the prostate in the male, forming an integral part of the outer muscular layer of the urethra. Some call this intramural portion the intrinsic rhabdosphincter. Although differences of opinion exist regarding the ultrastructure and physiologic type of striated muscle fibers at various points within the striated sphincter mechanism, there is agreement on the general concept of a gradual increase in activity in the striated sphincter during bladder filing, maintenance with the potential of increases in this activity during bladder storage, and virtual disappearance of this activity just prior to normal emptying/voiding.

B. Innervation and Receptor Function

1. *Autonomic nervous system (ANS).* The physiology and pharmacology of the LUT cannot be separated from those of the ANS. There are many differences between the ANS and the somatic nervous system (SNS), but the one easiest for clinicians to understand and remember is that the ANS includes all efferent pathways having ganglionic synapses outside the central nervous system (CNS). There are no synapses between the CNS and the motor end plates of peripheral structures (striated muscle) in the SNS.

2. *Sympathetic and parasympathetic.* The terms sympathetic and parasympathetic refer simply to anatomic divisions of the ANS. The sympathetic division consists of those fibers that originate in the thoracic and lumbar regions of the spinal cord, whereas the parasympathetic division refers to those fibers that originate in the cranial and sacral spinal nerves.

3. *Innervation and neuronal interaction.* The classic view of the peripheral ANS involves a two neuron system: preganglionic neurons emanating from the CNS and making synaptic contact with cells within ganglia, from which postganglionic neurons emerge to innervate peripheral

organs (Fig. 14-1). This relatively simply concept is still useful for the purposes of discussion but has undergone much expansion and modification. Most innervation of the lower urinary tract actually emanates from peripheral ganglia that are at a short distance from, adjacent to, or within the organs they innervate (the urogenital short neuron system). Additionally, the efferent autonomic pathways frequently do not conform to the classic two neuron model, as they are often interrupted by more than one synaptic relay. For many years, the only autonomic neurotransmitters recognized were acetylcholine and norepinephrine. It has become obvious that other transmitters are involved in various components of the ANS, and a once relatively simple concept of chemical neurotransmission has been expanded to include synaptic systems that involve modulator transmitter mechanisms, prejunctional inhibition or enhancement of transmitter release, postjunctional modulation of transmitter action, cotransmitter release, and secondary involvement of locally synthesized hormones and other substance. All of these are subject to neuronal and hormonal regulation, desensitization, and hypersensitization. Finally, these relationships may be altered by changes that occur secondary to disease or destruction in the neural axis, obstruction of the lower urinary tract, aging, and hormonal status.

4. *Bladder smooth muscle contraction and relaxation.* The classic model of smooth muscle contraction involves synaptic release of neurotransmitter in response to neural stimulation, with the transmitter agent subsequently combining with a recognition site, or receptor, on the postsynaptic smooth muscle cell membrane. The transmitter–receptor combination then initiates changes in the postsynaptic effector cell that ultimately results in what we consider the characteristic effect of that particular neurotransmitter on that particular smooth muscle.

Excitation–contraction coupling in bladder smooth muscle is mediated by a rise in cytosolic calcium, resulting from extracellular calcium influx and release from intracellular stores. The cytosolic calcium binds to calmodulin, initiating the cascade of events necessary to phosphorylate myosin and cause contraction. Relaxation is mediated by a decrease in intracellular calcium. This is accomplished by extrusion extracellularly or reuptake into intracellular stores. Smooth muscle relaxation can also be produced by causing intracellular potassium efflux, resulting in membrane hyperpolarization. Both of these latter actions are potential pharmacologic targets for decreasing bladder contractility. Unfortunately, there

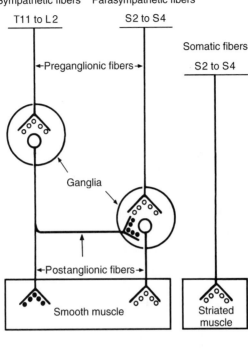

Sympathetic fibers   Parasympathetic fibers

T11 to L2   S2 to S4

Somatic fibers
S2 to S4

←Preganglionic fibers→

Ganglia

←Postanglionic fibers→

Smooth muscle   Striated
muscle

Nature of chemical transmitter

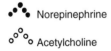 Norepinephrine

Acetylcholine

Figure 14-1 Classic neuroanatomic and neuropharmacologic description of the innervation of the smooth muscle of the bladder and urethra and the striated muscle of the external urethral sphincter. Note the termination of some postganglionic sympathetic (adrenergic) fibers of parasympathetic ganglion cells, providing the morphologic substrate for sympathetic inhibition of parasympathetic ganglion cell transmission. Note also the lack of ganglia in the somatic innervation.

are no bladder selective calcium channel blockers or potassium channel openers.

5. *Neurotransmitter terminology: cholinergic and adrenergic subtypes.* Clinicians are often confused because they assume that the terms sympathetic and parasympathetic

imply particular neurotransmitters. These terms imply only anatomic origin within the ANS. Other adjectives are used to describe the nature of the neurotransmitter involved (Fig. 14-1).

The term *cholinergic* refers to those receptor sites where acetylcholine is a primary neurotransmitter. Peripheral cholinergic fibers include somatic motor fibers, all preganglionic autonomic fibers, and all postganglionic parasympathetic fibers. The cholinergic receptor sites on autonomic effector cells are termed *muscarinic*. Atropine and its congeners competitively inhibit muscarinic receptor sites. Cholinergic receptor sites on autonomic ganglia and on motor end plates of skeletal muscle are designated *nicotinic*.

The term *adrenergic* is applied to those receptor sites where a catecholamine is the neurotransmitter. Most postganglionic sympathetic fibers are adrenergic receptor sites, including those to lower urinary tract smooth muscle, where the catecholamine responsible for neurotransmission is norepinephrine. Adrenergic receptor sites are further classified as alpha (α) or beta (β) on the basis of the differential effects elicited by a series of catecholamines and their antagonists. Classically, the term *α-adrenergic effect* designates vasoconstriction and/or contraction of smooth musculature in response to norepinephrine. These effects are inhibited by phentolamine, phenoxybenzamine, prazosin, and related compounds. The term *β-adrenergic effect* implies smooth muscle relaxation in response to catecholamine stimulation and also includes cardiac stimulation, vasodilation, and bronchodilation. These effects are stimulated most potently by isoproterenol (much more so than by norepinephrine), and antagonized by multiple β-blocker compounds, of which propranolol is the prototype.

Receptor subtyping is a relevant concept that explains why some neurotransmitters have differing effects in different organs or anatomic localizations. Subtyping can be based on functional assays, radioligand-binding affinity, or on cloning established genotypes. For instance, there are five different muscarinic receptor subtypes (M_1–M_5). Although it appears that the majority of these in human bladder smooth muscle are of the M_2 subtype, bladder smooth muscle contraction is mediated primarily by the M_3 subtype. There are multiple subtypes of α- and β-adrenergic receptors as well. Adding to the complexity is the fact that neurotransmitters may have differing (or no) effects at different sites (i.e., brain, pons, spinal cord, efferent ganglia, presynaptic and postsynaptic neural effector junction, sensory afferent fibers, and ganglia). In this chapter, we concentrate on peripheral smooth muscle actions.

6. *Other peripheral neurotransmitters.* Other nonadrenergic noncholinergic (NANC) peripheral neurotransmitters exist in the lower urinary tract and their role(s) in normal and abnormal states is the object of much current investigation. *Adenosine triphosphate* (ATP) has been postulated as the "other" excitatory neurotransmitter in some cases of atropine resistance (see I, B, 8). *Vasoactive intestinal polypeptide* (VIP) has been generally shown to have an inhibitory effect on bladder muscle contractility and postulated to act as a modifier of bladder activity during filling. *Nitric oxide* (NO) has been hypothesized to act to facilitate bladder neck and proximal urethral opening during bladder emptying. Other candidates for ganglionic and neural effector NANC transmitters include neuropeptide Y (NPY), leucine encephalin (ENK), endothelin, and substance P (SP). Sensory neurotransmitters, located in afferents projecting to the spinal cord dorsal root ganglia include glutamate and SP and could include VIP, ENK, cholecystokinin, NO, and calcitonin gene-related peptide (CGRP). Note, however, that the presence of a potential neurotransmitter and a laboratory tissue response to an agonist or/and antagonist does not necessarily imply physiologic function.

7. *Peripheral innervation.* The pelvic and hypogastric nerves supply the bladder and urethra with efferent parasympathetic and sympathetic innervation, and both convey afferent sensory impulses from these organs to the spinal cord. The *parasympathetic efferent supply* is classically described as originating in the grey matter of the interomediolateral cell column of sacral spinal cord segments S2–S4. This preganglionic supply is ultimately conveyed by the *pelvic nerve.* These fibers synapse with cholinergic postganglions in the pelvic plexus or in ganglia within the bladder wall. *Efferent sympathetic fibers* to the bladder and urethra are thought to originate in the interomediolateral cell column and nucleus intercalatus of spinal cord segments T11–L2 and are carried within the *hypogastric nerves.* Bilaterally, at a variable distance from the bladder and urethra, the hypogastric and pelvic nerves meet and branch to form the *pelvic plexus.* Divergent branches of this pelvic plexus innervate the pelvic organs. Efferent innervation of the striated sphincter is classically thought to be somatic and to emanate from *Onuf's nucleus* in sacral spinal cord segments S2–S4, exiting the spinal cord as the pudendal nerve. Some clinicians believe that the striated sphincter is innervated by branches of the ANS as well.

The *afferents* traveling in the pelvic nerve are responsible for the initiation of the micturition reflex in the normal state. *Myelinated A-delta fibers* normally subserve this function and convey mechanoreceptor input. *Unmyelinated C fiber afferents* are more prevalent, but remain relatively silent during normal filling and storage. These become "awakened" and functional under various conditions (i.e., responses to distention after spinal cord injury, to cold—the "ice water test," and to nociceptive stimuli). Myelinated somatic afferents from the striated sphincter travel in the pudendal nerve. Afferents also travel in the hypogastric nerve, but little is known about their specific function.

8. *Cholinergic innervation and parasympathetic stimulation.* Cholinergic innervation is abundant to all areas of the bladder of animals and humans. Although most researchers agree on the existence of a cholinergic innervation at least of the proximal urethra in animals, there is disagreement regarding the extent (and in some cases existence) of a similar innervation in humans. It is generally agreed that abundant muscarinic cholinergic receptor sites exist throughout the bladder body and base musculature of various animal species and of humans and that they are more numerous in the bladder body. A sustained bladder contraction is produced by stimulation of the pelvic nerves, and it is generally agreed that reflex activation of this pelvic nerve excitatory tract is responsible for the emptying bladder contraction of normal micturition and for the involuntary bladder contractions seen with various diseases of the neural axis and lower urinary tract obstruction. Whether acetylcholine is the sole neurotransmitter released during such stimulation is highly controversial. *Atropine resistance* refers to the incomplete antagonism produced by atropine of the bladder response to pelvic nerve stimulation or of isolated bladder strips to electrical field stimulation (producing intramural neural stimulation). This is in contrast to atropine's ability to completely block the response of bladder smooth muscle strips to exogenous acetylcholine. It is generally agreed that atropine resistance occurs in various experimental animal models, and the most logical explanation seems to be release of additional neurotransmitter(s) besides acetylcholine in response to nerve stimulation. Normally, atropine resistance does not occur in humans. However, one should not ignore the possibility that different types of atropine resistance may exist in various types of bladder hyperactivity, regardless of the normal state of affairs.

9. *Adrenergic innervation and sympathetic stimulation.* Adrenergic innervation of the bladder and urethral smooth musculature has been extensively demonstrated in animal studies. These studies have shown that the smooth musculature of the bladder base and proximal urethra possesses a rich adrenergic (norepinephrine containing) innervation, whereas the bladder body has a sparse but definite adrenergic innervation. The density of innervation seems, in all areas, to be less than that of the cholinergic systems. Considerable disagreement exists, however, as to even the presence of postganglionic sympathetic innervation in the human bladder and proximal urethra. There is general agreement that the smooth muscle of the human male bladder neck possesses a dense adrenergic innervation, but there is little consensus otherwise. Even those researchers who ascribe a significant influence on the micturition cycle to the sympathetic nervous system (SYNS) have difficulty demonstrating more than a sparse adrenergic innervation in other areas of the bladder and urethra. There is general agreement, however, that the smooth muscle of the bladder and proximal urethra in a variety of animals and in humans contains both α- and β-adrenergic *receptors*. α-Adrenergic contractile responses predominate in the bladder base and proximal urethra, whereas β-adrenergic relaxation responses predominate in the bladder body. Additionally, there is general agreement that there is a significant inhibitory influence exerted on parasympathetic ganglionic transmission by postganglionic sympathetic fibers (Fig. 14-1). Those who advocate a major role of the SYNS in the micturition cycle summarize the influences as primarily to facilitate the filling and storage phase of micturition by three mechanisms.

   a. Decreasing bladder contractility via an inhibitory effect on parasympathetic ganglionic transmission.
   b. Increasing outlet resistance by stimulation of the predominantly α-adrenergic receptors in the bladder base and proximal urethra.
   c. Increasing accommodation by stimulation of the predominantly β-adrenergic receptors in the bladder body.

   It should be noted, however, that some researchers are of the opinion that the SYNS plays a very minor role in the micturition cycle in the human.

II. CNS INFLUENCES ON MICTURITION

Micturition is basically a function of the peripheral ANS. However, the ultimate control of lower urinary tract function obviously resides at higher neurologic levels. There is general consensus that

Table 14-1 Potential Central Nervous System Neurotransmitter Other than Opiods and their Effects on the Micturition Reflex

NEUROTRANSMITTER	SITE	PREDOMINANT ACTION
Glutamate	Brain, SC	+
Glycine	Brain, SC	−
GABA (gamma amino butyric acid)	Brain, SC	−
Serotonin	SC	−
Acetylcholine	Brain	+
Dopamine (D-2)	Brain	+
Dopamine (D-1)	Brain	−
Norepinephrine (α-1)	SC	+ (?)
Norepinephrine (α-2)	SC	?
Norepinephrine	Brain	−

SC, Spinal cord

a micturition "center" in the spinal cord is localized to segments S2–S4, with the major portion at S3. Early workers believed that micturition was a simple sacral spinal reflex activity that was modulated by a number of central and peripheral reflexes. It is now acknowledged that the micturition cycle is coordinated in the *pontine mesencephalic reticular formation.* Input to this area is derived from the cerebellum, basal ganglia, thalamus, hypothalamus, and cerebral cortex. Bladder contraction elicited by stimulation at or above this area seems to occur with a decrease in activity of the periurethral striated musculature, as in normal micturition. In general, the tonic activity of the cerebral cortex and midbrain is inhibitory. The regions of the cerebral hemispheres primarily concerned with bladder function are the superomedial portion of the frontal lobes and the genu of the corpus callosum. The cerebral areas controlling bladder and striated sphincter activity are geographically separate.

Evidence exists that endogenous opioid peptides influence micturition by a tonic inhibitory effect on detrusor reflex pathways. These inhibitory effects could be mediated at several levels, including the peripheral bladder ganglia, sacral spinal cord, and brain stem micturition center. Different types of opioid receptors may be responsible, at different sites, for different types of effects on bladder contractility. Numerous other potential neurotransmitters can be found in various areas of the CNS. A partial list is in Table 14-1.

III. IMPORTANT FUNCTIONAL QUESTIONS

A. What Determines Bladder Response During Filling?

The normal adult bladder response to filling at a physiologic rate is an almost imperceptible change in intravesical pressure. During at least the initial stages of bladder filling, this very high compliance (Δ volume/Δ pressure) is due primarily to passive properties of the bladder wall. The elastic and viscous properties of the bladder wall allow it to stretch to a certain degree without any increase in tension exerted on its contents, and at physiologic filling rates, intravesical pressure remains virtually unchanged. In the usual clinical setting, filling cystometry shows a slight increase in intravesical pressure, but this pressure rise is a function of the fact that cystometry filling is carried out at a greater than physiologic rate. Compliance can also be decreased clinically by (1) any process that alters the viscoelasticity or elasticity of the bladder wall components; and (2) filling the bladder beyond its limit of distensibility.

The viscoelastic properties of the stroma (bladder wall less smooth muscle and epithelium) and the relaxed detrusor muscle account for the passive mechanical properties seen during filling. The main components of stroma are collagen and elastin. When the collagen component increases, compliance decreases. This can occur with various types of injury, bladder outlet obstruction, and neurologic decentralization. Once decreased compliance occurs because of a replacement by collagen or other components of the stroma, it is generally unresponsive to pharmacologic manipulation, hydraulic distention, or nerve section. Most often under those circumstances, augmentation cystoplasty is required to achieve satisfactory reservoir function.

At a certain level of bladder filling, spinal sympathetic reflexes are clearly evoked in all animals, and there is indirect evidence to support such a role in humans. An inhibitory effect on bladder contractility is thought to be mediated primarily by sympathetic modulation of cholinergic ganglionic transmission (see section I.B.9). Through this sympathetic reflex, two other possibilities exist for promoting filling and storage. One is neurally mediated stimulation of the predominantly α-adrenergic receptors in the area of the smooth sphincter, the net result of which would be to cause an increase in resistance in that area. The other is neurally mediated stimulation of the predominantly β-adrenergic receptors in the bladder body smooth musculature, causing a decrease in tension. Good evidence also seems to support a strong tonic inhibitory effect of endogenous opioids on bladder activity at the level of the spinal cord, the parasympathetic ganglia, and perhaps the brain stem as well. Finally, bladder filling and wall distention may release autocrine like factors which themselves influence contractility (e.g., nitric oxide, peptides, prostaglandins).

B. What Determines Outlet Response During Filling?

There is a gradual increase in urethral pressure during bladder filling, contributed to by at least the striated sphincter element and perhaps, by the smooth sphincter element. The rise in urethral pressure seen during the filling and storage phase of micturition can be correlated with an increase in efferent pudendal nerve impulse frequency. This constitutes the efferent limb of a spinal somatic reflex that is initiated when a certain critical intravesical pressure is reached. This is the so-called *guarding reflex,* which results in an increase in striated sphincter activity (Fig. 14-7).

Although it seems logical, and certainly compatible with neuropharmacologic, neurophysiologic, and neuromorphologic data, to assume that the muscular component of the smooth sphincter also contributes to the change in urethral response during bladder filling, it is extremely difficult to prove this either experimentally or clinically. The passive properties of the urethral wall undoubtedly play a large role in the maintenance of continence. Urethral wall tension develops within the outer layers of the urethra; however, it is a product not only of the active characteristics of smooth and striated muscle but also of the passive characteristics of the elastic collagenous tissue that makes up the urethral wall. In addition, this tension must be exerted on a soft, plastic inner layer capable of being compressed to a closed configuration—the "filler material" representing the submucosal portion of the urethra. The softer and more plastic this area is, the less the pressure required by the tension-producing layers to produce continence.

Finally, whatever the compressive forces, the lumen of the urethra must be capable of being obliterated by a watertight seal. This mucosal seal mechanism explains why a very thinwalled rubber tube requires less pressure to close an open end when the inner layer is coated with a fine layer of grease than when it is not, the latter case being analogous to scarred or atrophic urethral mucosa.

C. Why Does Voiding Ensue with a Normal Bladder Contraction?

It is intravesical pressure producing the sensation of distention that is primarily responsible for the initiation of voluntary induced emptying of the lower urinary tract. Although the origin of the parasympathetic neural outflow to the bladder, the pelvic nerve, is in the sacral spinal cord, the actual organizational center for the micturition reflex in an intact neural axis is in the brain stem, and the complete neural circuit for normal micturition includes the ascending and descending spinal cord pathways to and from this area and the facilitory and inhibitory influences from other parts of the brain.

The final step in voluntarily induced micturition initially involves inhibition of the somatic neural efferent activity to the striated sphincter and an inhibition of all aspects of any spinal sympathetic reflex evoked during filling. Efferent parasympathetic pelvic nerve activity is ultimately what is responsible for a highly coordinated contraction of the bulk of the bladder smooth musculature. A decrease in outlet resistance occurs, with adaptive shaping or funneling of the relaxed bladder outlet. Besides the inhibition of any continence promoting reflexes that have occurred during bladder filling, the change in outlet resistance may also involve an active relaxation of the smooth sphincter through a NANC mechanism mediated by nitric oxide. The adaptive changes that occur in the outlet are also in part due to the anatomic interrelationships of the smooth muscle of the bladder base and proximal urethra (continuity). Other reflexes elicited by bladder contraction and by the passage of urine through the urethra may reinforce and facilitate complete bladder emptying. Superimposed on these autonomic and somatic reflexes are complex modifying supraspinal input from other central neuronal networks. These facilitory and inhibitory impulses, which originate from several areas of the nervous system, allow for the full conscious control of micturition in the adult.

D. Why Does Urinary Continence Persist During Abdominal Pressure Increases?

During voluntarily initiated micturition, the bladder pressure becomes higher than the outlet pressure and certain adaptive changes occur in the shape of the bladder outlet with consequent passage of urine into and through the proximal urethra. Why do such changes not occur with increases in pressure that are similar in magnitude but produced only by changes in intra-abdominal pressure, such as straining or coughing?

First, a coordinated bladder contraction does not occur in response to such stimuli, clearly emphasizing the fact that increases in total intravesical pressure are by no means equivalent to emptying ability. For urine to flow into the proximal urethra, not only must there be an increase in intravesical pressure but the increase must also be a product of a coordinated bladder contraction, occurring through a neurally mediated reflex mechanism and associated with characteristic conformational and tension changes in the bladder neck and proximal urethral area.

Assuming the bladder outlet is competent at rest, a major factor in the prevention of urinary leakage during increases in intra-abdominal pressure is the fact that there is normally at least equal pressure transmission to the proximal urethra during such activity. Failure of this mechanism, generally associated with hypermobility of the bladder neck and proximal urethra (another way of describing pathologic descent with abdominal straining), is an almost invariable correlate of "genuine" stress urinary incontinence in the female. No such hypermobility occurs in the male. The increase in urethral closure pressure that is seen with increments in intra-abdominal pressure normally actually exceeds the extrinsic pressure increase, indicating that active muscular function due to a reflex increase in striated sphincter activity or other factors that increase urethral resistance, in addition to simple transmission of pressure, is also involved in preventing such leakage. A more complete description of the factors involved in sphincteric incontinence and its prevention can be found in the section on incontinence.

IV. OVERVIEW OF THE MICTURITION CYCLE: SIMPLIFICATION

Bladder accommodation during filling is a primarily passive phenomenon. It is dependent on the elastic and viscoelastic properties of the bladder wall and the lack of parasympathetic excitatory input. An increase in outlet resistance occurs via the striated sphincter somatic guarding reflex. In at least some species a sympathetic reflex also contributes to storage by (1) increasing outlet resistance by increasing tension on the smooth sphincter; (2) inhibiting bladder contractility through an inhibitory effect on parasympathetic ganglia; and (3) causing a decrease in tension of bladder body smooth muscle. Continence is maintained during increases in intra-abdominal pressure by the intrinsic competence of the bladder outlet and the pressure transmission ratio to this area with respect to the intravesical contents. A further increase in striated sphincter activity, on a reflex basis, is also contributory. Emptying (voiding) can be voluntary or involuntary and involves an inhibition of the spinal somatic and sympathetic reflexes and activation of the vesical parasympathetic pathways, the organizational center for which is in the brainstem. Initially, there is a relaxation of the outlet musculature, mediated not only by the cessation of the somatic and sympathetic spinal reflexes but probably also by a relaxing factor, very possibly nitric oxide, released by parasympathetic stimulation or by some effect of bladder smooth muscle contraction itself. A highly coordinated parasympathetically induced contraction of the bulk of the bladder smooth musculature occurs, with shaping or funneling of the relaxed outlet, due at least in part to a smooth muscle continuity between the bladder base and proximal urethra. With amplification and facilitation of the bladder contraction from other peripheral reflexes and from spinal cord supraspinal sources, and the absence of anatomic obstruction between the bladder and the urethral meatus, complete emptying will occur.

Whatever disagreements exist regarding the anatomic, morphologic, physiologic, pharmacologic, and mechanical details involved in both the storage and expulsion of urine by the lower urinary tract, we believe that agreement is found regarding certain points. First, the micturition cycle involves two relatively discrete processes: bladder filling and urine storage and bladder emptying. Second, whatever the details involved, these processes can be summarized succinctly from a conceptual point of view. Bladder filling and urine storage require the following.

1. Accommodation of increasing volumes of urine at a low intravesical pressure and with appropriate sensation.
2. A bladder outlet that is closed at rest and remains so during increases in intra-abdominal pressure.
3. Absence of involuntary bladder contractions.

Bladder emptying and voiding requires the following.

1. A coordinated contraction of the bladder smooth musculature of adequate magnitude.
2. A concomitant lowering of resistance at the level of the smooth and striated sphincter.
3. Absence of anatomic (as opposed to functional) obstruction.

Any type of voiding dysfunction must result from an abnormality of one or more of the factors listed above regardless of the exact pathophysiology involved. This division, with its implied subdivision under each category into causes related to the bladder and the outlet, provides a logical rationale for discussion and classification of all types of voiding dysfunction and disorders as related primarily to bladder filling and urine storage or to bladder emptying and voiding. There are some types of voiding dysfunction that represent combinations of filling and storage and emptying and voiding abnormalities. Within this scheme, however, these become readily understandable, and their detection and treatment can be logically described. Further, using this scheme, all aspects of urodynamic, radiologic, and video urodynamic evaluation can be conceptualized as to exactly what they evaluate in terms of either bladder or outlet activity during filling and storage or emptying and voiding. Treatments for voiding dysfunction can be classified under broad categories according to whether they facilitate filling and storage or emptying and voiding and whether they do so by acting primarily on the bladder or on one or more of the components of the bladder outlet. Finally, the individual disorders produced by various neuromuscular dysfunctions can be considered in terms of whether they produce primarily storage or emptying abnormalities or a combination.

V. OVERVIEW OF THE PATHOPHYSIOLOGY OF VOIDING DYSFUNCTION

The pathophysiology of the lower urinary tract's *failure to fill with or store urine adequately* must be secondary to reasons related to the bladder, the outlet, or both. *Overactivity of the bladder* during filling can be expressed as discrete involuntary contractions, low compliance, or a combination of both. *Involuntary contractions* are most commonly seen in association with neurologic disease or after neurologic injury but also may be associated with inflammation or irritation of the bladder wall, bladder outlet obstruction, or idiopathic. *Decreased compliance* may be secondary to neurologic injury or disease but may also result from any process that destroys the elastic or viscoelastic properties of the bladder wall. Storage failure may also occur in the absence of hyperactivity secondary to *hypersensitivity* or pain. The classic clinical example is interstitial cystitis. Irritation and inflammation can be responsible, as well as neurologic, psychologic, and idiopathic causes. *Decreased outlet resistance* can result from any process that damages the innervation or structural elements of the smooth or striated sphincter. This may be due to neurologic disease or injury, surgical or other mechanical trauma, or aging. Classic "genuine" stress urinary incontinence in women was historically associated with hypermobility-related failure of the normal transmission of increases in intra-abdominal pressure to the area of the bladder neck and proximal urethra. Whether or not all women with hypermobility-related incontinence have an additional component of decreased urethral resistance is unclear because there are many women with urethral hypermobility who do not demonstrate urinary incontinence. Nevertheless, this hypermobility is believed to accompany pelvic floor relaxation or weakness, which can be due to several causes. *Treatment* of filling and storage abnormalities is directed toward inhibiting bladder contractility, decreasing sensory input, or mechanically increasing bladder capacity; or/and toward increasing outlet resistance, either continuously or just during increases in intra-abdominal pressure.

Absolute or relative failure to empty results from decreased bladder contractility (a decrease in magnitude or duration), increased outlet resistance, or both. *Absolute or relative bladder contractility failure* can result from temporary or permanent alteration in one of the neuromuscular mechanisms necessary for initiating and maintaining a normal detrusor contraction. Inhibition of the voiding reflex in a neurologically healthy person can also occur, either by a reflex mechanism secondary to painful stimuli, especially from the pelvic and perineal areas, or by psychogenic means. Non-neurogenic causes can also include impairment of bladder smooth muscle function, which may result from overdistention, various drugs, severe infection, or fibrosis. Pathologically *increased outlet resistance* is much more commonly seen in men than women. Although it is most often secondary to anatomic obstruction, it may be secondary to a failure of coordination or active contraction of the striated or smooth sphincter during bladder contraction. Striated sphincter dyssynergia is a common cause of functional or non-anatomic (as opposed to fixed anatomic) obstruction in patients with neurologic disease or injury. *Treatment* of failure to empty generally consists of attempts to increase intravesical pressure or facilitate the micturition reflex, decrease outlet resistance, or both. If other means fail or are impractical, intermittent catheterization is an effective way to circumvent emptying failure.

VI. THE NEUROUROLOGIC EVALUATION
A. History

Symptomatology can be valuable in suggesting whether voiding dysfunction represents an abnormality of storage, emptying, or both (Table 14-2). A complete history of the symptoms and their onset, duration, time course, and relationship to neurologic disease or other neurologic symptoms is essential. *Incontinence* is generally a primary symptom of filling and storage failure and may be bladder or outlet related; however, it can also result from ureteral ectopy and

Table 14-2 Neurourologic Evaluation

History
Bladder diary
Quality of life assessment
Physical examination
Neurologic examination
Urine bacteriologic studies
Renal function studies
Radiologic evaluation
  Upper tract
  Lower tract
Urodynamic/video-urodynamic study
Endoscopic examination

congenital or acquired fistulae. Leakage that is associated only with increases in intra-abdominal pressure implies *genuine stress urinary incontinence,* at least in the female. Gravitational urethral incontinence that worsens on straining implies *intrinsic sphincter dysfunction.* *Precipitous incontinence* with a more sustained type of leakage similar to voiding is characteristic of involuntary bladder contractions. It can occur without urgency in the absence of sensation. Incontinence is not always, however, a primary symptom of filling and storage failure. *Overflow, or paradoxical incontinence,* can develop in a patient with insidious detrusor decompensation with emptying failure. The leakage in this case is generally most prominently associated with changes in position or sudden increases in intra-abdominal pressure and can mimic stress incontinence. *Urgency* is classically defined as a perceived need to void for fear of leakage. It can also be associated with pain or the anticipation of pain with further filling. The former is generally associated with bladder overactivity. A perceived need to void solely because of pain is generally secondary to inflammatory disease. An *increase in daytime urinary frequency* can be psychogenic, represent a response to pain on low volume bladder distention (usually indicative of inflammatory disease), due to detrusor overactivity, or simply due to increased fluid intake. Increased frequency can also result from emptying failure with a substantial residual urine volume and therefore a decreased functional bladder capacity. It can also exist in association with outlet obstruction induced detrusor overactivity. *Nocturia* usually accompanies nonpsychogenic urinary frequency and can be associated, on the same basis as increased daytime frequency, with either storage or emptying failure. It can also be due, however, simply to an increased nocturnal urine output (nocturnal polyuria syndrome). The symptom of *pressure* defies exact definition. It is not quite the urge to void but rather a feeling that the bladder is full or that the urge to void will occur shortly. There is often no discernible voiding dysfunction in patients who complain of this; however, such dysfunction can be due to an elevated intravesical pressure during filling, but one which is below the level necessary to elicit the sensation or distention or urgency. This symptom also may be representative of an accurate perception of inadequate emptying with a modest or large residual urine volume. A *bladder diary* is especially useful in accurately portraying symptoms due to a filling and storage abnormality. This should include at least the following: time and amount of voiding, association with urgency (or not), and leakage (or not), including type and amount. The diary will also allow estimation of the functional capacity, which should serve as a guide for filling volume during urodynamics.

Hesitancy, straining to void, and *poor stream* generally reflect a failure to empty adequately, but they can occur in an individual with frequency and urgency who, on toileting, simply has difficulty initiating a voluntary bladder contraction with a small intravesical urine content. A detailed history of prior medical and surgical treatment and the results should always be sought.

B. Physical and Neurologic Evaluation

Findings from a *general physical examination* are nonspecific. There may be cutaneous excoriation secondary to urinary leakage. A focused physical examination should include the lower abdomen, genitalia, and rectum in men and women. Prostate abnormalities must be detected. A careful pelvic examination in women is necessary to detect the presence and degree of pelvic organ prolapse: apical/uterine, anterior and posterior vaginal prolapse. The *neurologic examination* provides evidence of the presence or absence of a neurologic lesion and, if present, localizes it in an attempt to corroborate and explain a given voiding dysfunction. *Mental status* is determined by noting the level of consciousness, orientation, speech, comprehension, and memory. Mental status aberrations can be secondary to neurologic diseases that produce voiding dysfunction, such as senile and presenile dementia, brain tumors, and normal pressure hydrocephalus. Cranial nerve dysfunction, except when indicative of a brain stem lesion, has little specific relevance to voiding dysfunction. Careful examination of *motor function and coordination* and a sensory examination (including touch, pain, temperature, vibration, and position) can have anatomic and etiologic significance. *Sensory* or motor deficits may suggest specific levels of spinal pathology, either unilateral or bilateral. The abnormalities associated with spinal cord injury, Parkinson's disease, multiple sclerosis, and cerebrovascular disease are usually obvious. The presence of lateralizing signs suggests that only one side of the neural axis is affected. Quadriplegia suggests an abnormality of the cervical or high thoracic spinal cord, whereas true paraplegia indicates a cord lesion below the upper thoracic segments. Specific dermatomal sensory alterations or deficits suggest localized pathology at the spinal cord or nerve root level.

Evaluation of the *deep tendon reflexes* provides an indication of segmental spinal cord function as well as suprasegmental function. *Hypoactivity* of the deep tendon reflexes generally indicates a lower motor neuron (LMN) lesion (in this context, meaning from the anterior horn cells to the periphery), whereas *hyperactivity* generally indicates an upper motor neuron (UMN) lesion (between the brain and anterior horn cells of the spinal cord). These terms, UMN and LMN, refer, strictly speaking, only to the somatic nervous system. However, by convention, they are often applied by urologists and neurologists to the efferent portions of the ANS innervating the lower urinary tract. In this context, the terms are generally understood to mean the following: UMN, between the brain and anterior horn cells; and LMN, from anterior horn cells to the periphery, including al preganglionic and postganglionic fibers. Commonly tested deep tendon reflexes include the biceps (C5–C6), triceps (C6–C7), quadriceps or patellar (L2–L4), and Achilles (L5–S2). A pathologic toe sign (Babinski reflex) generally indicates a somatic UMN lesion but can be absent with a complete lesion and marked spasticity. A Babinski reflex may be present contralaterally with a unilateral lesion or may be present unilaterally with a bilateral lesion.

The generic term *bulbocavernosus reflex* (BCR) describes contraction of the bulbocavernosus and ischiocavernosus muscles after penile glans or clitoral stimulation, or stimulation of the urethral or bladder mucosa by pulling an indwelling Foley catheter. These reflexes are mediated by pudendal and/or pelvic afferents and by pudendal nerve efferents and, as such, represent a local sacral spinal cord reflex. Most clinicians would agree that the BCR reflects activity in S2–S4, but some believe that this may involve segments as high as L5. Motor control of the external anal sphincter (EAS) is variously described as being served by sacral cord segments S2–S4 or S3–S5. A visible contraction the EAS after pinprick of the mucocutaneous junction constitutes the *anal reflex,* and its activity usually parallels that of the BCR. EAS tone, when strong, indicates that activity of the conus medullaris is present, whereas absent anal sphincter tone usually indicates absent conal activity. Volitional control of the EAS indicates intact control by supraspinal centers. The *cough reflex* (contraction of the EAS with cough) is a spinal reflex that depends on volitional innervation of the abdominal musculature T6–L1. The afferent limb is apparently from muscle receptors in the abdominal wall that enter the spinal cord and ascend. As long as one of these segments remains under volitional control, the cough reflex may be positive. If a lesion above the outflow to the abdominal musculature exists, the cough reflex is generally absent.

In regard to lesions that affect the spinal cord, it must be remembered that the level of the vertebral lesion (such as in spinal cord injury or disk disease) usually differs from the spinal cord segmental level. Sacral spinal cord segments

S2–S4 are generally at vertebral levels L1–L2. Additionally, it must be remembered that after spinal cord trauma, descending degeneration of the cord may occur. In a complete spinal cord lesion above the conus medullaris (otherwise known as suprasegmental or UMN), there will generally be, after spinal shock has passed (see below), hyperactivity of the deep tendon reflexes, skeletal spasticity, and absent skin sensation below the level of the lesion; pathologic toe signs will exist. Following a complete spinal cord lesion at or below the conus (segmental or infrasegmental or LMN), after spinal shock has passed, there will generally be absent deep tendon reflexes, skeletal flaccidity, and absent skin sensation below the lesion level; pathologic toe signs will be absent.

C. Radiologic Evaluation

1. *Upper tracts* (See chapter 3). Many urologists believe that the intravenous urogram is the optimal screening study of the upper tracts (kidneys and ureters) in patients with significant voiding dysfunction. Ultrasonography can give adequate information about hydronephrosis, the presence of calculi, and occasionally, hydroureter. Isotope studies can be useful to evaluate renal blood flow and function and to establish the presence of renal or ureteral obstruction. Dilatation of the ureters or renal collecting system, or a decrease in function, can represent significant complications of lower urinary tract dysfunction and as such are absolute indications for intervention. Upper tract imaging, however, is generally recommended only in specific situations in the adult: (1) decreased bladder compliance; (2) neurogenic incontinence; (3) severe urethral obstruction; (4) incontinence associated with significant post void residual; (5) coexisting loin and flank pain; (6) severe untreated pelvic organ prolapse; and (7) suspected extra-urethral urinary incontinence.

2. *Lower tracts* (see Chapter 3). This portion of the chapter considers only basic cystourethrographic patterns that relate directly to voiding dysfunction caused by neuromuscular disease. Specific details and illustrations of complications caused by such voiding dysfunction (reflux, trabeculation, cellules, diverticula) of primary and secondary urethral pathology (stricture, fistulae, and diverticula) and of the cystourethrographic evaluation of female urinary incontinence can be found in the specific chapters covering these topics. The discussion here also serves as an introduction to the voiding patterns seen secondary to neuromuscular dysfunction and points out the essential nature of urodynamic studies in accurately diagnosing these dysfunctions.

There are only a few basic cystourethrographic radiologic configurations, but their significance can be fully ascertained only by concomitant urodynamic study. A *closed bladder neck* is normal in a resting individual whose bladder is undergoing either physiologic or urodynamic filling. However, it can also occur in an individual with an areflexic bladder who is straining to void and in an individual in whom a micturition reflex is occurring but whose smooth sphincter area is dysfunctional or dyssynergic. The closed appearance can sometimes be mimicked to a great degree by significant prostatic enlargement with bladder neck and urethral compression as well. An *open bladder neck* is normal during voluntarily induced micturition and during most involuntary bladder contractions as well. However, this appearance may also be due to intrinsic sphincter dysfunction (ISD), some types of neurologic illness, or to endoscopic or open surgical alteration, and it may be seen transiently in some females with genuine stress incontinence.

A *closed striated sphincter* is normal during physiologic or urodynamic filling and with an attempt to stop normal urination or to abort an involuntary bladder contraction. The sphincter also normally remains closed during abdominal straining. During voluntary micturition or during micturition secondary to an involuntary bladder contraction caused by neurologic disease at or above the brainstem, the striated sphincter should *open* unless the patient is trying to abort the bladder contractions by voluntary sphincter contractions.

A cystogram in the erect position at rest and during straining may be useful in quantitating the degree of classical "genuine" stress incontinence (bladder neck closed at rest, open with straining, associated with hypermobility) versus classical ISD (bladder neck open at rest, more leakage with straining, no hypermobility). Voiding cystourethrography is useful to diagnose the site of obstruction in a patient with proven urodynamic evidence of obstruction.

D. Endoscopic Evaluation

Endoscopy is recommended only in specific situations in the adult: (1) when initial testing suggests other types of pathology (microscopic gross hematuria; pain, discomfort, and persistent or severe symptoms of bladder overactivity; and suspected extra-urethral incontinence); (2) in patients who have previously undergone bladder, prostate, or other pelvic surgery; and (3) in men with incontinence. Bladder washings or a voided urine for cytology should be sent if symptoms suggest the possibility of neoplastic or preneoplastic changes in the bladder epithelium. The presence or absence of trabeculation (which is compatible with obstruction, involuntary bladder contractions, or neurologic decentralization) can also be determined. Endoscopic examination may likewise be confirmatory of or exclude anatomic obstruction at a particular site, but it should be recognized that not everything that appears obstructive endoscopically is obstructive urodynamically (all large prostates are not obstructive), and lack of a visually appreciated obstruction does not exclude functional obstruction (striated or smooth sphincter dyssynergia) during bladder emptying and voiding.

E. **Urodynamic/Video Urodynamic Evaluation**
1. *General* (Table 14-3). The studies that fall under the heading of lower urinary tract urodynamics consist simply of methods designed to generate quantitative data relevant to

Table 14-3 Urodynamics Simplified

PHASE	BLADDER	OUTLET
Filling and storage	P_{ves}[1] P_{det}[2] (FCMG[3]) DLPP[4]	UPP[5] VLPP[6] FLUORO[7]
Emptying	P_{ves}[1a] P_{det}[2a] (VCMG)[8]	MUPP[9] FLUORO[10] EMG[11]
	(_____ ‿ _____)	
	_____FLOW[12]_____	
	_____RU[13]_____	

[1,2]Total bladder (P_{ves}) and detrusor (P_{det}) pressures during a filling cystometrogram (FCMG).
[3]Filling cystometrogram.
[4]Detrusor leak point pressure.
[5]Urethral pressure profilometry.
[6]Valsalva leak point pressure.
[7]Fluoroscopy of outlet during filling/storage.
[1a,2a]Total bladder and detrusor pressures during a voiding cystometrogram (VCMG).
[8]Voiding cystometrogram.
[9]Micturitional urethral pressure profilometry.
[10]Fluoroscopy of outlet during emptying.
[11]Electromyography of periurethral striated musculature.
[12]Flowmetry.
[13]Residual urine.

This functional conceptualization of urodynamics categorizes each study as to whether it examines bladder or outlet activity during the filling and storage or emptying phase of micturition. In this scheme, uroflow and residual urine integrate the activity of the bladder and the outlet during the emptying phase.

events taking place in the bladder and bladder outlet during the two relatively discrete phases of micturition described previously: filling and storage and emptying and voiding. This conceptualization fits nicely with the concept of two phases of micturition and the description of each phase requiring three components to occur normally. Ideally, the urodynamic/video urodynamic evaluation should be able to answer the implied questions regarding the normality or abnormality of each of the components of the two phases of micturition. Combined video urodynamic or separate cystourethrographic study (referred to as fluoro in Table 14-3) also provides information regarding the presence or absence of vesicoureteral reflux. A simple formulation of the commonly utilized urodynamic studies, based on the two phases of micturition concept, is presented in Table 14-3, the individual studies characterized as to whether they evaluate aspects of bladder or outlet activity during filling and storage or emptying. Within this scheme, flow and residual urine are simply ways of integrating bladder and outlet activity during the emptying phase of micturition.

The *purpose* of urodynamic/video urodynamic evaluation is threefold: (1) determine the precise etiology(ies) of the voiding dysfunction; (2) identify urodynamic risk factors for upper and lower urinary tract deterioration; and, (3) identify factors that might affect the success of a particular therapy.

Certain very simple rules aid immeasurably in obtaining the maximum benefit from urodynamic and video urodynamic studies. Although these rules sound obvious, they are often ignored, sometimes even by experienced urodynamicists. The prime directive is that the study must reproduce the clinical symptomatology or clinical abnormality being investigated. If it does not, then, insofar as that particular patient is concerned, and despite the fact that the study may be perfectly done and the data beautifully reproduced, it may be worthless. Conversely, the appropriate study done to reproduce the symptoms always yields pertinent information. As a corollary, it is not necessary to perform the most complicated type of video urodynamic study with every patient. The simplest, most readily reproducible, and least invasive study that gives the information desired is always the best. The subject has become far more complicated than necessary. Up to 70 to 90 percent of voiding dysfunction problems can be diagnosed by a logical clinician using relatively simple urodynamic studies. As the complexity of the problem and the number of failed prior therapies increases, so does the need for combined video urodynamic studies. Finally, it must be remembered that urodynamics/video urodynamic evaluation must be an interactive process between the patient and examiner. Information must be constantly exchanged and the study sequence tailored to a given patient and his or her LUT symptoms and signs.

2. *Flowmetry.* Flowmetry is a way to integrate the activity of the bladder and outlet during the emptying phase of micturition. The flow *rate* and *pattern* represent the recorded variables; if these are both normal, it is unlikely that there is any significant disorder of emptying. A normal flow, however, does not entirely exclude obstruction, which is strictly defined on the basis of a relationship between detrusor pressure and simultaneous flow. Consistently low flow rates with adequate volumes voided generally indicate increased outlet resistance, decreased bladder contractility, or both. Flow rates considerably in excess of normal may indicate decreased outlet resistance. There are only a few abnormal flow patterns. An abnormally broad plateau with a low mean and peak rate generally indicates outlet obstruction or decreased detrusor contractility or both. Intermittent flow is generally secondary to abdominal straining or sphincter dyssynergia, but in rare instances, it can be due to undulating low amplitude detrusor contractions. An idealized normal flow curve is seen in Figure 14-2 and flow tracings from individuals with various characteristic abnormalities are seen in Figure 14-3.

The primary caveat in interpreting uroflow is to make sure that the flow event closely approximates the usual voiding event for that patient. In an adult, flow events of 100 mL or less should be interpreted with caution. An overfilled bladder may be accompanied by reduced flow rates as well, probably because of temporary dysfunction introduced by overstretching of detrusor fibers. Measurements of only one flow parameter, such as peak flow, may be misleading, as it is possible for patients with decreased outlet resistance to generate very high peak flows with straining. In comparisons of flow rates in a given individual from one time to another, either for the purposes of evaluating treatment or following a given condition, it is very important to standardize the rates to a given volume. Volume/rate nomograms can be useful in this regard. Most data from studies cite norms of 15 and 25 mL/sec for mean and maximum flow rates. However, flow rates should be standardized in terms of the minimum acceptable flow rates for given gender and age groups. Most "normal" data relate to flowmetry in patients below the age of 55 years.

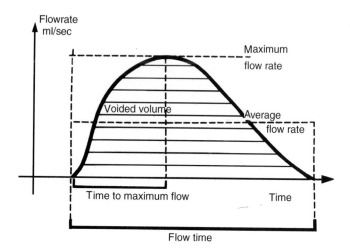

Figure 14-2 Terminology of the International Continence Society relating to the urodynamic description of urinary flow. *(Reproduced from Wein AJ, English WE, Whitmore KE: Office urodynamics. Urol Clin North Am 15:609, 1988.)*

3. *Residual urine volume.* Similarly, residual volume integrates the activity of the bladder and outlet during emptying. It can be measured directly or estimated by cystography or ultrasonography. A consistently increased residual urine volume that reflects the usual status of that patient generally indicates increased outlet resistance, decreased bladder contractility, or both. Negligible residual urine volume is compatible with normal function of the lower urinary tract but can also exist with significant disorders of filling and storage (i.e., incontinence) or emptying disorders in which the intravesical pressure is simply sufficient to overcome increases in outlet resistance up to a certain point. Generally, a significant residual urine volume is considered to be indicative of relative detrusor failure, with or without outlet obstruction.

4. *Filling cystometry.* Cystometry refers to the method by which changes in bladder pressure are measured. The test was designed originally to evaluate the filling and storage phase of bladder function and to measure changes in bladder pressure with slow progressive increases in volume. Strictly speaking, this is *filling cystometry,* as opposed to *voiding cystometry.* Unless the examiner clearly recognizes the distinction, erroneous conclusions regarding the activity of the bladder during the emptying phase

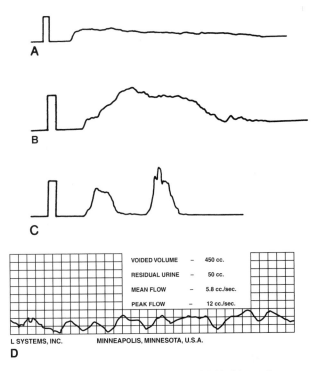

Figure 14-3 A. Flowmetry in a patient with bladder outlet obstruction. Height of bar represents a flow of 10 mL. Maximum flow is generally established soon after the onset of voiding. Peak and mean flow rates are decreased. Flow time is prolonged. Note that this diagnosis cannot be made from this flow event alone. However, this is most characteristic of bladder outlet obstruction in a patient with a normal detrusor. **B.** Uroflow event from a patient with impaired detrusor contractility. Maximum flow is established near the middle of the flow event. Mean and peak flow rates are decreased. Flow time is somewhat prolonged. To establish this diagnosis beyond doubt, especially since the therapeutic options differ, a pressure and flow study would be necessary to separate this entity from bladder outlet obstruction. **C.** Intermittent flow. This type of intermittent flow pattern is most commonly due to abdominal straining. In such a patient with decreased outlet resistance, the peak flow rate is often normal or may even be above normal. **D.** Another type of intermittent flow pattern. This can be due either to sphincter dyssynergia or low amplitude fluctuating detrusor contractions. With sphincter dyssynergia, the changes in flow usually occur faster and are more staccato-like. This is actually from a patient with low amplitude fluctuating detrusor contraction. (*Reproduced from Wein AJ, English WE, Whitmore KE; Office urodynamics. Urol Clin North Am 15:609, 1988.*)

of micturition may be made on the basis of what is commonly called a cystometrogram but which, in reality, represents only filling, and not voiding, cystometry. There is no single best method of performing cystometry, or any urodynamic study, for that matter. All have their shortcomings. The "experts" often differ significantly in their choice of testing sequences and catheters, but their conclusions about an individual patient are usually remarkably similar. Liquid is preferred as a medium for filling cystometry, but gas (carbon dioxide) can be used as well. Although quantitative measurements, such as first sensation and maximum cystometric capacity, decrease significantly when gas is used instead of liquid, the qualitative classification of abnormalities does not seem to change significantly when one is performing repetitive filling cystometry with one medium or the other. For full micturition studies (filling and voiding cystometry), the question of gas versus liquid cystometry is irrelevant because a liquid medium is obviously required.

The first sensation of bladder filling and the first sensation of fullness, as well as the urge to void and the feeling of imminent micturition, are important data to record. When a phasic involuntary detrusor contraction occurs, it is important to note whether this coincides with a sensation of urgency and whether suppression is possible. The pressure measured within the bladder is composed of that contributed by the detrusor plus intra-abdominal pressure. Thus, any pressure increment recorded on a simple cystometrogram may at least partially, and sometimes totally, reflect intra-abdominal pressure. To eliminate such artifactual problems, it is desirable to measure intra-abdominal pressure simultaneously, as reflected by a catheter mounted intrarectal pressure balloon, a vaginal catheter, or a catheter inserted next to the bladder. It is true that an experienced operator can very often tell the difference between a true detrusor contraction and an increase in bladder pressure caused by an increase in intra-abdominal pressure—by the configuration of the curve and by observation of the patient. However, if there is any question about this or if a significant decision is to be based on these data, electronic subtraction of the intra-abdominal pressure from the total bladder pressure (yielding detrusor pressure) is desirable.

The normal adult cystometrogram can be divided into four phases (Fig. 14-4).

1. Phase 1. The initial pressure rise represents the initial response to filling, and the level at which the bladder trace stabilizes is known as the initial filling pressure.

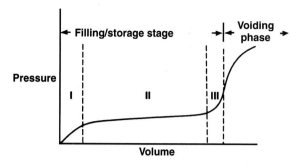

Figure 14-4 Idealized normal adult cystometrogram. (*Reproduced from Wein AJ, English WE, Whitmore KE: Office urodynamics. Urol Clin North Am 15:609, 1988.*)

The first phase of the curve is contributed to by the initial myogenic response to filling and by the elastic and viscoelastic response of the bladder wall to stretch, factors previously discussed. With liquid infusion, the initial filling pressure usually develops gradually and levels off between 0 and 8 cm of water in the supine position. With more rapid rates of filling, there may be an initially higher peak, which then levels off. This peak type of initial response is relatively common with gas cystometry. Although this is a detrusor response, its significance is not the same as that of an involuntary bladder contraction during phase 2.

2. Phase 2. Phase 2 is called the tonus limb, and compliance (Δ volume/Δ pressure) is normally high and uninterrupted by phasic rises. In practice, the compliance seen in the urodynamic laboratory is always lower than that existing during physiologic bladder filling. It must be remembered that if the filling rate with liquid is 2.4 times or less than the hourly diuresis rate, phase 2 will be perfectly flat. Normally, in the urodynamic laboratory, the rise is less than 6 to 10 cm of water. It is difficult to find stated values for normal compliance.

3. Phase 3. Phase 3 is reached when the elastic and viscoelastic properties of the bladder wall have reached their limit. Any further increase in volume generates a substantial increase in pressure. This increase in pressure is not the same as a detrusor contraction. If a voluntary or involuntary contraction occurs, phase 3 can be obscured by the rise in pressure so generated.

4. Phase 4. Ideally, involuntary bladder contractions do not occur during either phase 2 or 3; phase 4 consists

of the initiation of voluntary micturition. Many patients are unable to generate a voluntary detrusor contraction in the testing situation, especially in the supine position. This should not be called detrusor areflexia but, simply, absence of a detrusor contraction during cystometry, a finding that is not considered abnormal unless other clinical or urodynamic findings are present that substantiate the presence of neurologic or myogenic disease.

Involuntary bladder contractions during filling are always significant. Detrusor hyperreflexia and detrusor instability are both terms defined by the International Continence Society that relate to the generic term involuntary bladder contraction. *Detrusor hyperreflexia* refers to an involuntary contraction that is the result of associated neurologic disease; *detrusor instability* refers to an involuntary contraction seen in the absence of neurologic disease. Thus, a spinal cord injury patient with involuntary bladder contractions is said to have a detrusor hyperreflexia, whereas an elderly male with such a finding and prostatic obstruction is said to have detrusor instability. A number of representative adult filling cystometrograms (liquid) are diagrammed in Figure 14-5.

One of the most important urodynamic concepts to remember is that *adequate storage at low intravesical pressure* will avoid deleterious upper urinary tract changes in patients with bladder outlet obstruction and/or neuromuscular lower urinary tract dysfunction. McGuire and coworkers have clearly shown that upper tract deterioration is apt to occur when storage, even though adequate in terms of continence, occurs at sustained urodynamically generated intravesical pressures higher than 40 cm of water. Application of this concept to patients with storage problems and specifically those with decreased compliance and incontinence, has resulted in the concept of the *detrusor leak point pressure (DLPP)* as a very significant piece of urodynamic data. This is to be distinguished from the Valsalva leak point pressure (VLPP) described subsequently.

The DLPP is also known as the bladder leak point pressure (BLPP). It is important to understand the context in which this test was originally described and the astute intuitive reasoning that went into describing the original concept. In the early 1980s, McGuire and associates studied a group of myelodysplastic children with decreased compliance and incontinence. Those

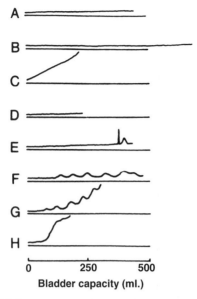

A. Normal filling curve in a patient with a bladder capacity of 450 mL, normal compliance, and no involuntary bladder contractions.

B

C

D

E

F

G

H

0   250   500
Bladder capacity (ml.)

Figure 14-5 Various representative adult filling cystometrograms. **A.** Normal filling curve in a patient with a bladder capacity of 450 mL, normal compliance, and no involuntary bladder contractions. Nothing can be said about bladder activity during the emptying phase of micturition from this tracing. **B.** Large capacity bladder with increased compliance at medium fill rate. This type of curve is characteristic of an individual with decreased sensation and bladder decompensation. Although most individuals will in fact have no or poor detrusor contraction, that conclusion cannot be made on the basis of this curve. **C.** Decreased compliance. **D.** Small capacity bladder secondary to hypersensitivity without decreased compliance or involuntary bladder contraction. **E.** Bladder contraction provoked by cough. This particular tracing represents total bladder pressure. To make this diagnosis from this tracing alone, the clinician would need to be either a very astute examiner or review separate recordings of intravesical pressure and intra-abdominal pressure (intra–rectal pressure). **F.** Low amplitude detrusor contractions. This is a subtracted bladder pressure, and this type of recording may be seen most characteristically in a patient with suprasacral neurologic disease or idiopathic detrusor instability. **G.** Decreased compliance and involuntary bladder contractions. **H.** High amplitude early involuntary bladder contraction. (*Reproduced from Wein AJ, English WE, Whitmore KE: Office urodynamics. Urol Clin North Am 15:609, 1988.*)

children who did not leak on filling cystometry until their detrusor pressures exceeded 40 cm of water exhibited upper urinary tract deterioration on subsequent follow up. Classically, the test was performed by passively filling the bladder through a small caliber urethral catheter with the patient at rest throughout the study, not attempting to volitionally void. The point at which leakage occurs around the catheter is measured as the DLPP. If the DLPP in such an individual with decreased compliance and incontinence is greater than 40 cm of water, the patient is felt to be at risk for upper tract deterioration. Thus, this test has become extremely useful in the management of such patients with neurogenic bladder dysfunction. An abnormal test dictates the necessity of reducing storage pressure to a point below which upper tract deterioration will subsequently be seen, even if this means combining measures to decrease bladder contractility and increase bladder capacity with intermittent catheterization. The concept has been extended to cover patients who have decreased compliance and who do not have incontinence, but whose measured detrusor pressure at bladder volumes they often "carry" exceeds 40 cm of water. Some apply the concept as well to patients with involuntary bladder contractions whose detrusor pressures exceed 40 cm of water. Whether this concept truly applies to this latter group of patients, except in instances where this occurs extremely frequently, or where the pressure is maintained once contraction has occurred, is unknown.

As a corollary, in patients with decreased compliance and incontinence, one must remember that to accurately measure compliance urodynamically the bladder outlet must be occluded. This is especially important if there is a plan to correct outlet related incontinence in an individual with neuromuscular dysfunction associated with decreased compliance (e.g., in the myelomeningocele patient). In other words, one may get a falsely reassuring sense of normal or only slightly decreased compliance in an individual with significant sphincteric insufficiency. Before correcting the sphincteric insufficiency, there needs to be an accurate idea of what bladder compliance will be when the outlet no longer leaks during filling and storage. This can be accomplished very simply by pulling a Foley balloon against the bladder outlet to occlude it during filling.

Cholinergic supersensitivity can be determined during cystometry (*bethanechol supersensitivity test*).

This test is based on Cannon's law of denervation, which implies that when an organ is deprived of its nerve supply, it develops hypersensitivity to a variety of substances, including those that are normally excitatory neurotransmitters for that organ. Originally devised by Lapides and associates, the test has remained virtually unaltered since 1962. It involves controlled liquid cystometry at an infusion rate of 1 mL/sec to a volume of 100 mL, when the bladder pressure is measured. After two or three such infusions, an average value is obtained, and this maneuver is repeated 10, 20, and 30 min after subcutaneous injection of 2.5 mg of bethanechol chloride. A normal bladder shows a response of less than 15 cm of water pressure above the control value at the 100 mL volume. Under these circumstances, a positive result strongly suggests an interruption in the peripheral neural and/or distal spinal pathways to and from the bladder. The more distal and complete the lesion, the more frequently positive the test seems to be. A negative result in an individual with a normal bladder capacity and no detrusor decompensation (admittedly sometimes hard to judge) and in whom the bethanechol is administered on a weight basis, strongly suggests that there is no such lesion. Known factors that can give a falsely positive test include urinary tract infection, azotemia, detrusor hypertrophy, and emotional stress. A falsely negative study may result from the decompensated bladder that cannot respond to cholinergic stimulation under any circumstances. False-negative results may also be due to an insufficient dose of the cholinergic agonist in a very heavy person, and it is useful to administer bethanechol on a weight basis (0.035 mg/kg) to obviate this. The test is not very useful in individuals with involuntary bladder contractions. Under such circumstances, the cholinergic agonist often simply raises bladder pressure sufficiently to make the involuntary contraction occur at a lower volume than usual. It has never been clear whether this was originally intended to be interpreted as a positive test. If one administers the bethanechol on a weight basis and infection, detrusor hypertrophy, stress, and azotemia have been excluded, there should be a few false-positive results.

The ice water test was originally described by Bors and Blinn in 1957. Methodology differs amongst practitioners, but the gist is this. Sterile 0 to 4°C water or saline is rapidly instilled into the bladder (100 mL within 20 sec or 200 mL per min to a volume of 30 to

50 percent of a previously determined cystometric capacity). A positive result is considered a detrusor contraction greater than 30 cm of water, with leakage around the catheter, expulsion of the catheter, or emptying immediately after removal of the catheter. The test has been described as a method of demonstrating a segmental reflex that is inhibited centrally in healthy subjects without neurologic lesions, but which appears when suprasacral lesions are present and normally occurs in infants and young children. The afferent fibers for the ice water test are thought to be unmyelinated C-fiber afferents, which are normally silent during filling and storage, but which become functional with various types of neurologic disease or injury (see I.B.7). Thus, a positive test can be considered indicative of a neurologic lesion, even though the neurologic lesion may not become manifest until a subsequent time. However, everyone with such a lesion may not have a positive ice water test.

5. *Voiding cystometry, combined pressure studies, video urodynamic studies.* Intravesical pressure, intra-abdominal pressure (generally reflected by intrarectal pressure), and flow are often measured simultaneously (Fig. 14-6). The purposes of pressure/flow studies are to be able to better define whether obstruction is present and to assess detrusor contractility more precisely. By assessing patterns of detrusor pressure and flow, thereby inferring resistance and patterns of increased resistance, the examiner can often ascertain the exact pathology (e.g., anatomic obstruction versus dyssynergia). The normal adult male generally voids with a detrusor pressure of between 40 and 50 cm of water. The normal adult female voids at a much lower pressure. Indeed, many women void with almost no detectable rise in detrusor pressure. This does not indicate that contraction is not occurring but simply that outlet resistance, lower in the female to begin with, drops to very low levels during bladder contraction. It should be remembered, however, as Griffiths, a pioneer urodynamicist, has pointed out, that detrusor pressure alone is insufficient to assess the strength of a detrusor contraction. This is because a muscle can use energy to either generate force or shorten its length. With respect to the bladder, a relatively hollow viscus, the force developed contributes to detrusor pressure while the velocity of shortening contributes to flow. With significant obstruction, detrusor pressure can rise to high levels. If resistance is very low, detru-

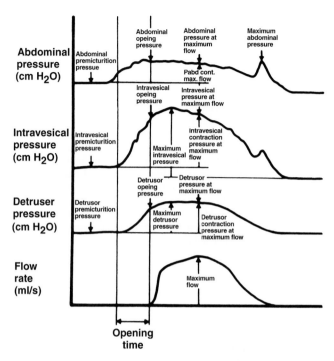

Figure 14-6 Recommended International Continence Society Registration of combined pressure(s) and flow recording. (*Reproduced from Wein AJ, English WE, Whitmore KE: Office urodynamics. Urol Clin North Am 15:609, 1988.*)

sor pressure may be undetectable but the contractility may be equal in the two instances.

Urodynamically, obstruction is generally defined only by the relationship between detrusor pressure and flow—high pressure and low flow. Once obstruction is diagnosed, it is necessary to determine the site, and in order to do this, simultaneous fluoroscopy is often used. This *video urodynamic study* combines the cystourographic imaging described previously with simultaneous urodynamic studies, permitting a generally accurate determination of the site of obstruction at the time high pressure and low flow coexist. The video urodynamic study is also extremely useful in assessing the etiology of complex cases of incontinence, as the precise pressure relationships existing in the bladder and urethra can be correlated with the cystourethrographic radiologic patterns, and a judgment, therefore, can be made of why involuntary leakage occurs at a particular time. In this case, the issue is generally whether the fluoroscopic demonstration of leakage occurs with or without detrusor overactivity or whether the incontinence is due in part to both detrusor and outlet related causes.

One of the most difficult problems in urodynamics is the clarification of whether contractile function is adequate; that is, whether it is sustained and coordinated. Phasic detrusor overactivity does not imply normal contractile function. There is a subset of patients with incontinence in whom detrusor hyperactivity and impaired contractile function coexist (so-called DHIC). The bladder is overactive in these patients but empties ineffectively because of diminished detrusor contractile function and not necessarily because of outlet obstruction. In some patients, obstruction coexists with impaired detrusor contractility, and this diagnosis cannot be made on the basis of simple pressure flow studies.

Several very sophisticated resistance formulas exist that attempt to calculate a number for outlet resistance utilizing data based on intravesical pressure, flow rate, and other mathematical factors. These formulas generally assume that the urethra is a rigid tube with a constant diameter and that the pressure always reflects that generated by a normal bladder, not a decompensated one. If a bladder has normal contractility and the pressure that it generates during contraction is high and if the corresponding flow rate that results is low, one does not need a formula to diagnose obstruction. On the other hand, if the bladder is decompensated and incapable of producing a significant rise in pressure, obstruction cannot be quantitated by these formulas. More sophisticated and innovative methods of defining the relationship between intravesical pressure and uroflow have been devised, and these methods are beyond the scope of this discussion of urodynamics. The global question surrounding all noncomputer-assisted and computer-assisted characterizations and interpretations of pressure flow data is, what do these add? Is the evaluation of the average older man with LUT symptoms more likely to lead to a better treatment outcome if pressure flow urodynamic studies are performed, including the analysis of results in various mathematical ways with computer assistance? Do sophisticated or unsophisticated urodynamic studies predict the outcome of various treatments for LUTS, including watchful waiting? Are patients with LUTS in whom outlet ablation fails as treatment the same patients as those in whom detrusor contractility is judged ineffective by the criteria under consideration? Unfortunately, those of us who perform urodynamics have not done a terribly good job of looking into these aspects of outcome analysis. Figure 14-6 displays the International Continence Society's recommended registration of combined pressure and flow recording. Kinesiologic electromyography (see following discussion) is often added as an additional channel, and some investigators record urethral pressure at one or various sites along the urethra simultaneously as well. The typical video urodynamic configuration includes this and a fluoroscopic lower tract image.

6. *Electromyography.* For the majority of urologists, electromyography is a urodynamic study that permits evaluation of the striated sphincter during the emptying phase of micturition. Kinesiologic electromyography is the term that describes this application, that is, the study of the activity of one group of muscles (the striated musculature of the outlet) with respect to another (the bladder). Normally, as the bladder fills with urine, there is a gradual and sustained increase in electromyographic activity recruited from the pelvic floor muscles. This reaches a maximum just before voiding. Compositely, this is known as the guarding reflex. The lack of a guarding reflex suggests neural pathology, as does the inability to produce a sphincter "flare" when given the command to "stop voiding." Voluntary voiding is normally followed by complete electrical silence—relaxation of the striated sphincter. There is a marked increase in electromyographic activity in response to a number of stimuli, including cough, Credé and Valsalva maneuvers, the BCR, and the request to stop voiding, a maneuver accomplished by most through forceful contraction of the pelvic floor musculature (Fig. 14-7). Kinesiologic electromyography enables the urodynamic examiner to ascertain whether the striated sphincter appropriately increases its activity in a gradual fashion during bladder filling (whether the "guarding reflex" is normal) and whether quiescence occurs normally before and during bladder contraction. Kinesiologic electromyography can be performed with either needle electrodes or surface or patch electrodes. Needle electrodes certainly permit more accurate placement and more accurate recording, but in many cases, surface electrodes seem perfectly adequate to obtain the necessary information.

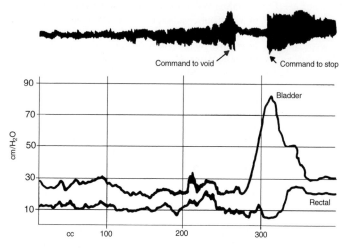

Figure 14-7 Normal pressure electromyographic tracing. Note the gradual increase in electromyographic activity during bladder filling with a decrease to control levels just before the onset of what is a voluntary bladder contraction. Note that the command to stop voiding evokes a pelvic floor striated muscle contraction reflected by a flare in sphincter electromyography. (*Reproduced from Wein AJ, English WE, Whitmore KE: Office urodynamics. Urol Clin North Am 15:609, 1988.*)

When electromyographic activity gradually increases during filling cystometry and then ceases prior to or at the onset of attempted voiding, this is normal and can be taken as a reflection of what goes on during actual bladder filling and emptying. However, a simultaneous increase of electromyographic activity with an increase in intravesical pressure during filling cystometry is not always indicative of detrusor-striated sphincter dyssynergia. Abdominal straining or attempted inhibition of a bladder contraction will yield an identical pattern. For a patient with normal sensation, no matter how cooperative, it is extremely difficult to maintain true relaxation during an involuntary bladder contraction. In fact, the appropriate response is to try to suppress such a contraction by voluntary contraction of the anal sphincter, the pelvic floor musculature, or both. All of these circumstances represent types of *pseudodyssynergia* and are extremely difficult to differentiate from true dyssynergia on the basis of any type of urodynamic study done solely during bladder filling. The term *detrusor-striated sphincter dyssynergia* should refer to obstruction to the outflow of urine during bladder contraction caused by involuntary contraction of the striated sphincter. This is most often seen in patients with discrete neurologic disease, such as suprasacral spinal cord transection after spinal shock has passed. Individuals suspected of having detrusor-striated sphincter dyssynergia but who lack identifiable neurologic disease should always be further investigated with sophisticated video urodynamic evaluation during a full micturition study. True detrusor-striated sphincter dyssynegia is extremely uncommon (some examiners say that it does not exist) in patients without neurologic disease, and such a diagnosis deserves exhaustive study before it is in fact confirmed.

7. *Urethral profilometry.* The term urethral profilometry refers to many entities utilized in various settings. The most common usage refers to a *static infusion urethral pressure profile.* In this study, a small catheter with radially drilled side holes is placed in the bladder and through it a medium, usually liquid, is infused. The catheter is then withdrawn at a constant rate, and the pressure required to push the medium through the side holes is recorded from inside the bladder to a site where the pressure becomes essentially isobaric with bladder pressure. The infusion profile curve is thus a result of a number of factors, including urethral wall compliance, resistance to inflow of the medium, resistance to runoff of the medium into the bladder and out the urethral meatus, and artifact generated by the apparatus. Because the study is usually done at rest and not during bladder filling or emptying, it is difficult to associate the recorded events with bladder– urethral interaction during filling or emptying. Specifically with relevance to neuromuscular dysfunction, the static infusion profile has been cited as useful at various times in diagnosing stress incontinence, detrusor sphincter dyssynergia, and obstruction. In our opinion, it is not very useful for the specific diagnosis of any of these. There is much overlap in maximum urethral pressures and functional urethral lengths between individuals with stress incontinence and normal individuals, especially in the elderly population. The rationale of diagnosing either smooth or striated sphincter dyssynergia on the basis of a static infusion profile is difficult to understand. A high pressure at a given point in the passage of

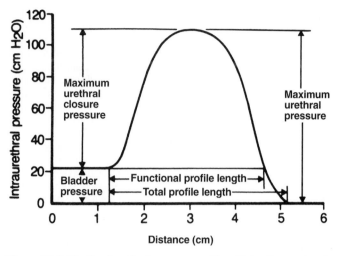

Figure 14-8 Idealized urethral pressure profile utilizing International Continence Society nomenclature (female). (*Reproduced from Wein AJ, English WE, Whitmore KE: Office urodynamics. Urol Clin North Am 15:609, 1988.*)

the catheter from the bladder through the urethra can be secondary to a number of phenomena, and this result by no means indicates that there will always be contraction in this area during voluntary or involuntary micturition. The static infusion urethral profile is certainly useful for testing the function of an artificial genitourinary sphincter. With specific relevance to neuromuscular dysfunction, it is useful for suspecting intrinsic sphincter dysfunction. In an individual with such an abnormality (Figs. 14-8 and 14-9), the proximal urethra is isobaric or almost isobaric with the bladder and the striated sphincter peak is generally lower than normal.

Stress urethral profilometry refers to a study done with a catheter with dual sensors, one in the bladder and one in the proximal urethra. With coughing or straining, the change in urethral pressure should always be equal to or greater than the change in bladder pressure. In patients with stress incontinence, along with much of the profile curve, the change in urethral pressure will be less than the change in bladder pressure. *Dynamic urethral profilometry* implies the use of a catheter with dual sensors—bladder and proximal

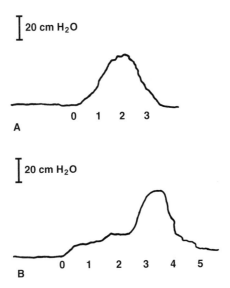

Figure 14-9 Actual urethral pressure profiles from normal female (**A**) and male (**B**) subjects. Numbers represent centimeters, with 0 representing the level of the bladder neck. The maximum urethral pressure in both males and females is normally at the level of the urogenital diaphragm. The initial portion of the curve in the male, from the bladder neck to the pressure rise culminating at the maximum urethral pressure, is sometimes called the prostatic plateau. The area under this portion of the curve corresponds roughly to prostatic size. (*Reproduced from Wein AJ, English WE, Whitmore KE: Office urodynamics. Urol Clin North Am 15:609, 1988.*)

urethra—with pressures recorded during bladder filling and emptying. An actual urethral pressure profile is not recorded. The interaction between bladder pressure and pressure in one area of the urethra, generally in the area of maximal closure pressure, usually at the level of the striated sphincter is recorded. *Micturitional urethral profilometry* refers to a study in which a catheter with dual or triple sensors, one of which is in the bladder, is withdrawn during voiding in a patient with known obstruction. In such a patient, the area of the maximal pressure drop is the site of obstruction. Micturitional profilometry generally requires fluoroscopic monitoring to identify the anatomic location of this maximal pressure decrease.

8. *Valsalva leak point pressure.* The Valsalva leak point pressure or abdominal leak point pressure (VLPP or ALPP) is a measure of the ability of the urethra to resist changes in abdominal pressure as an expulsive force. It has been popularized by McGuire as a clinically useful test, perhaps the most useful one, to differentiate the extremes of intrinsic sphincter deficiency from hypermobility-related stress incontinence. It is easy to see why the concept of this test appeals to straightforward logic: if straining or increases in intra-abdominal pressure produce incontinence, and a filling study shows normal compliance, there must be a problem with the bladder outlet. The amount of abdominal pressure necessary to cause leakage under such circumstances is inversely proportional to the amount of outlet dysfunction. A pressure catheter is placed in the bladder or rectum or both and the bladder filled to a predetermined volume, usually 150 to 200 mL. The patient is then asked to perform a graded Valsalva maneuver until leakage is seen per urethra. If Valsalva does not produce leakage, the patient is asked to cough. The pressure at which leakage is first seen is the VLPP. The higher the VLPP, the better the intrinsic sphincter function, and, conversely, the lower the VLPP, the worse the intrinsic sphincter function. There are still problems concerning standardization of technique, specification of variables, optimal location of pressure measurement, size of urethral catheter to be used, and the bladder volume at which the study is to be carried out. There is also disagreement about what "numbers" indicate a significant degree of intrinsic sphincter dysfunction. Originally, a VLPP of less than 65 cm of water was said to indicate ISD. One caveat to remember is that a large cystocele can invalidate the results, making the VLPP artificially higher.

9. *Ambulatory urodynamics.* An obvious limitation to routine or conventional urodynamic testing is the artificial environment and circumstances in which the test is conducted. Ambulatory urodynamics is an alternative technique in which the pressure transducing catheters are placed into the bladder and rectum but are attached to portable recording devices. The patient resumes his or her normal daily routine and cycles of natural bladder filling and storage. Emptying and voiding are recorded, while the patient writes down the time and qualitative nature of relevant subjective sensations. Provocative maneuvers such as coughing,

climbing, jumping, and hand washing can be performed in an attempt to reproduce the patient's symptomatology. At the conclusion of the study, the data is downloaded to a computer, compared with the written record of symptomatology, and analyzed. Advocates of this type of study cite the ability to objectively confirm the complaints of many patients in whom nonambulatory urodynamics have been unrevealing. However, limitations of this study include the following: (1) the triggering effect of a catheter in the bladder can cause a higher incidence of involuntary bladder contractions than in standard cystometry; (2) if one is recording urethral pressures as well, small movements of the catheter are unavoidable in an ambulatory patient, often resulting in artificial pressure dips; (3) measurement of actual leakage is difficult or near impossible; (4) the bladder filling rate depends on many factors that are still not controllable (such as intake, diuretic usage, congestive failure, etc.); (5) different states of rectal filling and rectal catheter stimulation in the ambulatory patient may exert reflex effects on the bladder; (6) it is difficult to simultaneously measure flow during ambulatory urodynamics, and so at present the study is more useful in the evaluation of filling and storage abnormalities than emptying/voiding abnormalities; (7) detrusor pressure values for certain parameters are different during ambulatory urodynamics as opposed to laboratory urodynamics (new agreed upon standards for normality and abnormality need to be developed); and (8) a certain percent of records will be uninterpretable because of artefacts. At present, ambulatory urodynamics are utilized primarily as a research tool, although the potential range of clinical applications, with some technological improvements, are numerous.

VII. CLASSIFICATION OF VOIDING DYSFUNCTION
A. General
There are many classification systems for voiding dysfunction, and these are based on neurologic, urodynamic, or functional considerations, or on a combination of these. That there are at least six to eight of these attests to the fact that none is prefect. The purpose of any classification system should be to facilitate understanding and management and to avoid confusion among those who are concerned with the problem for which the system was designed. A good classification should serve as intellectual shorthand and should convey, in a few key words or phrases, the essence of a clinical situation. Most

systems of classification for voiding dysfunction were formulated primarily to describe dysfunction secondary to neurologic disease or injury. The ideal system should be applicable to all types of voiding dysfunction.

In this section, we describe the classic system most frequently utilized, the functional type of classification that we
have found most useful, and the International Continence
Society classification.

B. Lapides Classification

Lapides, at the University of Michigan, contributed significantly to care of the patient with neuropathic voiding dysfunction by popularizing a classification scheme that remains
one of the most familiar to urologists and nonurologists. This
is because it describes in recognizable shorthand the clinical
and cystometric conditions of many types of neurogenic
voiding dysfunction (Table 14-4).

A *sensory neurogenic bladder* results from disease that
selectively interrupts the sensory fibers between the bladder
and spinal cord or afferent tracts to the brain. Diabetes mellitus, tabes dorsalis, and pernicious anemia are those most
commonly responsible. The first clinical changes are those
of impaired sensation of bladder distention. Unless voiding
is initiated on a timed basis, varying degrees of bladder
overdistention can result in hypotonicity. If bladder decompensation occurs, significant amounts of residual urine are
found and, at this time, the cystometric curve generally
demonstrates a large capacity bladder with a flat, high compliance, low pressure filling curve. The bethanechol supersensitivity test is usually positive in the early stages but later
may become negative as detrusor decompensation occurs.

A *motor paralytic bladder* results from disease processes
that destroy the parasympathetic motor innervation of the
bladder. Extensive pelvic surgery or trauma or herpes zoster
can produce this. The early symptoms can vary from painful
urinary retention to only a relative inability to initiate and
maintain normal micturition. Early cystometric filling is normal but without a voluntary bladder contraction at capacity.
Chronic overdistention and decompensation may occur in a

Table 14-4 Lapides Bladder Dysfunction Classification

Sensory neurogenic
Motor paralytic
Uninhibited neurogenic
Reflex neurogenic
Autonomous neurogenic

large capacity bladder with a flat, low pressure filling curve and a large amount of residual urine may result. The bethanechol test is positive early and remains so unless severe detrusor decompensation occurs.

The *uninhibited neurogenic bladder* was described originally as resulting from injury or disease to the "corticoregulatory tract." The sacral spinal cord was presumed to be the micturition reflex center, and this corticoregulatory tract was believed to normally exert an inhibitory influence on the sacral micturition reflex center. A destructive lesion in this tract would then result in overfacilitation of the micturition reflex. Cerebrovascular accident, brain or spinal cord tumor, and demyelinating disease are the most common causes in this category. The voiding dysfunction is most often characterized by frequency, urgency, and incontinence, and urodynamically by normal sensation with detrusor hyperreflexia at low filling volumes. The amount of residual urine is characteristically low unless anatomic outlet obstruction or true smooth or striated sphincter dyssynergia occurs. The patient generally can initiate a bladder contraction voluntarily but is often unable to do so during cystometry because sufficient urine storage cannot occur before detrusor hyperreflexia is stimulated.

Reflex neurogenic bladder describes the post-spinal shock condition that exists after complete interruption of the sensory and motor pathways between the sacral spinal cord and the brain stem. Most commonly, this occurs in traumatic spinal cord injury and transverse myelitis but can occur with extensive demyelinating disease or any process that produces significant destruction. Typically, there is no bladder sensation and there is inability to initiate voluntary micturition. Incontinence without sensation generally results because of low volume detrusor hyperreflexia. Striated sphincter dyssynergia is the rule.

An *autonomous neurogenic bladder* results from complete motor and sensory separation of the bladder from the sacral spinal cord. This can be caused by any disease that destroys the sacral cord or causes extensive damage to the sacral roots or pelvic nerves. There is inability to voluntarily initiate micturition, no bladder reflex activity, and no specific bladder sensation. This is the type of dysfunction seen in patients with spinal shock. The characteristic cystometric pattern is initially similar to the late states of the motor or sensory paralytic bladder, with a marked shift to the right of the cystometric filling curve and a large bladder capacity at low intravesical pressure. However, decreased compliance may develop, secondary to either chronic inflammatory change or the effects of denervation/defunctionalization with secondary neuromorphologic and neuropharmacologic changes. Emptying capacity can vary widely, depending on the ability of the patient to increase intravesical pressure and the resistance offered during this increase by the smooth and striated sphincter.

These classic categories in their usual settings are usually understood and remembered, and this is why the system provides an excellent framework for teaching some fundamentals of neurogenic voiding dysfunction to students and nonurologists. Unfortunately, many patients do not exactly fit into one or another category. Gradations of sensory, motor, and mixed lesions occur, and the patterns produced after different types of peripheral denervation and defunctionalization can vary widely from those that are classically described.

C. Functional Classification

Classification of voiding dysfunction can also be formulated on a simple functional basis, describing the dysfunction in terms of whether the deficit produced is primarily one of the filling and storage or emptying and voiding phase of micturition (Table 14-5). This type of system is an excellent alternative when a particular dysfunction does not readily lend itself to a generally agreed on classification elsewhere. This simple system assumes only that, whatever their differences, all "experts" would agree upon the two-phase concept of micturition (see IV) and on the simple formulation of the mechanisms underlying the normality of each phase.

Storage failure results because of bladder or outlet abnormalities or a combination of both. The bladder abnormalities very simply include involuntary bladder contractions, low compliance, and hypersensitivity. The outlet abnormalities can include only an intermittent or continuous decrease in outlet resistance.

Similarly, *emptying failure* can occur because of bladder or outlet abnormalities or both. The bladder side includes inadequate or unsustained bladder contractility, and the outlet side includes anatomic obstruction and sphincter(s) dyssynergia.

Table 14-5 Functional Classification

Failure to store
Because of the bladder
Because of the outlet
Failure to empty
Because of the bladder
Because of the outlet

Failure in either category generally is not absolute, but more often is relative. Such a functional system can easily be "expanded" and made more complicated to include etiologic or specific urodynamic connotations (Table 14-6). However, the simplified system is perfectly workable and avoids argument in those complex situations in which agreement on the exact etiology or urodynamic mechanism for a voiding dysfunction cannot be reached.

Table 14-6 Expanded Functional Classification

Failure to store
  Because of the bladder
    Detrusor hyperactivity
      Involuntary contractions
        Suprasacral neurologic disease
        Bladder outlet obstruction
        Idiopathic
      Decreased compliance
        Neurologic disease
        Fibrosis
        Idiopathic
    Detrusor hypersensitivity
      Inflammatory
      Infectious
      Neurologic
      Psychologic
      Idiopathic
  Because of the outlet
    Stress incontinence
    Intrinsic sphincter dysfunction, nonfunctional bladder neck and proximal urethra
Failure to empty
  Because of the bladder
    Neurologic
    Myogenic
    Psychogenic
    Idiopathic
  Because of the outlet
    Anatomic
      Prostatic obstruction
      Bladder neck contracture
      Urethral stricture
      Urethral compression
    Functional
      Smooth sphincter dyssynergia
      Striated sphincter dyssynergia

Proper use of this system for a given voiding dysfunction requires a reasonably accurate notion of what the urodynamic data show. However, an exact diagnosis is not required for treatment. It should be recognized that some patients do not have only a discrete storage or emptying failure, and the existence of combination deficits must be recognized to properly use this classification system. For instance, the classic T10 paraplegic patient after spinal shock generally exhibits a relative failure to store because of detrusor hyperreflexia and a relative failure to empty because of striated sphincter dyssynergia. To use this classification system, with such a combination deficit, the examiner must assume that one of the deficits is primary and that significant improvement will result from its treatment alone or that the voiding dysfunction can be converted primarily to a disorder either of storage or emptying by means of nonsurgical or surgical therapy. The resultant deficit can then be treated or circumvented. Using the same example, the combined deficit in a T10 paraplegic patient can be converted primarily to a storage failure by surgical procedures directed at the dyssynergic striated sphincter; the resultant incontinence (secondary to detrusor hyperreflexia) can be circumvented in a male with an external collecting device. Alternatively, the deficit can be converted primarily to an emptying failure by pharmacologic or surgical measures designed to abolish or reduce the detrusor hyperreflexia and/or increase bladder capacity. The resultant emptying failure can then be circumvented with clean intermittent catheterization. Other examples of combination deficits include impaired bladder contractility with sphincter dysfunction, bladder outlet obstruction with detrusor hyperactivity, bladder outlet obstruction with sphincter malfunction, and detrusor hyperactivity with impaired contractility.

D. International Continence Society Classification

The classification system proposed by the International Continence Society (ICS) is in many ways an extension of a urodynamic classification system (Table 14-7). The storage and voiding phases or micturition are described separately, and within each, various designations are applied to describe bladder and urethral function.

Normal bladder function during filling and storage implies no significant rises in detrusor pressure (stability). Overactive detrusor function indicates the presence of involuntary contractions. If due to neurologic disease, the term detrusor hyperreflexia is used; if not, the phenomenon is known as detrusor instability. Bladder sensation can be categorized only in qualitative terms as indicated. Bladder ca-

Table 14-7 International Continence Society Classification

STORAGE PHASE	VOIDING PHASE
Bladder Function	Bladder Function
Detrusor activity	Detrusor activity
Normal or stable	Normal
Overactive	Underactive
Unstable	Acontractile
Hyperreflexic	
Bladder sensation	Urethral Function
Normal	Normal
Increased or hypersensitive	Obstructive
Reduced or hyposensitive	Overactive
Absent	Mechanical
Bladder capacity	
Normal	
High	
Low	
Compliance	
Normal	
High	
Low	
Urethral function	
Normal	
Incompetent	

pacity and compliance (Δ volume/Δ pressure) are cystometric measurements. Normal urethral function during filling and storage indicates a positive urethral closure pressure (urethral pressure minus bladder pressure), even with increases in intra-abdominal pressure. Incompetent urethral function during filling and storage implies urine leakage in the absence of a detrusor contraction. This can be secondary to genuine stress incontinence, intrinsic sphincter dysfunction, or an involuntary fall in urethral pressure in the absence of a detrusor contraction (urethral instability).

During the voiding and emptying phase of micturition, normal detrusor activity implies voiding by a voluntarily initiated sustained contraction that also can be suppressed voluntarily. An underactive detrusor defines a contraction of inadequate magnitude or/and duration to empty the bladder within a normal time span. An acontractile detrusor is one that cannot be demonstrated to contract during urodynamic testing. Areflexia is defined as acontractility due to an abnormality of neural control, implying the complete absence of centrally coordinated contraction. Nor-

---

Condition					Comments
[illegible] Brain tumor	+	N	S	S	May have decreased sensation of lower urinary tract events; May not care about control
Dementia	+, N	N	S	S	
Cerebral palsy	+	N	S	S	
Parkinson's disease	+	N	S / ±VC / O	D (25%) / ±VC / S	
Shy-Drager syndrome	+	N	S	S	Striated sphincter may exhibit denervation
Multiple sclerosis	I / +	D / N	S	S / D (30–65%)	Dyssynergia figures refer to percent of those with detrusor hyperreflexia
Spinal shock	I	N	CNR	F	
Spinal cord injury	–(5–30%)				
Suprasacral	+	N	S	D	Smooth sphincter may dyssynergic if lesion above T7

mal urethral function during voiding indicates opening prior to micturition to allow bladder emptying. An obstructed urethra is one that contracts against a detrusor contraction or fails to open (nonrelaxation) with attempted micturition. Contraction may be due to smooth or striated sphincter dyssynergia. Striated sphincter dyssynergia is a term that should be applied only when neurologic disease is present. A similar syndrome, but without neurologic disease, is called dysfunctional voiding. Mechanical obstruction is generally anatomic and caused by BPH, urethral or bladder neck stricture, scarring or compression, or rarely, kinking of a portion of the urethra during straining.

Voiding dysfunction in a classic T10 level paraplegic patient after spinal shock has passed would be classified as follows.

- Storage phase: overactive hyperreflexic detrusor, absent sensation, low capacity, normal compliance, normal urethral closure function.
- Voiding phase: overactive obstructive urethral function, questionable normal detrusor activity (actually hyperreflexic).

The voiding dysfunction of a stroke patient with urgency incontinence would most likely be classified during storage as overactive hyperreflexic detrusor, normal sensation, low capacity, normal compliance, and normal urethral closure functions. During voiding, the dysfunction would be classified as normal detrusor activity and normal urethral function, assuming that no anatomic obstruction existed.

VIII. NEUROGENIC VOIDING DYSFUNCTION
A. Common Types
The more common types of voiding dysfunction secondary to neurologic disease, injury, or dysfunction are described. Table 14-8 classifies these dysfunctions on the basis of the most common type of problem that results from a given disease insofar as the activity of the bladder, smooth sphincter, and striated sphincter are concerned. The classification shown in this table does not mean that everyone who has a particular neurologic disease has the type of dysfunction listed, but simply indicates that, for the most part, individuals with the disease, who have voiding dysfunction because of it, have the type of dysfunction shown. Only some of these are further elaborated.

Discrete neurologic lesions generally affect the filling and storage and emptying and voiding phases of lower urinary tract function in a relatively consistent fashion, that fashion

being depe
function of
or irritative.
fect micturit
tractions wit
tion and vol
preserved. A
as a perman
of the spinal
they recover
tary bladder
ter synergy,
lesions abov
sphincter dy
p. 395, 400).
low S2 gener
tractions per
spinal shock,
rologic injury,
ing filling may
result, but wh
pathetic dece
neither) has ne
sphincter dysfu
tains a residual
as dyssynergia
functions that o
arc may be ver
Detrusor arefle
sult, the smoot
tent, and the str
ual tone not
peripheral neur
usual expected s

B. Cerebrovascula
Thrombosis, occ
mon causes of is
eas in the brain,
the initial acute
areflexia can occ
shock" is unclear
from the neurolo
parent over a few
term expression
cerebrovascular a
Sensation is varia

Table 14-8

DISORDER	DETRUSOR ACTIVITY	COMPLIANCE	SMOOTH SPHINCTER	STRIATED SPHINCTER	OTHER
Cerebrovascular	+	N	S	S	May be unable to forcefully contract striated sphincter

Lesion	Detrusor Activity	Compliance	Smooth Sphincter	Striated Sphincter	Comments
Sacral	−	N; D (may develop)	CNR; O (may develop)	F	Findings vary widely in different series: striated sphincter commonly shows some evidence of denervation
Autonomic hyperreflexia	+	D	O	F	—
Myelodysplasia	− or +	N or D	O	S	Primary problem is loss of function: detrusor may become decompensated secondary to overdistention
Tabes, pernicious anemia, sensa-	−	N	S	S	—
Disk disease	−	N	CNR	S	Striated sphincter may show evidence of denervation and fixed tone
Radical pelvic surgery	−	N or D	O	F	—
Diabetes	−	N	S	S	Sensory loss contributes but a motor neuropathy as well

Detrusor Activity: N, normal; I, Impaired; +, involuntary contraction; −, acontractile.
Compliance: N, normal; D, decreased; I, increased.
Smooth Sphincter: S, Dyssynergic; O, Open, competent at rest; CNR, Competent, non-relaxing.
Striated Sphincter: S, synergic; D, dyssynergic; ±VC, voluntary control may be impaired; F, fixed tone.
Typical voiding dysfunctions seen with various types of neurologic disease or injury. When dysfunction does occur, the most common pattern(s) is (are) noted.

urgency and frequency with hyperreflexia. Compliance is normal. The appropriate response is to try to inhibit the involuntary bladder activity by forceful voluntary contraction of the striated sphincter. If this is successful, only urgency and frequency result; if not, urgency with incontinence results. Patients with lesions in only the basal ganglia or thalamus have normal sphincter function. This means that when an impending involuntary contraction or its onset is sensed, they can voluntarily contract the striated sphincter in time to abort or considerably lessen the effect of the abnormal micturition reflex. The majority of patients with involvement of the cerebral cortex and/or internal capsule are unable to forcefully contract the striated sphincter under these circumstances. Detrusor hypocontractility or areflexia can also exist after CVA. True detrusor-striated sphincter dyssynergia does not occur following a CVA. Pseudodyssynergia may occur during urodynamic testing. Smooth sphincter function is generally unaffected by CVA. Poor flow rates and high residual urine volumes in a male with pre-CVA symptoms of prostatism generally indicate prostatic obstruction. A urodynamic evaluation is advisable before committing a patient to mechanical outlet reduction to exclude detrusor hyperactivity with impaired contractility (DHIC) as a cause of symptoms.

C. Dementia

Dementia is a poorly understood disease complex involving atrophy and the loss of grey and white matter of the brain, particularly the frontal lobes. When voiding dysfunction occurs, the result is generally incontinence. It is difficult to ascertain whether this is due to detrusor hyperreflexia with the type of disorder of voluntary striated sphincter control mentioned with CVA or whether it is a type of situation in which the individual has simply lost the awareness of the desirability of voluntary urinary control.

D. Cerebral Palsy

Cerebral palsy (CP) is the rubric applied to a nonprogressive injury of the brain in the prenatal or perinatal period (some say up to 3 years) producing neuromuscular disability and/or specific symptom complexes of cerebral dysfunction. The etiology is generally infection or a period of hypoxia. Most children and adults with only CP have urinary control and what seems to be normal filling and storage and normal emptying. The incidence of voiding dysfunction is vague because the few available series report mostly subcategorizations of those who present with symptoms.

E. Parkinson's Disease

This degenerative disorder primarily affects the pigmented neurons of the substantia nigra, resulting in a relative dopamine deficiency and a predominance of cholinergic activity in the corpus striatum. Voiding dysfunction occurs in 25 to 75 percent of patients. Preexisting detrusor or outlet abnormalities may exist, and the symptomatology can be affected by various types of treatment for the primary disease. When voiding dysfunction occurs, symptoms generally consist of urgency, frequency, nocturia, and urge incontinence. The most common urodynamic correlate is detrusor hyperreflexia. Impaired detrusor contractility may occur, either in the form of low amplitude or poorly sustained contractions, or a combination. The smooth sphincter is synergic. True striated sphincter dyssynergia does not generally occur, but pseudodyssynergia does occur, as well as a problem known as sphincter bradykinesia. This is a delay in the relaxation of the striated sphincter at the onset of voluntary or involuntary micturition and is most common in patients who exhibit significant skeletal muscle rigidity. This can also cause difficulty in rapidly and forcefully contracting the striated sphincter to try to prevent incontinence due to an involuntary bladder contraction. Detection of poor voluntary striated sphincter control is important because it will predispose to significantly increased incidence of post-prostatectomy incontinence.

One significant problem in dealing with voiding dysfunction in male patients with Parkinson's disease and after CVA is determining whether there is anatomic outlet obstruction secondary to prostatic enlargement and whether prostatectomy or other mechanical measures to decrease prostatic urethral resistance are indicated. Generally, detrusor contractility seems to be unimpaired in stroke patients with involuntary bladder hyperactivity, and, in the absence of dyssynergia (rare or nonexistent), poor flow rates and high residual urine volumes in the male generally indicate prostatic obstruction. Outlet reduction in these patients is generally beneficial because the functional bladder capacity improves, either as a result of a decrease in a residual urine volume or because the clinician feels more comfortable in treating these now unobstructed patients with agents to decrease bladder contractility. Male patients with Parkinson's disease and the identical symptoms and urodynamic findings do not fare as well after prostatectomy. Poorly sustained bladder contractions, and sphincter bradykinesia, may occur consequent to the neurologic disease, and in such individuals prostatectomy may result in no change or a worsening of the voiding symptoms.

F. Multiple Sclerosis (MS)

MS is due to focal neural demyelination, which causes impairment of nerve conduction. The slowing of nerve conduction results in varying neurologic abnormalities that are subject to exacerbation and remission. The demyelinating process most commonly involves the posterior and lateral columns of the cervical spinal cord, and, to a lesser extent, the lumbar and sacral cord. Of patients with MS, 50 to 80 percent complain of voiding symptoms at some time. Lower urinary tract involvement may constitute the sole initial complaint or be part of the presenting symptom complex in approximately 10 percent of patients, often in the form of acute urinary retention of "unknown" etiology or as an acute onset of urgency and frequency secondary to hyperreflexia. Detrusor hyperreflexia is the most common urodynamic abnormality detected, occurring in at least 50 percent of cases. Impaired detrusor contractility is not uncommon, complicating treatment of the hyperreflexia. Of the patients with hyperreflexia, 30 to 65 percent have coexistent striated sphincter dyssynergia. Sensation is usually intact and so the clinician must be careful to recognize and differentiate pseudo-dyssynergia. Some varieties of striated sphincter dyssynergia are more worrisome than others. For instance, in a female with MS, a brief period of striated sphincter dyssynergia (but one that does not result in excessive intravesical pressure during voiding, substantial residual urine volume, or secondary detrusor hyperactivity) may be relatively inconsequential, whereas those varieties that are more sustained—resulting in high bladder pressures of long duration—are most associated with urologic complications. Bladder areflexia can also occur; reports of its frequency as a urodynamic finding vary from 1 to 40 percent, but, of this number, a substantial proportion of cases progress to detrusor hyperreflexia. Generally, the smooth sphincter is synergic.

G. Spinal Cord Injury

1. *Spinal shock.* Following a significant spinal cord injury, a period of decreased excitability of spinal cord segments at and below the level of the lesion occurs. It is referred to as spinal shock. Somatic reflex activity is generally absent and flaccid muscle paralysis is found below this level. Spinal shock includes a suppression of autonomic as well as somatic activity, and the bladder is acontractile and areflexic with a closed bladder neck. The smooth sphincter mechanism seems to be closed and competent but nonrelaxing, except in some cases of thoracolumbar injury. Some electromyographic activity can generally be recorded from the striated sphincter, and the maximum

Table 14-7 International Continence Society Classification

STORAGE PHASE	VOIDING PHASE
Bladder Function	Bladder Function
Detrusor activity	Detrusor activity
Normal or stable	Normal
Overactive	Underactive
Unstable	Acontractile
Hyperreflexic	
Bladder sensation	Urethral Function
Normal	Normal
Increased or hypersensitive	Obstructive
Reduced or hyposensitive	Overactive
Absent	Mechanical
Bladder capacity	
Normal	
High	
Low	
Compliance	
Normal	
High	
Low	
Urethral function	
Normal	
Incompetent	

pacity and compliance (Δ volume/Δ pressure) are cystometric measurements. Normal urethral function during filling and storage indicates a positive urethral closure pressure (urethral pressure minus bladder pressure), even with increases in intra-abdominal pressure. Incompetent urethral function during filling and storage implies urine leakage in the absence of a detrusor contraction. This can be secondary to genuine stress incontinence, intrinsic sphincter dysfunction, or an involuntary fall in urethral pressure in the absence of a detrusor contraction (urethral instability).

During the voiding and emptying phase of micturition, normal detrusor activity implies voiding by a voluntarily initiated sustained contraction that also can be suppressed voluntarily. An underactive detrusor defines a contraction of inadequate magnitude or/and duration to empty the bladder within a normal time span. An acontractile detrusor is one that cannot be demonstrated to contract during urodynamic testing. Areflexia is defined as acontractility due to an abnormality of neural control, implying the complete absence of centrally coordinated contraction. Normal urethral function during voiding indicates opening prior to micturition to allow bladder emptying. An obstructed urethra is one that contracts against a detrusor contraction or fails to open (nonrelaxation) with attempted micturition. Contraction may be due to smooth or striated sphincter dyssynergia. Striated sphincter dyssynergia is a term that should be applied only when neurologic disease is present. A similar syndrome, but without neurologic disease, is called dysfunctional voiding. Mechanical obstruction is generally anatomic and caused by BPH, urethral or bladder neck stricture, scarring or compression, or rarely, kinking of a portion of the urethra during straining.

Voiding dysfunction in a classic T10 level paraplegic patient after spinal shock has passed would be classified as follows.

- Storage phase: overactive hyperreflexic detrusor, absent sensation, low capacity, normal compliance, normal urethral closure function.
- Voiding phase: overactive obstructive urethral function, questionable normal detrusor activity (actually hyperreflexic).

The voiding dysfunction of a stroke patient with urgency incontinence would most likely be classified during storage as overactive hyperreflexic detrusor, normal sensation, low capacity, normal compliance, and normal urethral closure functions. During voiding, the dysfunction would be classified as normal detrusor activity and normal urethral function, assuming that no anatomic obstruction existed.

VIII. NEUROGENIC VOIDING DYSFUNCTION
A. Common Types

The more common types of voiding dysfunction secondary to neurologic disease, injury, or dysfunction are described. Table 14-8 classifies these dysfunctions on the basis of the most common type of problem that results from a given disease insofar as the activity of the bladder, smooth sphincter, and striated sphincter are concerned. The classification shown in this table does not mean that everyone who has a particular neurologic disease has the type of dysfunction listed, but simply indicates that, for the most part, individuals with the disease, who have voiding dysfunction because of it, have the type of dysfunction shown. Only some of these are further elaborated.

Discrete neurologic lesions generally affect the filling and storage and emptying and voiding phases of lower urinary tract function in a relatively consistent fashion, that fashion being dependent on the area(s) affected, the physiologic function of the area(s), and whether the lesion is destructive or irritative. Neurologic lesions above the brainstem that affect micturition generally result in involuntary bladder contractions with smooth and striated sphincter synergy. Sensation and voluntary striated sphincter function are generally preserved. Areflexia may, however, occur, either initially or as a permanent dysfunction. Patients with complete lesions of the spinal cord between spinal cord level T6 and S2, after they recover from spinal shock, generally exhibit involuntary bladder contractions without sensation, smooth sphincter synergy, but striated sphincter dyssynergia. Those with lesions above T6 may experience, in addition, smooth sphincter dyssynergia and autonomic hyperreflexia (see p. 395, 400). Patients with significant spinal cord trauma below S2 generally do not manifest involuntary bladder contractions per se. Detrusor areflexia is the rule initially after spinal shock, and, depending on the type and extent of neurologic injury, various forms of decreased compliance during filling may occur. An open, smooth sphincter area may result, but whether this is due to sympathetic or parasympathetic decentralization/defunctionalization (or both or neither) has never been determined. Various types of striated sphincter dysfunction may occur, but commonly the area retains a residual resting sphincter tone, which is not the same as dyssynergia and is not under voluntary control. The dysfunctions that occur with interruption of the peripheral reflex arc may be very similar to those of distal spinal cord injury. Detrusor areflexia often develops, low compliance may result, the smooth sphincter area may be relatively incompetent, and the striated sphincter area may exhibit fixed residual tone not amenable to voluntary relaxation. True peripheral neuropathy can be motor or sensory, with the usual expected sequelae, at least initially.

B. Cerebrovascular Disease

Thrombosis, occlusion, and hemorrhage are the most common causes of ischemia and infarction of variably sized areas in the brain, usually around the internal capsule. After the initial acute episode, urinary retention due to detrusor areflexia can occur. The neurophysiology of this "cerebral shock" is unclear. Following a variable degree of recovery from the neurologic lesion, a fixed deficit may become apparent over a few weeks or months. The most common long-term expression of lower urinary tract dysfunction after cerebrovascular accident (CVA) is detrusor hyperreflexia. Sensation is variable but generally intact. The patient has

Table 14-8

DISORDER	DETRUSOR ACTIVITY	COMPLIANCE	SMOOTH SPHINCTER	STRIATED SPHINCTER	OTHER
Cerebrovascular accident	+	N	S	S	May be unable to forcefully contract striated sphincter
Brain tumor	+	N	S	S	May have decreased sensation of lower urinary tract events
Dementia	+, N	N	S	S	May not care about control
Cerebral palsy	+	N	S	D (25%) ± VC / S	—
Parkinson's disease	+	N	S ± VC	S	—
Shy-Drager syndrome	+	N	O	S	Striated sphincter may exhibit denervation
Multiple sclerosis	I + / I −(5–30%)	D / N	S	S / D (30–65%)	Dyssynergia figures refer to percent of those with detrusor hyperreflexia
Spinal shock	−	N	CNR	F	
Spinal cord injury					
Suprasacral	+	N	S	D	Smooth sphincter may dyssynergic if lesion above T7

Condition	Detrusor Activity	Compliance	Smooth Sphincter	Striated Sphincter	Comments
Sacral	−	N	CNR	F	
Autonomic hyperreflexia	+	D (may develop) / D	O (may develop) / D	F	
Myelodysplasia	− +	N or D	O	S	Findings vary widely in different series: striated sphincter commonly shows some evidence of denervation
Tabes, pernicious anemia sensa-	−	N	S	S	Primary problem is loss of [sensa-]tion: detrusor may become decompensated secondary to overdistention
Disk disease	− I	N	CNR	S	Striated sphincter may show evidence of denervation and fixed tone
Radical pelvic surgery	− −	N or D	O	F	—
Diabetes	− −	N	S	S	Sensory loss contributes but a motor neuropathy as well

Detrusor Activity: N, normal; I, Impaired; +, involuntary contraction; −, acontractile.
Compliance: N, normal; D, decreased; I, increased.
Smooth Sphincter: S, synergic; D, Dyssynergic; O, Open, competent at rest; CNR, Competent, non-relaxing.
Striated Sphincter: S, synergic; D, dyssynergic; ±VC, voluntary control may be impaired; F, fixed tone.
Typical voiding dysfunctions seen with various types of neurologic disease or injury. When dysfunction does occur, the most common pattern(s) is (are) noted.

urgency and frequency with hyperreflexia. Compliance is normal. The appropriate response is to try to inhibit the involuntary bladder activity by forceful voluntary contraction of the striated sphincter. If this is successful, only urgency and frequency result; if not, urgency with incontinence results. Patients with lesions in only the basal ganglia or thalamus have normal sphincter function. This means that when an impending involuntary contraction or its onset is sensed, they can voluntarily contract the striated sphincter in time to abort or considerably lessen the effect of the abnormal micturition reflex. The majority of patients with involvement of the cerebral cortex and/or internal capsule are unable to forcefully contract the striated sphincter under these circumstances. Detrusor hypocontractility or areflexia can also exist after CVA. True detrusor-striated sphincter dyssynergia does not occur following a CVA. Pseudodyssynergia may occur during urodynamic testing. Smooth sphincter function is generally unaffected by CVA. Poor flow rates and high residual urine volumes in a male with pre-CVA symptoms of prostatism generally indicate prostatic obstruction. A urodynamic evaluation is advisable before committing a patient to mechanical outlet reduction to exclude detrusor hyperactivity with impaired contractility (DHIC) as a cause of symptoms.

C. Dementia

Dementia is a poorly understood disease complex involving atrophy and the loss of grey and white matter of the brain, particularly the frontal lobes. When voiding dysfunction occurs, the result is generally incontinence. It is difficult to ascertain whether this is due to detrusor hyperreflexia with the type of disorder of voluntary striated sphincter control mentioned with CVA or whether it is a type of situation in which the individual has simply lost the awareness of the desirability of voluntary urinary control.

D. Cerebral Palsy

Cerebral palsy (CP) is the rubric applied to a nonprogressive injury of the brain in the prenatal or perinatal period (some say up to 3 years) producing neuromuscular disability and/or specific symptom complexes of cerebral dysfunction. The etiology is generally infection or a period of hypoxia. Most children and adults with only CP have urinary control and what seems to be normal filling and storage and normal emptying. The incidence of voiding dysfunction is vague because the few available series report mostly subcategorizations of those who present with symptoms.

urethral closure pressure is still maintained at the level of the external sphincter zone; however, the normal guarding reflex is absent. Because sphincter tone exists, urinary incontinence generally does not result unless there is gross overdistention with overflow. Urinary retention is the rule, and catheterization is necessary to circumvent this problem. Intermittent catheterization is an excellent method of management during this period.

If the distal spinal cord is intact but is simply isolated from higher centers, there is generally a return of detrusor contractility. At first, such reflex activity is poorly sustained and produces only low pressure changes, but the strength and duration of such involuntary contractions increase, producing involuntary voiding, usually with incomplete bladder emptying. Spinal shock generally lasts 6 to 12 weeks in complete suprasacral spinal cord lesions, but can last for as long as a year or two. It can last for a shorter period of time in incomplete suprasacral lesions and only a few days in some patients. In evolving lesions, every attempt should be made to preserve as low a bladder storage pressure as possible.

2. *Suprasacral spinal cord injury.* The characteristic fixed lesion that results when a patient has a complete lesion above the sacral spinal cord is detrusor hyperreflexia, smooth sphincter synergia (with lesions below the sympathetic outflow, usually T6), and striated sphincter dyssynergia. Neurologic examination shows spasticity of skeletal muscle distal to the lesion, hyperreflexic deep tendon reflexes, and abnormal plantar responses. There is impairment of superficial and deep sensation. Incomplete bladder emptying usually results. The neurologic center responsible for coordinating bladder and striated sphincter activity is in the pontine mesencephalic formation, and any lesion between this area and the sacral spinal cord can interfere with this coordination. Thus, true striated sphincter dyssynergia occurs. Once reflex voiding is established, it can be initiated or reinforced by the stimulation of certain dermatomes, such as by tapping the suprapubic area. The urodynamic consequences of striated sphincter dyssynergia vary with severity (complete lesions generally worse than incomplete, continuous contraction worse than intermittent) and anatomy (men worse than women).

From a functional standpoint, the voiding dysfunction most commonly seen in suprasacral spinal cord injury represents both filling and storage and emptying failure. Although the urodynamics are "safe" enough in some individuals to allow management consisting only of periodic stimulation of bladder reflex activity, many will require some treatment. If bladder pressures are suitably low or can be made suitably low with nonsurgical or surgical management, the problem can be treated primarily as an emptying failure, and intermittent catheterization can be continued when practical as a safe and effective way to satisfy many of the goals of treatment. Alternatively, external sphincterotomy can be used in males to lower the leak point to an acceptable level, thus treating the dysfunction primarily as one of emptying, and obviating the resultant storage failure either by timed stimulation or with an external collecting device. In the manually dexterous spinal cord injury patient, the former approach is becoming predominant. A combination of selective rhizotomy and electrical stimulation can result in a functional LUT, a reality once thought to be unattainable (see section on treatment). As with all patients with neurologic impairment, a careful initial evaluation and periodic follow up evaluation must be performed to identify and correct the following risk factors: bladder overdistention, high pressure storage, high detrusor leak point pressure, vesicoureteral reflux, stone formation (lower and upper tracts), and complicating infection, especially in association with reflux.

3. *Sacral spinal cord injury.* Following recovery from spinal shock, there is usually a depression of deep tendon reflexes below the level of the lesion with varying degrees of flaccid paralysis. Sensation is generally absent below the lesion level. Detrusor areflexia with high or normal compliance is the common initial result. Decreased compliance may develop, a change often seen with neurologic lesions at or distal to the sacral spinal cord and most likely representing a response to neurologic decentralization. The classical outlet findings are described as a competent but nonrelaxing smooth sphincter and a striated sphincter that retains some fixed tone but is not under voluntary control. Closure pressures are decreased in both areas. However, the late appearance of the bladder neck may be open. Attempted voiding by straining or Credé results in obstruction at the bladder neck (if closed) or at the distal sphincter area by fixed sphincter tone. Potential risk factors are those previously described, with particular emphasis on storage pressure, which can result in silent upper tract decompensation and deterioration in the absence of vesicoureteral reflux. The treatment of such a patient is generally directed toward producing or maintaining low pressure storage while circumventing emptying failure

with CIC when possible. Electrical stimulation may be useful in promoting emptying in certain circumstances.

4. *Neurologic and urodynamic correlation in SCI.* Although generally correct, the correlation between somatic neurologic findings and urodynamic findings in suprasacral and sacral SCI patients is not exact. A number of factors should be considered in this regard. First, whether a lesion is complete or incomplete is sometimes a matter of definition. A complete lesion, somatically speaking, may not translate into a complete lesion autonomically, and vice versa. Multiple injuries may actually exist at different levels, even though what is seen somatically may reflect a single level of injury. Even considering these situations, however, all such discrepancies are not explained. Management of the urinary tract in such patients must be based on urodynamic principles and findings rather than inferences from the neurologic history and evaluation. Similarly, although the information regarding "classic" complete lesions is for the most part valid, neurologic conclusions should not be made solely on the basis of urodynamic findings.

5. *Autonomic hyperreflexia.* Autonomic hyperreflexia (autonomic dysreflexia) occurs only in patients with transverse lesions of the cervical and thoracic spinal cord above the level of the T6 vertebra (above the sympathetic outflow from the spinal cord). Symptomatically, it is a syndrome of exaggerated sympathetic activity in response to stimuli below the level of the lesion. The pathophysiology is a nociceptive stimulation of afferent pathways that ascend through the cord and elicit reflex motor outflow, causing arteriolar, pilomotor, and pelvic visceral spasm. Normally, the reflexes should be inhibited by supraspinal modulation, but this does not occur because of the cord injury. Compensatory vasodilation occurs only above the lesion level. Striated sphincter dyssynergia invariably occurs, and smooth sphincter dyssynergia is generally a part of the syndrome in males. The symptoms are pounding headache, hypertension, and flushing, with sweating of the face and body above the level of the spinal cord lesion. Bradycardia is a usual accompaniment, although tachycardia may be present. Hypertension can be expressed in varying severity, from a mild headache before the occurrence of voiding to life-threatening hypertension and cardiac arrhythmia. Hypertension so severe as to cause seizure or cerebral hemorrhage occurs more frequently in patients with cervical rather than thoracic cord lesions. It does not occur

during spinal shock, and the first manifestation may not occur for 1 to 2 years following injury.

The stimuli for AH commonly arise from the rectum or bladder. Precipitation can be due to any instrumentation, catheter obstruction, or clot retention and, in such cases, resolves quickly if the stimulus is withdrawn. Other causes or exacerbating factors may include fecal impaction, long bone fracture, and pressure sores (decubitus ulcers). Ideally, any endoscopic procedure in susceptible patients should be done under spinal anesthesia or carefully monitored general anesthesia. Acutely, the hemodynamic effects of this syndrome can be managed with parenteral ganglionic or α-adrenergic blockade or with parenteral chlorpromazine. Oral nifedipine has been shown to be capable of lessening this syndrome when given prior to cystoscopy. Prophylactic α-1 blockade has also been advocated on a long-term basis.

6. *Spinal cord injury in women.* Special difficulty in this category of patients is encountered because of the lack of an appropriate external collecting device. Suitable bladder reservoir function can usually be achieved either pharmacologically or surgically, and paraplegic women can generally master CIC. Although a few quadriplegic women can be trained to self-CIC, for the majority, there is no practical alternative to indwelling urethral catheterization other than suprapubic urinary diversion.

H. Neurospinal Dysraphism

Although primarily a pediatric problem, certain considerations regarding the adult with these abnormalities should be mentioned. Secondary to progress in the overall care of children with myelodysplasia, urologic dysfunction often becomes a problem of the adult with this disease. The typical myelodysplastic patient shows an areflexic bladder with an open bladder neck. Decreased compliance may be present. The bladder generally fills until the resting residual fixed external sphincter pressure is reached, and then leakage occurs. Stress incontinence related to changes in intra-abdominal pressure occurs also. A small percentage of patients demonstrate detrusor-striated sphincter dyssynergia, but these individuals show normal bladder neck function which, if detrusor reflex activity is controlled, is associated with continence. After puberty most male myelodysplastic patients note an improvement in continence. In adult patients, the problems encountered in myelodysplastic children still exist, but are often compounded by prior surgery, upper tract dysfunction, and one form of urinary diversion or another. In adult females, the goal is to increase urethral sphincter efficiency without causing an undue enough increase in urethral closing pressure, which will result in a change in bladder compliance. Periurethral injection therapy to achieve continence may give as good a result as a pubovaginal sling or artificial sphincter in this circumstance. Continence in adult male myelodysplastic individuals follows the same general rules as in females, and injectable materials may give good results in this group as well, unless the outlet is widely dilated. Dry individuals, of course, will be on intermittent self-catheterization. Nowhere is the failure of a neurologic examination to predict urodynamic behavior more obvious than in patients with myelomeningocele.

I. Disk Disease

Most disk protrusions compress the spinal roots in the L4–L5 or L5–S1 interspaces. Voiding dysfunction occurs as a result, and when present, generally occurs with the usual clinical manifestations of low back pain radiating in a girdle-like fashion along the involved spinal root areas. Examination may reveal reflex and sensory loss consistent with nerve root compression. The incidence of voiding dysfunction in disk prolapse ranges from 1 to 18 percent. The most consistent urodynamic finding is a normally compliant areflexic bladder associated with normal innervation or incomplete denervation of the perineal floor muscles. There is a lower incidence of decreased compliance in root damage secondary to disk prolapse, as opposed to myelomeningocele. Occasionally, patients may show detrusor hyperreflexia, attributed to irritation of the nerve roots.

Patients with voiding dysfunction generally present with difficulty voiding, straining, or urinary retention. It should be noted that laminectomy may not improve bladder function, and prelaminectomy urodynamic evaluation is desirable because it may be difficult postoperatively to separate causation of voiding dysfunction due to the disk sequelae alone from changes secondary to the surgery.

J. Radical Pelvic Surgery

Voiding dysfunction following pelvic plexus injury occurs most commonly after abdominoperineal resection and radical hysterectomy. Neurologic dysfunction after these procedures is reported in 10 to 60 percent of patients, and in 15 to 20 percent, voiding dysfunction is permanent. The injury can occur consequent to denervation or defunctionalization, tethering of the nerves or encasement in scar, direct bladder or urethral trauma, or bladder devascularization. Any adjuvant treatment, such as chemotherapy or radiation, can play a role as well. The type of voiding dysfunction that occurs is dependent on the specific nerves involved, the degree of injury, and any pattern or reinnervation of altered innervation that results over time.

When permanent voiding dysfunction occurs, the pattern is generally one of a failure of voluntary bladder contractions, or impaired bladder contractility, with obstruction by what seems urodynamically to be residual fixed striated sphincter tone that is not subject to voluntarily induced relaxation. Often, the smooth sphincter area is open and nonfunctional. Whether this is due to parasympathetic damage or terminal sympathetic damage, or whether it results from the hydrodynamic effects of obstruction at the level of the striated sphincter, is debated and unknown. Decreased compliance is common in these patients, and this, with the "obstruction" caused by fixed residual striated sphincter tone, results in both storage and emptying failure. These patients often experience leakage across the distal sphincter area and, in addition, are unable to empty the bladder because, although intravesical pressure is and can be further increased, there is nothing that approximates a true bladder contraction. The patient often presents with urinary incontinence that is characteristically most manifest with increases in intra-abdominal pressure. This is usually most obvious in females because the prostatic bulk in males often masks an equivalent deficit in urethral closure function. Patients also present with variable degrees of urinary retention.

Urodynamic studies can show decreased compliance, poor proximal urethral closure function, loss of voluntary control of the striated sphincter, and a positive bethanechol supersensitivity test. Upper tract risk factors are related to intravesical pressure and detrusor leak point pressure. The therapeutic goal is always low pressure storage with periodic emptying. Performing a prostatectomy should be avoided unless a clear demonstration of outlet obstruction at this level is possible. Otherwise, prostatectomy simply decreases urethral sphincteric function and can result in the occurrence or worsening of sphincteric urinary incontinence.

Many of these dysfunctions will be transient, and the temptation to do something other than perform intermittent catheterization early after surgery in these patients, especially in those with little or no preexisting history of voiding dysfunction, cannot be too strongly criticized.

K. Diabetes Mellitus

The autonomic neuropathy of diabetes is secondary to a metabolic derangement of the Schwann cell, resulting in segmental demyelinization and impairment of nerve conduction. Neuropathy tends to develop in middle-aged and elderly patients with longstanding or poorly controlled diabetes. The exact incidence is uncertain, as patients not selected for examination and questioning generally do not complain of bladder symptoms. If specifically questioned, anywhere from 5 to 59 percent report symptoms of voiding dysfunction.

The classical description of the neuropathy and its lower urinary tract effects is of a primarily sensory neuropathy that first causes the insidious onset of impaired bladder sensation. A gradual increase in the time interval between voiding results, which may progress to the point at which the patient voids only once or twice a day without ever sensing any real urgency. If this continues, detrusor distention and decompensation ultimately occurs. Detrusor contractility, therefore, is diminished on this basis. Current evidence points to both a sensory and motor neuropathy as being involved in the pathogenesis, the motor aspect per se contributing to impaired detrusor contractility. The typical urodynamic findings include impaired bladder sensation, increased cystometric capacity, decreased bladder contractility, impaired uroflow, and later, increased residual urine. The main differential diagnosis is generally bladder outlet obstruction, as both conditions commonly produce a low flow rate. However, the flow pattern in diabetes is more commonly one of abdominal straining, and, of course, pressure and flow studies easily differentiate the two. Involuntary bladder contractions may also be seen. If due to diabetes and not to coincident pathology (bladder outlet obstruction, detrusor instability), the cause must be neuropathic change outside the bladder. Smooth or striated sphincter dyssynergia generally are not seen in diabetic cystopathy, but can easily be misdiagnosed on a poor or incomplete urodynamic study (abdominal straining alone will not open the bladder neck and will produce pseudodyssynergia). Early institution of timed voiding will avoid the portion of the impaired detrusor contractility due to chronic distention/decompensation. Some recent reports suggest that "classic" diabetic cystopathy may not be the predominant form of lower urinary tract dysfunction in this group but rather involuntary bladder contractions. The importance of urodynamic studies in diabetic patients before irreversible therapy is instituted cannot be overemphasized.

IX. COMMON NON-NEUROGENIC VOIDING DYSFUNCTIONS

A. Outlet Obstruction Secondary to BPH

This is probably the most common voiding dysfunction seen by the urologist (see Chapter 15). Classically, the patient complains of hesitancy and straining to void, with the urodynamic correlates of low flow and high intravesical pressure during attempted voiding. This situation represents a pure failure to empty. Approximately 50 percent of the time, the patient with significant prostatic obstruction develops detrusor hyperactivity secondarily, with resultant urgency, frequency, and, if the hyperactivity cannot be inhibited, urgency incontinence. Under such circumstances, the voiding dysfunction becomes a combined emptying and filling and storage problem. Treatment is relief of the obstruction either by reduction of prostatic bulk or tone. Relief of the outlet obstruction will result in the eventual disappearance of detrusor hyperactivity, where present, in approximately 70 percent of cases.

B. Bladder Neck Dysfunction

Also called smooth sphincter dyssynergia and proximal urethral obstruction, bladder neck dysfunction is characterized by an incomplete opening of the bladder neck during voiding. The dysfunction is found almost exclusively in young and middle-aged men, and characteristically they may complain of long-standing obstructive and irritative symptoms. It is not unusual for these patients to have been seen by many urologists. They have often been diagnosed as having psychogenic voiding dysfunction because of a normal prostate on rectal examination, a negligible residual urine volume, and a normal endoscopic bladder appearance. Objective evidence of outlet obstruction in these patients is easily obtainable by urodynamic study. Once obstruction is diagnosed, it can be localized at the level of the bladder neck by video urodynamic study, cystourethrography during a bladder contraction, or micturitional urethral profilometry (see section on urodynamics earlier). The diagnosis can also be made indirectly by the urodynamic findings of outlet obstruction in the typical clinical situation in the absence of a urethral stricture, of prostatic enlargement, or evidence of striated sphincter dyssynergia.

When prostatic enlargement develops in individuals with this problem, a double obstruction results, and Turner-Warwick has applied the term "trapped prostate" to this entity. A patient so affected generally has a life-long history of voiding dysfunction that has gone relatively unnoticed because he has always accepted this as normal, and exacerbation of these symptoms occurs during a relatively short and early period of prostatic enlargement. Although α-adrenergic blocking agents provide considerable relief in some patients with bladder neck dysfunction, greater and definitive relief in the male is almost always achieved by bladder neck incision (see treatment discussion that follows). In patients with bladder neck dysfunction and a trapped prostate, marked relief is generally afforded by a bladder neck incision and "small" prostatic resection. Such patients often note afterward that they have "never" voided as well as after their treatment.

Similar bladder neck obstruction in females is quite rare. This entity has been defined in a small number of women on the basis of videourodynamic criteria. Even then, surgical treatment of this problem should be obviously approached with caution, as incontinence with bladder neck incision is a significant risk in the female.

C. Low Pressure and Low Flow

Low pressure and low flow voiding occurs in younger men and is symptomatically characterized by frequency, hesitancy, and a poor stream. This entity is demonstrated on urodynamic assessment and with no endoscopic abnormalities. The patient generally notes marked hesitancy when attempting to initiate micturition in the presence of others, and some have therefore described this group has having an anxious or bashful bladder. Our experience has been similar to those reports stating that neither empirical pharmacologic treatment nor transurethral surgery has any consistent beneficial effect in this difficult to treat group of patients.

D. Dysfunctional Voiding

This syndrome, also known as non-neurogenic/neurogenic bladder, occult voiding dysfunction, or Hinman's syndrome, presents the unusual circumstance of what appears urodynamically to be involuntary obstruction at the striated sphincter level existing in the absence of demonstrable neurologic disease. It is very difficult to prove urodynamically that an individual has this entity. This requires simultaneous pressure flow electromyographic evidence of bladder emptying occurring simultaneously with involuntary striated sphincter contraction in the absence of any element of abdominal straining component, either in an attempt to augment bladder contraction or as a response to discomfort during urination. The etiology is uncertain and may represent a persistent transitional phase in the development of micturitional control or persistence of a reaction phase to the stimulus of lower urinary tract discomfort during voiding, long after the initial problem that caused this has disappeared. The preferred treatment is biofeedback. Intermittent catheterization may be useful, both as therapy and as an aid to facilitating the ability to voluntarily relax the striated sphincter.

E. Decompensated Bladder

This situation may occur after a longstanding bladder outlet obstruction or as a chronic response to neurologic injury. Attempts to produce emptying pharmacologically with a cholinergic agonist and an α-adrenergic antagonist have been generally unsuccessful, and the best treatment is intermittent catheterization. The temptation to surgically decease bladder outlet resistance in the hopes of "tipping the balance" in favor of emptying should be resisted. This approach is seldom effective unless it produces a form of stress incontinence.

F. Postoperative Retention

Urinary retention can occur postoperatively for a number of reasons. Nociceptive impulses can inhibit the initiation of reflex bladder contraction, perhaps through an opioid-mediated mechanism or sympathetic mediated inhibition. Transient overdistention of the bladder can occur under anesthesia or under the influence of analgesic medication. Purely neurologic injury during abdominal and pelvic surgery can also occur. Generally, in the absence of neurologic injury and with proper decompression, a patient's voiding status will return pretty much to what it was prior to the surgery and anesthesia. Therefore the optimal treatment is intermittent catheterization. Return of bladder function may be facilitated by the use of an α-adrenergic antagonist. Treatment with cholinergic agonists alone has been generally unsuccessful. A patient with prostatism on the borderline of significant voiding dysfunction may have his previously tenuous and abnormal ability to empty compromised. In these cases, prostatectomy may be justified.

X. Urinary Incontinence

Urinary incontinence is defined as the involuntary loss of urine. The term is used in various ways. It may denote a symptom, a sign, or a condition. The symptom is generally thought of as the patient's complaint of involuntary urine loss. The sign is the objective demonstration of urine loss. The condition is the underlying cause (pathophysiology). A simple classification of the various subtypes of urinary incontinence is seen in Table 14-9. The basic pathophysiology of incontinence and various related definitions are discussed in sections III, IV, and V.

There are situations in which urethral incontinence cannot be considered merely as an isolated abnormality of either bladder

Table 14-9 Classification of Incontinence

I. Extraurethral
   A. Fistula (vesicovaginal, ureterovaginal, urethrovaginal)
   B. Ectopic ureter
II. Urethral
   A. Functional
      1. Because of physical disability
      2. Due to lack of awareness or concern
   B. Bladder abnormalities
      1. Overactivity
         a. Involuntary contractions
         b. Decreased compliance
         c. Hypersensitivity with incontinence
   C. Outlet abnormalities
      1. Genuine stress incontinence
      2. Intrinsic sphincter deficiency
      3. Urethral instability
      4. Post-void dribbling
         a. Urethral diverticulum
         b. Vaginal pooling of urine
   D. Overflow incontinence

contractility or sphincter resistance. These situations, listed in Table 14-10, are more complicated to deal with, first, because they are more difficult to diagnose, and second, because one entity may adversely affect or compromise treatment of the other. The most common of these is detrusor hyperactivity with outlet obstruction. This occurs almost exclusively in the male. Outlet obstruction can cause detrusor instability; the incidence of detrusor instability in series of patients with outlet obstruction secondary to prostatism ranges from 50 to 80 percent. Treating only the detrusor hyperactivity in these patients could result in worsening the effects of the outlet obstruction if a significant decrease in detrusor contractility occurred. On the other hand, when the outlet obstruction is relieved in such patients, there is a high reversal rate of the bladder status to stable, although this reversion generally takes between 1 and 6 months and may take as long as 12 months. Resnick and Yalla described the phenomenon of detrusor hyperactivity with impaired contractility (DHIC), especially in frail, elderly, incontinent patients. They found that one third of such patients and one half of those with an overactive detrusor had bladders that were poorly contractile despite extensive trabeculation. Because bladder contractility is impaired, a vigorous pharmacologic approach usually used for involuntary bladder contractions may not be appropriate for this entity.

Table 14-10 Combined Problems Associated with Incontinence

Detrusor overactivity with outlet obstruction
Detrusor overactivity with impaired bladder contractility
Sphincteric incontinence with impaired bladder
Sphincteric incontinence with detrusor overactivity

Sphincter incontinence in an individual with impaired contractility should alert the clinician to the possibility of the requirement of permanent clean intermittent catheterization following surgical repair. Depending on the patient's ability and willingness to carry out intermittent catheterization, this may drastically alter an individual's usual treatment program for sphincter incontinence if the simpler, noninvasive therapeutic measures have failed. Sphincter incontinence can coexist with detrusor hyperactivity in a number of circumstances and with varying effects. Bladder instability or urge incontinence often occurs with stress incontinence. Such bladder hyperactivity has been cited as one of the most common causes of failure of a suspension operation for stress incontinence. Whether these urodynamic findings really do indicate that such an operation is likely to fail is an important question, as an affirmative answer would mandate a very careful urodynamic evaluation in all such patients and would doubtless decrease the enthusiasm for corrective surgery in such patients who have coexistent genuine stress incontinence. Patients with stress incontinence who also have decreased compliance do not seem to fare well after surgery to correct just the stress incontinence. The decreased compliance generally does not change, and if it was refractory to nonsurgical therapy before, it will remain that way, at least in our experience. A variant and more complicated form of such a combination may occur following radical pelvic surgery. Such patients may have a combination of decreased compliance with impaired bladder contractility (from the standpoint of emptying potential) with an open and nonfunctional smooth sphincter area and obstruction by residual striated sphincter tone that is not subject to voluntary induced relaxation. These patients often leak across the distal sphincter area and, in addition, are unable to empty their bladders, because, although they have an increased intravesical pressure, they have nothing that approximates a true bladder contraction. They often present with urinary incontinence, which is characteristically most manifest with increases in intra-abdominal pressure. This is usually most obvious in the female patient, as the prostatic bulk often masks a deficit in male urethral closure function.

One additional fact with respect to definition, however, bears mention. The traditional perspective on urinary incontinence fails to account for instances in which symptoms of urinary frequency and urgency are present without the involuntary loss of urine. "Overactive bladder" is a new term that is applied to the symptoms of frequency, urgency, urge, or reflex incontinence, alone or in any combination, when existing in the absence of local pathologic factors (urinary tract infection, bladder stone, bladder cancer, interstitial cystitis, etc.) explaining these symptoms. The management (evaluation and treatment) of overactive bladder should be the same as that of urgency incontinence or reflex incontinence.

In 1996, the Agency for Health Care Policy and Research reported urinary incontinence as affecting 10 million Americans in community and institutional settings, with an annual cost, estimated in 1994 dollars, of $16.4 billion. Reported prevalence rates of urinary incontinence vary considerably, depending on definition (how frequently, how much, how bothersome), how the information is obtained, and on the population studied. Reasonable estimates of the prevalence of urinary incontinence in the population between 15 and 64 years of age range from 1.5 to 5 percent in men and from 10 to 30 percent in women. For persons living in the community older than 60 years of age, prevalence estimates range from 15 to 35 percent, with women having twice the prevalence of men. Among the more than 1.5 million nursing facility residents, the prevalence of urinary incontinence is estimated at 50 percent or greater. In addition to the financial costs, urinary incontinence imposes a significant psychosocial impact on individuals, their families, and caregivers. Quality of life, as measured by both generic and lower urinary tract specific indices, is adversely affected to a significant degree. The primary spheres affected are (1) self-esteem; (2) ability to maintain an independent lifestyle; (3) social interactions with friends and family; (4) activities of daily life; and (5) sexual activity. A brief description of the more common types of urinary incontinence follows.

A. Outlet-Related Incontinence in the Female

Classically, sphincteric incontinence in the female patient had been categorized into (1) *genuine stress incontinence* (GSUI) and (2) what was originally described by McGuire and Woodside as type III stress incontinence, now referred to as *intrinsic sphincter dysfunction* (ISD). Genuine stress incontinence is associated with hypermobility of the vesicourethral junction due to poor pelvic support and an outlet that is competent at rest but loses its competence only during increases in intra-abdominal pressure. Intrinsic sphincter deficiency describes a non- or very poorly functional bladder neck and proximal urethra at rest. The division between these two situations, however, is not absolute, and virtually all "experts" agree that every case of sphincteric incontinence involves varying proportions of GSUI and ISD. The implication of classical ISD is that a surgical procedure designed to correct only urethral hypermobility will have a relatively high failure rate as opposed to one designed to improve urethral coaptation and compression. Stress urinary incontinence is a symptom that arises from damage to muscles and/or nerves and/or connective tissue within the pelvic floor. Urethral support is important; the urethra normally being supported by the action of the levator ani muscles through their connection to the endopelvic fascia of the anterior vaginal wall. Damage to the connection between this fascia and muscle, damage to the nerve supply, or direct muscle damage can therefore influence continence. Bladder neck function is similarly important, and loss of normal bladder neck closure can result in incontinence despite normal urethral support. In older writings, the urethra was sometimes ignored as a factor contributing to continence in the female, and the site of continence was thought to be exclusively the bladder neck. However, in approximately 50 percent of continent women, urine enters the urethra during increases in abdominal pressure. The continence point in these women is at the mid urethra, where urine is stopped before it can escape from the urethral meatus. With urethral hypermobility, there is weakness of the pelvic floor. During increases in intra-abdominal pressure, there is descent of the bladder neck and proximal urethra. If the outlet opens concomitantly, stress urinary incontinence ensues. In the classic form of urethral hypermobility, there is rotational descent of the bladder neck and urethra. However, the urethra may also descend without rotation (it shortens and widens) or the posterior wall of the urethra may be pulled open while the anterior wall remains fixed. It should be noted, however, that urethral hypermobility is often present in women who are not incontinent, and thus the mere presence of urethral hypermobility is not sufficient to make a diagnosis of a sphincter abnormality unless urinary incontinence is also demonstrated. The hammock hypothesis of DeLancey proposes that for stress incontinence to occur with hypermobility, there must be a lack of stability of the suburethral supportive layer. This theory proposes that the effect of abdominal pressure increases on the normal bladder outlet, if the suburethral supportive layer is firm, is to compress the urethra rapidly and effectively. If the supportive suburethral layer is lax and/or movable, compression is not as effective. ISD denotes an intrinsic malfunction of the urethral sphincter mechanism itself. In its most overt form, it is characterized by a bladder neck that is open at rest, a low Valsalva leak point pressure and urethral closure pressure, and is usually the result of prior surgery, trauma with scarring, or a neurologic lesion. *Urethral instability* refers to the rare phenomenon of episodic decreases in outlet pressure unrelated to increases in bladder or abdominal pressure. The term urethral instability is probably a misnomer, because many feel that the drop in urethral pressure represents the urethral component of a normal voiding reflex in an individual whose bladder does not measurably contract, either because of myogenic or neurogenic reasons.

B. Outlet-Related Incontinence in the Male

In theory at least, categories of outlet-related incontinence in the male are similar to those in the female. In reality, there is little if any information regarding the topic of urethral instability in the male. Sphincteric incontinence in the male is not associated with hypermobility of the bladder neck and proximal urethra, but is rather more similar to what is termed ISD in the female.

C. Bladder-Related Incontinence in the Female

Bladder-related abnormalities causing urinary incontinence consist of either detrusor overactivity or low bladder compliance. Detrusor overactivity is a generic term for involuntary bladder contractions. These can be either due to neurologic conditions (in which case detrusor hyperreflexia is the term applied) or non-neurologic in origin (in which case the term detrusor instability is employed). Neurologically, involuntary bladder contractions can be due to any lesion occurring above the sacral spinal cord. The cause(s) of detrusor instability in the female is (are) obscure. In addition to the etiologies noted previously (see neurogenic voiding dysfunction), one subject that should be mentioned is the simultaneous occurrence of bladder instability in stress urinary incontinence. The fact that minor components of detrusor instability, and sometimes major ones, often disappear after successful surgery for stress incontinence suggest that these two phenomena may be causally related in an as yet unknown fashion.

D. Bladder-Related Incontinence in the Male

The pathophysiology of bladder-related incontinence in the male is similar to that in the female except that there is no known association between detrusor instability and stress incontinence in the male. There is, however, a unique association of detrusor overactivity with bladder outlet obstruction in the male. The incidence of detrusor instability in males with outlet obstruction secondary to prostatism ranges from

50 to 80 percent. When the outlet obstruction is relieved in such patients, there is a high reversion rate of the bladder status to stability (approximately 70 percent), although this reversion generally takes between 1 and 6 months, and may take as long as 12 months.

E. Overflow Incontinence

This is a descriptive term that denotes leakage of urine associated with urinary retention. This is more common in the male than female. The primary pathophysiology is actually a failure of emptying, leading to urinary retention with "overflow" incontinence, resulting from either continuous or episodic elevation of intravesical pressure over urethral pressure. This generally results in outlet obstruction or detrusor inactivity, either neurologic or pharmacologic in origin, or may be secondary to inadvertent overdistention of the bladder.

F. Management of Incontinence

Management of incontinence includes the processes of evaluation and treatment. Various algorithms are available for each, ranging from the simplest to the most complicated. What is appropriate for one patient/health care provider combination may not be appropriate for another. The level of complexity of the evaluation and management depends, as it does for all types of voiding dysfunction, on the following.
1. The clinical problem at hand.
2. The prior treatment experience(s).
3. The patient's desire for treatment.
4. The patient's goals of therapy.
5. The patient's desire to avoid invasive procedures and/or complications.
6. The patient's ability and desire to follow instructions or carry out specific tasks.
7. The expected level of improvement under optimal circumstances.
8. The health care provider's level of expertise.
9. Environmental considerations.
10. Economic considerations.

XI. TREATMENT OF VOIDING DYSFUNCTION
A. General

There are only a discrete number of therapies available, and these are easily categorized on a functional "menu" basis according to whether they are used primarily to facilitate urine storage or emptying and whether their primary effect is on the bladder the outlet (Tables 14-11 and 14-12). Brief comments will be made about selected, more commonly used categories. Specific therapy for BPH is considered in Chapter 15.

Note that inclusion in the "lists" does not necessarily imply majority agreement on efficacy. Treatment should always begin with the simplest most reversible form(s) of therapy, proceeding gradually up the ladder of complexity, with the knowledge that it is only the patient (and/or family) who is (are) empowered to say when "enough is enough." A perfect result need not be achieved. Satisfaction and avoidance of adverse outcomes are the goals. At every step, the patient and/or family must understand the potential benefits, practicalities, and risks of further therapy.

B. **Therapy to Facilitate Bladder Filling and Urine Storage**
  1. Inhibiting bladder contractility/decreasing sensory input/ increasing bladder capacity (Table 14-11)
      a. *Behavioral therapy, behavioral modification, and bladder training.* These terms that are sometimes used interchangeably in describing nonmedical, nonsurgical methods to treat various types of voiding dysfunction. The term behavioral therapy includes: (1) patient education about lower urinary tract function; (2) information about lifestyle changes or dietary modification (e.g., fluid restriction, avoidance of irritants); (3) so-called bladder training or retraining, which includes instituting intervals of timed voiding and gradually increasing these intervals; (4) pelvic floor physiotherapy, with or without biofeedback, both to strengthen the pelvic floor musculature and to aid in the individual's ability to shut off an unwanted bladder contraction; and (5) for physically or mentally challenged individuals, scheduled toileting and/or prompted voiding. In patients with bladder overactivity, the pelvic floor physiotherapy is used primarily as an aid to patients in suppressing unwanted bladder contractions. They are taught to do "quick flicks" of the pelvic floor musculature in an effort to accomplish this. Putting all these things together involves establishing a regimen for the patient and combining all of these modalities, such that the patient voids according to a timed schedule that he or she can initially maintain. A bladder diary is useful in following the patient's progress. Periodically, the patient is asked to increase the intervals between micturition until an acceptable interval is reached without the symptoms of urgency or urge

Table 14-11 Therapy to Facilitate Urinary Storage and Bladder Filling

---

Bladder related (inhibiting bladder contractility, decreasing sensory input, and/or increasing bladder capacity)
  Behavioral therapy, including
    Education
    Bladder training
    Timed bladder emptying or prompted voiding
    Pelvic floor physiotherapy and/or biofeedback
  Pharmacologic therapy
    Anticholinergic agents
    Musculotropic relaxants
    Calcium antagonists
    Potassium channel openers
    Prostaglandin inhibitors
    β-Adrenergic agonists
    α-Adrenergic antagonists
    Tricyclic antidepressants
    Dimethylsulfoxide (DMSO)
    Polysynaptic inhibitors
    Capsaicin, resiniferatoxin, and similar agents
  Bladder overdistention
  Peripheral electrical stimulation (reflex inhibition)
  Acupuncture
  Neuromodulation
  Interruption of innervation
    Central (subarachnoid block)
    Peripheral motor: sacral rhizotomy, selective sacral rhizotomy
    Peripheral sensory: dorsal root ganglionectomy
    Perivesical (peripheral bladder denervation)
  Augmentation cystoplasty (bowel or auto)

---

incontinence interfering. *Biofeedback* is a technique that provides visual and/or auditory signals to an individual with respect to his or her performance of a physiologic process, in this case pelvic floor muscle contraction. Electromyography or vaginal pressure measurements are generally used. In spite of the logic of biofeedback, most comprehensive reviews have failed to demonstrate the superiority of pelvic floor muscle exercise instruction with biofeedback over pelvic floor exercise instruction alone. It is clear, however, that, whether considering stress, urge, or mixed urinary incontinence, and using the number of incontinence episodes or the amount of urine lost as

Table 14-11 (*continued*)

Outlet related (increasing outlet resistance)
  Behavioral therapy, including
    Education
    Fluid restriction
    Bladder training
    Timed bladder emptying or prompted voiding
    Pelvic floor exercises and/or biofeedback
  Peripheral electrical stimulation
  Pharmacologic therapy
    α-Adrenergic agonists
    Tricyclic antidepressants
    β-Adrenergic antagonists, agonists
    Estrogens
  Vaginal and perineal occlusive supportive devices; urethral plugs
  Nonsurgical periurethral compression
    Periurethral polytef, collagen, durasphere
  Vesicourethral suspension and/or prolapse repair (female)
  Sling procedures and/or prolapse repair (female)
  Bladder outlet reconstruction
  Artificial urinary sphincter
  Closure of the bladder outlet
Circumventing the problem
  Antidiuretic hormone-like agents
  Short-acting diuretics
  Intermittent catheterization
  External collecting devices
  Absorbent products
  Continuous catheterization
  Urinary diversion

---

primary outcome indicators, behavioral therapy is capable of causing a significant reduction. Quoted figures range from 40 to 80 percent. We think of behavioral therapy as an overall program that can be used for the treatment of urinary incontinence or bladder overactivity without urinary incontinence. With sphincteric related incontinence, obviously the patient should concentrate more on pelvic floor physiotherapy for the purpose of strengthening the pelvic floor musculature. With the overactive bladder, with or without urge incontinence, the patient should concentrate more on the behavioral modification, using pelvic floor physiotherapy more as a tool to abort

Table 14-12 Therapy to Facilitate Bladder Emptying and Voiding

Bladder related (increasing intravesical pressure or facilitating
  bladder contractility)
 External compression, Valsalva
 Promotion or initiation of reflex contraction
   Trigger zones or maneuvers
   Bladder "training," tidal drainage
 Pharmacologic therapy
   Parasympathomimetic agents
   Prostaglandins
   Blockers of inhibition
     α-Adrenergic antagonists
     Opioid antagonists
 Electrical stimulation
   Directly to the spinal cord
   Directly to the detrusor
   Directly to the nerve roots
   Intravesical (transurethral)
 Reduction cystoplasty
Outlet related (increasing outlet resistance)
 At a site of anatomic obstruction
   Pharmacologic therapy—decrease prostate size or tone
     α-Adrenergic antagonists
     5-α Reductase inhibitors
     LHRH agonists/antagonists
     Antiandrogens
   Prostatectomy, prostatotomy (diathermy, heat)

---

involuntary bladder contractions. Biofeedback is optional in either case.

b. *Pharmacologic therapy.* In general, drug therapy to inhibit bladder contractility is hindered by *uroselectivity.*
Uroselectivity exists on two planes. One is organ specificity and the other is function specificity. Organ specificity means that ideally only the bladder is affected.
Unfortunately, this is not the case, even with intravesical administration. *Anticholinergic agents* all possess,
in varying degrees, the disadvantage of affecting muscarinic receptors elsewhere. The most common troublesome side effects are dry mouth, blurred vision, and
constipation. Somnolence and cognitive dysfunction
can also be a problem, especially in the elderly patient.
It has been estimated that up to 40 to 50 percent of patients discontinue anticholinergic therapy because of
the side effects. *Calcium channel blockers* and *potas-*

Table 14-12 (*continued*)

Bladder neck incision or resection
Urethral stricture repair or dilation
Intraurethral stent
Balloon dilation of stricture and/or contracture
At the level of the smooth sphincter
  Pharmacologic therapy
    α-Adrenergic antagonists
    β-Adrenergic antagonists
  Transurethral resection or incision
  Y-V plasty
At the level of the striated sphincter
  Behavioral therapy and/or biofeedback
  Psychotherapy
  Pharmacologic therapy
    Skeletal muscle relaxants
    α-Adrenergic antagonists
    Botulinum A toxin (injection)
  Urethra overdilation
  Surgical sphincterotomy
  Urethral stent
  Pudendal nerve interruption
Circumventing the Problem
  Intermittent catheterization
  Continuous catheterization
  Urinary diversion (conduit)

---

sium channel openers would be ideal for the treatment of bladder overactivity if a receptor or channel could be found that was bladder specific. At this point, the dosages needed to affect lower urinary tract function are so high that undesirable side effects, primarily cardiovascular, are produced elsewhere. *Antidepressants,* the prototype of which is imipramine, have systemic anticholinergic side effects and a host of other potential side effects related to the mechanism of their antidepressant activity. The choice of a pharmacologic agent to decrease bladder contractility is often individual specific and institution specific. At the First International Consultation on Urinary Incontinence, the committee charged with reporting on drug therapy recommended the following agents as effective in the treatment of bladder hyperactivity (only those available in the United States are listed): propantheline, tolterodine, oxybutynin, imipramine, desmopressin.

i. *Anticholinergic agents.* The physiologic basis for the use of anticholinergic agents to decrease bladder contractility is that the major portion of the neurohumoral stimulus for physiologic and presumably involuntary bladder contraction is acetylcholine-induced stimulation of postganglionic parasympathetic cholinergic receptor sites on bladder smooth muscle. In patients with overactive bladder, the effects have been described as follows: (1) increase in the volume to the first involuntary bladder contraction; (2) decrease in the amplitude of involuntary bladder contractions; and (3) increase total bladder capacity. Symptomatology is decreased proportionally to these effects, although the "warning time" is not affected. In other words, although the threshold volume for an unsuppressible involuntary bladder contraction may be increased, the time between the signal that such a contraction is going to occur and its occurrence, with subsequent incontinence, is not changed. Thus, the rationale exists for combining drug therapy with behavioral therapy for optimum results. The fact that anticholinergic agents are able to increase bladder capacity and increase the volume to the first involuntary bladder contraction argues for some release of acetylcholine during filling and storage, rather than release only at the time of a bladder contraction. With respect to improving the use profile of anticholinergic agents, there is an argument about whether drugs that are specific for the M_3 receptor will ultimately prove to more effective than relatively nonselective anticholinergic agents. M_3 specificity would theoretically be an advantage, except for the fact that it is the M_3 receptor that is primarily responsible for salivary secretion, bowel contraction, and accommodation. Thus, organ specificity would seem to be preferable as a concept. Tolterodine is an agent that, at least in one experimental model, has selectivity for bladder contraction over the stimulation of salivation. This seems to have been translated clinically into an efficacy that is equivalent to oxybutynin, but with fewer side effects, especially dry mouth.

ii. *Agents with combined action.* There are number of agents that are grouped under the somewhat exotic term "musculotropic relaxant" or "antispasmodic" that are promoted as having more than an anticholinergic action. These additional actions include smooth muscle inhibition at a site metabolically distal to the cholinergic receptor mechanism and what are referred to as a local anesthetic properties. The former action may relate to some calcium channel blocking activity. It should be noted that these latter two activities can be demonstrated in vitro, but it is doubtful that when administered orally either of these activities contribute to the clinical efficacy of such agents, which is most likely due simply to the fact that they are good anticholinergic drugs. Oxybutynin falls into this category.

iii. *Tricyclic antidepressants.* The tricyclic antidepressants have been found by some to be useful agents for facilitating urine storage by both decreasing bladder contractility and increasing outlet resistance. There is disagreement about the latter function, but general agreement about their utility in decreasing bladder contractility. All of these agents possess varying degrees of three major pharmacologic actions: (1) they block the active transport system responsible for the reuptake of released amine neurotransmitters serotonin and norepinephrine; (2) they have central and peripheral anticholinergic effects at some, but not all, sites; and (3) they are sedatives, an action that occurs, presumably, on a central basis, but is perhaps related to antihistaminic properties. As histamine receptors, however, they also are antagonistic to some extent. Imipramine has prominent systemic anticholinergic effects, but only a weak antimuscarinic effect on bladder smooth muscle. This action could be mediated centrally, as an increase in serotonin concentration in the spinal cord could cause a decrease in bladder contractility, or it could be related to a direct inhibitory effect on bladder smooth muscle itself. In any case, the effects of imipramine on bladder smooth muscle do not appear to be mediated by an anticholinergic effect. There is a rationale for combining the use of such agents with an antimuscarinic drug before abandoning pharmaceutical treatment in cases where anticholinergic agents alone have not produced the desired effect.

iv. *Intravesical therapy to decrease bladder contractility.* One way of achieving a more bladder-selective response is to administer a drug intravesically. This has been easily done in the laboratory with multiple agents and has been done clinically with oxybutynin. Most series are small but report definite beneficial effects with seemingly fewer side effects. Although the drug is absorbed into the circulation and effective serum levels can be measured, the first-pass metabolism through the liver is less. It is thought that the primary metabolite of oxybutynin might well be responsible in large part for the side effects, and thus these would be less using this mode of administration. This is obviously cumbersome, requires catheterization to carry out, and there is no intravesical preparation. In addition, tablets must be dissolved in a vehicle to accomplish this. It may be, however, that with this mode of administration, those drugs with a theoretical combined action would be able to exert some direct effect on smooth muscle because of the high local concentration, whereas with oral administration they would not.

v. *Desmopressin.* This is a synthetic vasopressin analog that lacks significant vasopressor action. It does exert a pronounced antidiuretic effect. It is widely used as a treatment for primary nocturnal enuresis, and can be useful in adults with nocturia, particularly those who lack a normal nocturnal increase in plasma vasopressin (antidiuretic hormone).

vi. *Drugs affecting sensory neurotransmission.* One attractive modality of therapy for overactive bladder and bladder hypersensitivity, especially in an individual who retains the ability to voluntarily initiate a detrusor contraction, is to depress sensory neurotransmission. Theoretically, this would be effective only in neurogenically induced bladder overactivity and not that which is myogenic. *Capsaicin* is the active ingredient of red peppers and, in sufficiently high concentrations, causes desensitization of C-fiber sensory afferents by initially releasing and emptying the stores of neuropeptides, which serve as sensory neurotransmitters. C-fiber afferents act as the primary sensory pathway in patients with voiding dysfunction secondary to spinal cord injury and some other neurologic diseases (at least some cases of multiple sclerosis). C-fiber afferents may also be functional in patients with hypersensitivity disorders. Due to the initial release of neuropeptides after direct administration of the drug, capsaicin causes intense local symptomatology and often requires anesthesia for administration. In addition, although beneficial effects have been reported, these effects are not universal, although positive effects, when they result, have been reported to last for 2 to 7 months. *Resiniferatoxin* is a compound with effects similar to those of capsaicin, and is approximately 1000 times more potent than capsaicin in producing desensitization, but only 100 to 300 times more potent in producing inflammation. Resiniferatoxin is an interesting alternative to capsaicin, but the use of both can be considered works in progress. Further investigations are needed to explore and, perhaps confirm, the clinical utility of this type of agent.

c. *Peripheral electrical stimulation.* Electrical stimulation is mentioned in three areas under the category of treatment, reflecting its potential use to facilitate storage by both the inhibition of bladder contractility and an increase in sphincter resistance, and to facilitate emptying by stimulating a detrusor contraction. To inhibit bladder contractility, stimulation is generally applied to removable anal and vaginal devices, as well as peripherally through patch electrodes. The theory is that this induces an inhibitory pelvic to pudendal nerve reflex. Reported clinical results have been mixed, at best.

d. *Neuromodulation.* This word implies modification of sensory and/or motor function through electrical stimulation. For inhibition of bladder activity, electrical stimulation is applied to the S3 root, resulting in excitation of pudendal (and possibly other) afferents and possibly efferent nerves as well. The mode of action of neuromodulation is unclear. A precise definition of this concept is likewise unclear. "Modulation of reflex pathways to restore normal balance" is a general but deliberately vague summary statement that can be inferred from several reports. Bladder, sphincter, and pelvic floor function(s) can be favorably altered by electrical stimulation of S3. A temporary electrode is placed through the S3 foramen and attached to a stimulator that the patient wears for a short period of time. Those reporting improvement are suitable for permanent implantation of an electrode and a pulse generator operated by an external programming mechanism. Very promising results have been achieved to date in this difficult group of patients, all of whom have failed more conservative therapy, and for many of whom the next step would have been augmentation cystoplasty. Less invasive methods of gaining access to the S3 root are in development. One of these uses stimulation of the posterior tibial nerve, either through a very fine gauge needle or a small permanent subcutaneous implant. Initial reports have been provocative. Further testing is in progress.

e. *Interruption of innervation. Subarachnoid block* is no longer used for urologic indications. Historically, this was used to convert a state of severe somatic spasticity to flaccidity and to abolish autonomic hyperreflexia.

As a by-product, bladder hyperreflexia was acutely converted to areflexia. The obvious disadvantage of this type of procedure was a lack of neurologic selectivity. Additionally, the conceptually simple result of an areflexic bladder with normal compliance very often was not maintained, with decreased compliance occurring.

i. *Sacral rhizotomy, selective sacral rhizotomy.* Selective sacral rhizotomy was originally introduced as a treatment to increase bladder capacity by trying to abolish only the motor supply responsible for involuntary bladder contractions. Nonselective sacral rhizotomy often affected sphincter, and sexual, and lower extremity function. There was still a problem in obtaining a truly selective result, and this procedure has fallen out of favor. Deafferentation using a *dorsal* or *posterior rhizotomy* is generally used as a part of an overall plan to simultaneously rehabilitate storage and emptying problems in patients with significant spinal cord injury or disease. Electrical stimulation is used to produce bladder emptying as well. Dorsal root ganglionectomy has also been mentioned in this regard. Surgical treatment of bladder hyperactivity by peripheral bladder denervation was popularized in the early 1980s. There were a variety of techniques proposed to partially or totally denervate (or more correctly neurologically decentralize) the bladder. These have been largely abandoned because although some of these techniques had a high initial success rate in controlling bladder overactivity and related incontinence, the relapse rate was quite high. In addition, the long-term response to the neurologic procedure was sometimes associated with a type of neural plasticity, resulting in decreased bladder compliance.

f. *Augmentation cystoplasty.* Creation of a low pressure high capacity bladder reservoir by incorporation of a detubularized bowel segment is an important modality of treatment in lower urinary tract reconstruction and in the treatment of refractory filling and storage problems. Adequate reservoir function can generally be achieved by *augmentation enterocystoplasty.* Complications can arise including inadequate emptying or urinary retention, mucous accumulation and stones, electrolyte imbalance, recurrent infection, and the possibility of rare malignant change. Contraindications to augmentation enterocystoplasty include (1) urethral disease precluding intermittent catheterization; (2) unwillingness or inability to perform inter-mittent catheterization; (3) renal failure; (4) significant bowel disease; and (5) poor medical status precluding surgery. *Autoaugmentation* or *detrusor myomectomy* refers to a procedure whose purpose is to increase bladder capacity by, in essence, creating a large bladder diverticulum by removal of a section of the outer layer of the bladder wall down to the mucosa. This has the obvious advantage of not requiring bowel resection and anastomosis, but opinion is divided as to the efficacy of this procedure in increasing reservoir function in adults.

2. Increasing outlet resistance
   a. *Behavioral therapy.* Although behavioral therapy without pelvic floor physiotherapy has been shown to significantly reduce the incidence and amount of stress incontinence in females, the portion of a behavioral therapy program that has received most attention for sphincteric incontinence is the use of pelvic floor exercises. The literature is remarkably consistent in describing a significant improvement rate in 50 to 65 percent of patients treated with this modality of therapy, sometimes known as Kegel's exercises (after Arnold Kegel, a gynecologist). For hypermobility-related stress incontinence in the female and for stress incontinence in the male, it is certainly worthwhile to try pelvic floor exercise along with the rest of the behavioral therapy program as an initial or adjunctive form of treatment. For female patients with a significant element of intrinsic sphincter dysfunction, and for males with gross urinary leakage, it is conceptually doubtful whether significant improvement would occur in even a minority of such patients. However, it is also certain that such therapy would not hurt either, and such exercises may in fact allow the individual to be able to exert greater control over the detrusor reflex as well. As mentioned previously, it has never been objectively shown whether biofeedback, using either electromyographic or pressure displays, adds to careful and periodic personal instruction and supervision.
   b. *Electrical stimulation. Intravaginal* and *anal electrical stimulation* have been used to treat storage failure by increasing outlet resistance as well as decreasing bladder contractility. In this case, the mechanism is said to involve stimulation of the striated pelvic floor musculature through branches of the pudendal nerve. Most reviews have come to the conclusion that there is not consistent objective evidence supporting the value

of pelvic floor physiotherapy plus electrical stimulation over pelvic floor physiotherapy alone in the general population of patients with sphincteric incontinence. It may be that there are some subgroups that might benefit (i.e., those who cannot carry out pelvic floor exercises). *Sacral root stimulation,* by means of an implanted stimulator, has been described for the treatment of sphincteric weakness in patients with neurogenic difficulty. Long-term contemporary results are still forthcoming.

c. *Pharmacologic therapy.* The theoretical basis for pharmacologic therapy of sphincteric incontinence is the preponderance of α-adrenergic receptor sites in the smooth muscle of the bladder neck and proximal urethra. When stimulated, these should produce smooth muscle contraction. Such stimulation can alter the urethral pressure profile by increasing maximum urethral profile and maximum urethral closure pressure. Current *α-adrenergic agonists* in use (ephedrine and phenylpropanolamine) lack selectivity for urethra alpha receptors and may increase blood pressure and cause sleep disturbances, headache, tremor, and palpitations. Although there are reports in the literature of efficacy with these agents, the Committee on Pharmacology of the First International Consultation on Incontinence did not recommend any of these agents for the treatment of stress incontinence. The role of *estrogen* in the treatment of stress incontinence in the postmenopausal female has been controversial. Some studies have reported promising results, but this may be because they were observational, and not randomized, blinded, or controlled. There are several theoretic reasons why estrogen might be useful in the treatment of women with stress incontinence (and overactive bladder), but, although there are other valid reasons for hormonal supplementation in the post-menopausal female, there is no consistent body of objective evidence to prove its efficacy per se in the treatment of stress incontinence. Similarly, there is a theoretic basis for the use of imipramine in the treatment of stress incontinence (inhibition of the reuptake of norepinephrine with an α-adrenergic effect consequently produced in the smooth sphincter area), but objective, double blind, controlled, randomized studies are lacking.

d. *Vaginal and perineal occlusive and supportive devices; urethral plugs.* Support of the bladder neck in the female resulting in improved continence is possible with intravaginal devices that have not been reported to cause significant lower urinary tract obstruction or morbidity. Tampons, traditional pessaries and contraceptive diaphragms, and intravaginal devices specifically designed for bladder neck support have been used. Ideally, *support devices* would reduce any degree of vaginal prolapse and, by supporting the anterior vaginal wall and therefore the urethrovesical junction and bladder neck, control incontinence. Although most individuals would agree that information about vaginal support devices should be included in the treatment options when counseling women with stress urinary incontinence, most would also agree that studies performed on these devices in the acute laboratory setting demonstrate better performance than diary-based studies with respect to the amount and number of episodes of leakage. It is also generally agreed that such devices work best in individuals with minimal to moderate leakage. True pessary usage seems most effective and most common in the elderly woman with a major degree of anterior vaginal wall prolapse and hypermobility-related stress incontinence who is a poor surgical candidate.

Occlusive devices can be broadly divided into external and internal devices, referring to whether the device itself occludes the urethra or bladder neck from the outside or has to be inserted per urethra. There have been many patterns of external occlusive devices available for use in the *male,* but all seem to take the form of a clamp that is applied across the penile urethra. The Baumrucker and Cunningham clamps are basically double-sided foam cushions that squeeze the penile urethra between the two arms. The Baumrucker clamp uses a Velcro type system. Another type of compression device that is size adjustable encircles the penis and stops the flow of urine when it is inflated with air. Soft tissue damage by excess compression can occur with these clamps, and thus their use is extremely risky in patients with sensory impairment. Their prime use is in patients with sphincteric incontinence, although if applied tightly enough, the patient can occlude the urethra under any circumstances—although with a distinct danger of retrograde pressure damage.

Occlusive devices for *female sphincteric incontinence* have been mentioned (and mostly discarded) since the late 1700s. Multiple *intravaginal occlusive devices* have been described, all of which historically consisted of rather bizarre looking configurations of silicone and plastic with a dual purpose: to stay in the vagina and compress the urethra. None of these seem to have stood the test of time. Another interesting concept that proved to be poorly functional was an inflatable pad held firmly against the perineum by straps attached to a waistband, fitted to the individual patient. Inflation of the pad with a cuff resulted in an elevation and compression of the perineum. The simplest of the most recently introduced devices is a *continence control pad* or *external urethral occlusion device.* This Hydrogel-coated foam pad is placed by the patient over the external urethral meatus. Another type of device is a *meatal suction* or *occlusion device.* The concept is to create, by suction, a measured amount of negative pressure, causing coaptation of the urethral wall. *Intraurethral devices* are inserted into the urethra to block urinary leakage. Similarities among these devices include (1) a means to prevent intravesical migration (a meatal plate or tab at the meatus); (2) a mechanism to maintain the device in its proper place in the urethra (spheres, inflatable balloons, or flanges on the proximal end); and (3) a device or mechanism to permit removal for voiding (a string or pump). Most patients utilizing external meatal occlusive devices or intraurethral devices have reported dryness or improvement in the laboratory and on diaries. Long-term results, however, are limited, and the exact place of this therapy in the algorithm of conservative management of female sphincteric incontinence has not yet been determined. Certainly, the use of these devices is grossly out of proportion (lower) to the positive and optimistic reports in the literature.

The characteristics of an ideal occlusive or supportive device would include: (1) efficacy; (2) comfort; (3) ease of application/insertion/removal; (4) lack of interference with adequate voiding; (5) lack of tissue damage; (6) lack of infection; (7) no compromise of subsequent therapy; (8) cosmetic acceptance (unobtrusive); and (9) lack of interference with sexual activity. Ideally, such a device could be used continuously during waking hours (for the majority who do not have sphincteric incontinence after bedtime), but many people would obviously be happy with a device that functioned well for "spot usage"—that is, usage only during those activities most provocative of incontinence. The perfect patient for an occlusive device would be one who has pure sphincteric incontinence that is mild to moderate, who has neither severe involuntary bladder contractions nor decreased compliance, who desires active involvement in her treatment program, who desires immediate results, and who has the body habitus, manual dexterity, and cognitive ability to apply or insert the device and remove it. Many of the devices recently introduced are already off the market, a fact that is certainly at odds with the conclusions from the reports in the literature. Reasons for failure, in our opinion, include: (1) patients reluctance to "put anything inside me or on me"; (2) inconvenience (frequent removal/self-insertion with a requirement for periodic replacement by health care provider); (3) discomfort, real or perceived; (4) fear of infection and/or bleeding; (5) association of such devices by the patient with "last resort" remedies and the implications which that association raises; (6) nonwillingness to pay out of pocket for these (poor coverage for these devices); (7) perceived lack of long-term success; and (8) nonincentive for the health care provider to promote the devices, except in a capitated environment.

e. *Nonsurgical periurethral compression.* Periurethral bulking by the percutaneous or transvesical injection of polytetrafluoroethylene particles, purified bovine cross-linked dermal collagen, or carbon coated zirconium oxide beads to increase urethral resistance has been utilized in both women and men with sphincteric incontinence. In women, the results have ranged from quite good to not so good, with the best "success" and improvement rates ranging from 70 to 90 percent. Multiple therapy sessions may be necessary to achieve the desired result. The results obtained in men have not been as good, especially in patients with post radical prostatectomy incontinence. Originally, this therapy was recommended only for patients with intrinsic sphincter dysfunction and with a Valsalva leak point pressure of less than 60 cm of water. The technique has been used with success, however, in other categories of incontinent patients, including those patients, especially elderly ones, with what seems to be a combination of hypermobility-related incontinence (see previous discussion) and intrinsic sphincter deficiency. The procedure can be carried out under local anesthesia or sedation, making it simple and relatively noninvasive. It does not seem to compromise further therapy.

f. *Vesicourethral urethral suspension with or without prolapse repair (female).* Fixation of the vesicourethral junction in a physiologic position to prevent urethral hypermobility (posterior and inferior rotational descent with abdominal straining) has been observed to correct genuine stress incontinence in the female in 85 to 90 percent of those patients undergoing a first operation for this problem. There are over 150 varieties of this operation and the names attached to many of these read like an honor roll of urologic and gynecologic superstars (Marshall, Marchetti, Krantz, Lapides, Tanagho, Raz, etc.). Each practitioner has his or her favorite suspension procedure, generally based on the site of residency or fellowship training, or on some recent development or product that promises to achieve the same end with less time and morbidity. The use of bone anchors for suture fixation, stapling devices, and laparoscopic techniques have added to the seemingly endless variations available for vesicourethral suspension. If significant vaginal prolapse is present, this should be repaired at the same time, remembering that the pelvic floor in the female acts as a unit and that a surgical procedure should endeavor to correct all associated abnormalities. Suspension is rarely, if ever, used, in patients with other than stress incontinence, and these procedures should be utilized only after more conservative therapy types have at least been attempted or suggested.

g. *Sling procedures.* McGuire deserves, we believe, credit for popularizing the sling procedure, and, more importantly, concepts that relate to its utilization. McGuire was among the first to conceptualize, in logical fashion, the fact that there was a category of patients who leaked with stress who were not well repaired by standard suspension procedures. These were patients who had poor sphincter function, irrespective of mobility, and whose urethral function at that time could be semi-quantitated only with the urethral pressure profile. He later developed the concept of Valsalva leak point pressure to better quantitate sphincteric resistance in patients with stress incontinence. The noncircumferential compression afforded by the sling is optimal treatment for patients with poor urethral closure function and poor urethral smooth muscle function. Although originally described through a retropubic approach, these are done most commonly through a vaginal approach today. Success rates as high as 90 percent with the pubovaginal sling procedure for sphincteric incontinence have been reported. Initially, the use of the sling procedure was restricted to patients who satisfied the definition of intrinsic sphincter dysfunction and who did not have stress incontinence associated with urethral hypermobility.

However, as individuals have come to believe that genuine stress incontinence (hypermobility related) and intrinsic sphincter dysfunction were but two ends of the spectrum, and that the great majority of individuals had some combination of the two, the sling procedure became a logical choice for the correction of stress incontinence of all types. The sling provides an adequate suburethral supporting layer (see prior description of the hammock hypothesis) and thus corrects hypermobility-related incontinence as well as intrinsic sphincter deficiency. The use of the sling for the surgical correction of all types of female sphincteric incontinence has been popularized mostly by Blaivas, with increasing support from others. The sling itself can be autologous fascia (rectus or fascia lata) and, recently, a variety of other materials (cadaveric fascia, dura, synthetic materials) have been used, some with success and some with problems. The various new devices utilized for suspension procedures (bone anchors, stapling devices, laparoscopic approaches) are all applicable to the sling procedure. As with suspension procedures, significant prolapse should be repaired simultaneously in the female.

h. A relatively new procedure, *tension free vaginal tape* (TVT) is receiving notoriety as being successful for the treatment of stress incontinence in previously surgery naive patients. This is not quite a suspension or a sling procedure, but involves placing a polypropylene tape under the urethra and tunneling the ends through the retropubic space, but not tying these. The location of the tape is at approximately the mid urethra, thought to be the true site of continence in most females. Although high initial success rates have been reported in some centers, the results are small in number at this time, and further testing is ongoing, with longer term results awaited.

i. *Bladder outlet reconstruction.* This is primarily a historical treatment in adults. Reconstruction of the bladder outlet is one possible method of restoring sphincteric incontinence in patients with intrinsic sphincter deficiency. This technique was introduced by Young in 1907, was subsequently modified by Dees, Leadbetter, and Tanagho. Procedures utilizing the Young–Dees principle involve construction of a neourethra from the posterior surface of the bladder wall and trigone. In the male, the prostatic urethra affords additional substance for closure and increase in outlet resistance. The Leadbetter modification involves proximal reimplantation of the ureters to allow more extensive tubularization of the trigone. Tanagho described a procedure based on a similar concept, but using the anterior bladder neck to create a functioning neourethral sphincter. "Success rates" of between 60 and 70 percent were reported, but it is difficult to know what success means and what the real long-term success rates are.

j. *Artificial urinary sphincter.* Control of sphincteric urinary incontinence with implantable prosthetics has evolved rapidly over the last 30 years. Clearly, the most significant contribution was the introduction, by Scott and coworkers, of a totally implantable artificial sphincter mechanism that could be used in adults and children of both genders. This was originally introduced in the early 1970s. The current end result of the biomechanical evolution of this device currently is most frequently utilized for post prostatectomy incontinence, but use of the device has been championed by various clinicians for refractory sphincteric incontinence of virtually every etiology, assuming bladder storage is, or can be converted to, normal. The sphincter consists of an inflatable cuff that fits around the urethra (generally) or the bladder neck, a reservoir that generally is placed under the rectus muscle, and an inflate/deflate pump or bulb that transfers fluid from the cuff to the reservoir, allowing refilling of the cuff from the reservoir over a 3- to 4-min period. The pump is placed in the scrotum or the labia. High success rates have been achieved by experienced surgeons. The incidence of mechanical malfunction and infection, though initially high, is quite low in contemporary series.

k. *Closure of the bladder outlet.* This is generally an end-stage procedure suitable for an individual whose outlet is totally incompetent and uncorrectable by medical or conventional surgical means. It is also sometimes used in individuals who can be put into retention but who cannot catheterize themselves per urethra. In this latter condition and in the circumstance of an incompetent urethra in an individual with adequate hand control who desires to be dry, a continent catheterizable abdominal stoma can be created. Augmentation cystoplasty can be carried out at the same time. For individuals lacking adequate hand control or the cognitive facilities necessary for intermittent catheterization or who simply do not want to carry out catheterization, a "chimney" type conduit of bowel is created emanating from the bladder with an abdominal stoma that drains into an appliance.

3. Circumventing the problem

   Antidiuretic hormone-like agents have been mentioned under the category of pharmacologic therapy. Another "trick" utilized in an individual with significant nocturia is to try to adjust diuretic dosage, utilizing a *short-acting diuretic* some time in the afternoon, the object being to reduce the amount of fluid mobilized after the individual goes to bed.

   Popularization of *intermittent catheterization* as a treatment modality has made possible many of the other therapeutic options for the treatment of voiding dysfunction that are now commonplace. Originally introduced in the treatment of spinal cord injury patients as a method of reducing urinary tract infection by Guttman, credit needs to go to Lapides for advocating and popularizing the use of CIC (clean intermittent catheterization) for all types of voiding dysfunction where such circumvention of storage or emptying failure is necessary. The details (types of catheters, intervals, cleansing/sterilization regimens, prophylaxis/or not) are practitioner and institutional specific.

   Indwelling urethral catheters are generally used for short-term bladder drainage. The use of a small bore catheter for a short time, does not, with proper care, seem to adversely affect the ultimate outcome. Occasionally, more often in female patients, an indwelling catheter is a last resort type of therapy for long-term bladder drainage. A contracted fibrotic bladder may be the ultimate result; bladder calculi may form on the catheter; urethral complications in the female may include urethral dilation because of the temptation to replace each catheter with a larger bore one to prevent leakage around the catheter consequent to bladder spasm. A suprapubic catheter does not obviate urethral leakage and does not provide better drainage in patients with sphincteric incontinence. There is still some controversy as to whether long-term indwelling catheterization, especially in the female, in the neurologically challenged population, is associated with a poorer outcome with respect to either significant upper and lower tract complications or quality of life. It must be kept in mind that development of carcinoma of the bladder in patients with long-term indwelling catheter drainage is possible.

   External collecting devices are useful only in the male. A suitable external collecting device has not yet been devised for the female. Care must be taken in individuals with sensory impairment to avoid necrosis of the penis because of an inappropriately tightly fitting device. It is difficult to know whether to label *pads* and *absorbent products* as a treatment for refractory incontinence or as a convenient "bail-out." They are used for both. Approximately $2 billion is currently spent in the United States yearly for pads and absorbent products.

Urinary diversion is a last resort for these patients and is in a category known as "desperate measures." The diversion can utilize the patient's own bladder if the outlet is competent or closure can be accomplished, or a continent catheterizable reservoir can be constructed totally of bowel. Sometimes, the tried and true intestinal conduit (Bricker or bilateral ureteroileostomy) will represent, all things considered, the best choice for an individual patient. The usually listed standard indications for supravesical urinary diversion include: (1) progressive hydronephrosis or intractable upper tract dilatation (which may be due to obstruction at the ureterovesical junction or to vesicoureteral reflux that does not respond to conservative measures); (2) recurrent episodes of sepsis; and (3) intractable filling and storage or emptying failure when CIC is impossible.

C. Therapy to Facilitate Bladder Emptying and Voiding

1. Bladder related (increasing intravesical pressure or facilitating bladder contractility)

   a. *External compression, Valsalva.* Such voiding is unphysiologic and is resisted by the same forces that normally resist stress incontinence. Adaptive changes (funneling) of the bladder outlet generally do not occur with external compression maneuvers of any kind. Increases in outlet resistance may actually occur. The greatest likelihood of success with this mode of therapy (although some would say it should never be used) is in the patient with an areflexic and hypotonic or atonic bladder, and some outlet denervation (smooth or striated sphincter or both). Such a patient not uncommonly has stress incontinence as well. The continued use of external compression or Valsalva maneuver implies that the intravesical pressure between attempted voidings is consistently below that associated with upper tract deterioration. This may be an erroneous assumption, and close follow-up and periodic evaluation are necessary to avoid this complication.

   b. *Promotion or initiation of reflex contractions.* In most types of spinal cord injury characterized by detrusor hyperreflexia, manual stimulation of certain areas within sacral and lumbar dermatomes may provoke a reflex bladder contraction. The most effective classic method of doing so is rhythmic suprapubic manual pressure. If the pressure characteristics of such induced voiding are favorable, and induced emptying can be carried out frequently enough so as to keep bladder volume and pressure below the level dangerous for upper tract deterioration, the incontinence can be "controlled" and, conceptually, this amounts to a form of timed voiding in these neurologically impaired patients. Some clinicians still feel that the establishment of a rhythmic pattern of bladder filling and emptying by maintaining a copious fluid intake and by periodically clamping and unclamping an indwelling catheter or by intermittent catheterization can "condition" or "train" the micturition reflex. This concept, in our opinion, has yet to be proven, and it may be that the prime value of such programs is to focus attention on the urinary tract and ensure an adequate fluid intake.

c. *Pharmacologic therapy*

   i. *Parasympathomimetic agents.* Many acetylcholine-like drugs exist. However, only bethanechol chloride (Duvoid, Urecholine, Mytonachol) exhibits a relatively selective action on the urinary bladder and gut with little or no action at therapeutic dosages on ganglia or the cardiovascular system. It is cholinesterase resistant and causes a contraction in vitro of smooth muscle from all areas of the bladder. Although anecdotal success in rare patients with voiding dysfunction seems to occur, attempts to facilitate bladder emptying in series of patients where bethanechol chloride was the only variable have been disappointing. In adequate doses, bethanechol chloride is capable of eliciting an increase in tension in bladder smooth muscle, as would be expected from in vitro studies, but its ability to stimulate or facilitate a physiologic bladder contraction in patients with voiding dysfunction has been unimpressive. It is difficult to find reproducible urodynamic data that support a general recommendation for the use of bethanechol chloride in any specific category of patients.

   ii. *Other pharmacologic treatments.* One could construct a "wish list" of other potential pharmacologic avenues for facilitating bladder contractility or the micturition reflex. In the cat at least (see previous discussion) there is a sympathetic reflex elicited during filling that promotes urine storage partially by exerting an alpha adrenergic inhibitory effect on pelvic parasympathetic ganglionic transmission.

Alpha-adrenergic blockade, theoretically, then could facilitate transmission through these ganglia and thereby enhance bladder contractility. Alpha-adrenergic blockers are sometimes given for the "treatment" of urinary retention, using this rationale, but whether relief of retention occurs because of the use of these agents or simply simultaneously is unknown. Because endogenous opioids have been hypothesized to exert a tonic inhibitory effect on the micturition reflex at various levels, *narcotic antagonists* offer possibilities for stimulating reflex bladder activity. This concept has never been translated into successful clinical use. *Prostaglandins* contribute to the maintenance of bladder tone and bladder contractile activity. Some cause an in vitro and in vivo bladder contractile response and some cause a decrease in urethral smooth muscle tone. Intravesical prostaglandin use has been reported to facilitate voiding in postsurgical patients. A number of conflicting positive and negative reports exist, and double blind placebo studies are obviously necessary to settle this controversy.

d. *Electrical stimulation. Stimulation directly to the bladder or spinal cord* originated in the 1940s, but met with failure. Fibrosis related to the electrodes, bladder erosion, electrode malfunction, or other equipment malfunction was common. The spread of current to other pelvic structures with stimulus thresholds lower than that of the bladder resulted in undesirable stimulation of a number of bodily processes.

Stimulation to the nerve roots has been pursued for the last 30 years by Brindley, Tanagho and Schmidt for the treatment of voiding dysfunction. Anterior sacral root stimulation, in combination with dorsal rhizotomy or dorsal root ganglionectomy, has become a practicality and a reality, especially in patients with spinal cord injury. Prerequisites for such usage are (1) intact neural pathways between the sacral cord nuclei of the pelvic nerve and the bladder; and (2) a bladder that is capable of contracting. The champions of these techniques deserve much credit for pursuing and developing their ideas over the years, in the face of much negative opinion as to the possibility of their ultimate success. Although these techniques are still in a phase of evolution, they are currently practical and hold much promise for the future.

Intravesical electrostimulation is an old technique that has been resurrected with some very interesting and promising results. The mechanism of action is totally unknown, and it is similar to neuromodulation in two respects: the vague way in which it is defined, and the definition of its mechanism of action. Patients with incomplete central or peripheral nerve lesions and with at least some neural pathways between the bladder or cerebral centers are candidates for this technique. One conceptualization of the mechanism of efficacy invokes the involvement of an artificial activation of the micturition reflex, with repeated activation producing an "upgrade" of the micturition reflex.

e. *Reduction cystoplasty.* The problem of myogenic decompensation has suggested surgical reduction to some investigators, as the chronic overstretching affects mainly the upper free part of the bladder, and as the nerve and vessel supply enter primarily from below. Thus, resection of the dome (or doubling this over) does not influence the function of the spared bladder base and lower bladder body. This technique would seem to be most effective when the detrusor was underactive rather than acontractile, and measures to decrease outlet resistance might be required in addition to achieve adequate emptying. Anecdotal success stories aside, the risk–benefit of this procedure has not been established.

2. Outlet related (decreasing outlet resistance)
   a. At a site of anatomic obstruction
      These measures are all discussed in the chapters on benign prostatic hyperplasia and urethral stricture disease.
   b. At the level of the smooth sphincter
      i. *Pharmacologic therapy.* Krane and Olsson promoted the concept of a physiologic internal sphincter partially controlled by tonic sympathetic stimulation of contractile alpha adrenergic receptors in the smooth musculature of the bladder neck and proximal urethra. Further, they hypothesized that some obstructions at this level are a result of inadequate opening of the bladder neck and/or inadequate decrease in resistance in the area of the proximal urethra. They also theorized and presented evidence that α-adrenergic blockade could be useful in promoting bladder emptying in such a patient with an adequate detrusor contraction but without anatomic obstruction or detrusor-striated sphincter dyssynergia. Although most would agree that α-adrenergic blocking agents exert at least some of their favorable effects on voiding dysfunction by affecting the smooth muscle of the bladder neck and proximal urethra, other information in the literature suggests that they may affect

striated sphincter tone as well. These agents are also used to treat obstruction due to BPH by lowering prostatic "tone," and may have some secondary effects on bladder contractility in these patients as well, mediated through as of yet poorly characterized neurohumoral or neurological pathways.

ii. *Transurethral resection or incision of the bladder neck/smooth sphincter.* The prime indication for transurethral resection or incision of the bladder neck is the demonstration of true obstruction at the bladder neck or proximal urethra by combining urodynamic studies, with either fluoroscopic demonstration of failure of opening of the smooth sphincter area or a micturitional profile showing that the pressure falls off sharply at some point between the bladder neck and the area of the striated sphincter. Bladder neck or smooth sphincter dyssynergia has been previously discussed, and it is this entity (occurring almost exclusively in males) that is the most common indication for the current performance of transurethral incision or resection of the bladder neck. The preferred technique at this time is incision of the bladder neck at the 5 o'clock and/or 7 o'clock position, with a single full-thickness incision extending from the bladder base down to the level of the verumontanum. Most clinicians would place the incidence of retrograde or diminished ejaculation somewhere between the reported incidences of 10 and 50 percent.

iii. *Y-V plasty of the bladder neck.* This is recommended or suggested only when a bladder neck resection or incision is desired and an open surgical procedure is simultaneously required to correct a concomitant disorder. This is rarely carried out.

c. At the level of the striated sphincter

i. *Behavioral therapy with or without biofeedback.* Behavioral therapy in this case is used to facilitate emptying in an individual with occult voiding dysfunction (characteristics of striated sphincter dyssynergia, but neurologically normal). A urodynamic display of striated sphincter activity can facilitate clinical improvement in a strongly motivated patient capable of understanding the instructions of biofeedback assisted therapy.

ii. *Pharmacologic therapy.* There is no class of pharmacologic agents that selectively relaxes the striated musculature of the pelvic floor. Three different types of drugs have been used to treat voiding dysfunction secondary to outlet obstruction at the level of the striated sphincter: (1) the *benzodiazepines* [diazepam (Valium) is the most common]; (2) *baclofen* (Lioresal); and (3) *dantrolene* (Dantrium), all of which have been characterized under the general heading of antispasticity drugs. Baclofen and the benzodiazepines exert their actions predominantly within the CNS, whereas dantrolene acts directly on skeletal muscle. Unfortunately, there is no completely satisfactory form of therapy for alleviation of skeletal muscle spasticity. Although these drugs are capable of providing variable relief of spasticity in some circumstances, their efficacy is far from complete, and this, along with troublesome muscle weakness, adverse effects on gait, and a variety of other side effects, minimizes their overall usefulness. *Alpha-adrenergic blocking agents* have also been hypothesized to exert an inhibitory effect on the striated sphincter, and this may be especially pronounced in those cases where neuroplasticity with altered innervation of this area has occurred. Finally, *botulinum toxin* has been injected directly into the striated sphincter to reduce its tone. This is certainly an interesting and innovative therapy, but one that will require further observation and study.

iii. *Urethral overdilation.* Overdilation to 40 to 50 French in female patients can achieve the same objective as external sphincterotomy, but is rarely used because of the lack of a suitable external collecting device. It is sometimes used in young boys, when sphincterotomy is contemplated, and a similar stretching of the posterior urethra can be accomplished through a perineal urethrostomy. Observations indicate that in myelomeningocele patients treated by this method, compliance can be improved by decreasing the outlet resistance.

iv. *Surgical sphincterotomy.* The primary indication for this procedure is detrusor-striated sphincter dyssynergia in a male patient when other types of management have been unsuccessful or are not possible. A substantial improvement in bladder emptying occurs in 70 to 90 percent of cases. Upper tract deterioration is rare following successful sphincterotomy; vesicoureteral reflux, if present preoperatively, often disappears because of decreased bladder pressures and a reduced incidence of infection in a catheter-free patient with a low residual urine volume. An external collecting device is generally worn postoperatively, although total dripping incontinence or severe stress incontinence is unusual unless the proximal sphincter mechanism (the bladder neck and proximal urethra) has been compromised—by prior surgical therapy, the neurologic lesion itself, or as a secondary effect of the striated sphincter dyssynergia (presumably a hydraulic effect on the bladder neck itself).

The 12 o'clock sphincterotomy remains the procedure of choice for a number of reasons. The anatomy of the striated sphincter is such that its main bulk is anteromedial. The blood supply is primarily lateral, and thus there is less chance of significant hemorrhage with a 12 o'clock incision. There is some disagreement about the rate of postoperative erectile dysfunction in those individuals who preoperatively have erections. Estimates utilizing the 3 o'clock and 9 o'clock technique vary from 5 to 30 percent, but whatever the true figure is, it is clear that most would agree that this complication is far less common (approximately 5 percent) with incision in the anteromedial position. Other complications may include significant hemorrhage and urinary extravasation. Failure to attain satisfactory bladder emptying following external sphincterotomy may be due to inadequate or poorly sustained bladder contractility, a poorly done sphincterotomy, or persistent obstruction at the level of the bladder neck from unrecognized coexistent smooth sphincter dyssynergia. In these latter patients, bladder neck incisions, as described previously, may facilitate bladder emptying.

v. *Urethral stent.* Permanent urethral stents to bypass the sphincter area have been utilized and results have become available over the last 10 years. There is little question that a significant decrease in detrusor leak pressure and residual urine volume occurs. Certainly, compared to sphincterotomy, this would seem to be conceptually less morbid. The questions are long-term efficacy, ease of removal/replacement when required, and the true incidence of the development of bladder outlet obstruction.

vi. *Pudendal nerve interruption.* This procedure, first described in the last 1890s, is seldom if ever used today because of the potential of undesirable effects consequent to even a unilateral nerve section (impotence, fecal, and stress incontinence).

BIBLIOGRAPHY

Abrams P: *Urodynamics,* 2nd ed. London, Springer, 1997.

Andersson K-E, Appell R, Cardozo L, et al: Pharmacological treatment of urinary incontinence. In: Abrams P, Khoury S, Wein A, eds. *Incontinence.* 1st International Consultation on Incontinence, June 28–July 1, 1998, Monaco. Co-sponsored by World Health Organization and International Union Against Cancer. Health Publications Ltd., 1999, pp 449–486, distributed by Plymbridge Distributors, Ltd.

Brading AF, Fry CA, Maggi M, et al: *Cellular biology.* In: Abrams P, Khoury S, Wein A, eds. *Incontinence.* 1st International Consultation on Incontinence, June 28–July 1, 1998, Monaco. Co-sponsored by World Health Organization and International Union Against Cancer. Health Publications Ltd., 1999, pp 59–103, distributed by Plymbridge Distributors, Ltd.

deGroat WC, Downie JW, Levin RM, et al: Basic neurophysiology and neuropharmacology. In: Abrams P, Khoury S, Wein A, eds. *Incontinence.* 1st International Consultation on Incontinence, June 28–July 1, 1998, Monaco. Co-sponsored by World Health Organization and International Union Against Cancer. Health Publications Ltd., 1999, pp 107–154, distributed by Plymbridge Distributors, Ltd.

Nitti V: *Practical Urodynamics.* Philadelphia, Saunders, 1998.

Rovner ES, Wein AJ: Pharmacologic treatment for non-BPH induced voiding dysfunction: Facilitation of bladder emptying, part I. *AUA Update Series.* Houston, American Urological Association, Inc., vol. 17, lesson 33, pp 258–265, 1998.

Rovner ES, Wein AJ: Pharmacologic treatment for non-BPH induced voiding dysfunction: facilitation of urine storage, part II. *AUA Update Series.* Houston, American Urological Association, Inc., vol. 17, lesson 34, pp 266–272, 1998.

Steers WD: Physiology and pharmacology of the bladder and urethra. In: Walsh P, Retik A, Vaughan ED, Jr., Wein AJ, eds. *Campbell's Urology,* 7th ed. Philadelphia, Saunders, 1997, pp 870–916.

Steers WD, Barrett DM, Wein AJ: Voiding dysfunction: Diagnosis, classification, and management. In: Gillenwater JY, Grayhack JT, Howards SS, Duckett JW, eds. *Adult and Pediatric Urology.* St. Louis, Mosby-Yearbook, Inc., 1996, pp 1220–1326.

Wein AJ: Pathophysiology and categorization of voiding dysfunction. In: Walsh P, Retik A, Vaughan ED, Jr., Wein AJ, eds. *Campbell's Urology,* 7th ed. Philadelphia, Saunders, 1997, pp 917–926.

Wein AJ: Neuromuscular dysfunction of the lower urinary tract and its treatment. In: Walsh P, Retik A, Vaughan ED, Jr., Wein AJ, eds. *Campbell's Urology,* 7th ed. Philadelphia, Saunders, 1997, pp 953–1006.

Wein AJ, Barrett DM: *Voiding Function and Dysfunction: A Logical and Practical Approach.* New York, Year Book Medical Publishers, Inc., 1988.

Wein AJ, Rovner, ES: Adult voiding dysfunction secondary to neurologic disease or injury. *AUA Update Series.* Houston, American Urological Association, Inc., vol. 18, lesson 6, 1999, pp 42–27.

Wilson PD, Bø K, Bourcier A, et al: Conservative management in women. In: Abrams P, Khoury S, Wein A, eds. *Incontinence.* 1st International Consultation on Incontinence, June 28–July 1, 1998, Monaco. Co-sponsored by World Health Organization and International Union Against Cancer. Health Publications Ltd., 1999, pp 581–636, distributed by Plymbridge Distributors, Ltd.

Zderic SA, Levin RM, Wein AJ: Voiding function: Relevant anatomy, physiology, pharmacology and molecular aspects. In: Gillenwater JY, Grayhack JT,

Howards SS, Duckett JW, eds. *Adult and Pediatric Urology.* St. Louis, Mosby-Yearbook, Inc., 1996, pp 1159–1219.

SELF-ASSESSMENT QUESTIONS

1. Regardless of differences regarding physiologic and pharmacologic details, what would most experts agree are the requirements for normal bladder filling and storage? Discuss the main points relating to the anatomy, neurophysiology, and neuropharmacology of each of these factors.

2. Regardless of differences regarding physiologic and pharmacologic details, what would most experts agree are the requirements for normal bladder emptying and voiding? Discuss the main points relating to the anatomy, neurophysiology, and neuropharmacology of each of these factors.

3. Broadly generalize the differences between the autonomic and somatic nervous systems. Discuss the terms parasympathetic and sympathetic.

4. What are the primary neurotransmitters released at postganglionic, parasympathetic, and sympathetic effector sites in the lower urinary tract? Discuss the distribution and the results of activation of the cholinergic and adrenergic receptors in lower urinary tract smooth muscle.

5. Discuss the differences in organization of the micturition reflex in a normal adult and in an adult with a T10 spinal cord transection following spinal shock.

6. Categorize each urodynamic study (flowmetry, residual urine, filling and voiding cystometry, detrusor and abdominal [Valsalva] leak point pressures, urethral profilometry, and electromyography) as to what they characterize with respect to bladder and outlet activity during the filling and storage and emptying and voiding phases of micturition.

7. Characterize the most common types of voiding dysfunction seen with the following neurologic injury(ies) and disease(s) in terms of sensation, bladder activity, smooth sphincter activity, striated sphincter activity: (1) cerebrovascular accident; (2) Parkinson's disease; (3) multiple sclerosis; (4) suprasacral spinal cord injury; (5) sacral spinal cord injury; (6) radical pelvic surgery; and (7) diabetes.

8. Discuss the usual types of management employed in the treatment of the voiding dysfunctions in question 7.

9. Describe and discuss the use of pressure flow urodynamic studies and video urodynamic studies.

10. Excluding extraurethral incontinence and incontinence due to lack of concern or to cognitive dysfunction, discuss the basic pathophysiology of urinary incontinence in the adult.

11. Discuss the classic differentiation between genuine stress urinary incontinence and intrinsic sphincter deficiency and the therapeutic implications of each.

12. Discuss the normal support mechanism(s) of the bladder neck and proximal urethra in the female and the various theories of pathophysiology of hypermobility related stress incontinence.

13. Discuss the possibilities and practicalities of pharmacologic therapy for (1) bladder overactivity; (2) decreased outlet resistance; (3) increased outlet resistance; and (4) decreased bladder contractility.

14. Discuss the theory(ies) behind the use of peripheral and central electrical stimulation in the treatment of bladder overactivity.

15. Discuss the surgical options for treating sphincteric incontinence in adult men and women.

CHAPTER 15
Benign Prostatic Hyperplasia

Alan J. Wein
Eric S. Rovner

I. GENERAL CONSIDERATIONS

The evaluation and management of symptoms related to bladder outlet and urethral obstruction are responsible for a large portion of any given urology practice. An etiologic categorization is seen in Table 15-1. Although some of these entities may be associated with abnormalities of the urinary sediment or a characteristic finding on physical examination, most present only with symptoms of voiding dysfunction. These symptoms are remarkably nonspecific, and are associated more so with some entities rather than others strictly because of their prevalence.

This chapter considers the most common of these entities, benign prostatic hyperplasia (BPH). Bladder neck/smooth sphincter dyssynergia or dysfunction and striated sphincter dyssynergia are considered in Chapter 14, urethral stricture disease in Chapter 12.

II. DEFINITION

Benign prostatic hyperplasia (BPH) refers to a regional nodular growth of varying combinations of glandular and stromal proliferation that occurs in almost all men who have testes and who live long enough. Because of the anatomic localization of the prostatic growth that characterizes BPH—surrounding and adjacent to the proximal urethra—clinical problems can result. BPH can be defined in a number of ways, depending on the orientation of the user of the term. Microscopic BPH refers to the histologic evidence of cellular proliferation. Macroscopic BPH refers to organ enlargement due to the cellular changes. Clinical BPH refers to the lower urinary tract symptoms thought due to benign prostatic obstruction. BPH histopathologically is characterized by an increased number of epithelial and stromal cells in the periurethral area of the prostate, the molecular etiology of which is uncertain. The incidence of histologic or microscopic BPH is far greater than that of clinical or macroscopic BPH.

Table 15-1 Bladder Outlet and Urethral Obstruction: Etiology

Prostate
  Benign Prostatic Hyperplasia
  Cancer
  Other infiltrative processes
Bladder neck and proximal urethra
  Contracture, fibrosis, stricture, stenosis
  Dyssynergia/dysfunction
    Smooth sphincter
    Striated sphincter
  Secondary hypertrophy of bladder neck
  Compression
    Distended vagina and uterus
    Extrinsic tumors
  Calculus, mucous
  Ectopic ureterocele
  Polyp
  Posterior urethral valve
Distal urethra
    Contracture, fibrosis, stricture, stenosis
    Anterior urethral valve

BPH has also been referred to as hyperplasia, benign prostatic hypertrophy, adenomatous hypertrophy, glandular hyperplasia, and stromal hyperplasia.

III. EPIDEMIOLOGY, INCIDENCE, PREVALENCE, AND ECONOMICS

A.

Autopsy data indicates that anatomic (microscopic) evidence of BPH is seen in about 25 percent of men age 40 to 50 years, 50 percent of men age 50 to 60, 65 percent of men age 60 to 70, 80 percent of men age 70 to 80, and 90 percent of men age 80 to 90.

B.

Estimates of the prevalence of clinical BPH vary widely, probably because of the varying thresholds used to define the presence of BPH on the basis of symptoms and/or urodynamics (no uniform definition) or on the basis of the rate of prostatic surgery. It has been classically stated that from 25 to 50 percent of individuals with microscopic and macroscopic evidence of BPH will progress to clinical BPH. Depending on which definition is used, the prevalence of clinical BPH in an individual community in men ages 55 to 74 years may vary from less than 5 percent to more than 30 percent. Only 40 percent of this group, however, complain of lower urinary tract symptoms (LUTS), and only about 20 percent seek medical advice because of them. The number of individuals who receive treatment for BPH varies according to the threshold for providing such treatment, a threshold which can vary widely in different parts of the world and in different parts of the United States. As treatments become less invasive, this number can be expected to increase.

The total number of prostatectomies done yearly in the United States for what was originally diagnosed as benign prostatic disease was estimated at one point to be as high as 400,000 to 450,000. By 1993, the total number of prostatectomies in the United States was estimated by Barry and colleagues to have declined to 256,000. A better idea of the decline of surgery as first-line treatment in the United States can be gained by looking at the number of Transurethral Prostatectomies performed on Medicare patients in 1987 (258,000) compared with the number in 1996 (116,000). With the decline of surgery as first-line treatment, there has been a concomitant increase in the use of other management strategies for BPH. Most of these management options can be accomplished with a variable number of instruments (devices or drugs), each championed by a different manufacturer. In this environment, it is inevitable that each particular device and drug has its own team of "data doctors" to design and report efficacy studies in the best light possible. Comparisons can be quite confusing.

C.

No convincing evidence exists regarding a positive correlation for any factors other than age and the presence of testes in the development of BPH. Smoking has been suggested to be negatively associated with prostatectomy, but race (except for a lower incidence in Japanese men), dietary factors, body habitus, sexual or vasectomy history, and other diseases and medications have not been found to be positively associated either with the occurrence of clinical BPH or with prostatectomy. BPH does appear to have an inheritable genetic component, although the specifics are yet to be elucidated.

IV. PROSTATIC SIZE AND MORPHOLOGY PERTINENT TO BPH
A.

Although some prostatic growth occurs throughout life, the prostate changes relatively little in size until puberty, when it undergoes rapid growth. Autopsy studies indicate that the normal adult prostate plateaus at a weight of about 26 g at age 30 years. This remains relatively stable until approximately age 50, following which increasing weight is observed, such that the average prostatic weight is about 35 to 45 g at age 80. The Olmsted County (Minnesota) survey demonstrated an average 6 g per decade increase in prostate weight. Classical autopsy studies proposed a doubling time for weight of 4.5 years for men between ages 31 and 50, 10 years between ages 51 and 70, and of 100 years in men older than age 70. These observations are obviously inconsistent.

Throughout developmental life the prostate maintains its ability to respond to endocrine signals, undergoes rapid growth at puberty, and maintains its size and tissue androgen receptor levels. In some individuals, abnormal growth subsequently occurs, which may be either benign or malignant. The mechanisms of normal and abnormal growth have yet to be resolved, but are thought to involve multiple growth promoting and inhibiting factors ultimately controlling cell replication, cell cycle control, cell aging, cell senescence, and cell death, both necrosis and apoptosis.

The size of the prostate is not linearly correlated to either urodynamic evidence of bladder outlet obstruction or the severity of symptoms generally associated with clinical BPH. The adult prostate is a truncated cone with its base at the urethrovesical junction and its apex at the urogenital diaphragm. The prostate is pierced by the urethra, which angles forward at the verumontanum, and by the paired ejaculatory ducts, which join the urethra at its point of angulation.

B.

A lobar configuration of the prostate was originally described by Lowsley, based on studies of the human fetal prostate. A posterior, two lateral, an anterior, and a middle lobe were described. Although this description was used by urologists for years because it seemed to bear some relationship to endoscopic and gross surgical anatomy, distinct lobes do not exist in the prepubertal and normal adult prostate. The concept of a lobular structure has been replaced by one based on concentric zones that have morphologic, functional, and pathologic significance. McNeal and associates from Stanford have done the most to expand the understanding of adult prostate morphology, describing the zonal anatomy based on examination of the gland in different planes of section (Fig. 15-1). The urethra represents the primary reference point, dividing the prostate into an anterior fibromuscular and a posterior glandular portion. The anterior fibromuscular stroma comprises up to one third of the total bulk of the prostate. It contains no glandular elements. This fibromuscular stroma has not been linked to a specific pathologic

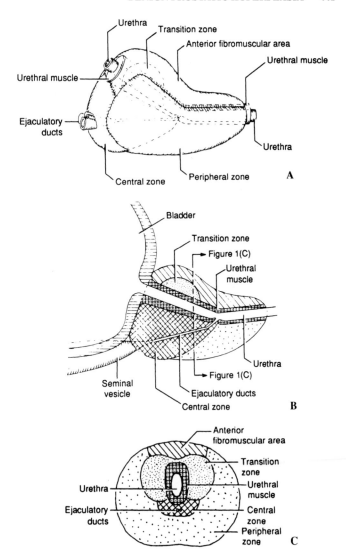

Figure 15-1 Prostatic zonal anatomy after McNeal. **A**. Schematic **B**. sagittal cross-section **C**. transverse cross-section

process. The two principal regions of the glandular prostate are defined as the peripheral zone (about 75 percent of total glandular volume) and the central zone, each morphometrically distinct. The central zone makes up about 25 percent of the functioning glandular prostate. It contacts the urethra only at the upper end of the veru, where its ducts open. Carcinoma is uncommon in this area. The peripheral zone is the site of origin of most prostate cancer. The glandular tissue that participates in BPH nodule formation is derived exclusively from the branches of a few small ducts representing about 5 to 10 percent of the glandular prostate, which join the urethra at or proximal to is point of angulation. Urethral angulation at the most proximal extent of the veru displaces the proximal urethral segment from the secretory gland mass anteriorly and into the anterior fibromuscular stroma. The resulting space between the urethra and glandular prostate accommodates a cylindrical smooth muscle sphincter that surrounds the proximal segment of the urethra from the base of the veru to the bladder neck. All nodules of BPH develop within or immediately adjacent to this smooth muscle layer, and this glandular tissue is subdivided by this muscle into two discrete regions. The transitional zone comprises less than 5 percent of the normal glandular volume and consists of two separate lobules of tissue immediately outside of the smooth muscle layer, located laterally and extending somewhat ventrally. A tiny periurethral region (less than 1 percent of the total glandular prostate) contains glands that are entirely confined within the smooth muscle layer from just proximal to the point of urethral angulation to the bladder neck. This periurethral zone is so small that it is not pictured in many other renditions of McNeal's zonal anatomy. The origin of BPH is confined exclusively to these areas, and some cancers may also originate here. Between the transitional and peripheral zones are the central zones, which have not been implicated in the origin of a specific pathologic process.

V. ETIOLOGIC THEORIES OF BPH: PATHOPHYSIOLOGY

A.

Clinically detectable BPH nodules arise from a variety of adenomas in the transitional and periurethral zones. As these grow, they may outwardly compress the anterior fibromuscular stroma and areas in the peripheral and central zones. A so-called surgical capsule develops between the hyperplastic nodules and the compressed glandular tissue. This serves as a plane of cleavage that is a useful landmark in the open or transurethral surgical removal of the adenoma. The etiologic factors responsible for BPH nodule induction and further development are unclear. However, there are a number of factors that are obviously involved, although the magnitude of their importance and their interactions remain to be fully elucidated. What follows is the briefest of descriptions of the possible major factors mentioned, gleaned mostly from the work of Walsh, Coffey, Partin, Isaacs, and their group at Johns Hopkins; Grayhack, Lee and the group at Northwestern; Lawson, and others.

B. Hormones

There is no question that a functioning testis is a prerequisite for the normal development of the prostate in animals and man. Patients castrated before puberty do not develop BPH. BPH is rare in males castrated before the age of 40. Androgen deprivation in the older male reduces prostatic size. Patients with diseases that result in impaired androgenic production or metabolism have reduced or minimal prostatic growth. Although other endocrine factors are doubtless involved, the androgenic influence on prostatic growth and function is obviously central, although endocrine evaluation of the aging male has disclosed no recognizable surge in androgen secretion. The prostate develops from the urogenital sinus during the third fetal month under the influence of dihydrotestosterone (DHT) produced from fetal testosterone (T) via 5 α-reductase. During development there is a close but as yet incompletely understood interaction between the stromal and epithelial components. DHT is produced from T in the stroma cell and has an autocrine effect there and a paracrine effect in the epithelial cell. These effects are thought to include induction of multiple growth factors and alterations in the extracellular matrix. Prostate growth and maintenance of size and secretory function is stimulated by serum T, converted within the prostate to DHT, a compound whose relative androgenicity is higher.

Originally, an abnormal accumulation of DHT in the prostate was hypothesized as a primary cause of BPH development. However, Coffey and Walsh showed that human BPH occurs in the presence of normal prostatic levels of DHT. Estrogen–androgen synergism has been postulated as necessary for prostatic growth, as well as other steroid hormones and growth factors. Although much remains to be elucidated regarding the hormonal interactions and necessities for the induction and maintenance of BPH, it is clear that, clinically, a reduction in prostatic size of approximately 20 to 30 percent can be induced by either interfering with the conversion of testosterone to DHT or by interfering with androgen receptor binding and metabolism.

C. Stromal–Epithelial Interaction Theory

This theory, first introduced by Cunha and associates, postulates that there is a delicate stromal–epithelial balance in the prostate and that stroma may mediate the effects of androgen on the epithelial component, perhaps by the production of various growth factors and/or autocrine and paracrine messengers.

D. Stem Cell Theory

This is attributed to Isaacs and associates, and hypothesizes that BPH may result from abnormal maturation and regulation of the cell renewal process. In simple terms, this postulates that abnormal size in an aged prostate is maintained not by an increase in the rate of cell replication but rather by a decrease in the rate of cell death. Hormonal factors, growth factors, and oncogenes all influence this balance of replication and cell death. The exact interaction of these, and possibly other factors, and what determines the setting points for the level of cells in the prostate and their rates of growth/replication/death are of major importance in understanding both BPH and prostate cancer.

E. Static and Dynamic Components of Prostatic Obstruction

It is extremely important to understand the concept of the two components contributing to bladder outlet obstruction caused by BPH. The static component implies bulk and includes elements of the stromal and epithelial cells as well as extracellular matrix. Androgen ablation, at least in short-term studies, affects primarily the epithelial cell population volume. Long-term effects on stromal and matrix volume and effects on aspects of stroma and matrix other than volume have not been excluded, however. Therapeutic modalities that reduce the size of the prostate or "make a hole" or enlarge one are directed towards this component.

The dynamic component refers to the obstruction to urine flow contributed by the prostatic smooth muscle. The tension of prostatic smooth muscle is mediated by the α_1-adrenergic receptor, 98 percent of which are in the prostatic stroma. Alpha$_1$-receptors also exist in the smooth muscle of the bladder neck and the prostatic capsule. Activation of these contractile receptors can occur either through circulating catecholamine levels or through adrenergic innervation. Prostatic intraurethral pressure can be reduced experimentally by as much as 40 percent after systemic administration of an α-receptor antagonist. This dynamic or active component may be responsible for the well-recognized variation in symptoms over time experienced by many patients, and it may account for the exacerbation of symptoms experienced by some individuals in response to certain foods, beverages, change in temperature, and levels of stress.

This two-component idea was first popularized by Caine, and later developed by Lepor and Shapiro, resulting in the successful application of selective α-adrenergic blocking agents for the treatment of BPH symptoms. The ratio of stroma to epithelium in the normal prostate is approximately 2:1, and in BPH is cited as approximately 5:1. This data for BPH is derived primarily from small resected prostates, however; the ratio for larger glands with epithelial nodules may be lower. Although the smooth muscle content of stroma has not been precisely determined, a significant proportion of the stroma is in fact smooth muscle.

VI. SYMPTOMS OF BPH
A. Lower Urinary Tract Symptoms
The symptoms related to bladder outlet obstruction due to BPH have in the past arbitrarily been described as a group as "prostatism" and further categorized as obstructive or irritative. Obstructive symptoms included impairment in the size/force of the urinary stream, hesitancy and/or abdominal straining, intermittent or interrupted flow, a sensation of incomplete emptying, and terminal dribbling, although the last by itself seems to have little clinical significance. Irritative symptoms included nocturia, daytime frequency, urgency, urge incontinence, and possibly dys-uria. Although these can result from an increased residual urine with consequent decreased functional capacity, they are generally thought to result from the effects of the obstruction itself on the bladder, producing either hyperactivity or hypersensitivity.

LUTS (lower urinary tract symptoms) is a rubric, introduced by Abrams, to replace the term "prostatism," which implied that the prostate was responsible for most (or all) symptomatic voiding complaints in men. LUTS with its subdivisions, filling and storage symptoms and voiding (emptying) symptoms, have replaced as well the terminology of "irritative" and "obstructive" symptoms, both rather imprecise terms that imply an etiology that may be incorrect. Another advantage of the term is that it can be applied to voiding symptoms in both men and women.

Although BPH is the most common etiology of significant voiding dysfunction seen by the urologist, the diagnosis cannot be made on the basis of symptoms alone, as these are very nonspecific. Symptoms are, however, what brings the patient to the doctor and their progression/regression/stability over time is important in determining the need for treatment, the aggressiveness of treatment once it is decided that treatment is necessary, and the results of treatment once instituted. The symptoms associated with BPH are not simply solely due to bladder outlet obstruction. Such symptoms are due, in varying proportions in different individuals, to anatomic obstruction, related changes in detrusor structure and function, age-related changes in detrusor structure and function, and changes in neural circuitry that may occur secondary to these factors.

VII. SIGNS OF BPH

A.

Detectable anatomic enlargement of the prostate on physical examination or imaging is generally, but not always, a correlate of symptom producing BPH. However, there is no clear relationship between the degree of anatomic enlargement and the severity of symptoms or the degree of urodynamic changes.

B.

Bladder changes secondary to obstruction can occur. These consist of bladder wall thickening, trabeculation (which are also associated with involuntary bladder contractions), and bladder diverticula (which could also be congenital). Bladder calculi can develop. Bladder decompensation can occur, and gross bladder distention can result. Chronically increased residual urine volumes may result and may contribute to frequency and urgency and persistent urinary infection. Acute urinary retention may supervene. Azotemia may result from upper tract changes. There is an increased incidence of lower urinary tract infections in obstructed patients.

C.

Upper tract changes of ureterectasis, hydroureter, and/or hydronephrosis can result. These can result either from secondary vesicoureteral reflux, sustained high pressure bladder storage without reflux, and/or sustained high pressure attempts at emptying. Ureteral obstruction can also occur secondary to muscular hypertrophy or angulation at the ureterovesical junction. Hematuria may arise from dilated veins coursing over the surface of the enlarged adenomatous prostate.

VIII. URODYNAMICS OF BPH

A.

The urodynamics of bladder outlet obstruction are described in the chapter on voiding function and dysfunction. Patients with clinical BPH characteristically exhibit decreased mean and peak flow rates, an abnormal flow pattern characterized by a long low plateau, and elevated detrusor pressures at the initiation of and during flow. They may or may not have residual urine. Approximately 50 percent of such patients are found to have bladder hyperactivity during filling. Pressure flow urodynamics are necessary to distinguish between patients with obstructive BPH and patients who have inadequate detrusor contractility, the symptoms of which may be identical. Specialized variations of urodynamic studies, either with or without video, are certainly helpful to separate BPH from other forms of outlet obstruction (see Chapter 14). However, argument exists among urodynamicists as to whether any urodynamic parameter(s) is (are) able to reliably predict those patients with BPH who will benefit from outlet reduction as opposed to those who will not. More promising indices have recently been proposed but bear further testing. In the past, the 10 to 30 percent of patients who did not experience symptomatic relief after Transurethral Resection prostate were either not categorized as to whether urodynamic obstruction existed prior, or such a correlation was found to be only minimally or moderately predictive. Some comments about specific studies follow.

B. Residual Urine Volume

If the residual urine volume is significant, its reduction is important in the evaluation of results of treatment of BPH. For many with a significant residual volume, it is impossible to differentiate deficient bladder contractility from outlet obstruction as the primary cause without a pressure-flow study. Most agree that a large residual urine volume reflects at least some bladder dysfunction, but it is difficult to correlate residual urine with either specific symptomatology or other urodynamic abnormalities. The most popular noninvasive method of measurement is ultrasonography. The error for ultrasound has been estimated at 10 to 25 percent for bladder volumes over 100 mL and somewhat worse for smaller volumes. Unfortunately for the BPH investigator, residual urine volumes in an individual patient at different times can vary widely. Reflux and large diverticula may complicate the accuracy of measurement. Abrams and colleagues, after a thorough review of the subject, conclude that elevated residual urine has a relation to prostatic obstruction, although not a strong one, as supported by the following observations.

1. Elevated residual urine is common in the elderly of both genders.
2. Elevated residual urine of greater than 50 mL is found in about 50 percent of patients with LUTS who have no urodynamically demonstrable obstruction.

3. The absence of residual urine does not rule out severe obstruction (one series is cited in which 24 percent of patients with severe obstruction had a residual urine volume of less than 50 mL).
4. Two studies are cited that show that elevated residual urine does not have a significant prognostic factor for a good operative outcome.
5. Of patients with a significant residual urine preoperatively, 30 percent retain this impairment postoperatively.

What constitutes an abnormal residual urine? Abrams and colleagues conclude that a residual urine volume of greater than 50 to 100 mL is abnormal.

C. Uroflowmetry

Significant disagreement exists regarding what constitutes an adequate urodynamic evaluation of prostatism and whether a urodynamically quantifiable definition of obstruction is necessary or desirable. Of all of these urodynamic studies, uroflowmetry seems to excite the least controversy. Although diminished flow may be caused by either outlet obstruction or impairment of detrusor contractility, and that outlet obstruction may certainly exist in the presence of a normal flow, it is acknowledged that most men with bladder outlet obstruction do have a diminished flow rate and altered flow pattern.

What is a normal flow rate? Abrams and Griffiths and Andersen proposed that, empirically, peak flow rates of less than 10 mL/sec were associated with obstruction; that peak flow rates greater than 15 mL/sec were not associated with obstructed voiding, and that peak flow rates between 10 and 15 mL/sec were equivocal. Although this proposal has been widely used, it is generally acknowledged that flow rates at any level may be associated with either obstruction or lack of obstruction. Studies are cited showing that 7 to 25 percent of patients referred with "prostatism" had high flow bladder outlet obstruction.

Potential problems related to uroflow include the following:

1. Many patients do not or will not void in a volume sufficient for accurate measurement.
2. Others void with an interrupted stream or with postvoid dribbling, which makes interpretation of the endpoint of micturition difficult, casting some element of subjectivity into the calculation of average flow rate.

3. Some patients are unable to relax sufficiently to void in the same manner in which they would in the privacy of their own bathroom.
4. A considerable discrepancy may exist between the first and subsequent measures of mean and peak flow.

Flow data changes can be expressed in terms of absolute change, percent change, or as a cumulative frequency distribution. Clearly important is the initial flow number, the value of which may make the absolute or percent change look better or worse. In other words, raw data must be expressed, as well as the other frills that may be added to embellish flow data. It should be noted as well that it is unknown what change in flow is necessary to give the impression of mild, moderate, or marked improvement.

Because voiding events may be different from point to point in an individual's life, a variety of flow nomograms have been constructed to facilitate comparison of them. It should be noted that there are many nomograms and tables of "acceptable flow rates" available for various age groups. Many believe that the Siroky nomogram, commonly used in the United States, overestimates peak and average flow rates for older men, and therefore underestimates the number of older men with bladder outlet obstruction. Other nomograms include the Drach peak flow nomogram and the Liverpool and Bristol nomograms. It is doubtful that consistency will be achieved among flow nomogram makers. However, one of the systems supported by at least a portion of urodynamicists should be utilized for comparisons following treatment of BPH.

D. Cystometry and Pressure-Flow Studies

Filling cystometry provides information on sensation, compliance, and the presence of and threshold for involuntary bladder contractions, and urodynamic bladder capacity. Compliance is generally not affected in patients with clinical BPH, but, as mentioned previously, approximately 50 percent of such patients will have involuntary bladder contractions.

On a logical basis, bladder outlet obstruction would seem to be defined by the relationship between flow rate and detrusor contractility. Outlet obstruction is best characterized by a poor flow rate in the presence of a detrusor contraction of adequate force, duration, and speed. With obstruction, detrusor pressure during attempted voiding generally rises, flow rates generally fall, and the shape of the flow curve becomes more plateau than parabola-like. There is, however, marked disagreement about the utility of pressure-flow uro-dynamic measurements in the evaluation of suspected out-let obstruction, in the prediction of success of a given treat-ment, and in the assessment of treatment results. Authorities who make an excellent case for the use of various types of pressure-flow studies in evaluating patients with prostatism and favorably affecting outcomes include Abrams and asso-ciates, Blaivas, Coolsaet and Blok, Jensen, Neal and col-leagues, Schafer and coworkers, and Rollema and Van Mas-trigt. Some add other mathematical means to augment the relationships observed on a simple plot of detrusor pressure versus flow. Equally forceful arguments against the utility of such measurements are made by Andersen, Bruskewitz and colleagues, Graverson and coworkers, and McConnell. Jensen did an exhaustive review of the subject of urody-namic efficacy in the evaluation of elderly men with prosta-tism. One conclusion was that in this group, interpretation of pressure-flow data using the nomogram of Abrams and Grif-fiths revealed a significantly better subjective outcome for surgery in patients classified as "obstructed" than in those classified as "unobstructed" (93.1% versus 77.8%, $P < .02$). Others have also demonstrated better outcomes for surgery in urodynamically obstructed men than in those with no obstruction.

Successful treatment of BPH by prostatectomy is gener-ally correlated with a reduction in the detrusor pressure (P_{DET}) during an increased uroflow. The maximum flow rate (Q_{MAX}) and the corresponding detrusor pressure at maxi-mum flow (P_{DET} at Q_{MAX}) are the most common and most important pressure-flow variables reported. Consideration of the entire pressure-flow plot or other complex mathematical manipulations and graphic representations may, in fact, prove to be more accurate and informative ways of looking at this relationship and may narrow further the diagnostic grey zone between bladder outlet obstruction and decreased detrusor function. The problem is that there is not just one such program, but a number of them, with intense competi-tion among their creators in the literature. We totaled 12 at last count.

E. Symptomatic versus Urodynamic Improvement

The data from pressure-flow studies can be reported either as raw changes in individual parameters (e.g., Q_{MAX}, P_{DET}, P_{DET} at Q_{MAX}), as a change in category or number designat-ing the grade or severity of obstruction, or by a visual demonstration of change on the nomogram itself. Aside from the utility (or nonutility) of these measurements in assessing the outcome of BPH treatment, the global question referable to these studies seems to be whether the evaluation of the average older man with LUTS is more likely to lead to a better treatment outcome if urodynamic studies are performed, including analyzing the results of these studies in the various mathematical ways described. In other words, can urodynamic studies predict the outcome of various treatments for LUTS, including watchful waiting? The critical question, when considering a given analysis of pressure-flow data, is, are patients with LUTS in whom treatment in the form of outlet ablation fails the same as those whose detrusor contractility is judged ineffective by the criteria under consideration? If the answer to this question is no, then the relevance of the analysis is in question, unless it can predict which patients will worsen or which patients will have undesirable sequelae, or it can predict which modalities are apt to be more successful in treatment than others. In our opinion, those who perform urodynamics have done a remarkably poor job of looking into this aspect of outcome analysis.

One final consideration should be mentioned—a seeming dissociation that may occur between symptomatic and urodynamic improvement. This has been most noticeable in data concerning pharmacologic agents. The fact that symptomatic improvement occurs that is seemingly out of proportion to the amount of urodynamic improvement may, in fact, indicate that a given treatment is not equal to the current gold standard of prostatectomy, or that the results will be of shorter duration. However, one important possibility to consider is that the actual symptoms of prostatism have much less to do with urodynamically defined obstruction than is thought, and their relief with these other types of treatment has to do more with the correction of some ill-defined mechanism within the prostate and/or prostatic urethra that is not directly related to the amount of mechanical obstruction. Alternatively, it may not be necessary to reduce outlet obstruction by the amount achievable by prostatectomy to significantly improve symptomatology and prevent bladder or upper tract deterioration.

IX. THE NATURAL HISTORY OF BPH AND ITS ALTERATION

A.

Although LUTS due to BPH are generally progressive over time, spontaneous improvement can occur in an untreated patient, and thus the course may be highly variable. Combining data from three reports of the natural history of untreated BPH, one can conclude that over a 1- to 5-year period, approximately 18 to 32 percent of patients with clinical BPH will experience subjective improvement, 15 to 52 percent will have no change, and 16 to 60 percent will experience a worsening in their symptomatology. Data suggest that over 3 to 5 years 15 to 25 percent of patients will show an increase in flow rates, 15 percent will have no change, and 60 to 70 percent will have a worsening. Placebo responses of 20 to 40 percent have consistently been reported over the years for drug therapy.

B.

Although BPH is rarely life-threatening, it is generally considered to be a slowly progressive disease. Although many patients may do perfectly well with watchful waiting over long periods of time, the natural history of the disease can include undesirable or even dangerous outcomes. More recently, attention has been focused not only on evaluating the acute positive effects of treatment but on stabilizing symptoms, reversing the natural progression of BPH, and avoiding acute or undesirable events. The outcome measures recorded generally include (1) progression of symptoms or signs, or both; (2) the occurrence of acute urinary retention; and (3) the need for surgical intervention. Progression can be measured in terms of any of the parameters used to assess outcome acutely or subacutely. A matched control group would obviously be valuable in this regard, as the use of historical control subjects is less than ideal. Acute urinary retention is probably the event most feared by men with BPH. Estimates of acute urinary retention in men with BPH as range from 0.004 to 0.13 episodes per person-year, with a 10-year cumulative incidence rate ranging from 4 to 73 percent. Others report the incidence of retention in 3 years to be 2.9 percent and cite incidences in the literature as low as 2 percent in 5 years and as high as 35 percent in 3 years. Progression to the point of requiring surgical intervention is an obvious undesirable outcome, but there are little data available regarding the incidence of this outcome, especially since the definitions of "surgery" and the indications for types of "make a hole" therapy other than prostatectomy are continually changing.

X. EVALUATION OF LUTS SUSPECTED TO BE DUE TO BPH

The essentials of the initial evaluation include history, digital rectal and focused physical examinations, urinalysis, urine cytology in those with significant irritative symptoms, serum creatinine, renal ultrasound (if creatinine abnormal), and a standardized symptom assessment, such as the AUA symptom index

(AUASS) (Fig. 15-2). "Routine PSA measurement" in this population has been a source of active debate. Our feeling is that PSA should be measured in men over 50 years of age with a life expectancy of 10 years or more and in whom prostate cancer would be treated. For African Americans or those with a family history (first-degree relative), we drop this age to 40. The AHCPR guidelines list PSA measurement as optional, whereas the International Consultation on BPH recommends it.

Men who do not have absolute or near-absolute indications for treatment (see the following discussion), and have an AUA symptom score of less than or equal to 7 (mild symptoms) do not need further evaluation or treatment. They should be followed on a watchful waiting program. In patients with more severe symptoms or who are being considered for active treatment, urodynamics may be desirable. The simplest of these, flowmetry and residual urine volume, are recommended by the International Consultation for all men presenting with lower urinary tract symptoms suggestive of benign prostatic obstruction but considered optimal by the AHCPR guidelines. Endoscopic examination of the lower urinary tract should be performed if other lower urinary tract pathology is suspected and is recommended prior to invasive treatment when the choice of treatment or changes of success or failure depends on the anatomic configuration and/or intraurethral size of the prostate. A reasonable algorithm by McConnell, combining both AHCPR and International Consultation recommendations is seen in Figure 15-3.

A. Symptoms and Symptom Scores

Symptoms have classically formed the initial database on which to formulate (1) evaluation of potential outlet obstruction, (2) indications for active treatment when obstructive BPH is present, and (3) evaluation of the results of treatment. Symptom quantitation is difficult, and meaningful comparison of symptoms before and after treatment is even harder. The concept of a symptom score or severity table for BPH was first developed by an ad hoc group formed by the Food and Drug Administration (FDA) in 1975; the initial recommendations were published in 1977. Investigators can and have evaluated every factor imaginable with such scoring tables, eliminating some symptoms and adding others, changing the weights and definitions of the severity of various symptoms, considering some symptoms separately, or dividing the symptoms into storage and voiding groups. There is generally no provision in a symptom score for considering specifically what actually changed most recently to bring the patient to the physician, what is in fact most annoying to him, and what he wants corrected most, or what effect the overall symptom complex, or any one symptom, has

Figure 15-2 A. AUA Symptom Index (range from 0 to 35 points).

	NOT AT ALL	LESS THAN 1 TIME IN 5	LESS THAN HALF THE TIME	ABOUT HALF THE TIME	MORE THAN HALF THE TIME	ALMOST ALWAYS
1. Over the last month how often have you had a sensation of not emptying your bladder completely after you finished urinating?	0	1	2	3	4	5
2. Over the last month, how often have you had to urinate again less than 2 hours after you finished urinating?	0	1	2	3	4	5
3. Over the last month, how often have you found you stopped and started again several times while urinating?	0	1	2	3	4	5
4. Over the last month, how often have you found it difficult to postpone urination?	0	1	2	3	4	5
5. Over the last month, how often have you had a weak stream while urinating?	0	1	2	3	4	5
6. Over the last month, how often have you had to push or strain to begin urinating?	0	1	2	3	4	5

Figure 15-2 Continued

7. Over the last month, how many times did you most typically get up to urinate from the time you went to bed until the time you got up in the morning?

0, none	1 time	2 times	3 times	4 times	5 or more times

AUA symptom index score: 0–7 mild; 8–18 moderate; 19–35 severe symptoms.

TOTAL ☐

QUALITY OF LIFE DUE TO URINARY SYSTEMS

	DELIGHTED	PLEASED	MOSTLY SATISFIED	MIXED ABOUT EQUALLY SATISFIED AND DISSATISFIED	MOSTLY DISSATISFIED	UNHAPPY	TERRIBLE
1. If you were to spend the rest of your life with your urinary condition just the way it is now, how would you feel about that?	0	1	2	3	4	5	6

QUALITY OF LIFE ASSESSMENT INDEX (QOL) = ·

B. Quality of life assessment recommended by the World Health Organization.

455

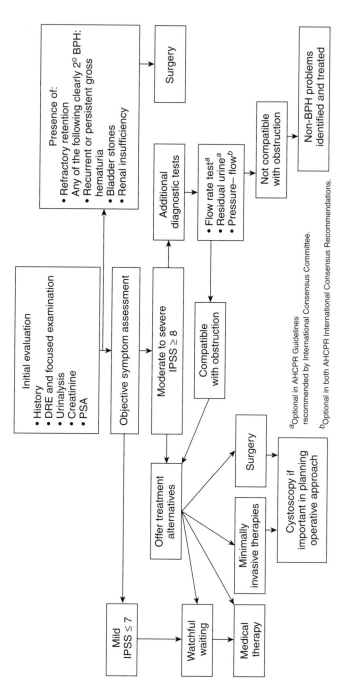

Figure 15-3

Initial evaluation
• History
• DRE and focused examination
• Urinalysis
• Creatinine
• PSA

Objective symptom assessment

Mild
IPSS ≤ 7

Moderate to severe
IPSS ≥ 8

Presence of:
• Refractory retention
Any of the following clearly 2° BPH:
• Recurrent or persistent gross hematuria
• Bladder stones
• Renal insufficiency

Surgery

Additional diagnostic tests
• Flow rate test[a]
• Residual urine[a]
• Pressure–flow[b]

Not compatible with obstruction

Non-BPH problems identified and treated

Compatible with obstruction

Offer treatment alternatives

Watchful waiting

Medical therapy

Minimally invasive therapies

Surgery

Cystoscopy if important in planning operative approach

[a]Optional in AHCPR Guidelines recommended by International Consensus Committee.

[b]Optional in both AHCPR International Consensus Recommendations.

456

on his quality of life, general activities of daily living, or any activity in particular, such as sexual activity.

Through its original Measurement Committee, the American Urological Association (AUA) formulated indices that address many of the issues relevant to symptom scores and produced a symptom index that has become widely utilized. (Fig. 15-2) This index correlates highly with the global rating by a subject of the magnitude of urinary problems attributed to BPH and has been reported to satisfy the requirements of validity, reliability, and responsiveness for BPH. The World Health Organization (WHO) Consultation on BPH has adopted this index, and in this context, it is referred to as the International Prostate Symptom Score (IPSS). This measure of voiding symptoms is useful to ascertain symptom severity and treatment response, or change over time without treatment. However, the AUA index (or score) does not make the diagnosis of BPH and it cannot be used to screen for BPH. A variety of primary and secondary bladder abnormalities and nonprostatic causes of obstruction can produce similar symptoms (to BPH) and high symptom scores. In our practice, the highest scores are generated by women with irritative LUTS. The AUA symptom score does not correlate with or predict urodynamically documented bladder outlet obstruction. Bothersomeness and effect on the quality of life are not addressed by the AUA questionnaire. Blaivas has questioned the accepted statements that the purpose of the AUA symptom score is to quantify severity of disease, document response to therapy, assess patient symptoms, follow them with time to determine disease progression, and allow comparison of the effectiveness of various interventions. He lists four reasons why, in his opinion, the AUA symptom score is not a good tool for accomplishing these purposes:

1. There is an undue emphasis on voiding compared with storage symptoms. In most series on LUTS in older men, urinary frequency and nocturia are the most common symptoms, and coupled with urge and urge incontinence, they seem to be the most troublesome. Only three of the seven questions relate to these symptoms.

2. There is no means of quantitating how badly the symptoms bother the patient. An example cited is that a man who voids every half hour during the day, has urgency and urge incontinence half of the time, and gets up three times a night to void, scores only 11 of 35 points, yet has severe symptoms. A man who voids three times daily, hesitates, stops and starts, and has a weak stream and sensation of incomplete emptying but no nocturia, urgency,

or incontinence, scores 20 of 35 points, even if he empties completely, yet has mild to moderate symptoms.

3. The symptom score does not consider the possibility that
   urinary frequency and nocturia may not reflect any dysfunction or may not be related to the lower urinary tract,
   because many persons void frequently by habit or by
   choice and do not consider daytime frequency or nocturia
   to be a symptom.

4. Changes in the symptom score are not necessarily a good
   measure of therapeutic efficacy because treatment of the
   most bothersome symptoms may be diluted by the response of symptoms that cause relatively no bother. An
   example cited is that in many of the original studies on
   drug treatment of BPH there was no effect whatever of
   drug versus placebo on the two most troublesome symptoms (nocturia and frequency) and yet there was a statistically significant effect on overall symptom score.

Changes in symptom scores are currently the most fea-
tured data in any clinical trial, but what constitutes a significant change may be viewed differently by patient, investigator,
gatekeeper or specialty physician, statistician, manufacturer,
and the FDA. In the original publication about the AUA
symptom score, the index was noted to decrease from a preoperative mean of 17.6 to 7.1 in 4 weeks after prostatectomy
and to 5 at 3 months. (Results of symptom scores can be reported in terms of absolute change or percent change from
the pretreatment value.) The higher the pretreatment symptom score, the lower the percent change of a given absolute
change. To compare symptom score changes, either absolute
numbers or percentages, between groups, the pretreatment
symptom scores clearly must be about the same. One obviously important question is, how much improvement in the
AUA symptom score is clinically significant? or, how much
of a change is sufficient in a patient to consider him "better"?
In a study by Barry and colleagues, subjects who rated themselves as being slightly improved had a mean decrease in
AUA symptom score of 3.1. Baseline scores strongly influence this relationship. Further inferences to be drawn from
this study would indicate that this group considers equal to or
greater than a symptom score improvement of 3 units a slight
improvement; equal to or greater than 6 units, moderate improvement; and equal to or 9 units, marked improvement.

B. Quality of Life Indices
Perhaps the softest, but maybe the most important, outcome
measure to gauge the overall effect of clinical BPH on an individual and the efficacy of treatment for BPH is quality of

life. Most men seek treatment for BPH because of the bothersome nature of their symptoms, which affect the quality of
their lives. Symptom severity does not necessarily correlate
with bothersomeness or quality of life indices. No consensus
has been reached as to the optimal tool to record and compare disease-specific quality of life measures in patient with
LUTS.

One question on the quality of life issue has been included
by the International Consensus Committee to assess the impact of symptoms on quality of life in clinical practice (see
Fig. 15-2). This has been a consistent recommendation since
the first WHO consultation on BPH in 1991. Although the
Committee recognized that this single question could not
capture the global impact of LUTS on quality of life, it was
believed that this might serve as a valuable starting point for
a physician–patient conversation concerning this issue.

XI. INDICATIONS FOR TREATMENT OF CLINICAL BPH

A.

Indications for surgery varied widely over time, and the current climate is much more conservative than existed 10 to 20
years ago. Certain absolute or near absolute indications exist; they are refractory or repeated urinary retention,
azotemia due to BPH, significant recurrent gross hematuria,
recurrent or residual infection due to BPH, bladder calculi, a
large residual urine, overflow incontinence, and large bladder diverticula due to BPH. All of these assume that the bladder is indeed contractile.

B.

Without an absolute or near absolute indication, or combinations of these, the bothersome nature of the symptomatology is generally what prompts the patient to request, or the
physician to suggest, treatment. Pathologic urodynamic
findings may certainly be influential as well. Once the option
of treatment is chosen, the risks and benefits of all applicable modalities must be discussed with the patient, and the patient must ultimately decide among these. General medical
status and comorbid conditions may significantly influence
this decision. In general, the more definitive the expectation
of a positive outcome is, the more invasive the procedure and
the greater the risk. The term "watchful waiting" has replaced "no treatment," and it is likely in the future that each
patient will be presented with a chart or other informational
medium that will describe each possible accepted treatment
in terms of the expected likelihood of improvement, the
magnitude of improvement, the likelihood of side effects (incontinence, impotence, retrograde ejaculation, and others),

the incidence of reoperation, and the incidence of death within 3 months of treatment.

XII. TREATMENT OF BPH
A.

The treatment options are summarized in Table 15-2. The natural history of prostatism determines the results that can be expected from watchful waiting. There are few studies

Table 15-2 Treatment Options for Benign Prostatic Hyperplasia

Watchful waiting (observation)
Pharmacologic
  Reducing prostate smooth muscle tone (the dynamic component)
    α-1 adrenergic antagonists
  Reducing prostate bulk (the static component primarily)
    Estrogen
    LHRH agonists/antagonists
    5-α-1 reductase inhibitors
    Antiandrogens
    Aromatase inhibitors
    Growth factor inhibitors (theoretical)
  Unknown
    Phytotherapy
    Other
Mechanical and Surgical
  Prostatic urethral stents
  Balloon dilation of the prostatic urethra
  Transurethral or transrectal hypothermia
  Transurethral thermotherapy
  Interstitial therapy
    Microwave thermotherapy (TUMT)
    Water induced thermotherapy
    Radiofrequency energy (TUNA)
    Laser energy
    High intensity focused ultrasound
    Ethanol injection
  Transurethral resection and incision by
    Laser (laser TURP, TUIBN-P)
    Electrosurgery (TURP, TUIBN-P)
    Electrovaporization (TUVP)
    Ultrasound aspiration
  Open prostatectomy

LHRH, leutinizing hormone releasing hormone; TUMT, transurethral microwave thermotherapy; TUNA, transurethral needle ablution; TURP, transurethral prostatectomy; TUIBN-P, transurethral incision bladder neck-prostate; TUVP, transurethral vaporization of prostate.

that actually describe the natural history of this condition, and only a few more that look at the long-term results of placebo treatment. It is clear that symptoms do tend to wax and wane and that a substantial number of men will have at least short-term stability or improvement of symptoms. The literature would suggest that, at least over a 5-year period, over 50 percent of patients are either improved or have exhibited no change on the basis of subjective criteria, and, even on the basis of objective criteria, 30 to 40 percent are stable or experience at least some improvement. Development of urodynamic parameters to predict those patients who will worsen is clearly paramount. The most commonly used, but not all, therapies are discussed.

B. Assessing the Results of Treatment

The outcome measures utilized to assess the results of treatment are seen in Table 15-3. Symptom scores and urodynamic parameters are most commonly used. Quality of life improvement and alteration of natural history are currently rarely utilized, an unfortunate state of affairs. It must be recognized, however, that different segments of the population will have different priorities and orientations and may draw different conclusions regarding relative value or efficacy from the same set of outcomes (Table 15-4).

C. Alpha-Adrenergic Antagonists

There are at least three α-1 adrenergic receptor subtypes in human tissues that have been identified by pharmacologic studies and receptor cloning. The current nomenclature recognizes α-1_A, α-1_B, and α-1_D. All three subtypes have been found in prostatic stromal tissue. The α-1_A receptor comprises 60 to 85 percent of the α-1 population. There is increasing evidence for an additional α-1 subtype with contractile properties but low prazosin affinity (α-1_L). Approximately 50 percent of total urethral pressure in patients

---

Table 15-3 Outcome Measures to Assess the Results of Treatment for Clinical Benign Prostatic Hyperplasia

Symptoms and symptom scores
Quality of life indices
Correction of undesirable sequelae (azotemia, e.g.)
Urodynamic Indices
Size (for bulk reducing therapy)
Alternation of natural history
Adverse effects
Cost and cost effectiveness

Table 15-4 Populations with Different Viewpoints on Evaluation of Outcomes Following Treatment

Patient
Family
Treater
Referrer
Friend
Manufacturer
Competitor
Person in the street
Agency for Health Care Policy and Research
Food and Drug Administration

with BPH is due to alpha receptor-moderated muscle tone. When discussing the treatment of BPH symptoms with alpha blockers, the extraprostatic actions of these drugs must be considered as well. Alpha receptors in the bladder base and proximal urethral smooth musculature affect urodynamic parameters, and receptors at the spinal cord and ganglionic level may do so as well. Alpha receptors in the vasculature and central nervous system may contribute to the potential side effects of these agents (hypotension, somnolence, fatigue, e.g.).

Alpha blockers for BPH treatment are classified according to the degree of α-1 receptor selectivity and by dosing requirements, the latter determined by serum half life. Phenoxybenzamine, a nonselective alpha blocker (blocks α-1 and α-2 receptors) was the first used to treat BPH. Prazosin was the next developed for use in the United States. It is a relatively selective α-1 blocker, but requires 3 times daily dosing. Terazosin and doxazosin are relatively selective α-1 blockers, with half lives that permit once daily dosing. All of the classic α-1 blockers appear to be very similar in terms of clinical efficacy and safety. Of the three molecularly cloned subtypes of the α-1 receptor, the α-1_A seems responsible for prostate smooth muscle tension. Whether superselective blockers for the α-1_A subtype (tamsulosin has some selectivity for the α-1_A receptor) will prove to be more effective for treatment with fewer vascular and central side effects is as yet not entirely clear. The maximal response to alpha blockade occurs within 2 weeks of dose escalation. Potential side effects include orthostatic hypotension (said to occur primarily in patients with hypertension), dizziness, fatigue, nasal stuffiness, and ejaculatory disturbances. Tamsulosin, perhaps because of the selectivity profile, may not cause somnolence or hypotension in excess of placebo. Mean treatment differences from placebo for alpha blockade therapy generally range from $+1.3$ to $+3.5$ mL/sec for peak flow (a 20 to 30 percent increase) and from -1.3 to -4.7 for symptom score (a 20 to 50 percent improvement, depending on the specific scoring system utilized and the pretreatment value).

D. 5-α Reductase Inhibitors

Finasteride is a competitive selective inhibitor of type II 5-α reductase. It does not reduce DHT levels to castrate values because circulating testosterone is still converted to DHT by type I 5-α reductase, which exists in skin and liver. It reduces prostatic DHT by 80 to 90 percent. It does not lower plasma testosterone. The multicenter double blind placebo studies to support the use of finasteride can be briefly summarized as follows. Finasteride reduces prostate volume approximately 20 percent; the overall treatment related improvement in symptom score varies from 0.6 units to 2.2 units. Peak flow rate improvement ranges from 0.2 to 1.8 mL/sec. These are statistically significant (with 5 mg dose) but modest numerically when compared to placebo. Finasteride reduces group mean serum PSA levels by approximately 50 percent but the effect on individual levels is highly variable. Approximately 12 percent of patients develop sexual side effects including decreased libido (3.4 to 4.7 percent), ejaculatory disorder (2.7 percent), and impotence (1.7 to 3.7 percent). The drug does seem to be effective in the management of BPH-related hematuria. Insofar as its effects on BPH associated voiding dysfunction are concerned, the drug is optimally effective in men with prostate volumes over 40 to 50 mL.

Does finasteride alter the natural history of BPH? Recent studies would suggest an advantage in this regard, using the outcome measures of acute urinary retention and the need for surgical intervention. Treatment with finasteride for up to 2 years compared to placebo resulted in a 75 percent reduction of acute urinary retention and an approximately one-third reduction in the need for surgical intervention in patients with "moderate" BPH. The actual numerical differences were small, however, much less impressive than the percentages. Although, this is one of the very few studies that attempts to examine this parameter.

Is combination therapy (alpha blocker plus finasteride) more effective than either alone? A Veterans Administration Cooperative Study by Lepor compared placebo, finasteride, terazosin, and finasteride plus terazosin. The mean group differences for all patients between finasteride and placebo were not statistically significant for AUA symptom index, symptom problem index, BPH impact index, and peak flow rate. The changes for terazosin were significant versus placebo and versus finasteride. The group mean differences between combination therapy and terazosin for all measures other than prostate volume were significantly in favor of terazosin. The volume decrease was 20 percent in the finasteride and combination groups. The AUA symptom index components were 2.6 units for placebo, 3.2 for finasteride, 6.6 for terazosin, and 6.2 for the combination. Finasteride supporters argue that the apparent lack of efficacy in this study was due to a relatively small mean prostate volume in the population studied. For the men with volumes larger than 50 mL, there was a mean increase in Q_{MAX} of 2.5 mL/sec and a mean decrease in AUA SS of 2.9, both significantly different from those of comparable men in the placebo group.

E. Balloon Dilation

Variable balloon lengths and diameters are available, and dilatation was carried out over 5 to 20 min with a pressure of 2 to 5 atmospheres. Treatment was performed under local or short general anesthesia and the balloon was positioned endoscopically, radiologically, ultrasonographically, or by rectal palpation. Improvement rates of 84 to 14.3 percent were reported. Lepor, using a sham control arm, concluded that improvement after balloon dilation was no greater than that after simple cystoscopy. This treatment has fallen out of favor.

F. Prostatic Urethral Stents

A bewildering array of prostatic urethral stents has become available. Many have been withdrawn from use. These are best implanted by endoscopic control. The stents may be biodegradable, temporary, or permanent. The optimal result would be a stent completely covered by urothelium, making encrustation impossible. Alleviation of voiding symptoms has periodically been reported in up to 85 percent of patients in the short term, with corresponding improvement in objective parameters as well. Biodegradable or temporary stents may be used to obviate retention resulting from various forms of BPH treatment. Currently, stents are thought to provide an alternative for patients for short-term management or for long-term management in patients unfit for surgical relief and who would otherwise have an indwelling Foley catheter. Removal of the stent can be difficult, and there is concern regarding potential long-term results and interference with subsequent procedures, if required. The consensus of the International Consultation on BPH is that the absence of randomized controlled clinical trials and cost effectiveness studies makes it difficult to offer recommendations for this mode of treatment.

G. Resection and Modalities Producing Vaporization or/and Coagulation Necrosis

Traditional electrocautery, laser, microwave, and radiofrequency energy can be utilized to resect, vaporize, or cause coagulation necrosis of prostatic tissue. At temperatures lower than 45°C, coagulation necrosis of normal tissue does not occur. Irreversible cellular damage begins to occur above 45°C. Coagulation can take up to an hour to occur at temperatures minimally above this level. At 60°C to 100°C, coagulation is rapid and at 100°C is virtually instantaneous. At temperatures higher than 100°C, tissue vaporization is produced.

H. Microwave Thermotherapy

This transurethral modality uses microwave energy to produce temperatures of 45°C to 60°C in the transitional zone of the prostate, resulting in coagulation necrosis occurring over an hour or so, the usual duration of treatment. The urethral urothelium is cooled via a "jacket" around the catheter, and the rectal temperature is continuously monitored. Variables include the microwave frequency and intensity and the shape and size of the microwave antenna. Temperatures of up to 60°C to 75°C have been recorded within the prostate. Necrosis is produced 15 to 20 mm from the urethra, with surrounding edema. Representative results include an increase in Q_{MAX} from 8 to 12 mL/sec, a decrease in AUASS from 22 to 12 and 17.5 to 9. Minimal erectile dysfunction, stricture, and incontinence have been reported. Mild ejaculation problems have been reported in 0 to 44 percent of treated patients. A higher power higher energy program (Prostatron 2.5 software) has resulted in Q_{MAX} increases of 9 to 15 mL/sec and AUASS decreases from 22 to 8.

I. Laser Usage

The tissue effects of laser energy are produced by the virtually instantaneous attainment of temperatures higher than 60°C to create coagulation necrosis and above 100°C to create vaporization. The types of laser utilized for clinical BPH treatment include:

1. Neodynium yytrium garnet (Nd:YAG). This is generally applied transurethrally through contact or noncontact fibers. At low power density, this laser penetrates deeply and produces coagulation necrosis. At higher energy levels, vaporization and coagulation occur. Interstitial fibers can also be placed to produce coagulation necrosis with

interstitial application; post procedure, the lesions result in secondary atrophy and regression of the prostatic "lobes." Internal scarring with retraction of the periurethral tissue also probably occurs.

2. Semiconductor diode. This can be used with either a free beam low energy technique or an interstitial technique.

3. Potassium titanyl phosphate laser (KTP). This uses a free beam treatment with high energy density to create vaporization without concurrent deep coagulation.

4. Pulsed holmiium:YAG. This causes thermomechanical vaporization and can be used as a cutting tool.

With the use of a transurethral right angle laser fiber, representative values for results include an increase in Q_{MAX} from 8 to 16 mL/sec and a decrease in AUASS from 21.3 to 7. There seems to be little difference in the results of coagulation versus vaporization, except for a slight advantage in Q_{MAX} improvement at 12 months following vaporization. In one trial comparing interstitial laser therapy to TURP, Q_{MAX} increased from 9 to 18 mL/sec following laser and from 9 to 25 mL/sec following TURP.

Advocates of laser therapy tout as advantages over electrosurgical TUR a shorter surgery, fewer complications including sexual dysfunction and stricture, a quicker recovery, and equivalent results. There is less bleeding, and this is definitely an advantage in anticoagulated patients. Less enthusiastic observers cite as disadvantages a lack of tissue for pathologic analysis (except for the Ho:YAG laser), a delayed time to voiding, postoperative filling and storage symptoms for up to 2 to 3 months, and a lower Q_{MAX} improvement.

J. Needle Electrode Delivered Radiofrequency

Interstitial placement of a radiofrequency delivery electrode creates tissue heating to the resistance to the current as it flow from an active electrode through the tissue to an indifferent electrode. Transurethral needle ablation TUNA creates temperatures of 60°C to 100°C during treatment times of 5 to 7 min to produce zones of coagulation necrosis. Representative results include Q_{MAX} changes from 7.8 to 14.4 and 8.8 to 15.5 mL/sec and AUASS changes from 24 to 11, 22 to 9, and 20 to 5.4. Although proponents cite no catheter requirement afterward as an advantage, 20 to 40 percent of patients experience urinary retention lasting 2 to 3 days. Hematuria is reported as minor. Sexual dysfunction and stricture are rare.

K. Electrosurgical Resection and Vaporization

This technique uses a resection loop and electrosurgical generator capable of delivering cutting and coagulating current.

The lower voltage continuous cutting wave form instanta-
neously vaporizes a path through the tissue and does not result in significant coagulation. The coagulation current consists of short segments of higher voltage lower current
energy, resulting in deeper penetrative heating and hemostasis. New resection loops have been developed that can be
used at higher cutting wattages to create increased hemostasis. For electrovaporization, a higher monopolar cutting
wattage is used to vaporize surface tissue and cause simultaneous coagulation beneath. The dessicated base, however, is
less susceptible to further vaporization.

TURP remains the standard for comparison for treatment.
The risk/benefit ratio of TURP was held up to significant
scrutiny by articles appearing in 1987 to 1989 that cited a
mortality rate of 2.5 percent within 90 days after surgery and
a requirement for reresection of about 2 percent per year or
16 percent at 8 years when compared with open prostatectomy. The relative risk of death was 1.45 at up to 5 years after TURP and the risk of reoperation was approximately
double. Since that time, a number of individuals have cited
significant problems with these data because of comorbidity
issues and because other populations have failed to confirm
these problems as sequelae of electrosurgical TURP.

L. Transurethral Vaporization (TUVP) of the Prostate

This technique uses familiar electrosurgical technology and
TURP-like maneuvers—a great advantage, because the
learning curve is short. Representative results include increases of Q_{MAX} from 9 to 24.3 mL/sec and 7.4 to 17 mL/sec
and decreases in AUASS from 24 to 8 and 23 to 5. Those
most familiar with the technique emphasize that the ease and
results are highly dependent on the generator utilized. As advantages, they cite decreased blood loss, decreased catheter
time, and decreased hospital stay. The operative time is
longer, however, and the technique is most applicable to
prostates weighing less than 50 g. Sexual side effects and incontinence rates are similar to those following TURP. Electrode design modifications are seemingly continuous, the
goal being to optimize tissue energy delivery with increased
vaporization efficiency.

**M. Electrosurgical Incision of the Bladder Neck and
Prostate (TUIBN-P)**

This transurethral technique is most useful in those patients
with a smaller prostate (weighing 30 g or less). It is quicker,
technically easier, and associated with less morbidity than
TURP. It is a definitely underutilized technique. In suitable
candidates, the improvement in Q_{MAX} is approximately the

same as with TURP (global improvement rates slightly less). The incidence of reported complications is certainly lower: incontinence 0 to 1 percent; impotence 0 to 4 percent; retrograde ejaculation 15 to 40 percent; and bladder neck contracture 1 percent. Based on historical statistics, nearly 80 percent of patients undergoing TURP in the United States have less than 30 g of tissue resected.

N. High Intensity Focused Ultrasound (HIFU)

This is a form of interstitial thermal ablation achieved by heating tissue to temperatures above 70°C. HIFU achieves this by directing ultrasonic energy with a transrectal probe. The technique involves creating an area of coagulation necrosis resulting from many overlapping focal lesions. Limited and selective experience has reported Q_{MAX} increases from 6.4 to 12.8 and 9.2 to 13.7 mL/sec along with AUASS decreases from 18 to 6.3, 20.3 to 9.6, and 26 to 14. Complications have included urinary retention, infection, and epididymitis. Clinical trials are ongoing.

O. Water-Induced Thermotherapy

This involves circulating 60°C water through a transurethral intraprostatic balloon and reportedly requires no anesthesia. Initial trials report a 71 percent increase in Q_{MAX} and a 24 to 11 reduction in AUASS. Clinical trials are ongoing.

P. Ethanol Interstitial Injection

This involves the transurethral injection of ethanol into the prostate to create an ovoid space of necrosis. Clinical trials are planned.

Q.

It is clear that the age of frequent surgery for clinical BPH is over. More data over longer periods of follow-up are necessary to fully describe the natural history, advantages, and disadvantages of the other methods of therapy, including watchful waiting. In the future, patients will likely be presented with a checklist of the advantages and disadvantages of each type of management. The number of surgical and mechanical therapies dictates, however, that no one practitioner will have expertise with all of these, but rather each will have his or her "favorites," hopefully based on sound reasoning and results. Patients with minimal to moderate symptoms and bother, who do not have an absolute indication for surgery, will doubtless choose less invasive therapy, at least initially. Finally, it remains to be seen how much, if anything, is "lost" by utilizing those surgical mechanical methods that do not yield tissue for pathologic analysis because prior to the PSA era, 10 to 12 percent of prostatectomy specimens were found to contain unsuspected cancer. Although this is probably less frequent since the advent of widespread PSA testing, it remains to be seen whether any noticeable delays in the diagnosis of cancer occur and, if so, whether outcome is adversely influenced.

BIBLIOGRAPHY

Abrams P: In support of pressure-flow studies for evaluating men with lower urinary tract symptoms. *Urology* 44:153–155, 1994.

Ball AJ, Fenely RCL, Abrams PH: The natural history of untreated "prostatism." *Br J Urol* 53:613–616, 1981.

Barry MJ: Epidemiology of benign prostatic hyperplasia. *AUA Update Series* 16:274–279, 1997.

Barry MJ, Fowler FJ, Bin L, et al: The natural history of patients with benign prostatic hyperplasia as diagnosed by North American urologists. *J Urol* 157:10–15, 1997.

Barry MJ, Fowler FJ, Jr., O'Leary MP, and the Measurement Committee of the AUA: The American Urological Association symptom index for benign prostatic hyperplasia. *J Urol* 148:1549–1557, 1992.

Barry MJ, Williford WO, Chang Y, et al: Benign prostatic hyperplasia specific health status measures in clinical research: How much change in the AUA symptom index and the BPH impact index is perceptible to patients? *J Urol* 154:1770–1774, 1995.

Blaivas J: The bladder is an unreliable witness. *Neurourol Urodyn* 15:443–445, 1996.

Denis L, Griffiths K, Khoury S, et al, eds. 4th *International Consultation on Benign Prostatic Hyperplasia (BPH).* Plymouth, United Kingdom, Plymbridge Distributors, Ltd., 1998.

   Chapter 3: Regulation of prostatic growth. Cockett ATK, Coffey D, DiSant Agnese A, et al.

   Chapter 5: Initial evaluation of LUTS. Artibani W, Correa R, Desgranchamps F, et al.

   Chapter 6: Quantification of symptoms, quality of life and sexuality. Adolfsson J, Barry M, Batista JE, et al.

   Chapter 7: The urodynamics of LUTS. Abrams P, Buzelin JM, Griffiths D, et al.

   Chapter 10: Interventional therapy. Altwein J, Baba S, Blute M, et al.

   Chapter 11: Endocrine treatment. Akaza H, Bartsch G, Calais daSilva F, et al.

   Chapter 12: Alpha-blocker therapy. AldoBono V, Andersson KE, Chapple C, et al.

   Chapter 15: BPH 1997—New treatment strategy. ElHilali M, Kirby R, McConnell J.

Lepor H, Williford WO, Barry MJ, et al: The efficacy of terazosin, finasteride, or both in BPH. *N Engl J Med* 335:533–539, 1996.

McConnell J: Why pressure flow studies should be optional and not mandatory for evaluating men with benign prostatic hyperplasia. *Urology* 44:156–158, 1994.

McConnell JD, Barry MJ, Bruskewitz R, et al: Benign prostatic hyperplasia: Diagnosis and treatment. *Clinical Practice Guideline,* no. 8, AHCPR publication No. 94-0582, Rockville, Md., Agency for Health Care Policy Research, Public Health Service, US Dept. Of Health and Human Services, 1994.

Walsh PC, Retik AB, Vaughan ED Jr., Wein AJ, eds: Campbell's Urology, 7th ed. Philadelphia, Saunders Company, 1998.

> Chapter 45: The molecular biology, endocrinology, and physiology of the prostate and seminal vesicles. Partin AW, Coffey DS.
>
> Chapter 46: Epidemiology, etiology, pathophysiology, and diagnosis of benign prostatic hyperplasia. McConnell JD.
>
> Chapter 47: Natural history, evaluation, and nonsurgical management of benign prostatic hyperplasia. Lepor H.
>
> Chapter 48: Minimally invasive treatment of benign prostatic hyperplasia. McCullough DL.
>
> Chapter 49: Transurethral surgery. Mebust WK.

Wasson JH, Reda DJ, Bruskewitz RC, et al: A comparison of transurethral surgery with watchful waiting for moderate symptoms of BPH. *N Engl J Med* 332:75–79, 1995.

Wein AJ: Criteria for assessing outcome following intervention for benign prostatic hyperplasia. In: Lepor H, ed. *Prostatic Diseases.* Philadelpha, Saunders, 1999, pp 210–231.

SELF-ASSESSMENT QUESTIONS

1. Discuss the varying definitions of BPH (microscopic, macroscopic, clinical) and the epidemiology of each.

2. Discuss the gross anatomy of the prostate as it relates to the origin of BPH and cancer.

3. Discuss the various theories of the initiation and maintenance of prostatic growth.

4. Discuss the concept of the dynamic and static component of prostatic urethral resistance and how these relate to the pharmacologic therapy of clinical BPH.

5. Discuss the origin and meaning of the term LUTS, the subdivisions of LUTS, and their potential etiologies.

6. Discuss the typical urodynamic changes seen in moderate to severe bladder outlet obstruction secondary to BPH.

7. Discuss the outcome measures for evaluating the efficacy of therapy for clinical BPH and their relative importance.

8. Discuss the relevant points related to the natural history of clinical BPH.

9. Discuss the pharmacologic therapy of clinical BPH, including expected changes in symptom scores and flowmetry.

10. Discuss ablative (resection, vaporization) and heat therapies for clinical BPH, including expected changes in symptom scores and flowmetry.

11. Formulate an algorithm for use by primary healthcare providers for the management of male patients with LUTS, with indications for specialist referral.

CHAPTER 16

Renal Physiology: Acute and Chronic Renal Failure

Roy D. Bloom
Robert A. Grossman

I. NORMAL RENAL ANATOMY AND PHYSIOLOGY

A. Anatomy

Each kidney contains about 600,000 nephrons. The nephron consists of a glomerulus with a capillary tuft that serves as a filter; each glomerulus is attached to a tubule that is unique for that glomerulus until the level of the collecting duct, where tubules from many glomeruli merge. The filtrate is extensively acted upon by the epithelial cells of the tubule.

B. Physiology

The kidneys receive about 20 percent of the resting cardiac output or about 1 L/min of blood. With a hematocrit of 40 percent, the renal *plasma* flow is about 600 mL/min. Normally, 20 percent of this plasma is filtered at the glomeruli, giving a glomerular filtration rate (GFR) of 120 mL/min or about 170 L/day. The filtrate is acted upon by the renal tubules, where over 99 percent is reabsorbed, leaving a final urine output of 1.0 to 1.5 L/day. The tubule consists of three parts.

1. *The proximal tubule.* Here, 70 percent of the filtrate is absorbed isosmotically (i.e., without substantial changes in the sodium or potassium concentrations or in the fluid pH.

2. *The loop of Henle.* In this region, 20 percent of the filtered sodium chloride is removed. Solute is removed in greater amounts than water so that filtrate leaving the loop is *hypo-osmolar* compared with plasma. The solute so removed is concentrated in the medulla by a countercurrent mechanism that renders the medulla *hyperosmolar* to plasma. This medullary hypertonicity provides the osmotic driving force needed to concentrate the final urine as it flows down the collecting duct.

3. *The distal convoluted tubule and collecting ducts.* Here, the final composition of the urine is attained. Water may be absorbed from the filtrate through the action of vasopressin, yielding a urine with an osmolality as great as 4 times that of plasma. Conversely, in the absence of vasopressin and with continued removal of solute, the urine may be diluted to an osmolality one fourth that of plasma. Potassium and hydrogen ions are actively and passively secreted; the final adjustment of sodium excretion is performed.

C. Clearance

If there were a substance s present in the blood at a stable level, freely filtered at the glomerulus, and neither absorbed nor secreted by the tubular cells, such a substance could be used to estimate the GFR by the following formula.

$$\text{GFR} \times P_s = U_s \times V \text{ (urine flow rate)}$$

or

The amount of s filtered $=$ the amount of s excreted

Rearranging the formula gives:

$$\text{GFR} = \frac{U_s \times V}{P_s}$$

This is the clearance equation; it can be used not only to estimate the GFR but also to assess the manner in which the kidney handles a multitude of substances.

1. *Clearance.* The theoretical amount of plasma from which a substance is completely removed by the action of the kidney in a defined period of time. It is usually expressed in milliliters per minute. Creatinine, for practical purposes, has all the characteristics of s mentioned in the previous equation. The creatinine clearance (C_{cr}) is used clinically to measure GFR.

$$C_{cr} = \frac{U_{cr}(\text{mg/dL}) \times V\,(\text{ml/min})}{P_{cr}(\text{mg/dL})}$$

A more practical method for calculating creatinine clearance, which is valid *only* for 24-hour collections follows.

$$C_{cr} = \frac{\text{24-hour urinary creatinine in grams} \times 70}{\text{serum creatinine level in milligrams per deciliter}}$$

The number 70 is not a "fudge factor"; it results from factoring of all the units used.

D. Fractional Excretion

Many substances are acted upon by the renal tubular cells. Substances that are predominately secreted by the tubular cells may have a clearance greater than C_{cr}; many drugs are handled in this manner. Conversely, substances that are substantially reabsorbed by the renal tubules may have a clearance much lower than C_{cr}. The renal handling of sodium is an example of the latter. At a GFR of 120 mL/min and a serum sodium concentration of 140 mEq/L, the normal kidneys filter about 24,000 mEq of sodium daily. Of this amount, only 120 to 240 mEq are excreted in the urine, for a fractional excretion of 0.5 to 1.0 percent. The fractional excretion of a substance is the amount of the substance excreted compared with the amount filtered expressed as percent. Clinically, the fractional excretion of a substance is calculated by dividing the clearance of the substance by the clearance of creatinine (the amount excreted/amount filtered) converted to percentage. The fractional excretion of sodium (FE_{Na}) is calculated as follows.

$$FE_{Na} = (C_{Na}/C_{Cr}) \times 100$$

Writing out the expression fully:

$$FE_{Na} = \frac{U_{Na}V/P_{Na}}{U_{Cr}V/P_{Cr}}$$

In the preceding equation, the Vs cancel, yielding:

$$FE_{Na} = \frac{U_{Na} \times P_{Cr}}{U_{Cr} \times P_{Na}} \times 100$$

Because the Vs cancel, a fractional excretion can be performed on any volume of urine; a 24-hour collection is not necessary. The clinical use of the FE_{Na} will be explained later.

E. Concentration, Dilution, and Oliguria

Through the countercurrent mechanism, the activity of the loop of Henle, and the action of vasopressin, the urine in a normal person can be concentrated to an osmolality of 1200 mOsm/kg H_2O (four times that of plasma). In the opposite direction, urine can be diluted to about 75 mOsm/kg H_2O, one fourth that of plasma. An adult eating a normal diet is obligated to excrete about 500 mOsm of solute per day;

half of this is sodium, potassium, and their anions, the other half is urea, the end-product of protein catabolism. If these 500 mOsm can be excreted in a urine concentrated to 1200 mOsm/kg H_2O, it will require a urine volume of slightly greater than 400 mL. By this definition, a urine volume of less than 400 mL/day is considered *oliguria*. However, in almost any disease state, the kidneys lose concentrating ability; additionally, in catabolic states, the obligatory solute load may far exceed 500 mOsm/day. Both of these conditions increase the volume of urine required. Nevertheless, the convention stands: a urine volume of less than 400 mL/day is considered oliguria.

II. ACUTE RENAL FAILURE (ARF)

ARF may be defined as a sudden deterioration of renal function resulting in the inability of the kidney to regulate fluid and solute balance. There is a rapid decline in glomerular filtration rate that is accompanied by an increase in serum creatinine level of at least 0.5 to 1.0 mg/dL. ARF is associated with a substantial increase in morbidity and mortality; it most commonly occurs in the in-hospital setting. Because about five percent of hospitalized patients develop ARF, early recognition and prompt intervention is essential.

ARF can be subclassified into three distinct clinical syndromes: (1) *Prerenal azotemia,* a reversible physiologic response to renal hypoperfusion where renal integrity is maintained; (2) *postrenal azotemia or obstructive uropathy,* a condition where glomerular filtration rate falls as a consequence of physical obstruction of urinary outflow; and (3) *acute intrinsic renal failure,* where ARF results from diseases of the renal parenchyma. A review of the history, physical examination, urinalysis, and urine and serum chemistry levels will commonly identify the syndrome that is implicated in the development of ARF.

A. Prerenal Azotemia

1. *Pathophysiology.* In prerenal azotemia (Table 16-1), the structure and function of the kidneys are normal but perfusion is poor because of decreased plasma volume or an "ineffective" plasma volume caused by vasodilitation or depressed plasma protein levels. Alternatively, the kidneys may be poorly perfused because of poor contractility of the heart. A reduction of true or "effective" blood volume stimulates neural and hormonal responses from cardiac and arterial baroreceptors. These responses include activation of the sympathetic nervous system, the renin–angiotensin–aldosterone axis, and the secretion of

Table 16-1 Cause of Prerenal Azotemia

Volume Depletion	Volume Shifts
Hemorrhage	Third space losses
Gastrointestinal losses	Vasodilating drugs
Vomiting	Early gram-negative sepsis
Diarrhea	
Renal losses	Volume Expansion
Excessive diuretics	Congestive heart failure
Addison's disease	Nephrotic syndrome
Salt-losing nephritis	Cirrhosis with ascites
Burns	Hepato-renal syndrome
Heat prostration	

vasopressin. The effector limb of these responses promote renal salt and water retention in an effort to preserve and restore the central circulation. Additionally, generalized vasoconstriction occurs, including within the renal vasculature, which results in a reduction of glomerular filtration rate. Because the kidneys are inherently normal, it would be expected that the urine is concentrated with a low sodium concentration and low FE_{Na}. The microscopic sediment should be benign.

2. History
  a. Fluid losses—vomiting or diarrhea are usually evident however, excessive use of diuretics or high insensible losses may be more subtle.
  b. Recent surgery or fevers.
  c. Drug history—many combination blood pressure medications contain thiazide diuretics.
  d. The degree of congestive heart failure or cirrhosis necessary to cause pre-renal azotemia is usually obvious in the uncomplicated patient.

3. Physical examination
  a. Low or relatively low blood pressure.
  b. Decreased skin turgor—the inner aspect of the thigh is a good place to check.
  c. Dry mouth or axillae.
  d. Orthostatic changes in pulse or blood pressure. This is an overly emphasized physical finding; substantial volume depletion may exist without orthostatic changes.
  e. The edematous states are usually self-evident.
  f. In complicated cases, measurement of central pressure and/or cardiac output may be necessary to define pre-renal azotemia.

4. Laboratory data (Table 16-2)
   a. Urinary concentration of sodium less than 20 mEq/L *prior to the administration of diuretics.*
   b. FE_{Na} less than 1 percent, again in the absence of diuretics.
   c. Urine osmolality greater than 130 percent of plasma osmolality.
   d. Little or no proteinuria.
   e. Benign microscopic urinary sediment.
   f. BUN:creatinine ratio often far greater than 20.
5. Therapy
   a. With volume depletion or shifts, expand the plasma volume with *isotonic* fluids (i.e. 0.9% saline, lactated Ringer's solution, albumin solutions, or blood).
   b. In edematous states, correct the underlying condition, if possible.
6. *Hepatorenal syndrome.* In the face of severe and worsening hepatic disease, renal failure is common and behaves as a pre-renal condition. It is thought to be a toxic phenomenon due to one or more substances that are not cleared by the diseased liver; however, the toxin(s) responsible have not been identified; endothelin-1, a potent vasoconstrictor has been implicated. It has been suggested that the kidneys may be responding in a physiologic manner to an abnormality of the circulatory system. Patients with hepatorenal syndrome exhibit severe peripheral vasodilitation, with a high cardiac output and low systemic vascular resistance. The kidneys respond to the low systemic pressure with oliguria, a decreased GFR, and an extremely low U_{Na}. The condition is uniformly fatal unless the liver recovers or a liver transplant is performed.

B. **Obstructive Uropathy or Postrenal Azotemia** (Table 16-3)
   1. *Pathophysiology.* Urinary tract obstruction accounts for less than 5 percent of cases of ARF. In obstructive uropathy, there is not an inflammatory process within the kidney; instead, there is increased back-pressure on the renal tubules causing tubular dysfunction. Almost all tubular functions are compromised: concentration and dilution of the urine, reabsorption of sodium and water, and secretion of potassium and hydrogen ions. Therefore, the urine produced is usually isotonic to plasma and has a high urinary sodium level and FE_{Na}. The microscopic sediment is usually benign unless infection has occurred.
   2. History
      a. The history is of little value, particularly when the site of obstruction is above the bladder neck. The process

Table 16-2 Urinalysis in Acute Renal Failure

	PRERENAL	AGN	ATN	OBSTRUCTION
Urine osmolality (mOsm/Kg H_2O)	> 350	> 350	< 350	< 350
Urine sodium level mEq/L	< 30	< 30	> 30	> 30
Qualitative urine protein	Negative-trace	3+ to 4+	Trace to 2+	Negative to trace
Urine microscopic sediment	Normal	Red cells and red cell casts	"Dirty"[a]	Normal
Fractional excretion of sodium	< 1%	< 1%	> 1%	> 1%

AGN, acute glomerulonephritis; ATN, acute tubular necrosis.

[a]Sediment contains red cells, white cells, renal tubular cells, and many types of casts including "broad" casts.

Table 16-3 Causes of Obstructive Uropathy

Bladder outlet
  Prostatic hyperplasia or carcinoma
  Uterine or cervical cancer
Bilateral ureteral obstruction
  Tumor invasion
  Retroperitoneal fibrosis
  Calculi
  Surgical accident
Renal pelvic or intrarenal obstruction
  Staghorn or other calculi
  Papillary necrosis
  Acute uric acid nephropathy (tumor lysis)
  Drugs, (e.g., acyclovir)

of obstruction of ureters is often asynchronous; one kidney is lost silently, then the process affects the opposite ureter and azotemia occurs.

  b. Bladder outlet obstruction—hesitancy, dribbling, frequency of urination, and decrease in the urinary stream.

  c. Obstruction above the bladder—the only historical fact occasionally found, is a change in voiding pattern. Remember, a partially obstructed kidney is *polyuric*; new nocturia and frequency may be noted. Rarely, a pattern of complete anuria alternating with polyuria may be found.

3. Physical examination

  a. Bladder outlet obstruction—palpable bladder after voiding; enlarged prostate on rectal examination.

  b. Obstruction above the bladder usually cannot be determined by physical examination.

4. Laboratory data

  a. *Urinalysis* (see Table 16-2.) The urine is usually bland microscopically, with little or no protein present. Because of tubular defects, it is usually isosmolar with plasma. It contains a high sodium concentration with a high FE_{Na}, often higher than 3 percent.

  b. *Diagnosis.* Bladder outlet obstruction can often be determined by the placement of a Foley catheter or the use of the now widely available ultrasonic "bladder scanners." Obstruction above the bladder is almost exclusively a radiologic diagnosis.

    1. Ultrasound examination
    2. Radionuclide scanning

    3. Computerized tomography
    4. Intravenous urography
    5. Magnetic resonance imaging
    6. Treatment
       a. Mechanical relief of obstruction
          1. Foley catheterization
          2. Percutaneous nephrostomy placement
          3. Retrograde ureteral catheterization
       b. Postobstructive diuresis
          i. Following relief of the obstruction, there may be a diuresis of several liters per day. The diuresis is due to the tubular defects mentioned above; in addition, at the time of the relief of the obstruction, the patient is often edematous, hypertensive, and has a high BUN level, all of which enhance the diuresis. The urine produced may be grossly bloody. During high pressure obstruction, small blood vessels within the collecting system may be torn. However, the high pressure itself causes tampanode of these vessels. With relief of obstruction (and pressure), bleeding occurs.
          ii. The urine usually contains 70 to 100 mEq of sodium and its anion plus only a small amount of potassium salts. Replace the urine with 0.45% saline with or without dextrose. Potassium chloride and sodium bicarbonate may be added to the intravenous solutions depending on the serum levels of the patient and measured urinary losses.
          iii. If the patient is edematous and/or hypertensive at the start of the diuresis, do not replace the full urine output until the patient has a near normal extracellular fluid volume; then replace the urine output fully until the BUN and creatinine levels become normal or reach a plateau. At that point, replace less than urine output so that urine flow is not being driven by the replacement fluids.

C. Acute Intrinsic Renal Failure (Table 16-4)
    1. Acute tubular necrosis (ATN)
       a. ATN causes more acute intrinsic renal failure than all of the other reasons combined and is potentially reversible. ATN usually occurs as a consequence of isch-emic or

Table 16-4 Causes of Acute Intrinsic Renal Failure

Acute tubular necrosis
  Ischemic injury (see Table 16-1)
  Toxic injury
    Endogenous toxins
      Heme pigments
      Bacterial endotoxins
    Exogenous toxins
      Aminoglycoside antibiotics
      Radiographic contrast dyes
      Ethylene glycol
      Heavy metals
      Organic solvents
      Herbicides and insecticides
Drug-induced interstitial nephritis
  Penicillins and cephalosporins
  Nonsteroidal anti-inflammatory drugs
Sulfonamides including diuretics
Cimetidine and other H_2 blockers
Allopurinol
Rifampin
Ciprofloxacin and other quinolones
Acute glomerulonephritis
  Isolated
    Post-streptococcal
    Idiopathic
  In systemic disease
    Lupus
    Abnormal proteins (cryo- or macroglobulins)
    Chronic bacteremia (SBE)
  Microvascular disease
    Vasculitis
    Malignant hypertension
    Scleroderma
Large Vessel Occlusion
    Atherosclerosis
    Renal artery or vein thrombosis in hypercoagulable states
    Tumor invasion
    Trauma
    Renal artery embolism

nephrotoxic injury. In contrast to prerenal azotemia, the ischemic injury does not immediately reverse with restoration of the circulation. Extreme ischemic injury can cause bilateral cortical necrosis which, by definition, is not reversible.

b. Pathophysiology

   i. The intimate mechanism causing and maintaining ATN remains a mystery although it has been studied for 50 years. Four theories have been proposed, no one of which entirely fits all the available data.

     1. Restriction of blood flow to filtering glomeruli at a local or regional level within the kidney. The mechanism may be by means of tubuloglomerular feedback whereby decreased solute delivery to the distal nephron results in constriction of the afferent glomerular arteriole and consequently, a reduction in glomerular filtration rate and renal blood flow.

     2. Decreased permeability, following injury, of the filtering basement membranes of the glomeruli.

     3. Tubular plugging with a mixture of necrotic cellular debris and protein.

     4. Disruption of the renal tubules and their basement membranes allowing glomerular filtrate to pass directly back into the blood stream. (Backleak Theory)

   ii. *Inciting events for ATN.* The event causing ATN may be ischemic, as listed in Table 16-1, or toxic, as shown in Table 16-4. Why an ischemic event that causes prerenal azotemia in one individual leads to ATN in another remains a mystery. There are several conditions that seem to predispose to the development of ATN of either toxic or ischemic cause including advanced age, pre-existing renal disease, hypovolemia, and recent administration of a nephrotoxic agent.

   iii. *Oliguric versus nonoliguric ATN.* With the inciting event, either toxic or ischemic, both GFR and renal blood flow fall dramatically to a few percent of normal. Over the next several hours, renal blood flow returns to 20 to 30 percent of normal but GFR remains severely depressed. The patient may be oliguric or nonoliguric with a urine output as great as a few liters per day. For example, if GFR falls to 4 mL/min and fractional excretion is 50 percent of that, filtered urine output will be 2 mL/min or almost 3 liters per day. With the same GFR, if fractional excretion of urine is 5 percent, urine output will be about 300 mL/day. In either case, the GFR is extremely low yet urine outputs differ dramatically. The mechanism whereby the urine output

differs with the same GFR is not clear; nevertheless, the nonoliguric patient seems to have a better
prognosis than the oliguric patient. The nonoliguric patient is less likely to develop problems with
fluid overload and electrolyte imbalance, particularly hyperkalemia.

c. *History.* A careful history will uncover an inciting
event for ATN in about 70 percent of patients, as listed
in Tables 16-1 and 16-4. However, in about 30 percent
of cases, no cause can be found.

d. *Physical examination.* There are no specific physical
findings in ATN. The examination is necessary to evaluate the volume status of the patient. Volume depletion
should be corrected. In the opposite direction, volume
expansion with severe hypertension or congestive
heart failure in the presence of oliguria may hasten the
need for dialysis.

e. *Laboratory examination.* There are no specific tests
for ATN; even a renal biopsy, which is rarely performed, is normal in almost half the cases.

  i. Urine (see Table 16-2)
    1. Osmolality of urine within 10% that of plasma
    2. Trace-2+ protein
    3. U_{Na} greater than 30 mEq/l, FE_{Na} greater than 1%
    4. Urine sediment shows renal tubular cells, white
       cells, red cells, broad "dirty brown" casts as
       well as fine and coarsely granular casts and of-
       ten white cell casts. Red cell casts are almost
       never found in ATN.
    5. If the patient is nonoliguric or more than a day
       or two has passed since the insult, the urine sed-
       iment may be bland.

  ii. Radiologic studies
    1. Ultrasound examination to exclude obstruction
       and measure the size and "density" of the kid-
       neys.
    2. Radionuclide scan to ensure renal blood flow.

f. *Treatment.* The treatment of ATN, including dialysis
when necessary, is beyond the scope of this chapter.
The text will be confined to early interventions, potential reversibility, and indications for dialysis.

  i. MAKE SURE THAT THE CIRCULATING
     PLASMA VOLUME IS ADEQUATE!
    1. Careful physical examination.
    2. In complicated cases, measurement of central
       pressures may be necessary.

  ii. Correct
    1. Volume depletion

    2. Congestive heart failure

    3. Severe plasma protein deficiency

iii. If volume correction fails to cause a diuresis or the blood volume is felt to be adequate, try furosemide. Initially, give 100 mg by IV infusion. If there is no increase in urine flow rate after 2 hours, give 200 mg by IV infusion. If there is no response, give 400 mg. At any dose if there is a brisk diuresis that gradually declines, that dose may be repeated as necessary. There is probably no advantage in using doses of furosemide greater than 400 mg. The risk of high-dose IV furosemide is very small if the drug is properly administered. Infuse furosemide at a rate not to exceed 1000 mg per hour (i.e., give 200 mg over 10 to 15 mins, 400 mg over 20 to 30 mins). At higher rates, flushing, vertigo, nausea, and *transient* deafness has been reported. Do *not* use IV ethacrynic acid in this setting. There is a 1 to 3 percent occurrence of *permanent* neural deafness following the administration of IV ethacrynic acid in the presence of acute renal insufficiency. If the patient is allergic to furosemide, equivalent doses of bumetanide may be used. There is no evidence that bumetanide is superior to equivalent doses of furosemide in the nonallergic patient and bumetanide is more expensive. There is no proof that the use of furosemide changes the course of the renal failure. However, there are many anecdotal reports where the use of furosemide, as outlined above, has converted an oliguric patient to polyuria.

iv. Indications for dialysis include:

    1. Uremia or impending uremia

    2. Volume overload

    3. Severe electrolyte abnormalities, usually hyperkalemia or hyponatremia

    4. Severe acidosis

v. *Outcome.* ATN of any form resolves by the development of a diuresis. During the early diuretic phase of ATN, before the diuresis reaches a peak, the BUN and creatinine levels may continue to rise with the patient becoming more uremic in spite of a rising urine output. As many as 25 percent of all the deaths during ATN occur during the diuretic phase. If the patient survives, 50 percent will undergo a diuresis within 2 weeks, 90 percent within 4 weeks. Of the remaining 10 percent, half will require more than 4 weeks to resolve while the remaining 5 percent will never resolve. The resolution of ATN is usually complete in that the patient's renal function is certainly adequate to maintain life and seems "normal." However, if careful studies are performed on patients who have recently recovered from ATN, it will be found that they have abnormalities in GFR, concentrating ability, acid and potassium excretion. These defects resolve in a period of months to years, with younger patients more rapidly returning to normal than older persons. Subtle defects in renal function may never resolve in the elderly.

vi. *Mortality of ATN.* ATN is a serious condition with a surprisingly high mortality rate, as with many diseases, the death rate rises with the age of the patient. An estimate of death rates follows:

Polyuric ATN	25–35%
Oliguric ATN	
Surgical causes	50–70%
Medical causes	30–50%

vii. *Causes of death in ATN.* With the availability of dialysis, patients die *with* renal failure but not *of* renal failure. Common causes include:
1. The disease process causing renal failure
2. Infections
3. Hemorrhage
4. Electrolyte abnormalities
5. Cardiovascular disease

2. Acute Glomerulonephritis (AGN)
   a. *Pathophysiology.* In AGN, the principal abnormality is inflammation of the glomeruli, with relative sparing of the tubules. As a result, the glomerular blood flow and GFR are low, because the circulation to the tubules is a "portal" system, with blood flowing through the glomeruli and then to the peritublar capillaries, renal blood flow is decreased. For this reason, the kidney behaves as though it is prerenal, with the urine having a high osmolality and low U_{Na}. However, with damage to the glomerular filtering membrane, the urine contains a good deal of protein, red cells, and the hallmark of AGN, red blood cell casts.
   b. *History.* The history is often not terribly helpful. An antecedent strep infection of the pharynx or skin can rarely be found in an adult. Signs of serosal inflammation, rashes, fever, or weight loss may point toward a systemic vasculitis, lupus, or endocarditis.

  c. *Physical examination.* Edema and hypertension are common. Skin lesions, arthritis, pleural or pericardial rubs may suggest vasculitis. A changing or new murmur can imply bacterial endocarditis.

  d. *Laboratory data* (Table 16-2). The urinalysis is the key for diagnosis of AGN. As noted previously, the urine is concentrated, has a low FE_{Na}, and a large amount of protein. Microscopic examination shows red cells and red cell casts. Further tests include blood cultures for endocarditis, serologic tests for lupus, vasculitis, and other idiopathic glomerulonephritides. The diagnosis is usually confirmed by renal biopsy.

  e. *Treatment.* Details of therapy for the various forms of AGN is, again, beyond the scope of this chapter but includes control of blood pressure, proper antibiotics for endocarditis, and steroids and/or immunosuppressive agents for other conditions causing AGN.

3. Allergic Interstitial Nephritis (AIN)

  a. *Pathophysiology.* A wide variety of drugs are associated with an acute decrement in renal function in sensitive individuals (Table 16-4). Histologically, the kidneys show an intense interstitial infiltrate with mononuclear cells and eosinophils.

  b. *History.* Almost any drug can cause AIN, the list grows longer as the condition is more widely recognized. It may be a new drug or a drug the patient has taken for years. An unexplained fever and/or a maculopapular eruption (drug rash) is present in many patients but is not necessary for the diagnosis.

  c. *Physical examination.* The presence of fever or a drug rash are the only clues from examining the patient.

  d. Laboratory data. Eosinophilia is found in a small majority of patients. Eosinophils are found in the urine in 40 to 80 percent of patients with AIN and are suggestive, but not specific for the diagnosis. Urine is difficult to stain with Wright's or Giemsa stain. However, Hansel's stain, used commonly in cytology labs, stains eosinophils in the urine well. Most hospital laboratories will now stain urine for eosinophils. Renal biopsy may be necessary for the diagnosis.

  e. *Treatment.* Cessation of the presumed offending drug; any drug not absolutely necessary for the patient's care should be stopped. Although they are commonly used, it is unclear whether corticosteroids alter the course of the disease.

4. *Large vessel occlusion.* Occlusion of the major artery or veins of a kidney is an extremely rare cause of renal failure. Renal failure only occurs if a single functioning kidney

is present. If the occlusion is sudden, it may be accompanied by gross hematuria, flank pain, fever, or ileus. More commonly, the occlusion is gradual without any symptoms. At present, the "gold standard" for the diagnosis of renal vascular occlusion is angiography. However, MR angiography is rapidly assuming this role since the diagnosis may be made without vascular catheterization or the injection of radiographic contrast material.

V. RECOGNITION OF CHRONIC INSTEAD OF ACUTE RENAL FAILURE

Patients will often be found to have renal insufficiency without a history of renal disease and no available prior laboratory values. The differentiation of acute renal failure from "acute discovery of chronic renal failure" is usually important and often difficult. Short of a renal biopsy, which is often impractical, there are clues that point in the direction of chronic disease.

1. Small or "dense" kidneys on ultrasound examination.
2. The absence of anemia argues for acute disease, patients with chronic renal failure are usually anemic.
3. Serum calcium and phosphate levels are difficult to interpret; however, the presence of renal osteodystrophy in x-rays of the hands or clavicles makes a strong case for chronic disease.
4. Stable renal insufficiency: acute renal failure usually gets better or worse.

BIBLIOGRAPHY

Greenberg A, Cheung AK, Coffman TM, Falk RJ, Jennet JC, eds: *Primer on Kidney Diseases,* 2nd ed. San Diego, Academic Press, 1997.

Schrier RW, ed: *Renal and Electrolyte Disorders,* 5th ed. Philadelphia, Lippincott-Raven, 1997.

UpToDate: clinical reference on CD-ROM, Wellesley, MA, UpToDate, Inc. A CD-ROM now covering much of internal medicine, updated 3 to 4 times per year.

CHAPTER 17
Adult Genitourinary Cancer

S. Bruce Malkowicz
Ricardo F. Sánchez-Ortiz
Alan J. Wein

I. **CARCINOMA OF THE KIDNEY**
   A. **General Considerations**

   Although renal cell carcinoma (RCC) is primarily a surgical disease, its diagnosis may involve several medical specialists since these tumors have multiple presenting signs and symptoms. In the era of contemporary imaging, however, the initial diagnosis is most commonly made incidentally during an ultrasound or CT scan performed for other reasons. Tumors are radioresistant and unresponsive to traditional forms of chemotherapy. Complete responses to immunotherapeutic agents are rare in advanced disease.

   B. **Incidence**
   1. United States incidence is 30,800 new cases annually (12,100 cancer-related deaths).
   2. Incidence has risen in the past 20 years. Represent 2 to 4 percent of human neoplasms.
   3. The majority of tumors (85 to 90 percent) are renal parenchymal lesions, most commonly clear cell adenocarcinoma.
   4. Thirty percent of patients present with metastatic disease.

   C. **Epidemiology**
   1. Male-to-female ratio is roughly 2:1.
   2. The majority of patients present in the fifth to seventh decades of life.
   3. Racial distribution is equal.
   4. The highest incidence is in Scandinavia; the lowest is in Asia.
   5. It is more common in urban settings.

6. Most cases are sporadic but it is also seen in families with von Hippel-Lindau disease (VHL) and less commonly with the tuberous sclerosis complex (TSC). Familial RCC without VHL mutations have also been described. VHL disease is a rare multiorgan syndrome of autosomal dominant inheritance associated with RCC (40 percent), renal cysts (75 percent), cysts of the epididymis and pancreas, as well as cerebellar hemangioblastomas, retinal angiomas, and pheochromocytoma (14 percent). It occurs in 1/36,000 live births. The protein produced by the VHL gene (3p25-26) has been isolated and found to bind to the cellular transcription protein elongin, inhibiting transcriptional activity in vitro via RNA polymerase II dysfunction.

D. Etiology

1. The strongest risk factor is tobacco use (twofold increased relative risk).
2. Industrial exposure (except coke oven workers) is not a significant risk.
3. Acquired renal cystic disease in dialysis patients with 4 to 9 percent incidence. It occurs in both patients undergoing hemodialysis or peritoneal dialysis. Experts recommend yearly ultrasound screening examinations.

E. Pathology: Renal Tumors

1. Renal cell carcinoma
   a. Represents up to 90 percent of solid renal tumors.
   b. Classic histologic patterns include conventional (clear cell) RCC (60 to 75 percent), papillary RCC (15 percent), chromophobe RCC (5 percent), collecting duct carcinoma (less than 1 percent), and unclassified carcinoma (up to 5 percent). Arise from proximal tubular renal cells. Occurs in familial and sporadic forms.
   c. *Conventional (clear cell) RCC.* Most common histology. Associated with a point mutation or allelic loss of the von Hippel-Lindau (VHL) gene, which maps to 3p25-26. Grossly, tumors appear yellow or gray-tan in color with variable areas of hemorrhage, necrosis, or cystic change. Microscopically, they are composed predominantly of cells with clear eosinophilic or granular cytoplasm. These tumors are usually unilateral but may be bilateral in 1 to 2 percent of cases. Prognosis is worse in patients with metachronous as opposed to synchronous presentation.
   d. *Papillary RCC.* Comprise 5 to 15 percent of renal carcinomas. May occur in both inherited and noninherited

forms, but the VHL gene mutation is not involved. Hereditary papillary renal cell carcinoma is related to a defect in c-met on the long arm of chromosome 7. Other genetic alterations identified include Y-chromosome loss and trisomies of chromosomes 7, 16, and 17. Age and gender predilections are similar to conventional RCC. It is multifocal in up to 40 percent of cases and bilateral in up to 6 percent of patients.

e. Chromophobe tumors are associated with multiple chromosome losses excluding 3p. Age and gender distribution are similar to conventional RCC. Grossly, appear well-circumscribed, tan or beige in color. Microscopically, an admixture of clear and eosinophilic cells is common. It may be confused with oncocytoma, a benign renal lesion. They are multifocal in less than 10 percent of cases. Bilaterality is exceedingly rare.

f. *Collecting duct carcinoma.* Seen in less than 1 percent of patients. May mimic renal pelvic transitional cell carcinoma.

2. *Oncocytoma.* Renal oncocytomas, accounting approximately 5 percent of all renal parenchymal tumors, are well-circumscribed parenchymal masses composed of densely acidophilic cells that show mitochondrial hyperplasia on electron microscopy. Bilaterality has been reported in up to 5 percent of cases. They may also be seen in the adrenal, thyroid, parathyroid, and salivary glands. In contrast to RCC, the principal genetic alteration appears to involve changes in mitochondrial DNA and translocation of chromosome 14. Grossly, they are usually mahogany brown in color, encapsulated, and contain a dense central scar extending in a stellate pattern (seen in one third of cases). Angiographically, there is often a "spoke wheel" appearance to the vessels that surround the tumor. Several case reports in the 1980s reported the potential for metastasis before the realization that, histologically, oncocytoma is difficult to distinguish from chromophobe renal cell carcinoma. Oncocytomas are benign and merit conservative treatment, but unfortunately, their preoperative diagnosis based on imaging is unreliable, and a definitive diagnosis cannot be made on frozen section. Radical nephrectomy is the safest method of treatment unless other factors argue for a conservative approach.

3. *Angiomyolipoma (renal hamartoma).* These benign lesions composed of fat, muscle, and blood vessels can usually be definitively diagnosed by the presence of fat on

computed tomography (negative Hounsfield CT attenuation units). Lesions also appear hyperechoic on renal sonography due to their high fat content and may demonstrate arterial microaneurysms detected on angiography. Isolated angiomyolipomas usually present at a mean age of 50 years with a 4:1 female predominance. Although they are generally noted as incidental radiographic findings, they may present dramatically with acute flank pain or shock due to spontaneous renal or retroperitoneal hemorrhage. Multiple and often bilateral AMLs are seen in the TSC, a condition of autosomal dominant inheritance associated with seizures, mental retardation, and adenoma sebaceum. Eighty percent of patients with the TSC will develop angiomyolipomas. Patients with pulmonary lymphangiomyomatosis, a progressive global pulmonary condition, also exhibit renal angiomyolipomas in 40 percent of cases. Treatment is based on tumor size and patient symptoms. Asymptomatic tumors smaller than 4 cm may be followed closely with serial imaging. However, symptomatic tumors or those greater than 4 cm should undergo selective embolization or tumor enucleation by partial nephrectomy.

4. *Sarcoma.* Sarcomas constitute 2 to 3 percent of malignant renal parenchymal tumors. They are more common in women. Differentiation from RCC is difficult. The predominant subcategory is leiomyosarcoma. The treatment of choice is radical nephrectomy, since chemotherapy does not improve survival in adults.

5. *Hemangiopericytoma.* These rare, usually small, renin-secreting lesions are profusely vascular and may have regional or distant metastases in 15 percent of cases. They may produce severe hypertension.

6. *Lymphoblastoma.* Reticulum cell carcinoma, lymphosarcoma, and leukemia are uncommon and rarely present as a primary renal lesion.

7. *Metastasis.* The most common tumors that metastasize to the kidneys are carcinomas of the lung, breast, and uterus. Metastatic melanoma is often noted on autopsy. Metastatic lesions appear poorly vascularized and display irregular borders on imaging studies. Although we do not recommend diagnostic percutaneous biopsy of renal masses, it may be indicated in this setting.

8. *Xanthogranulomatous pyelonephritis (XGP).* XGP is a rare renal infection that may mimic a renal tumor. It is more commonly seen in women (3:1) in the fifth to seventh decade of life. Diabetes mellitus is found in up to fifteen percent of patients. Usually infection (*Escherichia*

coli or *Proteus mirabilis*) and obstructing renal calculi are present. The lesions demonstrate lipid-laden macrophages that resemble clear cell RCC. Patients are generally best treated with nephrectomy rather than incision or drainage.

F. Grading and Staging
1. Fuhrman system generally used in the United States (I–IV).
2. General classification systems include the Robson system and TNM system (Tables 17-1 and 17-2).

G. Clinical Presentation
1. An increasing number of renal cell tumors are found as incidental asymptomatic masses on imaging studies obtained for another purpose.
2. *"Classic triad."* Only 11 percent of RCC patients present with the classic triad of hematuria, flank pain, and a palpable mass. These patients generally have advanced disease. Gross or microscopic hematuria is classically quoted as present in 40 to 60 percent, flank pain in 40 to 50 percent, and a flank mass in 20 to 35 percent. These numbers need downward revision in view of the increasing number of unanticipated discoveries (see previous discussion).
3. *General symptoms.* Weight loss (33 percent), fever (15 percent), anemia (33 percent), and night sweats (7 percent) are common systemic manifestations. The lesion may present by a manifestation of metastasis. Growth along the

Table 17-1 Robson Staging System for Renal Cell Carcinoma (RCC)

Stage I	Tumor is confined to the kidney; perinephric fat, renal vein, and regional nodes show no evidence of malignancy.
Stage II	Tumor involves the perinephric fat but is confined within's Gerota's fascia; renal vein and regional nodes show no evidence of malignancy.
Stage III	Tumor involves the renal vein or regional nodes, with or without involvement of the vena cava or perinephric fat.
Stage IV	Distant metastases secondary to RCC are evident on presentation or there is histologic involvement of contiguous visceral structures by tumor.

Table 17-2 Tumor Node Metastasis (TNM) Staging System for Renal Tumors American Joint Commission for Cancer (AJCC) 1997

Primary Tumor (T)

TX	Primary tumor cannot be assessed
T0	No evidence of primary tumor
T1	Tumor 7 cm or less in dimension limited to the kidney
T2	Tumor more than 7 cm in dimension limited to the kidney
T3a	Tumor invades adrenal gland or perinephric tissues but not Gerota's foscia
T3b	Tumor grossly extends into renal vein or vena cava below diaphragm
T3c	Tumor grossly extends into vena cava above diaphragm

Regional Lymph Nodes (N)

NX	Regional lymph nodes cannot be assessed
N0	No regional lymph node metastasis
N1	Metastasis in a single regional lymph node or nodes
N2	Metastasis in more than one regional lymph node

Distant Metastasis (M)

MX	Distant metastasis cannot be assessed
M0	No distant metastasis
M1	Distant Metastasis

Staging Grouping

I	T1	N0	M0
II	T2	N0	M0
III	T1	N1	M0
	T2	N1	M0
	T3a	N0	M0
	T3a	N1	M0
	T3b	N0	M0
	T3b	N1	M0
	T3c	N0	M0
	T3c	N1	M0
IV	T4	N0	M0
	Any T	N2	M0
	Any T	Any N	M1

left renal vein or vena cava can block the testicular vein, producing a varicocele. The sudden appearance of a right-sided varicocele or a varicocele in a man over 40 (especially if it does not disappear on recumbency) warrants renal and retroperitoneal imaging.

4. *Paraneoplastic syndromes.* Hypercalcemia secondary to the production of a parathormone-like substance is not

uncommon (5 percent); this may also be due to metastatic bone destruction. Stauffer's syndrome (14 percent) refers to abnormal liver function studies with hepatomegaly but no metastasis. These values revert to normal after nephrectomy in the majority of patients (88 percent). Recurrent or persistent hepatic dysfunction suggests tumor recurrence or unrelated hepatic disease. Less common syndromes include protein-wasting enteropathy, erythrocytosis, neuromyopathy, and gonadotropin production. Amyloidosis is present in approximately 2 percent of patients.

H. Imaging Evaluation
The majority of renal masses (90 percent) are benign renal cysts. These exist in approximately 5 percent of all patients over the age of 55. A mass not demonstrating ultrasound criteria for a simple cyst requires a dedicated renal CT scan or MRI with thin cuts. The study should be performed with and without contrast for better definition. Other imaging tests may serve as the starting point for the detection of a renal mass.
1. Diagnostic studies
   a. *Intravenous excretory urography.* Usually the starting point of the hematuria evaluation to identify parenchymal renal masses as well as calyceal, renal pelvic, and ureteral urothelial abnormalities. The scout film may give information regarding the position, size, and outline of the kidneys. Mottled central calcifications indicate a carcinoma with more than 90 percent specificity. Peripheral or rim calcifications are associated with RCC in 10 to 20 percent of cases. After the administration of intravenous contrast media, nephrotomographic views are obtained to evaluate the renal parenchyma. Findings suggestive of a renal mass include renal enlargement, elongation, displacement of the renal pelvis, indistinct or irregular renal borders, or changes in cortical density. Radiographs during contrast excretion are used to evaluate the renal calyces, renal pelvis, and ureters for urothelial lesions.
   b. *Renal sonography.* Ultrasound is used to distinguish cystic from solid renal masses. A classic cyst will be smooth with a definite border of imperceptible thickness, be absent of internal echogenicity, and should display acoustic enhancements beyond the posterior wall. In certain cases ultrasound may be employed with cyst puncture, cytology, and contrast injection to better define complex lesions. This is rarely employed with the advent of newer CT or MRI techniques.

    c. *Computed tomography.* CT scans can evaluate the renal parenchyma both with and without the injection of intravenous contrast material. CT is also an excellent staging modality and provides superior data on lymph node involvement, perinephric extension, and renal vein or vena caval involvement. CT is probably the single most accurate imaging study to diagnose renal masses, especially to identify angiomyolipomas, due to the presence of fat (negative Hounsfield units).

      Bosniak classification of cystic masses.
        I Very rarely malignant, usually do not need surgery.
       II Hyperdense cyst, generally nonsurgical.
      III Thicker regular nodular walls with thicker regular calcifications and septations: RCC in up to 40 percent.
      IV Nodular or solid component: 90 percent demonstrate RCC.

    d. *Magnetic resonance imaging (MRI).* This imaging modality is most effective in demonstrating the presence and extent of renal vein or vena caval tumor thrombi. It can also provide excellent renal imaging, especially with gadolinium enhancement for difficult to diagnose cases. It is especially useful in patients with iodinated contrast allergy, renal insufficiency, a nondiagnostic CT scan, or questionable venous invasion.

    e. *Angiography.* Classic angiography has been supplanted by magnetic resonance angiography in the preoperative planning for surgery on solitary kidneys or before partial nephrectomy. Renal angioembolization is considered useful by some in tumors greater than 10 cm to facilitate dissection during nephrectomy.

    f. *Radionuclide imaging.* This is most useful in defining "pseudomasses." A normal variant such as a hypertrophied column of Bertin can be distinguished from a tumor by the uniform distribution of radioisotope uptake. Both benign cysts and tumors will appear as photon-deficient areas of uptake.

    g. *Percutaneous biopsy.* Not recommended due to the high incidence of false-negative biopsies (sampling errors). May be indicated when lymphoma is suspected, in patients with a history of another primary malignancy to rule-out metastatic disease, or in complex cysts for cytologic examination.

2. *Clinical staging.* Clinical staging consists of a history, physical examination, and the following.

    a. Chest x-ray (CXR) (chest CT with pulmonary symptoms or abnormal CXR).

b. CT scan of abdomen and pelvis or MRI.

c. CBC, liver function tests, alkaline phosphatase, calcium, BUN and creatinine.

d. Bone scan with plan films as indicated (patients with elevated alkaline phosphatase or bone pain).

I. Treatment

1. T1 and T2 disease

   a. Radical nephrectomy is the gold standard treatment for localized RCC with a normal contralateral kidney. Components of a radical nephrectomy include early vascular ligation and en bloc removal of the kidney, Gerota's fascia, ipsilateral adrenal, upper ureter, and, for some, lymph nodes from the crus of the diaphragm to the aortic bifurcation. Although recent data suggest that a thorough lymphadenectomy may provide a small (10 to 15 percent) benefit in micrometastatic disease, its value remains controversial to most physicians. Occasionally, very large vascular tumors (larger than 10 cm) may be preoperatively embolized to make the procedure technically easier. Recent data confirm that adrenal glands appearing normal on CT or MRI associated with smaller renal tumors may be left intact. The most common surgical approaches include an 11th or 12th rib extraperitoneal flank incision or thoracoabdominal (large upper pole tumors). Other approaches include transabdominal and subcostal.

2. *Laparoscopic radical nephrectomy.* Introduced in 1990 by Clayman and colleagues, it is now frequently performed for stages T1 and T2 RCC in specialized centers. Offers the advantages of a smaller incision, shorter length of stay, and shorter convalescence with the drawback of a longer operative time and the potential for complications given the steep learning curve. Approaches include transperitoneal (hand assisted or pure with morcellation) or retroperitoneal. The latter offers expeditious access to the renal pedicle, but with limited working space. The efficacy and safety of laparoscopic radical nephrectomy was recently addressed by a large retrospective multicenter report of 157 patients with T1-2 tumors. No renal fossa or port-site recurrences were identified at a mean follow-up of 19.2 months. However, larger prospective studies with longer follow-up are needed to compare disease-free survival with open surgery.

3. Nephron sparing surgery

   a. Absolute indications include a solitary kidney, bilateral tumors, and VHL disease (although some believe bilateral nephrectomy is more appropriate). Relative indications include poor bilateral or contralateral renal function.

b. Acceptable option in smaller tumors (4 cm or smaller) with a normal contralateral kidney.

c. Approaches include segmental polar nephrectomy, heminephrectomy, wedge resection, or tumor enucleation (preferred for multiple tumors).

d. Local recurrence is generally less than 10 percent (nearly zero over 5 years in incidental lesions 4 cm or less).

e. The morbidity is similar to radical nephrectomy, but with the potential for slightly greater blood loss and the development of a urinary fistula. Although significant urinary fistulae may require prolonged internal ureteral stenting and Foley catheter drainage, over 90 percent will heal with conservative management, avoiding the need for reoperation.

f. Large or central lesions may require renal cooling and complete arterial occlusion to minimize warm ischemic damage.

g. Intraoperative ultrasound is paramount to ensure adequate margins (ideally 1 cm of normal renal tissue).

4. Stage T3 tumors

a. Inferior vena cava extension occurs in 4 to 10 percent of patients. In the absence of vessel wall invasion or metastasis, nephrectomy with tumor thrombectomy is recommended given a 5-year survival (pT3b or pT3c) of 40 to 60 percent. Advanced surgical techniques can be very successful, usually with thoracoabdominal, bilateral subcostal, or midline approaches to ensure complete vascular control above and below the kidneys. Cardiopulmonary bypass with or without hypothermic cardiac arrest can be used in bulky intrahepatic and suprahepatic lesions. Preoperative and intraoperative transesophageal echocardiography is recommended for tumors with proximal thrombi.

b. Operative mortality ranges from 1.4 to 14 percent, with 30 to 40 percent postoperative complications such as sepsis, retroperitoneal hemorrhage, or hepatic dysfunction.

c. Tumor subclassification is based on the extent of thrombus (Fig. 17-1). A different classification has been proposed as follows.

   i. Level I—into the IVC less than 2.5 cm from the renal ostia.

   ii. Level II—extending cranially more than 2.5 cm but below hepatic veins.

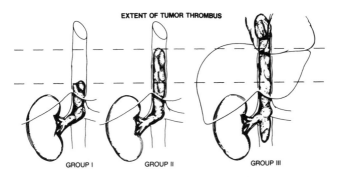

EXTENT OF TUMOR THROMBUS

GROUP I   GROUP II   GROUP III

Figure 17-1 The different classifications of renal tumors with inferior vena caval involvement. Each presentation requires implementation of specific surgical techniques. (*Reproduced from Skinner DG, Lieskovsky G, eds: Diagnosis and Management of Genitourinary Cancer, 1988, p 697.*)

       iii. Level III—up to the hepatic veins but below the diaphragm.
       iv. Level IV—thrombus extending above diaphragm.
  5. Metastatic RCC
    a. The role of radical nephrectomy in metastatic RCC is limited to those individuals with an excellent performance status who will undergo adjuvant immunotherapy, or local symptoms which are severe or unremitting, although these patients are rare and generally, these situations are amenable to angioinfarction as well.
    b. *Management of solitary metastases.* Seen in 1.5 to 3.5 percent of patients. Surgical removal is recommended given a 5-year survival rate between 30 and 50 percent. Solitary pulmonary lesions have the best prognosis.
  6. *Chemotherapy.* No single agent or combination of chemotherapeutic agents is consistently effective against RCC. Five to 15 percent response rates have been reported in multiple trials. Very few patients demonstrate a sustained complete response (CR).
    a. *Interferons.* Interferon alpha provides a 15 percent partial response rate and 1 percent CR. It is a component of immunotherapy in combined chemotherapy trials.
    b. *Interleukin-2.* The only drug approved by the FDA specifically for metastatic carcinoma. A partial response rate of 14 percent with 5 percent CR and a mean duration of 22 months. Continuous infusion or

subcutaneous injections are less toxic. Its major toxicity is Acute Respiratory Distress Syndrome (ARDS) due to the capillary leak syndrome.

7. *Management of angiomyolipoma.* Symptomatic lesions or those greater than 4 cm should undergo angioinfarction or partial nephrectomy. Smaller asymptomatic lesions may undergo surveillance.

J. Tumor Stage is the Most Important Predictor of Prognosis

1. Disease-specific survival rate (percent) after radical nephrectomy (5 and 10 years)

   a. Stage I   85/82
   b. Stage II   70/80
   c. Stage IIIA   57/50
   d. Stage IIIB   46/34
   e. Stage IIIC   22/16
   f. Stage IVA   5/3

2. Extension through the renal capsule and into perinephric fat occurs in 25 percent of patients.

3. The phenomenon of spontaneous tumor regression is extremely rare and estimated at less than 1 percent.

4. Metastatic disease presents most commonly to the lung (50 percent), lymph nodes (35 percent), liver (30 percent), bone (30 percent), and adrenal (5 percent). Only one third of patients with metastases present with symptoms.

K. Follow-up of Renal Cell Carcinoma after Nephrectomy or Renal Sparing Surgery

a. Traditionally, most patients with sporadic RCC are followed every 6 months or yearly with a history and physical examination (H&P), liver function studies, serum chemistry (including alkaline phosphatase), CXR, and abdominal cross-sectional imaging.

b. However, contemporary series from M.D. Anderson and the Cleveland Clinic suggest that recurrence is generally a rare event for T1 and T2 lesions. In addition, pulmonary metastasis are most common and usually can be diagnosed by chest radiography. Stage-specific follow-up guidelines have been proposed as follows.

1. T1: H&P, serum chemistry, and CXR yearly for 5 years

2. T2: H&P, serum chemistry, and CXR every 6 months; abdominal CT scan at 2 and 5 years for 5 years

3. T3: H&P, serum chemistry, and CXR at 3 months, then every 6 months; abdominal CT scan at 2 and 5 years

II. UROTHELIAL TUMORS OF THE RENAL PELVIS, COLLECTING SYSTEM, AND URETER

A. General Considerations

The urinary system lined by transitional cell epithelium (urothelium) extends from the most proximal calyces to the proximal urethra. In this section, attention is given to the tumors of the renal collecting system and the ureter. It is important that they be understood in the broad context of transitional cell carcinoma (TCC), which is discussed in greater detail in the section on bladder cancer.

B. Incidence

a. Account for 7 percent of all renal tumors.

b. Overall, urothelial tumors are distributed as follows: the bladder (90 percent), urethra (7 percent), and ureter or renal collecting system (3 percent).

c. Patients with a history of bladder cancer have 2 to 4 percent chance of developing upper tract tumors (synchronous or asynchronous). This figure increases up to 25 percent in patients with bladder carcinoma in situ.

d. Patients with a history of an upper tract tumor have a 15 to 50 percent chance of eventually developing TCC of the bladder. Such patients also have a 2 to 4 percent chance of developing a contralateral lesion.

e. After cystectomy, there is an approximately 7 percent chance of developing upper tract TCC. The risk is highest with the presence of carcinoma in situ (CIS) in the cystectomy specimen. The highest risk is within 3 to 4 years following cystectomy.

f. There is evidence to suggest that patients with high-grade superficial bladder tumors undergoing bacillus Calmette-Guérin (BCG) intravesical therapy have an increased tendency to develop upper tract lesions. Thus, the entire urothelium must be routinely surveyed for the development of cancer once any part has undergone malignant transformation.

C. Pathology

Upper urinary tract tumors include the same pathologic types as those of the bladder. Tumors may be papillary or nodular, muscle invasive or noninvasive. Staging systems are less well defined than for other malignancies but are analogous to the bladder TNM system.

1. Stage T0: mucosal lesion without invasion
2. Stage T1: involvement of the lamina propria

3. Stage T2: muscularis propria invasion
4. Stage T3:extension beyond the renal pelvis or ureter
5. Stage T4: adjacent organ involvement, usually associated with positive lymph nodes
6. Histologic subtypes
   a. *Transitional cell carcinoma.* Approximately 85 percent of renal pelvic tumors and almost all ureteral tumors are transitional cell lesions. The male-to-female ratio is 3:1.
   b. *Squamous cell carcinoma* (10 to 17 percent of tumors). Primarily associated with chronic irritation and renal calculi. These lesions are usually of more advanced stage and associated with leukoplakia and metaplastic changes.
   c. *Adenocarcinoma.* This is a very rare (less than 1 percent) upper tract tumor. It occurs predominantly in females and is usually associated with chronic infection or irritation and is often seen in conjunction with pyelitis cystica or pyelitis glandularis.
   d. The differential diagnosis of upper urinary tract filling defects includes papilloma, malakoplakia, sloughed papilla, secondary metastasis, uric acid or matrix calculi, extrinsic compression (vessels, adenopathy, retroperitoneal fibrosis), urinary tuberculosis, ureteritis or pyelitis cystica, inverted papilloma, and sarcoma.

D. Etiology and Natural History

Chemical carcinogenesis is the leading factor in the development of TCC in the upper urinary tract. Probably because of the relative short transit time of urine through the upper tracts, lesions of the upper tract occur much less often than bladder lesions. Tobacco use is associated with at least a twofold increased relative risk for the disease (two- to sixfold). Two conditions more commonly associated with upper tract lesions are Balkan nephropathy (an inflammatory lesion of the renal interstitium edemic to the Balkan region) and phenacetin abuse. In addition, the nephrotoxic Chinese herb *Aristolochia fangchi* has recently been associated with the development of upper tract urothelial carcinoma.

Papillary tumors of the renal pelvis or ureter tend to be of low grade, whereas nodular or flat lesions tend to be of higher grade. Patients with low-grade lesions (grade 1) have a nearly 100 percent 5-year disease-specific survival, whereas patients with high-grade lesions (grade 3) display a 20 percent 5-year survival.

E. Clinical Presentation

Sixty to 90 percent of patients present with microscopic or gross hematuria. Only 10 percent are noted in conjunction with testing for other conditions. Almost one third of patients with a renal pelvic lesion will complain of flank pain, as will one sixth of patients with ureteral tumors. Physical examination is usually unrevealing.

F. Diagnosis
1. Radiologic studies
   a. *Intravenous excretory urography.* Either a fixed radiolucent defect or nonvisualization of part or all of the collecting system is noted. Stippled calcifications may also be seen on the plain film.
   b. Retrograde pyelography is indicated to evaluate pyelocalyceal and ureteral segments not adequately visualized on excretory urography, given its greater sensitivity. With this technique, upper tract tumors demonstrate filling defects in up to 75 percent of cases.
   c. CT scan of the retroperitoneum may help to differentiate a renal parenchymal mass from a renal pelvic mass. Its role in ureteral lesions is limited.
   d. Ultrasound delineates nonopaque calculi from soft tissue density.
2. *Brush biopsy and cytology.* This is usually performed during pyeloureterography and may be done by a urologist or radiologist. The combination of an upper tract filling defect and a positive renal wash cytology in the same side is enough evidence for definitive treatment, most commonly with nephroureterectomy or distal ureterectomy with reimplantation (in the case of tumors in the distal third of the ureter). However, a renal wash cytology positive for transitional cell carcinoma without the presence of urothelial filling defects on urography mandates further evaluation with ureteroscopy.
3. Ureteroscopy allows direct visualization and biopsy of the upper tract urothelium. In addition, laser photocoagulation of the lesion may be performed in patients with small, low-grade lesions, a solitary kidney, or in the setting of compromised renal function.

G. Treatment
1. TCC of the renal pelvis
   a. *Nephroureterectomy.* The classic therapy for upper tract TCC is nephroureterectomy with excision of a bladder cuff. The procedure may be performed via a single thoracoabdominal incision or a two-incision approach (flank and infraumbilical midline). If the ureteral stump is left in place, there is a 20 percent chance for recurrence at a site that is difficult to monitor. Less aggressive surgery has been performed in

patients with solitary renal units, bilateral lesions, or compromised renal function. Stage and grade are often stronger predictors of long-term survival than treatment choice. For this reason, more conservative treatments have been advocated. Even with improvements in ureteroscopy, this treatment philosophy requires persistent, often difficult, and perhaps less than adequate active observation of the remaining urothelium. Endoscopic evaluation and treatment can be employed in lower grade lesions.

b. *Laparoscopic nephroureterectomy.* In specialized centers, this has now become a feasible option. The bladder cuff is excised around the ureter by transurethral ureteral unroofing using a Collins knife prior to the laparoscopic procedure. Nephroureterectomy may then be performed transperitoneally (hand assisted or pure) or retroperitoneally. The kidney and ureter are then removed en bloc and delivered via a subcostal, lower midline, or low flank incision. Bladder cuff closure can be performed with a laparoscopic stapler or left open with Foley catheter drainage for 2 weeks. Recent experience has shown that laparoscopic nephrourete-rectomy requires twice the operating time of open nephroureterectomy. However, analgesic requirements and hospital length of stay were reduced by approximately 60 percent. Overall cancer-specific survival was similar at a mean follow-up of 2 years. There have been no reports to date of trocar site or peritoneal seeding after laparoscopic nephroureterectomy.

c. *Antegrade (percutaneous) or retrograde nephroscopy.* Indicated only in patients with a solitary kidney, compromised renal function, or very small low grade lesions. Treatment may involve endoscopic resection with diathermy, cold-knife, or laser tissue destruction.

2. TCC of the ureter

a. Nephroureterectomy with excision of a bladder cuff is still the classic treatment for this condition given its multifocal nature, especially in tumors of the upper two thirds of the ureter. However, in cases of tumors of the distal third of the ureter or in patients with compromised renal function, distal ureterectomy and ureteroneocystostomy has been proven as effective as a nephroureterectomy.

b. Indications for endoscopic percutaneous or retrograde treatment include: a single low-grade ureteral lesion, high-risk surgical candidates, solitary kidney, bilateral disease, and renal insufficiency. Strict compliance with follow-up is paramount in these patients.

   c. A less favored option includes ureteral resection with ileal interposition.

3. Chemotherapy

   a. *Topical therapy.* Not standard of care, but indicated for patients with compromised renal function, a solitary kidney, high risk surgical candidates, or patients with carcinoma in situ of the ureter or the renal pelvis. Refer to the section on superficial bladder cancer for the most commonly used agents (BCG, thiotepa, mitomycin, adriamycin, and interferon), their indications, and side-effect profiles.

   b. *Systemic chemotherapy.* The standard of care for the management of metastatic TCC is MVAC chemotherapy (methotrexate, vincristine, adriamycin, cis-platinum). Chemotherapy with paclitaxel and carboplatin may be better tolerated by patients with compromised renal or cardiac function. Prospective trials are ongoing to evaluate the long-term efficacy of adjuvant chemotherapy in patients with positive lymph nodes or unfavorable pathology.

4. *Surveillance after definitive treatment.* No strict guidelines exist for follow-up after nephroureterectomy or distal ureterectomy. At our institution, we generally follow these patients with a history, physical examination, cystoscopy, urinalysis, and cytology every 3 months for a year, then every 6 months for 2 to 5 years, then yearly. We obtain a CXR, intravenous urogram, and abdominal cross-sectional imaging yearly or as indicated based on pathologic stage or clinical symptoms.

III. CARCINOMA OF THE BLADDER
A. General Considerations

Bladder cancer is the second most common urologic malignancy after prostate carcinoma. The most common histologic diagnosis is transitional cell carcinoma (TCC). Sixty to 75 percent of these lesions are noninvasive, superficial tumors, but 10 to 20 percent of these tumors will progress to muscle-invasive disease, especially patients with high-grade disease and transitional cell carcinoma in situ. However, the majority of muscle-invasive tumors (over 80 percent) initially present as invasive tumors in patients without a prior history of transitional cell carcinoma. Intravesical chemotherapy has been used for superficial disease in an attempt to decrease tumor recurrence and possibly decrease tumor progression. The most effective agent is bacillus Calmette-Guérin (BCG) intravesical immunotherapy, which decreases tumor recurrence by 40 to 70 percent. In the case of transitional cell carcinoma in situ (CIS), it may reduce tumor progression. Muscle-invasive tumors are classically and best treated by radical exenterative surgery and some form of urinary diversion. Advanced TCC responds to platinum- and paclitaxel-based chemotherapy regimens, but sustained complete responses are rare.

B. Incidence

1. In the United States, there will be 53,400 new cases diagnosed in the year 2001, accounting for 6 percent of new cancer cases in men and 2 percent in women. In addition, there will be 12,400 annual cancer-related deaths.

2. It is the fourth most common form of cancer in men.

C. Etiology

1. *Industrial carcinogens.* In 1895, the initial link was made between bladder cancer and exposure to aniline dyes. Further connections have been established with the rubber manufacturing and textile printing industries. Exposure to aromatic amines is the common event, and substances such as 2-naphtylamine, 4-aminobiphenyl, and 4-nitrobiphenyl are believed to be potent carcinogenic elements. The latency period may be several decades.

2. *Tobacco exposure.* A two- to threefold relative risk for developing bladder cancer exists for cigarette smokers. The relationship is less well-established for other tobacco products.

3. *Chemotherapeutic agents.* As high as a ninefold relative risk may exist for patients exposed to cyclophosphamide or ifosfamide chemotherapy. The presence or absence of hemorrhagic cystitis does not correlate with the likelihood of developing carcinoma. The major toxic metabolic agent is acrolein, and most lesions present as muscle-invasive tumors. Administration of Mesna at the time of therapy reduces the urothelial injury by acrolein.

4. *Schistosomiasis. Schistosoma haematobium* is endemic in Egypt, where 70 percent of bladder cancers have squamous cell pathology. The disease characteristically results in bladder wall calcification, polyposis, ulcers,

and urothelial hyperplasia leading to an end-stage contracted bladder. The presence of high concentrations of N-nitroso compounds has been implicated as a possible etiologic factor for the development of bladder cancer, which usually presents with an early onset (fifth decade of life). More than 40 percent of squamous cell carcinomas associated with schistosomiasis are well-differentiated and typically carry a good prognosis, unlike squamous cell carcinomas of other etiologies.

5. *Pelvic irradiation.* A two- to fourfold increase in bladder cancer incidence has been noted in women treated for cervical malignancy.

6. *Chronic irritation and infection.* Patients with indwelling urinary catheters for many years are subject to chronic bacterial infection, stone formation, and foreign body reactions. A 15- to 20-fold increase in bladder cancer (primarily squamous) has been noted in some series. Malignant or premalignant changes have been noted in 2 to 8 percent of patients with Foley catheters indwelling for more than 10 years. A yearly cystoscopic examination is recommended in these patients.

7. *Phenacetin.* The N-hydroxy metabolite of phenacetin is the probable active metabolite that causes urothelial tumors. Upper tract lesions are most common. A long latency period and massive ingestion (5 to 10 kg) are characteristic of this condition.

8. *Bladder exstrophy.* This rare midline closure defect is associated with bladder adenocarcinoma. It occurs in patients who underwent late closure and is thought to result from chronic irritation.

9. *Coffee.* Coffee and tea have been implicated in a few studies. The relationship is not strong and is further weakened by the confounding occurrence of associated smoking.

10. *Saccharin.* Artificial sweeteners have been shown to result in bladder cancer in experimental animals. No association has been proven in humans.

D. Epidemiology

1. *Age.* Peak incidence is in the sixth to eighth decades. It is rare before the age of 40 and extremely rare in the first two decades of life.

2. *Race.* Bladder cancer is diagnosed twice as frequently in white American men as in African American men. A 50 percent increase in bladder cancer has been reported in

white American women versus African American women. Much of this difference may be attributed to inadequate detection and reporting in African Americans. Asians have a lower reported incidence than white Americans do.

3. *Gender.* The male-to-female ratio is approximately 3:1.

4. *Genetics.* The genetic aspects of bladder cancer pathology are under intense investigation. The loss of genetic material on the long arm of chromosome 9 ($p16^{ink/arf}$) appears to be one of the earliest developments in superficial TCC. Alterations in p53, p21, and PRb may play a significant role in development of the invasive metastatic phenotype.

5. *Demography.* The incidence appears higher in the United States compared to Japan and Scandinavia.

6. *Relative impact.* Bladder cancer is the 7th most common cause of cancer death in men and the 10th to 12th most common cancer-related death in women. The disease has displayed an almost 50 percent increase in incidence over the past 40 years.

7. *Screening.* The role of population screening for hematuria is uncertain at present. The detection rate for bladder cancer is approximately 1 to 3 percent in most study groups. Newer molecular markers for bladder cancer have not been demonstrated to be appropriate screening tools at this time.

E. Symptoms

1. *Hematuria.* Either gross or microscopic hematuria is present in 85 percent of cases. The amount of hematuria is not necessarily proportional to the severity of the lesion, and intermittence is not a reason to exclude an evaluation. Hematuria in older patients may result in the diagnosis of a urologic malignancy in 10 percent of patients, with the majority of these lesions being TCC. Microscopic or gross hematuria indicates cancer until proven otherwise and must be evaluated.

2. *Irritative voiding symptoms.* Increased frequency of urination, dysuria, and urgency may be present in up to 20 percent of patients with bladder cancer, particularly CIS.

3. *Bladder filling defect on urography.* This is not a true positive finding on all occasions, since the urinary bladder is usually not maximally distended. More importantly, the absence of a defect on an intravenous urogram, cystogram, or CT scan does not rule out the presence of a lesion.

4. *Unanticipated finding at cystoscopy.* Bladder carcinoma may be discovered at the time of cystoscopy for totally unrelated reasons, such as an evaluation for outlet obstruction.

F. Diagnosis

1. *Transurethral resection (TUR).* The lesion in question is usually excised by classic TUR. An effort to resect into the bladder muscle (muscularis propria) is made to fully establish the diagnosis of superficial or invasive disease.

2. *Random bladder and posterior urethral biopsies.* Biopsies from sites adjacent to the tumor, other parts of the bladder, and the prostatic urethra are obtained to detect any associated CIS or tissue dysplasia. Such findings suggest potentially more aggressive disease. In addition, it is important to document the absence of CIS or TCC in the urethra if an orthotopic urinary diversion is planned. Some concerns do exist, however, that this practice has the possibility of seeding primary tumor to other sites.

3. *Urinary cytology.* Urinary cytology is highly specific (81 percent) for the diagnosis of TCC but it is fairly insensitive (30 to 50 percent). Its sensitivity increases with bladder barbotage (60 percent) and with poorly differentiated tumors and CIS (70 percent). It is a useful component of the hematuria evaluation but it is notoriously poor in detecting low-grade lesions.

4. *Flow cytometry.* This technique consists of an automated method of determining bladder cell DNA content. It has not proven to be superior to conventional cytology in managing patients with bladder cancer given that many tumors that progress are diploid and some aneuploid tumors do not progress.

5. *Tumor markers.* The criteria for an ideal tumor marker includes perfect sensitivity and specificity, the prediction of natural history or treatment outcome, the perfect detection of recurrence, and technical ease. Multiple candidate bladder tumor markers have been reported in the past few years. These include NMP-22, BTA stat, BTA trak, hyaluronic acid-Haase, telomerase activity, and microsatellite analysis. In general, these offer higher sensitivity than cytology even for lower-grade tumors (65 to 70 percent). Their most promising initial role would appear to be in monitoring those patients diagnosed and treated for superficial TCC. Exact guidelines for their use have yet to be established. The BTA test is a qualitative latex

agglutination assay that detects basement membrane antigens characterized from patients with TCC. The BTA trak assay quantitatively assesses human complement factor H-related protein produced by TCC. The NMP22 test quantitatively measures a non-chromatin nuclear protein shed in cells with rapid turnover. Although these tests offer higher sensitivity than urine cytology, their main limitation is a high false-positive rate when used in patients with history of calculi, lower urinary tract symptoms, cystitis, or incorporated bowel segments.

a. *NMP-22.* Nuclear matrix protein-22 measures a nuclear mytotic apparatus protein that is expressed at an increased level in transformed urothelial cells. The test is an ELISA assay. It provides greater sensitivity than urine cytology. The absolute normal cutoff value has not been determined. This marker may have value in monitoring patients with diagnosed disease.

b. *H-related protein test (BTAstat/trak).* The hCFRrp antigen demonstrates greater sensitivity but lower specificity than urine cytology. The antigen can be measured in a point of contact test or in a quantitative ELISA assay. Current data suggests that they may have a role in the monitoring of patients with diagnosed disease.

c. *Hyaluronic acid hyaluronidase.* The HA test is an ELISA-like assay measuring the production of these products in the urine of patients with bladder cancer. Its operating characteristics suggest that it may have a role in monitoring patients with bladder cancer.

d. *Telomerase activity.* Telomerase is an enzyme that may play a role in maintaining two limer sequences at the end of chromosomes. Its activity may reflect the presence of a mortal or cancer cell. Recent investigations suggest it is a potential tumor marker for bladder cancer.

e. *Microsatellite analysis.* Microsatellite repeat sequences can be measured at multiple gene loci, which in effect provides loss of heterozygosity (LOH) data on multiple key genes associated with bladder cancer progression. Early analysis suggests further potential of this technology in diagnosing and monitoring bladder cancer.

G. Pathology

TCC accounts for approximately 90 percent of bladder cancers, squamous cell carcinoma for 7 to 9 percent, and adenocarcinoma for 1 to 2 percent. Cytologic grade is an important component of tumor pathology, but no method of grading is uniformly accepted. Generally, lesions are graded on a 1 to 3 system of well, moderate, or poorly differentiated histology, respectively. Tumor grade does provide some independent prognostic information distinct from tumor stage.

1. *Epithelial dysplasia.* Dysplasia exhibits irregular urothelial and nuclear changes in a gradation toward carcinoma. High-grade dysplasia is difficult to distinguish from CIS. This is distinct from atypia, which is defined as an increase in cell layer number without changes in tissue structure or nuclear appearance.

2. *Carcinoma in situ.* This lesion is considered by many investigators to be the progenitor lesion for the majority of muscle-invasive tumors. When associated with diagnosed tumors, the potential for tumor recurrence and progression is thought to be higher. Its behavior is heterogeneous, however, since CIS can also be persistent yet indolent. It is often associated with irritative symptoms and must be ruled out in patients before diagnosing interstitial cystitis. These cells display little cell–cell adhesion and are readily identified on urine cytology obtained via barbotage.

3. *Superficial TCC.* These lesions are usually papillary but may also be nodular. The majority of lesions are mucosal only (Ta), but they may invade the lamina propria (T1). Superficial lesions may be high or low grade. In general, approximately 10 to 20 percent of patients with superficial lesions will display progression to muscle-invasive cancer on subsequent recurrent lesions. High-grade stage T1 tumors have a greater propensity to recur and progress to muscle-invasive lesions (30 percent).

4. *Muscle-invasive TCC.* The majority of these lesions tend to be nodular or sessile. Tumor infiltration of the muscularis propria is generally noted, but the invasion may be nodular or "pushing" rather than tentacular. Invasion may be noted through the entire detrusor layer and into the perivesical fat. The majority of these lesions are of high cytologic grade.

5. *Squamous cell carcinoma.* This is distinct from squamous metaplasia of the trigone only, which is noted in 20 to 30 percent of bladders of normal females. The lesion is probably secondary to chronic irritation. In Egypt, the majority of squamous cell carcinomas are associated with schistosomiasis infection. Patients with squamous cell carcinoma without a history of schistosomiasis usually present with high clinical stage lesions with a prognosis generally worse than TCC.

6. *Adenocarcinoma.* This accounts for 1 to 2 percent of bladder carcinomas and is noted at the bladder dome when associated with the urachus or at the bladder base near the trigone. Patients with bladder adenocarcinoma should undergo a complete work-up to rule-out other primary sources such as the gastrointestinal tract or breast.

7. *Sarcoma of the bladder.* Embryonal rhabdomyosarcoma or botryoid tumors may arise in the urinary bladder, vagina, prostate, or spermatic cord of infants and young children. Sarcoma of the bladder is rare in adults.

8. *Small cell carcinoma.* Rarely seen in the bladder or prostate, it consists of tumors of poorly differentiated cells with neuroendocrine features histologically undistinct from oat cell lung carcinoma. These tumors show rapid progression carry a poor prognosis. They are usually treated with a combination of radiotherapy and chemotherapy with etoposide (VP-16) and cis-platinum.

H. Natural History

Bladder tumors display a great deal of heterogeneity and often have a less than predictable natural history. Tumor development does not follow a linear progression from atypia to muscle invasion, and the genetic and biochemical events responsible for tumor progression are incompletely understood. General clinical patterns of tumor progression and therapeutic response can be predicted with greater confidence, but the future behavior of an individual tumor cannot easily be predicted.

1. *Superficial TCC.* These lesions comprise approximately 70 percent of bladder tumors. Only 10 to 20 percent of patients with these lesions display tumor progression to higher clinical stages over time. After resection, there is a cumulative 70 percent lifetime risk of tumor recurrence. Although most of these occur in the first year, it can be decreased with the use of intravesical chemotherapy. Tumor grade and size, multifocality, and associated CIS are associated with a greater chance for tumor recurrence.

2. *Carcinoma in situ.* CIS is a flat lesion displaying no tissue polarity. It can occur alone or in association with other lesions. It may or may not be associated with irritative symptoms; thus, this diagnosis must be ruled out before treating a patient for interstitial cystitis. Early series reported a progression rate as high as 80 percent to muscle-invasive carcinoma. This finding has been tempered by more recent reports suggesting lower progression rates

(20 to 50 percent) in patients with pure CIS without the presence of other tumors.

3. *Muscle-invasive TCC.* This form of bladder cancer is generally very aggressive. Older studies suggested a greater than 90 percent mortality rate within 2 years in untreated patients. The muscle spread may be tentacular or nodular. Survival has been correlated to stage. Overall survival after cystectomy is slightly higher than 50 percent at 5 years. Patients with node-positive disease have poorer survival rates than patients with node-negative disease, yet patients with a few (1 to 3) microscopic nodes can display reasonable survival rate (20 to 35 percent) at 5 years with the use of adjuvant chemotherapy.

4. *Pattern of progression.* Patients with invasive disease will display a 3 to 15 percent local recurrence rate after radical cystectomy. The usual sites for metastatic spread include the lungs, liver, and bones. Most recurrences occur within 18 to 24 months after definitive treatment.

I. Staging

1. The major staging systems are the Jewett-Strong-Marshall system (American) and the TNM system (UICC) (Fig. 17-2 and Table 17-3).

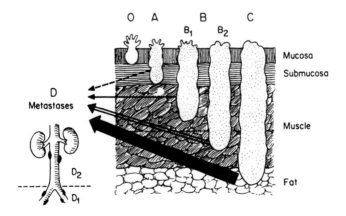

Figure 17-2 The American (Strong-Jewett-Marshall) staging system of bladder carcinoma serves as a conceptual basis for staging bladder cancer. (*Reproduced from Skinner DG: Current state of classification and staging of bladder cancer. Cancer Res 37:2838–2842, 1977.*)

Table 17-3 Bladder Cancer TNM Staging System 1997

Primary Tumor (T)

TX	Primary tumor cannot be assessed
Ta	Noninvasive papillary carcinoma
Tis	Carcinoma in situ
T1	Tumor invades subepithelial connective tissue
T2a	Tumor invades superficial detrusor muscle
T2b	Tumor invades deep detrusor muscle
T3a	Tumor invades perivesical tissue microscopically
T3b	Tumor invades perivesical tissue macroscopically
T4a	Tumor invades prostate, uterus, vagina
T4b	Tumor invades pelvic wall, abdominal wall

Regional Lymph Nodes (N)

NX	Regional lymph nodes cannot be assessed
N0	No regional lymph node metastasis
N1	Metastasis in a single lymph node, 2 cm or less in greatest dimension
N2	Metastasis in a single lymph node > 2 cm but < 5 cm, or multiple lymph nodes, none > 5 cm
N3	Metastasis in a lymph node > 5 cm in greatest dimension

Distant Metastasis (M)

MX	Distant metastasis cannot be assessed
M0	No distant metastasis
M1	Distant metastasis

Stage Grouping

0a	Ta	N0	M0
0is	Tis	N0	M0
I	T1	N0	M0
II	T2a	N0	M0
	T2b	N0	M0
III	T3a	N0	M0
	T3b	N0	M0
	T4a	N0	M0
IV	T4b	N0	M0
	Any T	Any N	Any M

2. Staging procedures

   a. *Cystourethroscopy with resection or excisional biopsy.* This is the standard initial method of staging. Superficial tumors should be completely removed, whereas obvious muscle-invasive lesions should be resected adequately to provide an unequivocal diagnosis. It is important to resect underlying muscle of a lesion to stage it appropriately. Additional random biopsies may be valuable to detect any carcinoma in situ. These should include the prostatic urethra since it can be the site of TCC and/or CIS and could affect the decision with regard to methods of treatment and urinary diversion.

  b. *Bimanual examination under anesthesia.* This is generally carried out at the time of endoscopy and TUR. Pelvic fixation generally denotes disease that has extended through the bladder wall (T3).

  c. *Excretory urography.* This is a component of the hematuria evaluation and is essential to the initial evaluation of newly diagnosed bladder cancer to rule out concomitant upper tract involvement or obstruction. As many as 4 percent of patients with bladder cancer will have or develop upper tract TCC.

  d. Chest x-ray or chest CT (T2 disease)

  e. Biochemical profile

  f. *Bone scan.* This is essential in a patient with T2 or greater disease.

  g. *CT of the abdomen and pelvis.* Cross-sectional imaging cannot accurately determine the level of detrusor invasion. It is useful in grossly assessing the lymph nodes and the liver.

  h. *Magnetic resonance imaging.* This technique provides equivalent information to that obtained with CT scanning. The role of endorectal coil MRI technology in staging this disease is under investigation.

  i. *Accuracy of staging.* Clinical staging can be quite imprecise with understaging occurring in 30 to 45 percent of patients and overstaying in 20 to 50 percent of patients. The most important issue in pretreatment clinical staging is the presence or absence of muscle invasion. Accurate and complete pathologic assessment is of vital importance, however, in assessing the cystectomy specimen.

J. Treatment
  1. Superficial bladder cancer
    a. *Transurethral resection of bladder tumor (TURBT).* This is the initial and standard therapy for these lesions. The tumor should be removed as completely, with inclusion of muscle in the specimen for adequate staging. Random biopsies are also obtained to detect CIS. The potential for further tumor seeding is debated. Intravesical chemotherapeutic agents may be given early after TURBT to abrogate this process.
    b. *Laser photocoagulation.* The neodymium–yttrium–aluminum–garnet (Nd-YAG) laser can be employed in

the treatment of superficial bladder cancer. Its principal disadvantage is the lack of available tissue for pathologic diagnosis. Advantages include less discomfort for the patient, minimal bleeding, and tissue denaturation, which reduces the possibility of tumor implantation.

c. *Intravesical therapy.* Due to the high rate of tumor recurrence and the chance for tumor progression, intravesical chemotherapy has evolved. The drugs are usually administered for a set course of weekly treatments. Continuous prophylactic therapy has been employed with mixed results. Most intravesical agents will decrease tumor recurrence from the baseline of 70 percent to 30 to 40 percent. There are no data to support the role of intravesical chemotherapy to reduce tumor progression.

  i. *Mitomycin C.* A dosage of 40 mg (1 mg/mL) is administered intravesically weekly for 6 to 8 weeks. It reduces tumor recurrence to 30 to 40 percent, but has not been shown to decrease tumor progression. It has been reported to possibly be more effective in higher grade lesions. Systemic effects are uncommon due to a lower level of absorption (high molecular weight: 329 kDa). Particular side effects include local skin irritation and the potential for chemical cystitis. Of note, it is the most expensive agent available.

  ii. *Adriamycin.* This drug has been used successfully for both prophylactic and definitive treatment. Response rates are standard. It is relatively well tolerated and exhibits few systemic side effects.

  iii. *Thiotepa.* This is the classic intravesical agent introduced in the 1960s. Between 30 and 60 mg (1 mg/mL) are administered according to various schedules. Myelosuppression with leukopenia and thrombocytopenia may occur in between 10 and 50 percent of patients due to the low molecular weight (198 d), which permits systemic absorption. Therefore, all patients should have complete blood counts monitored weekly while undergoing therapy. Treatment should be delayed with platelet counts lower than 100,000/mm^3 or white blood cell count lower than 4,000/mm^3. It has a minor role today in the treatment of bladder cancer.

  iv. *Bacillus Calmette-Guérin (BCG).* BCG is not a chemotherapeutic agent but an attenuated strain of *Mycobacterium bovis* that effects an inflammatory and immune response in the bladder. Its use in treating bladder cancer was first described in 1976. Several strains of BCG exist, Tice and Connaught being the most frequently employed. The efficacy of BCG is related to the number of colony-forming units per milligram of vaccine. Its exact mechanism is unknown but it appears to work through a T-cell mediated interaction. Efficacy is in part determined by the contact of BCG to the tumor surface. BCG is effective in reducing tumor recurrence (0 to 40 percent versus 70 percent of controls). It induces a complete response rate in as many as 72 percent of CIS patients (better than any other agent does). Contrary to other intravesical agents, evidence also suggests that BCG can delay disease progression in CIS patients. The optimal treatment course with BCG has not been established, but six weekly treatments are usually employed. A repeat course may be administered with an increase in the overall response rate. Nonresponders, however, have the potential (5 to 10 percent) to progress during therapy.

The major side effect of BCG is bladder irritability consisting of dysuria, frequency, and urgency in up to 90 percent of patients. Co-existent bacterial cystitis should be ruled-out in these patients. Care should be taken when treating bacterial urinary tract infections empirically, since quinolone antibiotics have been shown to decrease the effectiveness of the bacillus. Nitrofurantoin and sulfa-based antimicrobials are recommended, given the resistance of BCG to these antibiotics. Approximately 2 percent of patients will develop systemic symptoms (BCGosis) accompanied by fever longer than 48 hours. Triple-drug antituberculosis therapy should be instituted with isoniazid (300 mg), rifampin (600 mg), and ethambutol (1200 mg) daily. Approximately 0.4 percent of patients can develop frank BCG sepsis. Deaths have been reported with BCG use. Cycloserine should be added in life-threatening sepsis given its faster onset of action. BCG should not be administered in the presence of hematuria, urinary tract infection, or following a traumatic catheterization.

  v. *Other agents.* Interferons (INF-α2b) have been tested as possible intravesical agents with positive responses. Other cytokines are also being investigated. Keyhole limpet cyanin (a mollusk-derived, nonspecific immune stimulant) has also displayed promise as a therapeutic agent. Photodynamic therapy with different agents is also under investigation.

d. *Monitoring.* There is no evidence-based schedule for patient follow-up. A reasonable approach consists of cystoscopy with cytology every 3 months for a year, followed by an examination every 6 months for a variable period in the absence of any recurrence. After a long tumor-free interval, the frequency of examinations may be reduced. The newly described tumor markers may play some role in the future in modulating this schedule, perhaps decreasing the cystoscopy interval. The development of upper tract tumors in these patients, although classically felt to be low, may be higher than previously suspected (10 to 30 percent up to 15 years), especially for those patients treated for carcinoma in situ. Therefore regular periodic intravenous urograms are necessary. There is no established schedule for this monitoring test.

2. Muscle-invasive TCC

a. *Radical cystectomy.* This is the standard of care in treating muscle-invasive bladder cancer. A radical cystectomy entails en bloc removal of the bladder, prostate, seminal vesicles, and proximal urethra. Indications for radical cystectomy include muscle invasion, low-stage tumors that are unresectable or multicentric, high-grade tumors associated with CIS, and rapidly recurring multifocal tumors or CIS after transurethral resection and intravesical therapy. Patients with high-grade superficial disease who recur after two courses of intravesical BCG in less than 1 year should be offered radical cystectomy. Recent studies have shown that as many as 30 percent of these patients will have muscle invasion in the cystectomy specimen.

The most important predictor of recurrence in the urethra is prostatic involvement, followed by multifocal bladder or prostatic carcinoma in situ. In these patients, recurrence rates range between 17 and 37 percent, as opposed to a 1 to 4 percent recurrence rate in patients without prostatic involvement. Prostatic stromal invasion is most ominous. Therefore, in males, urethrectomy is generally recommended in the presence of prostatic urethral involvement, prostatic stro-

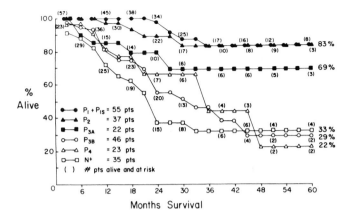

Figure 17-3 Kaplan Meyer survival curves are presented for nonirradiated patients undergoing cystectomy alone for treatment of bladder carcinoma. At present, patient survival is better stage for stage with surgery compared to more conservative forms of therapy. (*Reproduced from Skinner DG, Lieskovsky G, eds: Diagnosis and Management of Genitourinary Cancer, 1988, p 697.*)

mal invasion, diffuse bladder or prostatic CIS, or a positive margin at the time of cystectomy.

In females, an anterior exenteration is performed that includes removal of the bladder, entire urethra, anterior vaginal wall, a total abdominal hysterectomy, and bilateral salpingoophorectomy. This is justified given that the recurrence rate in the anterior vagina is 28 percent when it is left in situ. An en bloc pelvic lymph node dissection starting at the aortic bifurcation or common iliac vessels is performed in both genders. Survival for patients with radical cystectomy alone is shown in Figure 17-3. Urinary diversion is an integral component of the procedure and accounts for most of the long-term postoperative morbidity. The physiologic and technical aspects of this are discussed fully in Chapter 18. The major forms of diversion include a standard ileal conduit, colon conduit, or continent urinary diversion, which may be cutaneous or orthotopic.

Operative mortality for radical cystectomy and urinary diversion is roughly 1 to 3 percent. Early and late postoperative complications range from 10 to 30 percent. Early complications include wound infection (3 to 5 percent), intestinal obstruction (5 to 10 percent), deep vein thrombosis, and rectal injuries (1 to 4 percent). Notable late complications include fecal–urinary fistulas (4 percent), pyelonephritis, ureterointestinal anastomotic strictures, renal deterioration, and erectile dysfunction. Ureterointestinal anastomotic stricture rates have decreased considerably, with the use of silastic stents. Strictures shorter than 2 cm are best managed by antegrade balloon dilatation. Success rates with percutaneous techniques are poor for longer strictures. These patients may require open anastomotic revision.

b. *Partial cystectomy.* This technique may be employed on a very selective basis for circumscribed lesions, usually in the dome of the bladder, where a 1- 2-cm free margin can be obtained without requiring a further procedure such as ureteral reimplantation. In addition, it may be indicated in patients with papillary TCC within a bladder diverticulum. Some centers advocate the use of low-dose neoadjuvant external beam radiation therapy immediately before partial cystectomy to decrease the incidence of wound implantation. Partial cystectomy can be overextended in the hope of preserving a normal lower urinary tract. This should not be the case in the present era of continent urinary diversion.

c. *Radiation therapy.* Definitive radiation therapy has been employed in invasive bladder cancer. Overall durable complete responses are 40 percent and are much poorer stage for stage than those obtained with surgery. Interstitial radiation therapy (iridium needles) has been employed primarily in Europe. Careful patient selection is necessary to obtain success.

d. *Transurethral resection (TUR).* In the case of patients who are severely medically compromised, TUR can be an appropriate form of therapy for invasive lesions. Laser photocoagulation can be employed in addition in this situation. A complete response may be obtained in as many as 20 to 30 percent of patients with the use of intravesical therapy. Reports of greater success also incorporate salvage cystectomy as part of the therapy.

e. *Combined modality therapy.* TUR, platinum-based combination chemotherapy, and external beam radiation therapy have been employed on a protocol basis (the so-called bladder salvage regimen). Select patients have experienced good short-term complete responses while preserving their bladders. Long-term follow-up is necessary to gauge duration of response and side effects on lower tract urinary function.

f. *Adjuvant therapy.* Invasive TCC is responsive to several cytoreductive agents. It is debatable whether chemotherapy in an adjuvant or neoadjuvant setting provides a greater sustained complete response to radical cystectomy alone. Please refer to the chapter on chemotherapeutic drugs for an in-depth discussion.

g. *Metastatic disease.* Almost 50 percent of patients with muscle-invasive TCC will suffer a distant or local recurrence of disease. The classic therapy regimen methotrexate, vinblastine, adriamycin, and cis-platinum (MVAC) can effect 50 to 70 percent response rates but less than 15 percent sustain complete responses. Other agents such as paclitaxel, carboplatin, and gemcitabine are also being studied. The role of molecular markers such as p53 in directing or predicting response to chemotherapy is being actively evaluated.

h. *Palliative therapy.* Aggressive intervention is occasionally necessary without intent to cure. Intractable hemorrhage is the most common indication. It can be treated by several methods including salvage cystectomy, hypogastric infarction, supravesical diversion, and intravesical formalin instillation (in the absence of reflux).

2. *Follow-up after cystectomy.* Although there are no established guidelines for surveillance after cystectomy, a reasonable schedule proposed by the Memorial-Sloan Kettering Cancer Center group includes a history and physical examination (H&P), chest x-ray, urine cytology, and serum laboratories (CBC, SMA-6, and alkaline phosphatase) every 3 months for 1 year, every 4 months for 2 years, and then every 6 months thereafter. In addition, they recommend yearly cross-sectional imaging (CT scan or MRI) and intravenous urography to rule out visceral metastases, lymphadenopathy, ureteral obstruction, and upper tract recurrence. Because approximately 10 percent of patients will develop a urethral recurrence after cystectomy, patients who do not meet the criteria for urethrectomy at the time of cystectomy will need life-long follow-up. An intact urethra is best monitored by routine urethral cytology performed 4 to 8 weeks after cystectomy, with decreasing frequency thereafter. This is most

important early on because most urethral recurrences will manifest in the first 3 years after cystectomy. Patients with positive cytology, hematuria, or symptoms should undergo urethroscopy. In the case of a urethral recurrence after an orthotopic continent urinary diversion, patients should undergo urethrectomy with some form of urinary diversion.

Swanson and colleagues at M.D. Anderson Cancer Center proposed a cost-effective follow-up schedule based on pathologic stage, given that 5-year recurrence rates for pT1, pT2, and pT3 disease were 5, 20, and 40 percent, respectively. Since no patients with pathological stage T1 disease developed pelvic recurrences, they recommend a yearly H&P, laboratories (CBC, SMA-6, liver function tests), upper tract evaluation (intravenous urogram, loopogram, or renal ultrasound), and urine cytology. Patients with pathological stage 2 disease undergo an H&P, laboratories, and CXR every 6 months for 3 years, then yearly. Urine cytology and upper tract imaging (intravenous urogram or renal ultrasound) are recommended on a yearly basis. Patients with pathological stage 3 disease undergo the same surveillance as patients with pT2, with the addition of abdominal CT scans at 6 months, then yearly.

IV. ADENOCARCINOMA OF THE PROSTATE
A. General Considerations

Adenocarcinoma of the prostate is the most common cancer in men and the second most common cause of cancer-related death after lung cancer. The addition of serum prostate-specific antigen (PSA) determinations to digital rectal examination for detection strategies has caused a significant stage migration in prostate cancer. Ultrasound-guided needle biopsy has become the principal method of diagnosis and information gained from these tissue cores in conjunction with the serum PSA level provides the majority of staging information required for therapeutic decisions. The choice of therapy for localized disease must be based on many factors including the grade and stage of disease, personal preference, patient age, and performance status. Appropriate therapy for organ-confined disease is controversial, with radical surgery and external beam radiation therapy as the major treatment modalities. Prostate tumors are generally androgen sensitive, and advanced disease is most often treated by single or combined androgen ablation. Those patients with clinically advanced disease (extensive lymphadenopathy or bony metastasis) are still initially treated with androgen ablation. This is generally palliative. Although hormone refractory of prostate cancer may be responsive to newer chemotherapy regimens, few patients experience sustained complete response. However, the largest group of patients with "advanced disease" includes those patients with a detectable or rising PSA after therapy for organ-confined disease (biochemical failure). Novel therapy for advanced disease is an active area of investigation. Treatment for hormone refractory disease is at present limited.

B. Incidence

Approximately 180,000 new cases of prostate cancer will be diagnosed in 2000, and prostate cancer will account for approximately 31,000 cancer-related deaths occurred in 2000. Since the introduction of PSA as a screening tool, there has been a large incidence increase in prostate cancer, which has now subsided. This "cull defect" demonstrates the harvesting of prevalent disease after the introduction of this new test. The death rate from prostate cancer has decreased nearly 10 percent over the past 15 years and is indirect evidence for the positive impact of screening strategies.

C. Etiology

The specific genetic and biochemical alterations responsible for the development of prostate cancer are under intense investigation, but a specific cause for this disease has yet been detected. Prostate cancer is unevenly distributed geographically and among ethnic groups, suggesting certain risk factors for disease.

1. *Age.* Prostate cancer is generally detected after the age of 50. It can be seen earlier in African Americans and in men with a family history. The autopsy incidence of prostate cancer is at least 30 percent in men over the age of 50 and climbs to over 70 percent by the 8th decade of life. A majority of these lesions may be otherwise undetectable and clinically insignificant.

2. *Family history.* Active research has disclosed a twofold risk for prostate cancer if an individual has a first-degree relative with prostate cancer. This climbs to almost ninefold if three first-degree relatives are affected. Risk also exists if second-degree relatives have a diagnosis of prostate cancer. Multiple putative loci for heredity prostate cancer genes have been suggested on the short and long arms of chromosome 1, the short arm of chromosome 17, and the X chromosome.

3. *Ethnic origin.* African American men have the highest related risk of prostate cancer of any group in the world. They also suffer higher age-specific mortality, diagnosis at an earlier age, and higher age-specific incidence. Their rate of disease is nearly twice that of white men. Asian men have a very low risk of prostate cancer, which rises after migration to the United States.

4. *Androgens.* Studies on androgen levels have been conflicting but have suggested higher testosterone levels or dihydrotestosterone–colon testosterone ratios in African American men. Mutations or alterations in the androgen receptor (CAG repeats) may also be unequally distributed among individuals in populations affecting response to testosterone.

5. *Diet.* High intake of animal fat is associated with increased prostate cancer risk. Conversely, the intake of soy products (isoflavenoids, phytoestrogens, bowman-birk inhibitor) may inhibit the development and progression of prostate cancer. Studies in other tumor systems on vitamin E and selenium showed a one- to two-third decrease in prostate cancer incidence, respectively. Carotenoids such as lycopene (responsible for the red color of tomatoes) may be associated with the decrease prostate cancer risk.

6. *Vasectomy.* The overwhelming majority of studies measuring the effect of vasectomy and the development of prostate cancer have failed to confirm any association between this procedure and prostate cancer.

7. *Environmental exposure.* Although a weak association to cadmium exposure is often cited, no causative agents have been identified.

8. *Insulin-like growth factors.* Several recent studies have demonstrated that elevated levels of insulin-like growth factor 1 (IGF-1) are associated with a higher risk of prostate cancer.

D. Epidemiology

1. *Autopsy incidence.* The same autopsy incidence of prostate cancer described earlier is noted in several more contemporary studies in European, Asian, and African populations. This suggests that other factors have an impact on a similar baseline predisposition to the disease.

2. *Race.* There is a striking difference in the racial distribution of prostate cancer. African Americans have the highest incidence of the disease followed by white Americans and Europeans. The rate of prostate cancer in native Asian

populations is 15 times lower than American white populations. African Americans have twice the incidence and death rate from prostate cancer compared to whites, even when studies are controlled for socioeconomic status.

3. *Geography.* Newer data suggest an inverse relationship between latitude and the incidence of prostate cancer. Northern populations have a greater level of disease, and it is hypothesized that it is related to the lower vitamin D levels secondary to less exposure to ultraviolet radiation. Migration studies of Asians moving west demonstrate an increase in prostate cancer incidence compared to that of white populations in the same area, perhaps due to dietary changes or other factors. Native black populations in Zaire have lower levels of prostate cancer compared to ethnic Zairians living in Belgium.

E. Pathology

1. *Benign.* Cystadenoma.
2. *Prostatic intraepithelial neoplasia (PIN).* Proliferation of acinar epithelium displaying varying grades of cytologic abnormalities. Patients with high-grade PIN (2 and 3) have a 30 to 40 percent chance of developing prostate carcinoma in the future, not necessarily at sites of prior PIN. Therefore, these patients should undergo repeat biopsies from different areas of the prostate. Since its natural history is poorly understood, patients with negative repeat biopsies should be closely monitored.
3. Malignant
   a. *Conventional adenocarcinoma (small acinar carcinoma).* The vast majority (95 to 97 percent) of prostate cancer is adenocarcinoma derived from acinar epithelium. The majority of lesions arise in the peripheral zone of the prostate gland. Approximately 20 to 25 percent of adenocarcinomas arise from the transitional zone. Classically, these tumors are discovered after TURP and described as stage 1a or 1b disease. The grading and staging of this entity is discussed elsewhere.

   Histologic variants include the following.
   1. *Ductal or endometriod carcinoma.* Displays exuberant papillary growth into prostatic ducts, which may be seen endoscopically. Usually present at advanced stages. May have a poor prognosis, stage for stage, than conventional adenocarcinoma.
   2. *Mucinous adenocarcinoma.* More than 25 percent of the tumor must be composed of mucing

containing glands to qualify for this diagnosis. Prognosis may be equal or worse than with conventional prostatic adenocarcinoma.

3. *Signet cell carcinoma.* Very poor prognosis. Most patients die with 40 months of diagnosis.

4. *Small cell carcinoma.* Neuroendocrine carcinoma of the prostate is rare and has been confused with poorly differentiated adenocarcinoma. The precursor cells, however, secrete different neuropeptides and may play a role in the hormonal refractory phenotype of prostate cancer. The diagnosis carries a very poor prognosis, although some patients show a partial response to radiotherapy and chemotherapy with VP-16 (etoposide) and cis-platinum.

5. *Squamous and adenosquamous carcinoma.* Very aggressive.

6. *Basaloid and adenoid cystic carcinoma.*

b. *Transitional cell carcinoma (TCC).* TCC of the prostate may be derived from major ducts of the prostate near the urethra. It is seen as the direct extension of a bladder tumor or as separate foci of cancer in the prostate. The worst prognosis is seen in patients with stromal invasion. Patients with isolated CIS of the prostatic urethra should undergo TURP and subsequent BCG intravesical therapy.

c. Sarcomas of the prostate are rare. In the adult population, leiomyosarcomas predominate. Prognosis is poor with an average 5-year survival rate of 40 percent. Rhabdomyosarcomas, which have a worse 5-year survival rate (0 to 10 percent), are generally seen in pediatric patients.

d. Metastatic tumors (colorectal, melanoma, lung, etc.)

e. Hematologic malignancies (lymphoma, plasmacytoma, leukemia involvement)

5. *Patterns of spread.* Prostate tumors can spread by direct extension into the seminal vesicles and extracapsularly through the periprostatic nerve routes. Direct extension into the rectum is uncommon. Ureteral obstruction can occur in 10 to 35 percent of patients during the course of their disease. Lymphatic spread is not uncommon and occurs to the hypogastric, obturator, external iliac, presacral, common iliac, and paraaortic nodes in roughly that order. Skip metastases are rare. Ninety percent of distant metastases are osseous. Visceral metastases to the lung, liver, and adrenals are less common and are rarely seen without bone involvement.

Age at Diagnosis, y

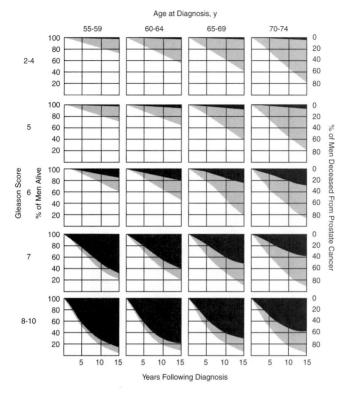

Figure 17-4 Connecticut tumor registry data on natural history of prostate cancer. Shaded area represents death from all causes. Blackened area represents death from prostate cancer.

F. Natural History

1. Selection bias and higher risk factors for competing forms of mortality seriously confound a majority of the data on natural history. In general, those patients with low-grade disease have a 10 percent or less chance of mortality over 10 years of follow-up. However, those patients with high-grade disease have a 60 percent probability of a prostate cancer-related death. The average patient with moderate grade prostate cancer has a 13 percent mortality, yet a 40 percent chance of tumor progression over 10 years.

2. The most accurate assessment of the natural history of prostate cancer is derived from the Connecticut tumor registry and is depicted in Figure 17-4. The blackened

area represents the risk of a prostate cancer related death. The shaded area represents death from all causes. The risk increase in those patients demonstrating Gleason pattern 4 disease is striking.

3. Natural history of advanced disease is best understood with a median survival of 30 to 33 months, 75 percent mortality at 5 years, and 90 percent mortality at 10 years.

G. Grading and Staging Systems

1. *Gleason grade.* This is a system based on the degree of glandular differentiation and growth pattern. Five patterns are described. A "score" is given for each tumor that represents the sum of the two most common patterns displayed. The scores range from 2 to 10 and have some prognostic predictive value at the very low or very high ranges.

2. *Mostofi grade.* This system is based on the degree of nuclear irregularity. The lesions are graded as well, moderately, or poorly differentiated.

3. *Staging systems.* The American Joint Committee on Cancer has a modified TNM system. This is depicted in Table 17-4.

H. Signs and Symptoms

Prostate cancer has few dramatic primary signs or symptoms. It can be associated with urinary obstructive symptoms or hematuria, although these findings are usually due to other causes. Bone pain can unfortunately be an initial symptom, but it represents very advanced disease. A prostatic nodule or induration of the gland is a hallmark sign on physical examination. It is not always specific for a carcinoma and can underestimate the extent of disease when it does represent a carcinoma.

I. Diagnosis and Staging

1. *Digital rectal examination (DRE).* This is a classic component of the physical examination that, by itself, is not as sensitive or specific for prostate cancer as one might think. Any palpable irregularity has an approximately 50 percent chance of being a carcinoma. Conversely, a normal DRE does not exclude the possibility of prostate cancer.

2. *Transrectal ultrasound (TRUS).* Multiple studies have shown TRUS to be a very sensitive but nonspecific method of detecting prostate cancer. The classic finding is a hypoechoic lesion that, in general, has a 30 percent

Table 17-4 Prostate Cancer TNM Stating System AJCC 1997

Primary Tumor (T)

TX	Primary tumor cannot be assessed
T1a	Normal DRE; incidental tumor $\leq$ 5% of total surgical specimen and of low to medium grade
T1b	Normal DRE: incidental tumor $\geq$ 5% of specimen, any grade, or $\geq$ 5% of specimen with any high grade
T1c	Normal DRE; tumor identified by prostate needle biopsy (e.g. elevated PSA)
T2a	Organ-confined limited to one lobe of the prostate
T2b	Organ-confined; involves both lobes
T3a	Extracapsular (unilateral or bilateral)
T3b	Tumor invades seminal vesicles
T4	Tumor is fixed or invades adjacent structures other than seminal vesicles (e.g., bladder, rectum)

Regional Lymph Nodes (N)

NX	Regional lymph nodes cannot be assessed
N0	No regional lymph node metastasis
N1	Metastasis in regional lymph node or nodes

Distant Metastasis (M)

MX	Distant metastasis cannot be assessed
M0	No distant metastasis
M1a	Nonregional lymph node metastasis
M1b	Bone metastasis
M1c	Other metastatic sites

Stage Grouping

I	T1a	N0	M0	G1
II	T1a	N0	M0	G2, 3-4
	T1b	N0	M0	Any G
	T1c	N0	M0	Any G
	T1	N0	M0	Any G
	T2	N0	M0	Any G
III	T3	N0	M0	Any G
IV	T4	N0	M0	Any G
	Any T	N1	M0	Any G
	Any T	Any N	M1	Any G

DRE, digital rectal examination; PSA, prostate specific antigen.

chance of being positive for carcinoma. Because prostate cancer can also present as isoechoic or hyperechoic lesions, transrectal ultrasonography should not be used as a screening tool for prostate carcinoma. The most important use of TRUS is in aiding transrectal needle biopsies of the prostate gland.

3. *Serum markers.* The classic marker for prostate cancer was acid phosphatase. The enzymatic test was elevated in 70 percent of patients with extracapsular and metastatic prostate cancer. The more sensitive radioimmunoassay of this enzyme is not as useful for detecting extracapsular disease and has no value as a screening test for prostate cancer. PSA is the most useful marker in the detection and monitoring of prostate cancer and is discussed in detail separately.

4. *Prostate needle biopsy.* A spring-loaded gun is used to obtain prostate needle biopsy cores. The classic approach is to obtain sextant biopsies. However, recent data suggest that more biopsies should be obtained (8 to 12 cores) to increase sampling of the peripheral zone, and thus prostate cancer detection. There is a lesser role for sampling the transitional zone or mid zone. The percentage of positive cores, line length, or percentage of cancer per core can provide further predictive information with regard to staging and outcome. The procedure is well tolerated with the major side effect being prolonged hematospermia. Severe hematochezia and sepsis are rare complications. Lower gastrointestinal tract cleansing enemas and prophylactic antibiotics are routine.

5. *Bone scan.* Given the propensity of prostate cancer to metastasize to bone, radionuclide imaging is routinely used to evaluate for disseminated disease. Before a lesion can be seen on a conventional radiograph, it must have replaced bone mass by 30 to 50 percent and must be at least 10 to 15 mm in diameter. Plain radiograph correlates usually clarify any suspicious areas. In some cases, dedicated MRI or CT imaging can resolve equivocal cases. Recent studies have shown that the likelihood of a positive bone scan in patients with a PSA value less than 10 ng/mL and no bone symptoms is 1 per 1000. Although most experts agree that the positive predictive value of a bone scan in men with organ-confined disease and a PSA less than 10 ng/mL is very low, some still advocate its role in this setting as a baseline study.

6. *Computed tomography and magnetic resonance imaging (MRI).* CT scans and body surface coil MRI of the pelvis have poor performance characteristics for assessing metastatic disease and are not part of standard staging. However, endorectal MRI may provide additional staging information in those patients with intermediate PSAs and greater than 50 percent positive needle core biopsies to assess the presence of extracapsular disease.

7. *Bilateral pelvic lymphadenectomy.* This procedure is usually performed at the time of radical prostatectomy. In cases with a higher likelihood of positive nodes (Gleason score 7 or higher or PSA higher than 10), most urologists await frozen section analysis before proceeding with the prostatectomy. However, disease stage migration due to widespread screening has significantly decreased the probability of positive pelvic lymph nodes at the time of prostatectomy. Since these are found in less than 5 percent of most newly detected cases, most urologists will proceed with the prostatectomy without frozen section analysis if the nodal tissue feels benign on palpation in patients with a serum PSA lower than 10 and Gleason score 6 or less. Some centers advocate a staging pelvic lymphadenectomy (laparoscopic or open) in patients undergoing external beam radiation therapy who are at higher risk of recurrence due to a high Gleason score or PSA (e.g., higher than 10 ng/mL) or in the presence of presumed extracapsular disease. In the setting of positive nodes, some radiotherapists may elect to widen the radiation field or treat the patient with androgen ablation for a longer time. The role of laparoscopic pelvic lymphadenectomy, however, remains controversial.

8. *Multimodal staging.* Pioneering work by Partin has demonstrated that multivariant analysis of easily obtainable parameters such as serum PSA, Gleason score, and digital rectal examination can be used to give a reasonable preoperative estimate of tumor stage. Such systems may be helpful when counseling patients.

J. Cancer Screening

1. The major goal of any screening test is to decrease the number of deaths caused by that particular cancer. Because of the long time to progression and death from prostate cancer, it is not known whether present screening strategies are absolutely effective. The continuing decrease in the death rate from prostate cancer is indirect proof for the efficacy of serum PSA.

2. *Digital rectal examination (DRE-based screening).* In patients whose cancer was detected by DRE alone, over two thirds had extraprostatic disease at the time of surgery. Strategies incorporating PSA and DRE can detect more prostate cancer, and it appears that both tests provide independent unique information.

3. *PSA.* In general, 5 to 8 percent of a screening population will demonstrate an abnormal PSA. A serum PSA

between 4 to 10 ng/mL suggests a 16 to 25 percent chance of a positive needle biopsy in the setting of a normal DRE. A serum PSA greater than 10 ng/mL is associated with a 67 percent chance of a positive biopsy. In general, 1 to 3 percent of participants are found to have cancer (significantly lower than the incidental pathologic incidence). This is indirect evidence suggesting PSA does not over detect prostate cancer. Using a cutoff value of 4.0 ng/mL, the positive predictive value of PSA alone, DRE alone, and the combination of PSA and DRE for the detection of prostate cancer is 42, 34, and 61 percent, respectively. The sensitivity and specificity for PSA as a detection tool is 80 percent and 65 percent, respectively.

a. *Free PSA.* PSA is a serine protease that can exist free in the serum or bound to alpha-1-antichymotrypsin and alpha-2-macroglobulin. Because patients with prostate cancer have lower levels of free PSA, the percentage free PSA may be used as a screening strategy to increase specificity. If a 25 percent free PSA cutoff value is employed, 90 percent of all prostate cancers can be detected by reducing the number of unnecessary biopsies by 31 percent. With this strategy, however, specificity is enhanced at a cost of decreased sensitivity. Therefore, although its use as a primary screening tool is controversial, many urologists use free PSA in evaluating the need for repeat biopsies in men with a history of prior negative biopsies.

b. *PSA velocity.* Several studies suggest that if the serum PSA increases greater than 0.75 g/mL per year the potential for prostate cancer is greater. Unfortunately, since PSA variability can be as high as 23.5 percent per reading, three separate readings 6 months apart are necessary to establish a true trend. In addition, no added benefit has been demonstrated in patients with a PSA level between 4 and 10 ng/mL.

c. *PSA density.* Because the volume of the normal prostate is directly proportional to serum PSA, it is logical to assume that higher PSAs associated with smaller glands would have a greater potential for cancer. An optimal cutoff of 0.15 ng/mL^3 has been suggested. Unfortunately, the variability of ultrasound volume determination ranges between 20 and 30 percent.

d. *Age-adjusted PSA.* Strategies to lower the "normal" PSA for younger patients and raise it for older patients has been suggested to increase sensitivity in younger patients and specificity in older patients. This strategy carries a 15 to 20 percent "miss rate" in older population groups. Similar race-based age-specific PSA scales have been developed.

4. *Bias.* Length time bias consists of detecting a case at an earlier time in its history and suggesting a longer survival period from treatment, which is actually just a longer period of observation. Lead-time bias consists in part of selecting cases from a disease population with good survival traits and thus suggesting an apparent survival benefit that does not exist.

5. *Beneficence.* Active detection can have a negative effect by causing more morbidity and mortality through detection and treatment of disease that is clinically insignificant.

6. *Cost.* The cost of screening and treatment can be tremendous, yet many of these estimates are based on very high compliance rates that do not usually occur in a general population.

7. Advocates of screening point to the high percentage of patients who present initially with organ-confined disease as a reason for screening. Additionally, most clinical detection programs have a discovery rate of 2 to 5 percent, not the 30 to 50 percent seen in pathologic series, suggesting that important clinical disease is being detected by such strategies. In addition, cancers detected by PSA screening are clinically significant as defined by Catalona (i.e., PSA does not detect insignificant lesions).

8. The American Cancer Society now recommends that a serum PSA and DRE be performed yearly in men over the age of 50 years. Confirmation of this recommendation as an efficient screening tool is pending. African Americans and individuals with a family history of prostate cancer may benefit from detection strategies starting at age 40.

K. Prostate Specific Antigen

1. *Biochemical characteristics.* PSA is a 240 amino acid single chain glycoprotein that has a molecular weight of 34 kd. It is coded on chromosome 19 (6 Kb: 4 introns, 5 exons), is homologous to members of the kallikrein gene superfamily, and is designated human kallikrein3 (hK3). It behaves as a serine protease.

2. *Physiology.* PSA liquifies the seminal coagulum that is formed after ejaculation. A substrate produced in the seminal vesicles has been identified. PSA has chymotrypsin- and trypsin-like activity. Its half-life is 2.2 to 3.2 days.

3. *Marker properties.* The generally used monoclonal assay (2 murine MAbs for two specific epitopes) suggests a normal serum value of 4.0 ng/mL. Serum values are not generally altered by DRE, but can be affected by urologic instrumentation, ejaculation, and prostate biopsy. Benign conditions that can raise PSA levels include prostatitis, prostate infarction, and benign prostatic hypertrophy.

4. *General clinical use.* PSA is most useful as a surveillance tool to monitor patients after radical prostatectomy because postoperative baseline values should be in the undetectable range. Residual disease is suggested by detectable postoperative levels greater than 0.4 ng/mL. Rising PSA levels after surgery imply disease recurrence at least 6 months prior to other clinical modalities. PSA values nadir after radiation therapy, and should be at or less than 0.5 within 12 months of treatment. Three consecutive elevations after the PSA nadir suggest failure after radiation therapy. After androgen ablation, PSA levels do not necessarily represent disease volume.

5. Cancer detection and PSA (see screening).

L. Treatment for Localized Disease

1. *General considerations.* In discussing treatment for prostate cancer, it is important to consider patient factors such as age and general performance status as well as tumor factors such as Gleason score, initial serum PSA, and estimated clinical volumes/stage of the tumor. If a patient has less than a 50 percent chance of surviving 10 years, it is difficult to measure the positive effect of treatment. The side effects of different therapies also have to be considered. It is optimal when patients come to a treatment decision based on consultation and input from both surgical and radiation oncology services.

2. *Radical or complete prostatectomy.* This is the treatment choice for patients with organ-confined disease and a life expectancy of more than 10 years. Generally, age 70 is used as a relative cutoff for strongly recommending surgery. Using an anatomical retropubic approach, Walsh has shown that the carvernosal nerves that mediate erectile function can be identified and avoided, reducing postoperative erectile dysfunction considerably. This can be done in greater than 50 percent of men under the age of 60 but is less successful in men as they approach and surpass the age of 70. Significant urinary incontinence may be encountered in up to 4 to 8 percent of patients, and bladder

neck contractures can occur in 2 to 6 percent of patients. Surgical mortality is less than 0.2 percent but 1 to 2 percent of patients may develop pulmonary emboli. The radical perineal prostatectomy is associated with reduced blood loss as the dorsal venous complex is not divided. It may be the preferred approach in very obese men or in those with a history of abdominal or pelvic surgery where significant retropubic scarring and fibrosis are suspected.

3. Radiation therapy
   a. *External beam radiation therapy.* This is an option for localized prostate cancer and is the treatment of choice for T3 disease. This modality is discussed in greater depth in Chapter 20. In general, it is administered in divided doses ranging from 70 to 80 Gy and is well tolerated. Approximately 3 to 5 percent of patients will experience persistent rectal or bladder symptomatology and greater than 50 percent of patients develop erectile dysfunction within 2 years. Hematuria or hemorrhagic cystitis is a late development in a small percentage of patients. Techniques of conformal therapy have reduced unwanted radiation to the bladder and rectum.
   b. *Interstitial brachytherapy.* Ultrasound-guided transperineal brachytherapy has become an accepted modality for the treatment of localized prostate cancer using ^{125}I or ^{103}Pd radiation sources. Recommended minimum dosing is 144 Gy. Optimal candidates have a serum PSA of less than 10 ng/mL and a Gleason score of 6 or lower. Many centers utilize short-term neoadjuvant hormonal blockade given the difficulty in treating prostate glands larger than 50 g. Conversely, glands smaller than 20 g are difficult to implant. Short-term complications include urinary retention, urethritis, and irritative voiding symptoms, especially in patients with a history of lower urinary tract obstructive symptoms. Long-term major complications include stricture or contracture development and proctitis. Incontinence is uncommon but averages 20 percent in men with a history of transurethral resection of the prostate. Short-term results (5 years) suggest similar outcomes to surgery or external beam radiation therapy, but long-term data are lacking. Results are not as encouraging for men with tumors of Gleason grade 7 or higher. Newer protocols include combination of brachytherapy and external beam radiation therapy.

4. Follow-up after treatment for localized disease
   Serum PSA is the single most important follow-up parameter in evaluating patients after definitive treatment

with either surgery or radiation. A reasonable surveillance schedule should include a history and physical examination and serum PSA every 3 months during the first year, every 6 months for 4 years, and yearly thereafter. Bone scans and CT scans should be obtained only as indicated.

a. In patients who are managed surgically, the serum PSA should nadir to an undetectable level. Occasionally, very low persistent PSA levels that do not progress are noted. In most cases, if the serum PSA becomes detectable and rises above 0.4 ng/mL, the patient continues to show disease progression. Biochemical failure can predate clinical failure by 4 to 6 years. Newer data suggest that biochemical failure is a surrogate marker for ultimate clinical failure and survival. The incidence of a detectable PSA 5 years after radical prostatectomy depends on pathologic stage, being approximately 5 percent for patients with organ confined disease, 11 percent with capsular penetration, 66 percent for seminal vesicle involvement, and 76 percent in patients with lymph node involvement. Patients with high-grade disease who fail early and display a short doubling time may have a survival as early as 7 years, while late failures in low to moderate grade disease who are progressing slowly may live as long as 19 years. The overall 10- to 15-year recurrence rate for localized disease is approximately 20 percent. Further follow-up is necessary to truly define the true impact of clinical failure.

b. There is a role for external beam radiation therapy after postsurgical biochemical failures due to local recurrence. Success rates are highest when therapy is instituted before the PSA is greater than 1.0 ng/mL. Percentage for cure ranges between 30 and 50 percent in different series.

c. In general, response to external beam radiation therapy as a primary form of therapy depends on the pretreatment PSA and can be predicted by the PSA nadir after treatment. In other words, overall outcome is best in patients with the lowest post-treatment PSA nadir. Biochemical failure is defined by three consecutive elevations in the PSA level above the nadir. These patients may be candidates for salvage prostatectomy or cryosurgery if they have no evidence of systemic disease or extracapsular extension. The major side effect is significant incontinence in as many as 50 percent of patients. Please refer to the section on radiation therapy for an in-depth discussion.

M. Treatment of Advanced Disease

Prostate cancer is an androgen-sensitive tumor. Ninety to 95 percent of circulating androgens are produced by Leydig cells of the testis and consist of testosterone. The remaining circulating androgens come from adrenal sources and peripheral fat conversion. In initial advanced prostate cancer, 40 percent of tumors will regress, 40 percent will stabilize, and 20 percent will progress if androgen withdrawal is initiated. Methods of androgen ablation are listed in Table 17-5. Diethylstilbesterol has significant cardiovascular side effects, and its use has been virtually eliminated. The luteinizing hormone (LHRH) agonists and castration are the preferred methods of androgen ablation.

1. *Castration.* Simple orchiectomy is easily accomplished, relatively inexpensive, well-tolerated, and almost free of complications. Vasomotor instability (hot flashes), loss of libido, and erectile dysfunction are the major side effects. Issues regarding body image are of concern with this form of therapy.

2. *LHRH agonists.* These peptide agents stimulate luteinizing hormone release, causing an initial flare of serum testosterone, followed by a drop to castrate levels after receptor downregulation. Long-term effects on bone mineralization may be severe. They are as effective as castration with similar side effects and are administered subcutaneously on a monthly or trimonthly basis. The major drawback of such therapy is its expense.

3. *Antiandrogens.* Flutamide and bicalutamide act by blocking the dihydrotesterone receptor. As a form of monotherapy, they are not as effective as castration or LHRH therapy. They do not lower the serum testosterone level so they do not generally cause impotence or decreased libido. Side effects include diarrhea and liver function

Table 17-5 Methods of Androgen Ablation

Bilateral simple orchiectomy
Diethylstilbesterol
DHT receptor blockade (flutamide, bicalutamide)
LHRH agonist (leuprolide)
Aminoglutethimide
Ketoconazole

DHT, Dihydrotestosterone, LHRH, Leutinizing hormone release hormone

abnormalities. Liver function tests should be checked within 1 month of instituting therapy. Ketoconazole will result in castrate testosterone levels very rapidly by inhibiting steroid synthesis. It is indicated in patients with spinal cord compression due to vertebral metastasis.

4. *Timing of therapy.* It is debatable whether early versus late therapy provides better outcomes. There are data to support both perspectives. With early therapy the potential advantages of treatment must be weighed along with the side effects of androgen blockade, which have been described.

5. *Combined androgen blockade.* Multiple clinical trials have addressed the value of androgen suppression by an LHRH agonist or castration alone versus the addition of an oral antiandrogen. There appears, at best, to be a minimal (3 percent) advantage in patients receiving this therapy and is generally not recommended as an initial form of treatment.

6. *Androgen withdrawal effect.* Those patients experiencing a clinical or biochemical failure while on antiandrogens can experience a regression on withdrawal that may last from several months to a year. PSA levels may decrease by as much as 50 percent within days (flutamide) or months (bicalutamide).

7. *Hormone refractory disease.* Patients who develop symptomatic progression of disease after androgen ablation have a very poor prognosis, with a mean survival of 11 months. Prostate cancer is responsive to certain cytoreductive chemotherapy agents including platinum cyclophosphonide, paclitaxel, and estramustine. Prolonged responses are seen in a minority of patients. Refer to the section on chemotherapy for an in-depth discussion.

V. URETHRAL CANCER
A. Carcinoma of the Female Urethra

1. *Anatomy.* The female urethra measures 2.5 to 4 cm in length and is lined with transitional epithelium in its proximal third and stratified squamous epithelium in its distal portion. However, boundaries between these types are not discrete, and areas of pseudostratified and stratified columnar epithelium may also be present. The wall of the urethra also contains glands and smooth muscle bundles. The lymphatics of the proximal urethral segment primarily drain to the internal and external iliac nodes, whereas distal lymphatics drain to the inguinal and subinguinal lymph nodes.

2. *Epidemiology.* Carcinoma of the urethra is a rare tumor. It is more common in older, Caucasian women, with most cases occurring in patients over 50 years of age. Urethral strictures and diverticula are thought to have some association with urethral carcinoma.

3. *Pathology.* Squamous cell carcinoma is the most prevalent histologic pattern, accounting for 60 to 70 percent of cases. Transitional cell carcinoma may be present in up to 20 percent of cases as a direct continuation of a bladder cancer or as part of a multifocal process. Adenocarcinoma (10 to 18 percent of cases) may be seen in association with urethral diverticula or in the rare occurrence of prostate cancer of the female urethra. Melanomas and lymphomas may occur in less than 1 percent of cases.

4. *Presentation.* Urethral bleeding or spotting is the most common symptom. Other symptoms can include urinary frequency, dysuria, and obstruction. The possibility of malignancy should at least be considered with any urethral mass or stricture.

5. *Diagnosis.* Physical examination, urinalysis, and urine cytology, endoscopy, and biopsy are usually sufficient to make the diagnosis. Differential diagnosis includes caruncle, urethral prolapse, leukoplakia, structure, fistulas, erosion, and, rarely, nephrogenic adenoma. Spread is by local infiltration followed by lymphatic spread. Staging is similar to that of the American bladder system (ABCD).

6. *Management.* Caruncles of the female urethra can mimic carcinoma but are best managed conservatively given their benign nature. Only caruncles that develop erosion or bleeding should be biopsied. Distal third carcinomas can be managed by distal urethrectomy (preferably) or by radiation therapy (external beam or brachytherapy) with excellent results. Proximal or advanced lesions have a very poor prognosis and are best managed by anterior exenteration with adjuvant radiation therapy.

7. *Urethral diverticula.* Less than 50 cases of carcinoma arising in female urethral diverticula have been reported. Five of these cases were associated with a calculus within a urethral diverticulum. The association with urethral diverticula must be considered rare given the relatively high rate of urethral diverticula in the general population. Any filling defect within a diverticulum, however, demands exploration.

B. Carcinoma of the Male Urethra

1. *Anatomy.* The male urethra is approximately 20 cm in length and is divided into prostatic, bulbomembranous,

and penile segments. The prostatic segment is lined by transitional epithelium. The remaining urethra is covered by pseudostratified columnar epithelium, and the meatus is lined by stratified squamous epithelium. The lymphatics of the prostate and posterior urethra are drained by the internal and external iliac nodes.

2. *Epidemiology.* The incidence of urethral carcinoma in males is only one-third to one-half that in females. Chronic inflammation and urethral strictures may have an etiologic role. Patients are generally over 50 years old.

3. *Pathology.* As many as two thirds of these tumors originate in the bulbar or bulbomembranous urethra. Most anterior lesions are at the fossa navicularis. The most common histologic type is squamous cell carcinoma, followed by transitional cell carcinoma. Adenocarcinoma is rare and usually found in the bulbomembranous urethra.

4. *Presentation.* This carcinoma is usually a locally invasive lesion. Symptoms include urethral obstruction, stricture, bloody discharge, perineal mass, abscess or fistula, perineal pain, or adenopathy. Distant metastases are rare at initial presentation.

5. *Diagnosis.* Endoscopic biopsy under anesthesia is the mainstay of diagnosis. All suspicious or recurrent urethral strictures should undergo biopsy. Urinary or urethral cytology may also be useful. Imaging modalities include retrograde urography and CT scanning. The staging evaluation is similar to bladder cancer as is the ABCD grading system. The differential diagnosis includes benign stricture disease, periurethral abscess, and inflammatory phlegmon.

6. *Management.* Therapy is dependent on tumor location. Low-grade lesions in any part of the urethra may be managed by transurethral resection, whereas higher-grade distal urethral tumors may require a partial or total penectomy. Invasive proximal lesions require an aggressive en bloc resection of the urethra and rim of the pubis and an anterior exenteration. There may be a role for adjuvant radiation therapy.

VI. PENILE AND SCROTAL CANCER
A. General Considerations

The incidence of penile cancer in the United States is approximately 1 per 100,000 males per year. However, in underdeveloped countries or in areas where circumcision is not practiced, it may account for up to 20 percent of all tumors in men and up to 45 percent of genitourinary tumors. The disease is almost nonexistent in populations practicing infant circumcision. Because of its rarity, there are few controlled trials to direct therapy. Therapeutic decisions can also be difficult because surgery can be disfiguring or cause significant morbidity.

B. Penile Cancer
1. Premalignant lesions
    a. *Condylomata acuminata.* These lesions are caused by human papillomavirus (HPV) infection and can involve the glans, prepuce, or shaft of the penis. Five percent of patients have urethral involvement. Although over 65 different HPV subtypes have been identified, subtypes 6 and 11 have been specifically associated with benign lesions, whereas subtypes 16 and 18 have been isolated from invasive penile carcinomas. Condyloma acuminata are usually treated topically with podophyllin, imiquimod, or 5-fluorouracil (5-FU) cream. Patients with refractory lesions are candidates for laser photocoagulation or diathermy.
    b. *Buschke-Lowenstein's tumor.* This lesion is also known as giant condyloma accuminatum. It does not metastasize but can cause local tissue destruction as it enlarges. It can be treated by wide local excision or partial penile amputation.
    c. *Leukoplakia.* This term describes a white cutaneous plaque that can be hypertrophic or atrophic. It may coexist with or precede the development of squamous cell carcinoma. It is usually secondary to chronic irritation. Circumcision, surgical excision, and irradiation have all been used in treatment. Close follow-up to detect malignant degeneration is essential.
    d. *Balanitis xerotica obliterans.* A subcategory of lichen sclerosus et atrophicus limited to the male genitalia associated with destructive inflammation, phimosis, urethral stenosis, and squamous cell carcinoma. These hypopigmented, papular, or atrophic lesions typically involve the glans and urethral meatus in uncircumsized men. Treatment involves circumcision or high-potency topical steroids.
    e. *Bowenoid papulosis.* Uncommon genital dysplasia now considered to be a sexually transmitted disease probably caused by human papillomavirus type 16. Clinically, it usually resembles persistent warts, but histologically it resembles squamous cell carcinoma in situ. Unlike Bowen's disease, it does not progress to invasive squamous cell carcinoma. Management with

topical 5-fluorouracil cream, laser photocoagulation, or cryoablation suffices.

2. Carcinoma in situ and other malignant lesions

   a. *Queyrat's erythroplasia and Bowen's disease.* Histologically, these conditions are carcinoma in situ of the skin of the glans penis. The former presents as a localized, velvety red lesion on the glans or prepuce. The latter can develop on the skin anywhere on the penis and may be associated with internal carcinomas. Circumcision and biopsy will confirm the diagnosis. Topical 5-FU and external radiation have been used to treat these lesions. Up to 10 percent of these patients will progress to invasive carcinoma.

   b. *Kaposi sarcoma.* Penile or genital involvement of Kaposi sarcoma as painless, raised, bluish lesions can be an early manifestation of the acquired immunodeficiency syndrome. In patients who have failed systemic chemotherapy, radiation therapy offers the best chance for palliative control.

3. Invasive squamous cell carcinoma

   a. *Pathology.* Various subtypes of penile carcinomas have been identified, including:

      i. *Verrucous carcinoma.* Comprise approximately 10 percent of all penile carcinomas. Typically present as large, well-differentiated, fungating lesions that have a tendency for local extension and recurrence, but low metastatic potential. Wide local excision is recommended. Radiation therapy is ill advised as it may result in tumor dedifferentiation and progression.

      ii. *Basaloid carcinoma.* Poorly differentiated variant usually presenting with advanced disease.

      iii. *Spindle cell (sarcomatoid) carcinoma.* Very rare but associated with a better prognosis that conventional squamous cell carcinoma.

      iv. *Penile malignant melanoma.* Less than 1 percent of penile carcinomas. Depth of invasion important.

   b. *Etiology.* The development of penile carcinoma has long been associated with poor hygiene and exposure to irritants, carcinogens, or possible viral pathogens. In particular, the organism *Mycobacterium smegmatis* has been shown to convert sterols present in smegma to substances that have been shown to be carcinogenic in mice. In addition, infection with HPV-16 or HPV-18 has been associated with up to 60 percent of penile and cervical carcinomas, suggesting a venereal basis for both malignancies. Penile and urethral condyloma has been identified in up to 55 percent of sexual partners of women with cervical carcinoma. On the other hand, sexual partners of men with penile carcinoma have a three-fold higher incidence of cervical carcinoma. Malignant transformation of HPV-infected cells is thought to result from the inactivation of tumor suppressor gene proteins (p53 and Rb) by viral gene products E6 and E7.

c. *Natural history.* Carcinoma of the penis usually begins as a small lesion on the glans or prepuce, which may be exophytic or ulcerative and accompanied by secondary infection. Invasion is usually direct and capable of destroying surrounding tissue. Exophytic lesions tend to be better differentiated than ulcerative lesions, which may also exhibit spindle cell morphology and tend to metastasize earlier. Regional inguinal and iliac nodes are the earliest sites of dissemination, in that order. The right and left lymphatic drainage systems are interconnected. The lymphatic drainage of the prepuce terminates in the upper inner group of superficial inguinal lymphatics. In the glans, however, lymphatics divide to follow the femoral canal and drain to superficial inguinal nodes, the nodes of Cloquet (or Rosenmuller), and retro-femoral nodes. Distant metastases can involve the abdominal lymph nodes, liver, and lungs. Death is usually secondary to involvement of regional nodes, which results in skin necrosis, chronic infection, sepsis, or hemorrhage secondary to erosion into the femoral vessels.

d. *Clinical features.* Carcinoma of the penis generally begins as a painless nodule, wart-like growth, ulceration, or vesicle. Phimosis is present in as many as 50 percent of patients. Since the patient usually ignores the lesion until it reaches a considerable size, the mean time lag for diagnosis is 1 year after initial recognition. Lymph nodes are palpably enlarged in almost 50 percent of patients, but in many cases the adenopathy is secondary to infection.

e. *Diagnosis and staging.* Diagnosis depends on tissue biopsy. Tumor size, location, fixation, and involvement of the corporal bodies should be assessed. Careful bilateral palpation of the inguinal areas is of extreme importance. The Jackson and AJCC staging systems are commonly employed (Table 17-6 a, and b). Metastatic evaluation should include a chest x-ray, bone scan, and CT scan to assess regional node involvement.

Table 17-6a Jackson Classification for Squamous Penile Carcinoma

Stage I	Tumor confined to glans or prepuce
Stage II	Invasion into shaft or corpora; no nodal or distant metastases
Stage III	Tumor confined to penis; operable inguinal nodal metastases
Stage IV	Tumor involves adjacent structures; inoperable inguinal nodes and/or distant metastasis(es)

Table 17-6b AJCC Staging System for Penile Carcinoma

Primary Tumor (T)

TX	Tumor stage cannot be assessed
T0	No evidence of primary tumor
Tis	Carcinoma in situ
Ta	Noninvasive verrucous carcinoma
T1	Tumor invades subepithelial connective tissue
T2	Tumor invades corpus spongiosum or cavernosum
T3	Tumor invades urethral or prostate
T4	Tumor invades other adjacent structures

Regional Lymph Nodes (N)

NX	Regional lymph nodes cannot be assessed
N0	No regional lymph node metastasis
N1	Metastasis in a single, superficial, inguinal lymph node
N2	Metastasis in multiple or bilateral superficial inguinal lymph nodes
N3	Metastasis in deep inguinal or pelvic lymph nodes

Distant Metastasis (M)

MX	Presence of distant metastasis cannot be assessed
M1	No distant metastasis
M1	Distant metastasis

    f. Treatment

        1. *Primary lesion.* All penile lesions present for more than 3 weeks should undergo biopsy with a deep margin to ensure proper staging. Simple circumcision may treat lesions confined to the prepuce. Patients with superficial tumors (stages Tis and T1) can be managed with penile-salvage techniques using Mohs microresection, laser photocoagulation (CO_2 or Nd-YAG), or radiation therapy (external beam or brachytherapy) with approximate recur-

rence rates of 6 percent, 25 percent, and 21 percent, respectively. Large stage T1 tumors and T2 lesions of the glans or penile shaft should be treated by partial penile amputation, ensuring a 2-cm tissue margin proximal to the tumor, since local wedge resection has a 50 percent recurrence rate versus 0 to 8 percent with partial penectomy. In bulky T3 and T4 tumors or if tumor location is such that amputation would leave a penile stump inadequate for voiding or sexual activity, a total penectomy with perineal urethrostomy is preferred.

2. *Inguinal lymph nodes.* The presence of inguinal metastases is a more important prognostic factor than tumor grade. Although approximately 55 percent of patients present with palpable inguinal nodes, half of these are tumor free on histologic examination. Therefore, all patients with inguinal adenopathy should be treated with 6 weeks of oral antibiotics after undergoing penectomy to segregate those patients with true metastases. One quarter of patients without palpable adenopathy will have nodes containing metastases. Patients with palpable inguinal lymphadenopathy despite oral antibiotic therapy should undergo superficial and deep ipsilateral ilioinguinal lymphadenectomy. When lymph nodes are positive on one side, the contralateral nodes are involved in 50 percent of cases, and iliac nodes involved in one third of cases. Therefore, these patients should also undergo a contralateral superficial inguinal lymphadenectomy. In addition, many experts would argue for the performance of an ipsilateral pelvic lymph node dissection. The timing of surgery (simultaneous versus asynchronous) remains controversial. Although approximately 20 percent of patients with nonpalpable inguinal lymph nodes harbor microscopic metastasis, considerable controversy exists regarding the performance of a prophylactic inguinal lymphadenectomy due to its significant morbidity. Nevertheless, recent reports indicate that survival is significantly improved in patients who undergo a prophylactic (5-year survival, 88 percent) versus delayed (38 percent) inguinal lymphadenectomy. Although no strict criteria have been established, indications for prophylactic superficial inguinal lymphadenectomy in patients with a normal inguinal physical examination include invasive T1-T3 lesions or high tumor grade.

The margins of dissection of the inguinal lymphadenectomy include the inguinal ligament, adductor longus, sartorius, and the base of the femoral triangle. The fascia lata separates the superficial from the deep inguinal lymph node compartments. The development of modified dissections involving limited surgical margins and the preservation of the saphenous vein may incur less morbidity. The sartorius muscle can be detached from the anterior superior iliac spine and repositioned more medially to protect the femoral vessels. Alternatively, a gracilis or rectus muscle flap can be used to fill large defects after resecting large masses, thus preventing vessel erosion and skin necrosis. The presence of pelvic node disease portends a very poor outcome.

g. *Prognosis.* The 5-year survival rate in patients without palpable adenopathy is 65 to 80 percent. Patients with positive lymph nodes have 5-year survival rates of 20 to 50 percent, with the poorest survival noted in patients with iliac metastasis. As many as 90 percent of patients with pathologically negative inguinal nodes survive 5 years. Chemotherapy regimens for metastatic disease include single-agent therapy with cis-platinum, methotrexate, bleomycin, or cyclophosphamide. Combination therapy regimens include bleomycin, vincristine, and methotrexate; and methro-trexate, bleomycin, and cisplatin; and cis-platin and 5-fluorouracil. Up to thirty percent of patients will exhibit a partial response but complete responses are rare. Radiation therapy may be effective for T1 and T2 lesions but has been traditionally poor for higher stage lesions.

C. Carcinoma of the Scrotum

Carcinoma of the scrotum, initially identified in chimney sweeps by Sir Percival Pott, was one of the first environmentally related carcinomas described. Mule spinners also suffered from scrotal carcinoma, as their clothes became saturated with lubricating oil from the spinning jenny. Squamous cell carcinoma arose from exposure to the aromatic hydrocarbons in soot, tars, and petroleum products. These tumors are exceedingly rare. They present as ulcerated or exophytic growths. Wide local excision with or without ipsilateral ilioinguinal lymphadenectomy is the treatment of choice. Nonoccupational tumors of the scrotum include reticulum cell carcinoma, rhabdomyosarcoma, leiomyosarcoma, liposarcoma, and melanoma.

VII. TESTICULAR TUMORS

A. General Comments

Testicular tumors are uncommon but are the most curable form of urologic cancers. More than 95 percent of lesions are derived from germinal tissue, whereas the rest arise from nongerminal or stromal cells. Germ cell tumors of the testicle are classified as pure seminoma or as nonseminomatous. Seminomas are exquisitely sensitive to radiation therapy, whereas nonseminomatous germ cell tumors (NS-GCT) are very responsive to platinum-based combination chemotherapy. Retroperitoneal lymphadenectomy plays a very important role in the treatment of nonseminomatous lesions. The tumor markers beta-human chorionic gonadotropin (beta-hCG) and alpha-fetoprotein (AFP) are extremely useful in diagnosing and monitoring disease.

B. Incidence

The general incidence of testicular cancers (4.5 per 100,000 per year) appears to be slowly rising; 6600 new cases of testicular cancer are estimated per year. Only 350 deaths from this disease are expected. This mortality statistic is almost tenfold lower than it was 15 years ago due to the ability of platinum-based chemotherapy to cure this disease.

C. Etiology

No definitive cause of testicular cancer has been identified. Testicular maldescent has been associated with the disease, and a five- to 15-fold relative risk for developing a testicular tumor exists if this condition is present. Of patients with testicular cancer, 7 to 12 percent have a prior history of cryptorchidism. In patients with unilateral cryptorchidism and testicular cancer, the tumor occurs in the contralateral testicle in 5 to 15 percent of cases. There is a slight predilection for testis tumors on the right side. This coincides with the slightly greater involvement of the right testis with cryptorchidism.

D. Epidemiology

Testicular cancer occurs most frequently in young men and is the most common solid tumor in men between the ages of 20 and 34 years. Smaller peak incidences exist for men over 60 and boys under the age of 10. The cumulative life-time risk of developing testicular cancer is 1 in 500. The incidence of testicular cancer in African Americans is approximately one fourth to one third of that in whites. A higher incidence of disease has been noted in Scandinavia.

E. Natural History

Intratubular germ cell neoplasia in situ initially grows beyond the basement membrane to eventually replace some or all of the testicular parenchyma. Because 50 percent of patients with testicular carcinoma in situ will progress to a germ cell tumor, patients with this finding on testis biopsy (usually performed as part of an infertility evaluation) should undergo radical orchiectomy. Epididymal and cord involvement is hindered by the tunica albuginea.

1. Whereas pure seminoma is confined to the testis at initial presentation in two thirds to three fourths of cases, up to two thirds of patients with NSGCT may present with metastasis. Lymphatic spread can occur early and usually precedes vascular invasion. Early vascular invasion is noted frequently in pure choriocarcinoma. Sites of hematogenous spread include the lungs, liver, and bones.

2. In patients with organ-confined disease after orchiectomy (stage I or A), failure will ultimately occur in 30 percent of patients (80 percent retroperitoneal; 20 percent distant). If a retroperitoneal lymph node dissection is performed for stage I disease, 5 to 8 percent of such patients will have a recurrence, almost exclusively at an extra retroperitoneal site, usually in the chest.

3. All germinal cell testis tumors in adults should be treated as malignant. Spontaneous regression of this disease is extremely rare. The majority of patients who die from testicular cancer do so within 3 years of diagnosis.

F. Pathology

Several classifications of testicular carcinoma have been proposed. The Dixon-Moore classification is presented as follows.

1. Germinal neoplasms
   a. Seminoma
      i. *Classic.* Pure or "classic" seminoma accounts for approximately 85 percent of seminomas and 30 percent of all testicular germ cell tumors. Approximately 15 percent will also contain syncytiotrophoblastic elements, which can produce human chorionic gonadotropin. Peak incidence is seen in the 4th and 5th decades of life, one decade later than nonseminomatous germ cell tumors (NSGCT). Grossly, seminomas appear as well-defined, yellow-tan tumors.
      ii. *Anaplastic.* Account for approximately 10 percent of seminomas. Characterized by increased mitotic activity. Although they usually present at higher stages than classic seminoma, stage for stage, these tumors carry the same prognosis. These tumors account for 30 percent of mortalities due to seminoma.

       iii. *Spermatocytic.* Classically seen in an older age group (50 percent are older than 50 years old), it accounts for 1 to 2 percent of all testicular tumors. Only one case of metastasis has been reported, so inguinal orchiectomy is sufficient treatment.

  b. *Embryonal carcinoma.* Represent approximately 3 percent of pure germ cell tumors, but may be a component of up to 25 percent of mixed germ cell tumors.

  c. *Teratoma (with or without malignant transformation).* These tumors can be comprised of endodermal, mesodermal, or ectodermal elements. It is the second most common testicular tumor in children after yolk sac tumor. Treatment is surgical because response to radiotherapy and chemotherapy is poor. Many arise from malignant transformation of NSGCT after chemotherapy.

       i. *Mature.* Cystic areas lined by epithelium that may contain respiratory epithelium, blood vessels, cartilage, or squamous epithelium.

       ii. *Immature.* As above but with primitive elements.

  d. *Choriocarcinoma.* Represent less than 1 percent of all NSGCT. Usually present with advanced clinical stage and very high serum levels of hCG.

  e. *Yolk sac tumor.* Also referred to as endodermal sinus tumor, it is the most common NSGCT in children. It accounts for roughly 2 percent of all germ cell tumors in its pure form, but may be present in up to 25 percent of mixed germ cell tumors. Cells produce alpha fetoprotein that can be measured in serum.

 2. Nongerminal neoplasms

  a. Gonadal stromal tumors include Leydig cell tumor and gonadoblastoma.

  b. Miscellaneous neoplasms include carcinoid, adrenal rests, and mesenchymal neoplasms.

G. Staging

 1. Different systems for staging testicular tumors are not uniform but are based on the basic subdivisions proposed by Boden and Gibb: stage A (I): confined to the testicle; stage B (II): retroperitoneal node involvement; and stage C (III): extranodal metastasis.

 2. Stage II disease has been subdivided by Skinner and others to more accurately express its clinical manifestations.

   IIa Less than six positive nodes, none more than 2 cm in any dimension

   IIb More than six positive nodes, any more than 2 cm in any dimension

   IIc Massive retroperitoneal disease (larger than 5 cm)

Table 17-7 AJCC Staging System for Testis Carcinoma

Primary Tumor T Stage (pT)

pT0   No evidence of tumor in testis (scar may be present)

pTis   Intratubular germ cell neoplasia (CIS)

pT1   Tumor limited to the testis/epdidymis without vascular or lymphatic invasion; tumor may invade the tunica albuginea but not the tunica vaginalis

pT2   Tumor limited to the testis/epididymis with vascular or lymphatic invasion or tumor extending to and involving the tunica vaginalis

pT3   Tumor invading the spermatic core $\pm$ vascular or lymphatic invasion

pT4   Tumor invading the scrotum $\pm$ vascular or lymphatic invasion

Regional Nodes (N)

pNX   Regional lymph nodes cannot be assessed

pN0   No regional lymph node metastasis

pN1   Metastasis with a lymph node mass, 2 cm or less in greatest dimension and less than or equal to 5 nodes positive, none more than 2 cm in greatest dimension

pN2   Metastasis with a lymph node mass, more than 2 cm but not more than 5 cm in greatest dimension; or more than 5 nodes positive, none more than 5 cm; or evidence of extra-nodal extension of tumor

pN3   Metastasis with a lymph node mass more than 5 cm in greatest dimension

Distant Metastasis (M)

MX   Distant metastasis cannot be assessed

M0   No distant metastasis

M1   Distant metastasis

M1a   Nonregional nodal or pulmonary metastasis

M1b   Distant metastasis other than to nonregional lymph node and lungs

(continued)

3. *Seminoma.* There is a wide variance in the representative staging systems. Stage 1: limited to the testis; stage 2A: positive retroperitoneal nodes on imaging examination; stage 2B: palpable abdominal mass; stage 3: supradi-aphragmatic adenopathy, mediastinal, and/or cervical; and stage 4: visceral metastases.

4. The most recent staging system by the AJCC includes a separate category for tumor marker status to aid in iden-tifying patients with high risk for relapse (Table 17-7).

Table 17-7 (*continued*)

Serum Tumor Markers (S)

SX   Marker studies not available

S0   Markers within normal limits

S1   LDH < 1.5 × Normal **AND** hCG < 5000 mIu/mL **AND** AFP < 1000 ng/mL

S2   LDH 1.5–10 × N **OR** hCG 5,000 to 50,000 mIu/mL **OR** AFP 1000–10,000 ng/mL

S3   LDH > 10 × N **OR** hCG > 50,000 mIu/mL **OR** AFP > 10,000 ng/mL

Definitions of Clinical Stages for Testis Cancer

I or A Tumor	Tumor confined to the testicle or cord structure
II_A or B_1	Microscopic regional lymph node involvement in < 6 nodes
II_B or B_2	Microscopic involvement in > 6 regional lymph nodes or gross nodal involvement < 6 cm
II_C or B_2	Gross nodal involvement > 6 cm in one lymph node or as an aggregate of lymph nodes
III or C	Disease above the diaphram or involving abdominal organs

(Regional Nodes) Clinical

NX   Regional lymph nodes cannot be assessed

N0   No regional lymph node metastasis

N1   Metastasis with a lymph node mass 2 cm or less in greatest dimension; or multiple lymph nodes, none more than 2 cm in greatest dimension

N2   Metastasis with a lymph node mass, more than 2 cm but not more than 5 cm in greatest dimension; or multiple lymph nodes any one mass greater than 2 cm but not more than 5 cm in greatest dimension

N3   Metastasis with a lymph node mass more than 5 cm in greatest dimension

---

H. Clinical Presentation

Because this disease affects a younger age group not generally aware of the possible diagnosis, a 4 to 6 month delay in diagnosis is not uncommon. The most common symptom is a painless testicular mass. In some series, however, pain has been associated with almost one half of the presentations. Between 5 and 25 percent of patients may be initially misdiagnosed and treated for epididymitis. Gynecomastia can be present and is secondary to the effect of tumor estradiol synthesis. This is classically associated with Leydig cell tumors. Cough, abdominal mass, back pain, and supraclavicular or other a lymphadenopathy can present in cases of advanced disease.

1. Diagnosis
   a. Transcrotal ultrasound can confirm the presence of an intraparenchymal testicular mass, rule out benign processes such as a hydrocele or epididymitis, and effectively evaluate the contralateral gonad.
   b. *Inguinal (radical) orchiectomy.* The primary lesion is best handled by early clamping of the spermatic cord near the internal ring and complete removal of the gonad. Only in very rare circumstances is exploration and frozen biopsy performed. The extent of the tumor, any vascular invasion, and the subtype composition of the lesion (i.e., mixed germ cell) should be noted. A scrotal approach should not be employed as this may theoretically increase the risk of inguinal nodal metastasis and recurrence. Nevertheless, there is no need for a hemiscrotectomy or prophylactic inguinal lymph node dissection in the rare patient who has undergone a scrotal orchiectomy for testicular cancer.
   c. Imaging is best conducted with a standard chest x-ray and a CT scan of the retroperitoneum. There is a 20 to 30 percent chance of understaging lesions by this method. Chest CT detects many small nodes, which are usually benign. Pedal lymphangiography is no longer performed on a regular basis.

2. Tumor markers
   a. *Human chorionic gonadotropin (hCG).* hCG is a heterodimeric protein with immunologically distinct chains. Circulating levels are extremely low (1 ng/mL) in normal males. The syncytiotrophoblastic tissue of some germ cell tumors produces this substance. It can, therefore, be detected in almost all choriocarcinomas, 40 to 60 percent of embryonal cell carcinomas, and 5 to 10 percent of pure seminomas. In seminoma, the level is rarely elevated above twice-normal. The half-life for this substance ranges between 24 and 36 hours, but the beta subunit alone has a half-life of 1 hour. Since beta-hCG shares structural homology with luteinizing hormone, spurious elevations can occur in patients with inadequate testosterone production from the contralateral testis (thus higher LH).
   b. *Alpha-fetoprotein.* AFP is an oncofetal protein detected in testis and liver tumors. It is produced by yolk sac elements that may or may not be histologically recognized. This substance is not produced in pure

choriocarcinoma or pure seminoma. The presence of elevated AFP in a patient with histologic seminoma precludes the diagnosis of pure seminoma. The half-life of AFP is 5 to 7 days.

c. *Lactate dehydrogenase.* This general cellular enzyme is not particularly specific for testicular lesions but provides a correlation to tumor bulk. It may have some role in monitoring patients with advanced seminoma and in marker-negative patients with NSGCT and persistent disease.

d. *Placental alkaline phosphatase.* This substance can be elevated in patients with advanced stage testicular cancer. It can be spuriously raised by tobacco use.

e. Over all stages, 90 percent of patients with nonseminomatous tumors will have an elevation of one or both markers. Fifty to 70 percent will display an elevation of AFP and 40 to 60 percent will have an elevation of β-hCG. In stage I lesions, two thirds of patients will have an elevation of one or both major markers. After therapy, tumor markers should display a logarithmic pattern of decrease in accordance with their half-lives. Sustained elevation of markers or slower decrease after orchiectomy or retroperitoneal lymph node dissection (RPLND) suggests residual disease. Normalization of markers is not definite evidence of complete surgical cure.

J. Treatment (After Orchiectomy)

1. *Seminoma.* The majority of seminomas are confined to the testis and are very sensitive to external beam radiation therapy. Adjuvant low-dose (1500 cGy) radiation to the retroperitoneum and ipsilateral pelvis is recommended for patients with stage I seminoma given that approximately 15 percent of patients on surveillance will relapse. In the era of platinum-based chemotherapy, prophylactic mediastinal radiotherapy is no longer recommended. The 5-year actuarial cure rates approach 97 percent in low-stage disease. Patients may elect to forego radiotherapy and choose surveillance with the understanding that up to 17 percent will relapse within 5 years. These patients should be committed to intense monthly follow-up and may be salvaged in up to 80 percent of cases by platinum-based chemotherapy. Proponents in favor of adjuvant radiotherapy argue that some patients who elect surveillance may never be salvaged given the bulk of disease at presentation. Some debate exists with regard to treatment for intermediate stage disease, whereas most agree that chemotherapy should be employed in bulky or advanced

disease (stage IIb and III). Although anaplastic seminoma usually presents at a higher stage than classic seminoma, it carries the same prognosis stage for stage and should be treated as such. The use of RPLND in the treatment of postchemotherapy residual disease is controversial.

2. Nonseminomatous germ cell tumors

   a. *Stage I.* Clinical stage I NSGCT are best treated with a retroperitoneal lymph node dissection (RPLND). This can be performed by a transabdominal or thoracoabdominal approach. Only 10 percent of patients treated this way will relapse, and virtually all recurrences will occur in the chest, which is easily monitored and treated. The cure rate for this approach is roughly 99 percent. If a patient decides against surgery and undergoes intensive surveillance after orchiectomy, relapse will occur in 30 percent of cases (chest and retroperitoneum) as late as 4 years post-orchiectomy. Due to noncompliance with surveillance and the potential for presentation with bulky metastatic disease, the cure rate with platinum-based chemotherapy is approximately 95 percent. Given the inherent risks of RPLND, the International Germ Cell Cancer Collaborative Group developed a prognostic factor-based staging system to assess risk of recurrence. Patients in the good prognosis group (AFP less than 1000 ng/mL, hCG less than 5,000 mIu/L, and LDH less than 1.5 × normal) may be better candidates for surveillance, given that a minority of these patients will relapse in the retroperitoneum, thus saving the morbidity of RPLND. This issue, however, remains controversial. The major long-term complication of RPLND is disruption of ejaculatory function as a result of damage to the sympathetic nerve fibers to the pelvis. Decreased morbidity has been obtained by mapping the metastatic deposits of NSGCT and developing surgical templates specific for the involved testicle (Fig. 17-5). Lymphatics draining the right testicle drain primarily to retroperitoneal nodes in the interaortocaval region. In addition, metastatic disease from right-sided tumors may cross over to the left side. For this reason, a modified right-sided template RPLND should include a complete dissection above the level of the inferior mesenteric artery (IMA) up to the renal vessels, laterally up to both ureters, and caudally (below the IMA) down to the aortic bifurcation on the ipsilateral side. Left-sided tumors, however, primarily metastasize to the para-aortic lymph nodes and rarely cross over to the right side. A modified left-sided RPLND is the mirror

Modified RPLND
for Right–Sided Tumor
En bloc Dissection

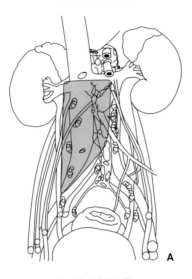

A

Modified RPLND
for Left–Sided Tumor
En bloc Dissection

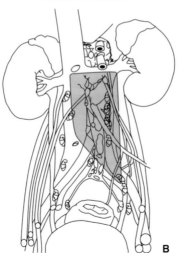

B

Figure 17-5 Modified templates for (**A**) right- and (**B**) left-sided retroperitoneal lymph node dissections for testicular carcinoma.

image of a modified right-sided template, except that the right-sided border only extends near the right margin of the inferior vena cava, and not the ureter. Using a nerve-sparing technique, ejaculation is preserved in 75 to 90 percent of patients with little potential compromise of surgical cure.

b. *Early stage 2 disease can be treated with surgery.* Advanced stage 2 and 3 disease is best treated by chemotherapy first, followed by a postchemotherapy RPLND for suspected residual disease. Postchemotherapy tumor histology may show only necrotic tumor (40 percent), mature teratoma (40 percent), or residual carcinoma (20 percent).

3. *Chemotherapy.* This modality is discussed in Chapter 19. Platinum-based combination chemotherapy has revolutionized the treatment of this disease. Present clinical research efforts are now being directed at salvage chemotherapy and the combined use of chemotherapy and bone marrow transplant in patients with advanced disease. Patients who have a residual retroperitoneal mass after chemotherapy with normalization of serum tumor markers should be considered for retroperitoneal lymphadenectomy, given that histology will demonstrate fibrosis (10 percent), teratoma (40 percent), or residual carcinoma (50 percent). Resection of the entire mass is required as teratomas are not radiosensitive or chemosensitive. Patients with residual tumor should undergo salvage chemotherapy, usually with standard bleomycin, etoposide, and cis-platinum plus ifosfamide.

4. Patient surveillance

a. *Seminoma.* Patients with recurrent disease after radiotherapy may be salvaged by platinum-based chemotherapy so careful patient follow-up is essential. These patients should be followed with a monthly H&P, chest x-ray, and serum tumor markers for 1 year, then every other month for 1 year, and then annually for several years.

b. *Nonseminomatous germ cell tumors.* These patients should be monitored with a monthly H&P, chest x-ray, and serum tumor markers for 1 year, then every other month for 1 year, and every 3 to 6 months thereafter. In addition, they should undergo a CT scan of the retroperitoneum every 2 to 3 months for the first 2 years, then every 6 months thereafter for a minimum of 5 years and up to 10 years post-orchiectomy.

K. Other Testis Neoplasms

1. Leydig cell tumors

a. Constitute 1 to 3 percent of testis tumors.

  b. Ten percent are malignant. They are never malignant in prepubertal patients.
  c. Malignancy is diagnosed by presence of metastases.
  d. Histologic determination of malignancy unreliable.
2. Sertoli cell tumors
  a. Less than 1 percent of testis tumors.
  b. Ten percent are malignant (determined by presence of metastases).

SELF-ASSESSMENT QUESTIONS
I. Carcinoma of the Kidney

1. What is von Hippel-Lindau disease? What nonurological abnormalities are part of the condition? What genetic abnormalities are associated with it?
2. What are the different histologic subtypes in renal cell carcinoma?
3. What paraneoplastic syndromes are associated with renal cell carcinoma?
4. What are the indications for treatment in patients with renal angiomyolipomas?
5. What are the indications for renal sparing surgery in renal cell carcinoma?
6. Are there any indications for a diagnostic percutaneous biopsy of a renal mass?
7. What renal lesions are associated with the tuberous sclerosis complex?
8. What are the advantages and disadvantages of a laparoscopic radical nephrectomy when compared to open nephrectomy?
9. What is acquired renal cystic disease? What histologic type of renal tumors is associated with it?
10. Under what circumstances can the adrenal gland be spared during a radical nephrectomy for renal cell carcinoma?

II. Bladder Carcinoma and Urothelial Tumors of the Renal Pelvis and Ureter

1. What are the risk factors for development of bladder carcinoma?
2. What are the indications for intravesical therapy for bladder carcinoma?
3. Which intravesical agent is the most effective?
4. What is the most serious side effect of thiotepa intravesical therapy? How should patients be monitored during treatment?
5. A patient with history of a mitral regurgitation and multifocal superficial bladder cancer presents for BCG intravesical therapy. Which antibacterial agents should be used to prevent endocarditis while maximizing BCG efficacy?
6. A patient develops high fever and chills one day after receiving his third course of BCG immunotherapy. Urine culture is negative. What antimicrobial agents should be used?
7. A 63-year-old with renal insufficiency undergoes cystoprostatectomy for muscle invasive TCC of the bladder and pathology shows node-positive disease. Given his renal function, he is not a candidate for standard MVAC chemotherapy. What other chemotherapeutic drugs could be used?
8. A 53-year-old woman with high-grade T1 bladder carcinoma develops a recurrence after 6 courses of BCG intravesical therapy. Six months after undergoing tumor resection and 6 repeat courses of BCG, she develops another grade 3, T1 recurrence. What do you recommend?
9. A male patient with muscle-invasive bladder cancer is interested in a continent urinary diversion. What are his options?

10. What are the indications for radical cystectomy?
11. Why is a meticulous lymphadenectomy at the time of radical cystectomy so important?
12. What is the risk of developing ureterointestinal strictures after urinary diversion? What are the different management strategies?
13. What are the indications for urethrectomy in patients with muscle-invasive bladder cancer?
14. In patients with an intact urethra, what is the best method of urethral surveillance after cystectomy?
15. What percentage of patients with muscle-invasive bladder cancer will develop upper tract transitional cell carcinoma?

III. Prostate Cancer

1. A 55-year-old man undergoes transrectal prostate needle biopsy for an elevated PSA showing prostatic intraepithelial neoplasia. What is his risk of developing carcinoma? How will you follow him?
2. What is endometriod or ductal prostatic carcinoma? What is its presentation and prognosis?
3. What are the indications for a staging laparoscopic pelvic lymphadenectomy in prostate cancer?
4. What are the most important factors predicting biochemical failure after definitive treatment for localized prostate cancer?
5. How is biochemical failure defined after radical prostatectomy? After external beam radiotherapy?
6. What are the potential complications of interstitial radiation therapy for prostate cancer? How can these be minimized?
7. A 75-year-old man with known metastastic prostate cancer presents with symptoms of cord compression. The radiation oncology team is consulted. What antiandrogen will lower serum testosterone to castrate levels most rapidly?
8. What are differences in side-effect profile between oral antiandrogens and LHRH agonists?
9. What is the best predictor of biochemical survival after external beam radiation therapy for prostate cancer?
10. What are the most common complications after radical prostatectomy?

IV. Testicular Cancer

1. What are the different histologic subtypes of seminoma? How do they differ in prognosis?
2. List the serum tumor markers used to monitor testis tumors. What are their half-lives?
3. A 31-year-old male is referred with embryonal carcinoma after left transcrotal orchectomy. You are concerned about his potential for metastasis to the inguinal lymph nodes. Is there a role for prophylactic inguinal lymphadenectomy?
4. What is the standard of care for stage I pure seminoma following orchiectomy?
5. A 35-year-old man with stage I embryonal carcinoma elects watchful waiting over retroperitoneal lymph node dissection. What is his risk of relapse? If he does relapse, what is his chance of cure with chemotherapy?
6. What are the most commonly used chemotherapeutic agents in testicular cancer?

7. What are the surgical boundaries of a modified left-sided RPLND for Stage I NSGCT? How is this different for right-sided tumors?
8. A 30-year-old male undergoes primary chemotherapy for a NSGCT metastatic to the retroperitoneum (6 cm) with a reduction in size of 40 percent. His tumor markers are negative and he undergoes RPLND. What is the pathology likely to show?
9. What are possible complications after RPLND?
10. How should patients with seminoma be followed? Is this different from patients with NSGCT?

V. Penile, Urethral, and Scrotal Carcinoma

1. What are the treatment options for Tis and T1 penile carcinoma?
2. What are the indications for total penectomy with perineal urethrostomy in penile carcinoma?
3. What are the anatomic boundaries of the inguinal lymphadenectomy for penile cancer?
4. What are the indications for inguinal lymphadenectomy in penile cancer?
5. What are the most commonly used chemotherapeutic drugs in metastastic penile carcinoma?
6. What types of muscle flaps can be used to prevent skin necrosis or vessel erosion after inguinal lymphadenectomy?
7. Is urethral carcinoma more common in men or women?
8. What is the standard of care for carcinoma in the distal third of the urethra in a female?
9. What acquired urethral abnormality is associated with adenocarcinoma of the female urethra?
10. What occupational risk is classically associated with scrotal cancer?

SUGGESTED READING

Penile, Urethral, and Scrotal Carcinoma

Carroll PC, Dixon CM. Surgical anatomy of the male and female urethra. *Urol Clin North Am* 19:339–346, 1992.

Catalona WJ: Modified inguinal lymphadenectomy for carcinoma of the penis with preservation of saphenous vein: Technique and preliminary results. *J Urol* 140:836, 1988.

deKernion JB, Abi-Aad AS: Controversies in ilioinguinal lymphadenectomy for cancer of the penis. *Urol Clin North Am* 19:319–324, 1992.

Forman JD, Lichter AS: The role of radiation therapy in the management of carcinoma of the male and female urethra. *Urol Clin North Am* 19:383–390, 1992.

Gerbaulet A, Lambin P: Radiation therapy of cancer of the penis: Indications, advantages, and pitfalls. *Urol Clin North Am* 19:325–332, 1992.

Johnson DE, Ames FC: *Groin Dissection.* Chicago, Yearbook Medical Publishers, 1985.

Lowe FC: Squamous cell carcinoma of the scrotum. *J Urol* 130:423, 1983.

Russo P, Gaudin P: Carcinoma of the penis: Diagnosis and staging. *Cont Urol* 4:12–31, 2000.

Schellhammer PF, Jordan GH, Schlossberg SM: Tumors of the penis. In: Walsh PC, Retik AB, Stamey TA, Vaughan ED, eds. *Campbell's Urology,* 6th ed. Philadelphia, Saunders, 1992, pp 1264–1298.

Skinner EC, Skinner DG: Management of carcinoma of the female urethra. In: Skinner DG, Lieskovsky G, eds. *Diagnosis and Management of Genitourinary Cancer.* Philadelphia, Saunders, 1988, pp 490–497.

SUGGESTED READINGS
Prostate and Bladder Cancer

Albertson PC, Hanley JA, Gleason DR, Barry MJ: Competing risk analysis of men aged 55 to 74 years at diagnosis managed conservatively for clinically localized prostate cancer. *JAMA* 280:975–980, 1998.

D'Amico AV, Whittington R, Malkowicz SB, et al: Biochemical outcome after radical protatectomy, external beam radiation therapy, or interstitial radiation therapy for clinically localized prostate cancer. *JAMA* 280:969–974, 1998.

Droller MJ: Bladder: Anatomical overview in surgical management of urologic disease: An anatomic approach, MJ Droller, St. Louis, Mosby Yearbook, p 575, 1992.

Eastham JA, Scardino PT: Radical prostatectomy. In: Walsh PC, et al, eds: *Campbell's Urology,* 7th ed. Philadelphia, Saunders, 1998, pp 2547–2564.

Eisenberger MA, Blumenstein BA, Crawford ED, et al: Bilateral orchiectomy with or without flutamide for metastatic prostate cancer. *N Engl J Med* 339:1036–1042, 1998.

Herr HW, Schwalb DM, Zhang ZF, et al: Intravesical bacillus Calmette-Guérin therapy prevents tumor progression and death from superficial bladder cancer: Ten-year follow-up of a prospective randomized trial. *J Clin Oncol* 13:1404, 1995.

Lamm DL: Complications of bacillus Calmette-Guérin immunotherapy. *Urol Clin North Am* 19:565, 1992.

Malkowicz SB: Superficial bladder cancer: The role of molecular markers in the treatment of high-risk superficial disease. *Semin Urol Oncol* 15:169–178, 1997.

Messing EM, Catalona W: Urothelial tumors of the urinary tract. In: *Campbell's Urology* 7th ed. PC Walsh, AB ED Vaughan, AJ Wein, Vol 3, Chap 77, 2327, 1998.

Partin AW, Kattan MW, Subong EN, Walsh PC, Wojno KJ, Oesterling JE, Scardino PT, Pearson JD. Combination of prostate-specific antigen, clinical stage, and Gleason score to predict pathological stage of localized prostate cancer. A multi-institutional update. *JAMA* 277:1445–1451, 1997.

Polascik TJ, Oesterling JE, Parting AW: Prostate specific antigen: A decade of discovery—What we have learned and where we are going. *J Urol* 162:293–306, 1999.

Ragde H, Blasko JC, Grimm PD, et al: Interstitial iodine-125 radiation without adjuvant therapy in the treatment of clinically localized prostate carcinoma. *Cancer* 80:442–453, 1997.

Spruck CH, Ohneseit PE, Gonzalez-Zulueta M, et al: Two molecular pathways to transitional cell carcinoma of the bladder. *Cancer Res* 54:784–788, 1994.

Walsh PC, Partin AW, Epstein JI: Cancer control and quality of life following anatomical radical retropubic prostatectomy: Results at 10 years. *J Urol* 152:1831–1836, 1994.

Zincke H, Oesterling JE, Blute ML, et al: Long-term (15 years) results after radical prostatectomy for clinically localized (stage T2c or lower) prostate cancer. *J Urol* 152:1850–1857, 1994.

Testis Cancer

Baniel J, Foster RS, Rowland RG, Bihrle R, Donahue JP: Testis cancer: Complications of post-chemotherapy retroperitoneal lymph node dissection. *J Urol* 153:976–980, 1995.

Donohue JP, Thornhill JA, Foster RS, Bihrle R, Rowland RG, Einhorn LH: The role of retroperitoneal lymphadenectomy in clinical stage B testis cancer: The Indiana University experience (1965 to 1989). *J Urol* 153:85–89, 1995.

Einhorn LH: Salvage therapy for germ cell tumors. *Semin Oncol* 21:47–51, 1994.

Einhorn LH, Donohue JP: Advanced testicular cancer: Update for urologists. *J Urol* 160:1964–1969, 1998.

Moller H, Skakkeback NE: Testicular cancer and cryptorchidism in relation to prenatal factors: Case control studies in Denmark. *Cancer Causes Control* 8:904–12, 1997.

Nichols C, Loehrer P Sr: The story of second cancers in patients cured of testicular cancer: Tarnishing success of burnishing irrelevance. *J Natl Cancer Inst* 89:1304–1305, 1997.

Wegner HEH, Hubotter A, Andresen R, Miller K: Testicular microlithiasis and concomitant testicular intraepithelial neoplasia. *Int Urol Nephrol* 30:313–315, 1998.

Renal Cell Carcinoma

Bostwick DG, Eble JN: Diagnosis and classification of renal cell carcinoma. *Urol Clin N Am* 26:627–635, 1999.

Caddeddu JA, Ono Y, Clayman RV, et al: Laparoscopic nephrectomy for renal cell cancer: Evaluation of efficacy and safety: A multicenter experience. *Urology* 52:773–777, 1998.

Levy DA, Slaton JW, Swanson DA, Dinney CP: Stage specific guidelines for surveillance after radical nephrectomy for local renal cell carcinoma. *J Urol* 15:1163–1167, 1998.

Montie JM: Lymphadenectomy for renal cell carcinoma. *Semin Urol* 7:181–185, 1989.

Motzer RJ, Bander NH, Nanus DM: Renal-cell carcinoma. *N Engl J Med* 335:865–875, 1996.

Novick AC: Renal-sparing surgery for renal cell carcinoma. *Urol Clin North Am* 20:277–282, 1993.

Sagalowsky AI, Kadesky KT, Ewalt DM, Kennedy TJ: Factors influencing adrenal metastasis in renal cell carcinoma. *J Urol* 151:1181–1184, 1994.

Skinner DG, Pritchett RT, Lieskovsky G, Boyd SD, Stiles QR: Vena caval involvement by renal cell carcinoma. Surgical resection provides meaningful long-term survival. *Ann Surg* 210:387–394, 1989.

Sufrin G, Cashon S, Golio A, Murphy GP: Paraneoplastic and serologic syndromes of renal adenocarcinoma. *Semin Urol* 7:158–171, 1989.

Yang JC, Topalian SL, Parkinson D, et al: Randomized comparison of high-dose and low-dose intravenous interleukin 2 for the therapy of metastatic renal cell carcinoma: An interim report. *J Clin Oncol* 12:1572–1576, 1994.

CHAPTER 18
Urinary Diversion

S. Bruce Malkowicz

I. GENERAL CONSIDERATIONS

Urinary diversion is an integral part of urinary reconstruction and urologic oncology. Such surgery can be technically advanced and is associated with potential long-term as well as short-term complications. Additionally, careful consideration must be given to the physiologic costs of diverting the urinary tract and the appropriate selection of patients for a particular procedure. Urinary diversion can consist of simple diversion of the ureters to the skin, diversion of urine into the alimentary tract, or diversion of urine into an isolated segment of bowel serving as a conduit or reservoir for urine. There is no one preferred method of performing urinary diversion, therefore, fundamental principles of reconstruction must be understood to appropriately apply these techniques in a given situation.

II. HISTORY

During the mid- and late 19th century, many efforts were made to divert urine into the alimentary tract in an attempt to treat congenital malformations such as bladder exstrophy or conditions such as bladder cancer. Although innovative, multiple complications occurred due to technical limitations in the preantibiotic era. The ureterosigmoidostomy of Coffey provided one of the first reasonable methods of diverting the urinary system. Metabolic complications and the development of adenocarcinoma at the ureter–bowel junction discouraged further widespread use of this technique. The ileal loop urinary conduit described by Bricker in 1950 became the standard form of urinary diversion over the next several decades. Different techniques of continent urinary diversion have since been developed and modified by multiple individuals. The application of continent diversion has been further aided by the acceptance of clean intermittent catheterization as an appropriate form of urinary drainage.

III. GENERAL PHYSIOLOGIC CONSIDERATIONS

A. Renal Function

Approximately 30 percent of patients will experience long-term (5 to 15 years) renal deterioration after urinary diversion. It must be remembered, however, that not all renal units associated with a diversion are normal preoperatively. This deterioration can be hastened by high static pressures within the reconstructed urinary tract, reflux, or chronic infection. Many of the metabolic abnormalities described first became manifest or are exacerbated by patients displaying a serum creatinine greater than 2 ng/dL. Care must, therefore, be taken when considering such patients for urinary diversion.

B. Infection

The majority of patients with a urinary diversion will display urine colonized with bacteria. In general, there is no concomitant symptomatic infection, and this situation is best left untreated. Repeated therapy for asymptomatic colonization can lead to infection with stone formation or severely resistant strains of bacteria. This may necessitate the use of parenteral antibiotics. Classically, 4 to 6 percent of patients with urinary diversions may eventually die of urosepsis.

C. Urolithiasis

This may occur in 2 to 10 percent of patients with urinary diversions. The presence of foreign bodies, especially staples, provides a nidus for stone formation. Stones also have a greater tendency to form in patients with *Proteus* urinary tract infections and in patients with hyperchloremic metabolic acidosis.

IV. METABOLIC CONSIDERATIONS

A. Electrolyte Abnormalities

These occur secondary to the interaction of urine with a particular bowel epithelium. The altered transport of different ions gives rise to particular metabolic abnormalities.

1. *Colon.* The classic abnormality seen in ureterosigmoidostomy is hyperchloremic metabolic acidosis. It was first recognized by Ferris and Odel in 1950. The condition can be seen in as many as 80 percent of patients and is exacerbated by the large surface area of the colon exposed to urine. Essentially, a significant amount of bicarbonate equivalents are lost into the colonic urine with the absorption of chloride from the urine. This condition can lead to a severe acidosis that is exacerbated by compromised baseline renal function. Another less recognized complication can be total body potassium depletion and

hypokalemia. Furthermore, elevated ammonia levels may develop in patients secondary to bacterial overgrowth. This is best treated by adequate urinary drainage and/or treatment with neomycin or lactulose.

2. *Ileum.* Hyperchloremic metabolic acidosis is also seen in patients with ileal conduits. Although the findings are less severe, they can be present in as many as 70 percent of patients with ileal conduits. Again, patients with impaired baseline renal function will display a greater propensity toward metabolic derangement.

   a. *Monitoring.* McDougal and Koch emphasize the potential implications of long-term subtle metabolic abnormalities such as growth retardation and osteomalacia. The exact timing for intervention in subtle acidosis is not clear (especially in elderly adults treated for cancer), yet these issues are of great concern in the pediatric and young adult population.

   b. *Treatment.* Hyperchloremic acidosis is treated by alkalizing agents such as oral sodium bicarbonate, polycitra, or Shohl's solution. If a sodium cannot be tolerated, cAMP inhibitors such as nicotinic acid and chlorpromazine may be employed. Although sodium overload is avoided with such therapies, potential side effects such as peptic ulcer disease and tardive dyskinesia can occur.

3. *Jejunum.* Use of this bowel segment is associated with a hyponatremic, hypochloremic, hyperkalemic, metabolic acidosis. This is due to a loss of salt and an increase in potassium and hydrogen ions. A feed-forward mechanism is established by the initial loss of salt and water, followed by a renin-aldosterone response to the hypovolemia. The permeable jejunal epithelium is presented with a low-sodium, high-potassium urine, which facilitates further body loss of sodium into the conduit and reabsorption of potassium. Initial management requires fluid resuscitation followed by long-term sodium chloride supplementation.

4. *Stomach.* This bowel segment has been employed in urinary diversion or bladder augmentation in several different configurations. It has been employed predominantly in the pediatric population. The advantages of using stomach include compensation for pre-existing metabolic acidosis, conversation of gastrointestinal absorptive area, and decreased mucous production. The most common metabolic side effect is a hypokalemic, hypochloremic, metabolic alkalosis such as that seen with prolonged nasogastric suction. It is best managed with good oral fluid intake.

V. OTHER CONSIDERATIONS

A. Neoplasia

Reports of adenocarcinoma in patients with ureterosigmoidostomies were first made in 1929. This event will occur in approximately 10 percent of such patients with a latency period of 10 to 20 years. Since serial screening was not performed, original reports displayed generally advanced disease with up to a 36 percent mortality rate. Although the lesion is usually at the ureter–colon junction, it is difficult to discern the issue of origin. The etiology of these carcinomas is poorly understood. Cases of carcinoma have been reported in ileal conduits and cystoplasties. The long-term implications for continent diversion are unknown.

B. Drug Absorption

A large bowel segment provides a significant reabsortive area for many chemicals. This is important because many patients undergoing chemotherapy for bladder cancer may be at risk for intoxication. Methotrexate, which is employed in the methotrexate, vinblastine, adriamycin, cisplatin (MVAC) regimen, has reported to cause toxicity. Anticonvulsant agents may also be reabsorbed by the bowel of a urinary diversion.

C. Vitamin B$_{12}$ Metabolism

Vitamin B$_{12}$ is absorbed primarily in the terminal ileum, which is often isolated from the alimentary tract when constructing a continent reservoir. Since usual body reserves are adequate for approximately 5 years, this is not an immediate postoperative concern, but it must be addressed with regard to replacement therapy in patients over the long term. The 15- to 20-cm segment employed in a standard ileal conduit usually does not deplete the absorptive distal ileum still in continuity with the alimentary tract.

D. Hematuria-Dysuria Syndrome

This is a complex of symptoms in patients with a diversion or bladder augment from a gastric segment which includes bladder spasm, urethral pain, gross hematuria, and skin irritation. The etiology is incompletely understood yet is probably related to the secretion of gastric acid. The activation of pepsinogen to pepsin at a low pH has been proposed as the urothelial irritant. It is best treated by oral hydration and histamine blockade. This syndrome is partially related to hypergastrinemia, which can be demonstrated in gastric segment diversions. Ulceration is another possible problem with these segments.

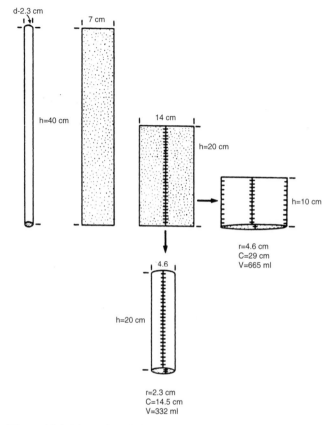

Figure 18-1 Illustration of the principle of maximizing the volume of a given surface area. By detubularizing a segment of bowel and approximating a spherical shape, a high-volume, low-pressure urinary reservoir may be constructed. (*Reprodced from Hinman F Jr: Selection of intestinal segments for bladder substitution: Physical and physiological characteristics. J Urol 139:519–523, 1988.*)

VI. MECHANICAL CONSIDERATIONS

A. Neuromuscular Activity

Bowel segments have an intrinsic coordinated contractile activity that must be taken into consideration when constructing conduits. It is a physiologic property that is disadvantageous for the active storage of urine. For continent reconstruction, the splitting of bowel on its antimesenteric border and its reconfiguration are meant to cause a zero net resultant pressure vector, thus preventing directional flow of urine. Additionally, a general discoordination of contraction activity occurs and thus lowers intraluminal pressure. This discoordination is the primary mechanical effect of reconfiguration, but its long-term efficacy is questionable because several studies suggest the return of coordinated activity fronts over time.

B. Geometric Aspects

Much of the effectiveness in creating high-volume, low-pressure reservoirs by bowel reconfiguration can be accomplished by the fact that detubularization essentially approximates a sphere. This is the maximized volume for a given surface area, and the sphere has a larger radius than the tube of the bowel Fig. 18-1). The law of Laplace states that for a given wall tension, a larger radius will result in lower intraluminal pressure, which is the goal of a continent pouch with regard to continence and the prevention of upper tract deterioration.

VII. FORMS OF URINARY DIVERSION (NON-CONTINENT)

A. Ileal Conduit

Since its introduction in 1950, the ileal conduit has become reference standard for urinary diversion. Approximately 15 to 20 cm of terminal ileum are isolated bowel continuity, allowing this bowel segment to server as an conduit or passageway to the skin (Fig. 18-2). General complications are listed in Table 18-1.

1. *Cutaneous considerations.* The loop may be matured at the skin as a Brooke ostomy or as a Turnbull loop (Figs. 18-3 and 18-4). The latter is useful in patients with a thick abdominal wall. One of the several ostomy appliances are attached to this site. Appropriate preoperative marking on the abdominal wall and care in constructing the stoma bud are important to avoid difficulties with patient comfort and skin care. Stomal stenosis is the most common long-term complication of cutaneous urinary diversion.

2. *Ureteral considerations.* The ureteral–enteral anastomosis is a potential site for complications. A direct anastomosis between the bowel and ureter with mucosa-to-mucosa apposition is the preferred method of construction. Early ureteral leakage was a significant and morbid complication of this procedure that has been reduced by greater attention to technique and the use of ureteral diversion stents in the perioperative period. Ureteral stenosis is not uncommon and may require balloon dilatation or reanastomosis.

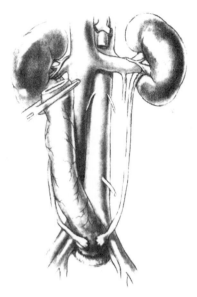

Figure 18-2 An isolated segment of distal ileum serves as an excellent straightforward urinary conduit after cystectomy. The Leadbetter technique shown avoids extensive mobilization of the ureters. (*Reproduced from Skinner DG, Lieskovsky G, eds: Diagnosis and Management of Genitourinary Cancer, 1988, p. 635.*)

Table 18-1 General Complications of Heal Loop Diversion

COMPLICATION	PERCENT
Renal deterioration	20–50
Ureteral obstruction	5–22
Pyelonephrosis	4–20
Stomal stenosis	5–40
Loop stenosis	2–8
Renal calculi	3–10
Stomal hernia	2–5

B. Colon Conduit

A portion of colon can be employed as a urinary conduit. The potential for hyperchloremic acidosis exists but is reduced if short segments of colon are used. When employed in conjunction with a full pelvic exenteration, a bowel anastomosis may be avoided. A transverse colon conduit is a very useful

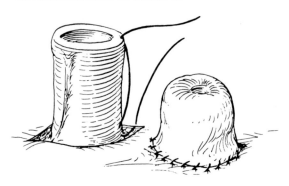

Figure 18-3 The distal end of an ileal conduit can be brought to the skin and fashioned in a simple Brooke stoma (rose bud). (*Reproduced from Walsh PC, et al., eds: Campbell's Urology, 5th ed. 1986, p. 2611.*)

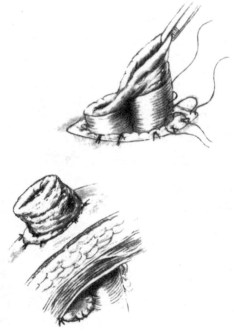

Figure 18-4 In patients with a thick abdominal wall or short mesentery, a Turnbull loop may be fashioned to provide a good cutaneous stoma. (*Reproduced from Skinner DG, Lieskovsky G, eds: Diagnosis and Management of Genitourinary Cancer, 1988, p. 650.*)

alternative in patients with heavily irradiated bowel. This segment is usually away from most radiation fields and provides a healthy alternative to possibly damaged ileum. Nonrefluxing ureteral anastomoses may be constructed with the use of tinea coli, but the potential for ureteral obstruction exists.

C. Jejunal Conduit

The jejunum has been employed as an alternative segment in cases of irradicated bowel. Due to its permeability characteristics, it is prone to the severe metabolic complications previously described and is not generally employed in urinary diversion.

D. Cutaneous Ureteral Diversion

This is a direct form of urinary diversion generally complicated by stenosis at the level of the skin and by potential difficulties with collection appliances.

VIII. CONTINENT URINARY DIVERSION

A. General Goals

1. Adequate capacity reservoir
2. Low-pressure reservoir
3. Urinary continence during normal activities
4. Volitonal emptying

B. General Construction

1. Cutaneous urinary diversion
2. Orthotopic urinary diversion

C. Continence Mechanisms

1. Intussuscepted nipple valve
2. Fixed resistance
3. Flap valve—Mitrofanoff principle
4. Pelvic floor external sphincter (orthotopic)

D. Ureterosigmoidostomy

This is one of the original forms of urinary diversion and can be considered continent urinary diversion in the broad sense (Fig. 18-6). It is rarely applied in developed countries due to the metabolic and neoplastic complications previously described. Recent modifications of this procedure have included J-pouch alteration of the sigmoid colon or the use of detubularized ileal patches to increase local capacity and decrease tenasmus.

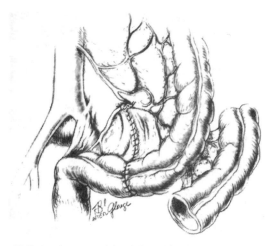

Figure 18-5 A urinary conduit of sigmoid colon may be constructed when terminal ileum is not an appropriate choice of bowel. In pelvic exenterations the use of this bowel segment can avoid the need for a bowel anastomosis. In a heavily radiated pelvis, the use of transverse colon is a preferred bowel segment due to its usual exclusion from the radiation field. (*Reproduced from Skinner DG, Lieskovsky G, eds: Diagnosis and Management of Genitourinary Cancer, 1988, p. 642.*)

E. **Cutaneous Continent Diversion**

In this form of diversion, a reservoir or ileum, colon, or a combination of both is constructed from detubularized bowel and brought to the skin as a discrete flush, catheterizable stoma. The site may be paraumbilical of just above the pubic hairline. In the case of a thick or distorted abdominal wall, the umbilicus is the preferred site. The site must be catheterized every 4 to 6 hours to avoid overdistention. In addition to the standard complications of urinary diversion, patients may develop eccentricity of the catheterization pathway or incontinence, requiring revision of the site. Initial series reported revision rates of 25 to 30 percent but these have decreased to a 5 to 15 percent range.

1. *Indiana pouch.* A detubularized segment of cecum and colon acts as a storage reservoir whose continence is maintained by fixed resistance established at the ileocecal valve and distal ileum (Figs. 18-7, 18-8). The tapered distal ileum serves as the catheterizable limb. Ease of construction and a low complication profile make this a popular form of diversion. Capacity is lower than that seen with ileal pouches, and a potential for chronic diar-

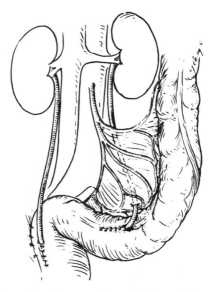

Figure 18-6 Illustration of a ureterosigmoidostomy. This was one of the earliest forms of urinary diversion and employs the rectal sphincter for continence. Metabolic abnormalities can occur through the contact of urine with the extensive colon surface area. Adenocarcinoma may occur at the ureterocolonic anastomosis. (*Reproduced from Walsh PC, et al., eds: Campbell's Urology, 5th ed. 1986, p. 2602.*)

rhea exists (5 percent) due the removal of the ileocecal valve and colonic tissue.

2. *Penn pouch.* In this form of diversion, the appendix is used in a tunneled method and acts as a flap valve (Mitrofanoff principle) to provide urinary continence (Fig. 18-9). This recapitulates the natural course and mechanism of the ureter as it enters the bladder. Issues of pouch capacity and diarrhea are similar to those seen in the Indiana pouch. The appendix may not be suitable catheterizable limb in all adults.

3. *Monti procedure.* The use of a transversely tubularized bowel segment (TTBS) increases the range and flexibility for the construction of a catheterizible limb in a cutaneous continent urinary reconstruction (Fig. 18-10). A 2.5-cm segment of small bowel can be detubularized and transversely retubularized to create long, relatively narrow bowel segments, which can be implanted in a urinary reservoir and brought to the skin. When necessary, two

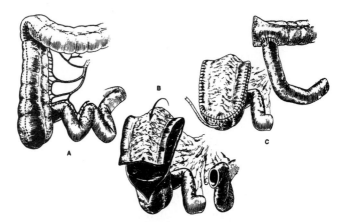

Figure 18-7 Basic steps in the construction of the Indiana pouch. A large reservoir is constructed from a segment of the ascending and transverse colon along with a portion of distal ileum. An ileocolic anastomosis restores bowel continuity. (*Reproduced from Rowland R: A straightforward surgical approach to urinary diversion. Contemp Urol 3:13–19, 1990.*)

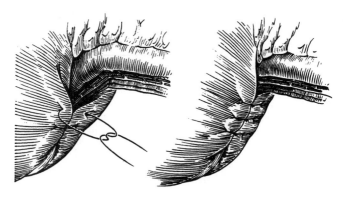

Figure 18-8 Continence is established in the Indiana pouch by constructing an area of fixed resistance at the cecal junction of the tapered distal ileum. The patient remains dry since the pouch pressures are lower than the pressure at this site. The pouch is emptied by clean intermittent catheterization at the flush cutaneous stoma. (*Reproduced from Rowland R: A straightforward surgical approach to urinary diversion. Contemp Urol 3:13–19, 1990.*)

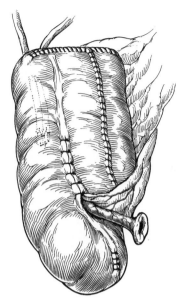

Figure 18-9 The Penn pouch uses a segment of colon for pouch construction and the Mitrofanoff principle as a continence mechanism. In this instance the appendix is tunneled obliquely into the pouch in a flap-valve manner. As the pouch fills, the fluid pressure closes the appendix against the pouch wall providing continence. This is similar to the natural arrangement as the ureters tunnel into the native bladder. (*Reproduced from Duckett JW, et al: New life for the appendix as a continence mechanism. Contemp Urol 5:53–70, 1993.*)

segments can be attached in series to gain additional length. This is an extension of the Mitrofanoff principle, which uses a small diameter tube implanted in a flap valve fashion to provide continence.

4. *Pouch hygiene.* As previously stated, forms of urinary diversion are subject to bacterial colonization. In continent reservoirs, this may proceed to frank "pouchitis" and pyelonephritis if emptying is inefficient or incomplete. Furthermore, most bowel segments continue to produce mucus for at least 1 year, which can be a source of obstruction leading to dysfunction and infection. The potential for such difficulties can be reduced by simple maneuvers such as daily pouch irrigation with saline solution by the patient after a routine catheterization.

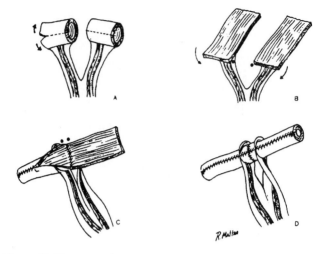

Figure 18-10

F. Orthotopic Continent Diversion

This is a form of continent reconstruction based on the striated external sphincter as the primary continence mechanism (Fig. 18-11). A high-capacity, low-pressure system is essential for an optimal result. Potential complications include enuresis in 5 to 10 percent of patients (due to relaxation of the pelvic floor during deep stages of sleep) and tumor recurrence at the urethral margin necessitating major surgical revision. Pouches may be constructed of pure ileum (hemiKock pouch, ileal neobladder) or mixed segments of large and small bowel (Mainz pouch).

1. *Urodynamics.* Functional studies reveal excellent capacity and storage as well as efficient emptying with a combination of pelvic floor relaxation and abdominal straining. The potentially large capacity of these pouches can make a patient inattentive to the need for voiding. If the reservoir is chronically overdistended, the ability to empty is compromised and may necessitate the need for intermittent catheterization. Upper tract deterioration is primarily avoided by having low static pressures in the pouch and avoiding pouch–ureter reflux. Reflux may be further prevented by an intussuscepted nipple.

2. *Female orthotopic diversion.* The technique of orthotopic diversion has recently been extended to female pa-

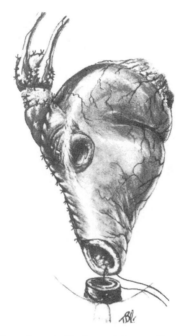

Figure 18-11 The orthotopic Kock pouch is one of several forms of orthotopic continent diversion. The native external sphincter is employed as the continence mechanism and voiding is in a near-normal manner. In this particular pouch, the ureters are implanted into an afferet limb. Advantage is taken of the nipple-valve mechanism and the flap-valve placement of the nipple against the pouch wall to prevent urine reflux. (*Reproduced from Boyd S, et al: Kock pouch bladder replacement. Urol Clin North Am 18:641–648, 1991.*)

tients. Careful pathologic studies have suggested that the absence of carcinoma in situ or lack of tumor involvement in the trigone or bladder neck are associated with a lack of tumor in the female urethra. Although a concern for urinary incontinence was an initial issue, it has been noticed that many of these patients will develop partial or complete urinary retention. Patients tend to be equally divided: one third void normally with or without occasional catheterization, one third experience complete urinary retention, and one third have stress urinary incontinence. No significant problems with urethral recurrence have been reported.

SUGGESTED READINGS

Benson MD, Olsson CA. Urinary diversion. In: Walsh PC, Retik AB, Stamey TA, Vaugh ED Jr, eds. Campbell's urology, 6th ed. Philadephia: WB Saunders, 1992:2654-2720.

Hall MC, Koch MO, McDougal WS: Metabolic consequences of urinary diversion through intestinal segments. Urol Clin North Am 18:725-736, 1991

Klein EA, Montie JE, Montague DK, et al. Jejunal conduit urinary diversion. J. Urol. 135:244-246, 1986.

McDougal WS. Use of intestinal segments in the urinary tract: basci principles. In: Walsh PC, Retik AB, Stamey TA, Vaughn ED, eds. Campbell's Urology, 6th ed. Philadephia WB Saunders, 2596-2629, 1992

Skinner DG, Lieskowsky G, Boyd S. Continent urinary diversion. J Urol 1989;141:1323-1327.

Rowland RG, Mitchell ME, Bihrle R, et al. The Indiana continent urinary reservoir. J Urol 1987;137:1136-1139.

Studer UE, Zingg EJ. Ileal orthotopic bladder substitutes. What we have learned from 12 years' experience with 200 patients. Urol Clin North Am 1997;24:781-793.

Skinner DG, Boyd SD, Lieskovsky G, Bennett C, Hopwood B. Lower urinary tract reconstruction following cystectomy: experience and results in 126 patients using the Kock ileal reservoir with bilateral ureteroileal urethrostomy. J Urol 1991;146:756-760.

SELF-ASSESSMENT QUESTIONS

1. What are the potential consequences of diverting the urinary stream directly into the sigmoid colon?
2. Describe the electrolyte abnormalities associated with an ileal loop diversion and a jejunal loop diversion.
3. What is the Mitrofanoff principle.
4. How does detubularization of a bowel segment optimize the properties of a continent urinary reservoir?
5. What are the significant short term complications encountered when performing a urinary diversion?
6. How can particular electrolyte disturbances associated with urinary diversion be corrected?
7. What are the basic differences between cutaneous and orthotopic continent diversion?
8. What are the significant long term complications associated with urinary diversion?
9. What are the particular complications associated with the use of stomach in urinary diversion?
10. What is the difference between urinary colonization and urinary infection?

CHAPTER 19
Radiation Therapy

Richard Whittington

The role of radiation in the management of genitourinary malignancy is one of the more controversial topics in clinical oncology. Radiation may be used alone in the curative management of some tumors or in combination with other therapies as an adjuvant to surgery or chemotherapy. It also can be used as a salvage therapy after failure of surgical therapy, or as a palliative therapy to alleviate symptoms in patients with advanced disease. Appropriate utilization of radiation requires knowledge of its mechanisms and techniques to understand the potential and limitations of this modality.

X-rays and gamma rays, the two types of electromagnetic energy used to treat cancer, were discovered during the last decade of the 19th century, and the effects on tumors and normal tissues were quickly described. The first use of external beam radiation was reported by Pratt in 1896. In 1904, Alexander Graham Bell suggested that radioactive sources should be planted "directly into the heart of the tumor." This was brought to reality in 1912 when the first patient was treated with interstitial brachytherapy. Other modalities such as electrons, protons, neutrons, and π-mesons have been investigated. Thus far, only protons have shown potential utility in managing prostate cancer.

I. PHYSICS

Both x-rays and gamma rays are electromagnetic radiation. Gamma rays are radiation produced by the decay of radioactive isotopes, either natural or produced. X-rays are artificially produced when charged particles strike a target. Gamma rays have well-defined energies characteristic of the isotope that emits them, whereas x-rays have a broader spectrum that is determined by the energy of the machine that produced them. The energy of the electromagnetic radiation determines the ability of the radiation to penetrate tissue, with higher energy allowing deeper penetration. Higher energies scatter their energy in a more forward direction, so that with high-energy machines, the maximum energy is deposited below the skin surface. For this reason, a low-energy machine operating at a peak energy of

140,000 volts (140 kVp) would be preferable in treating superficial tumors such as skin cancer because the maximum dose is deposited in the skin and the dose decreases exponentially to less than 25 percent of the maximum dose at a depth of 4 cm. For tumors deeper in the body, a more penetrating beam such as one operating at a peak energy of 10 to 15 million volts (10 to 15 MV) is preferable. A 15-MV beam deposits its maximum energy at a depth of 2.8 cm and is still able to deliver 50 percent of its' maximum dose at a depth of 20 cm. Electrons deposit their maximum dose at or near the surface, penetrate to a predictable depth with a relatively constant dose, and then decrease rapidly. A sample of the depth dose curves of a variety of beams is shown in Figure 19-1.

In some situations, it is preferable to deliver radiation to the tumor from an internal source. Radiation dose is determined by the ability of the radiation to penetrate tissue and the distance from the source of the radiation. Similar to visible light, the intensity of the radiation decreases in proportion to the square of the distance from the source ($1/d^2$). Since doubling the distance from the source of radiation will decrease the intensity by 75 percent and tripling the distance will decrease the intensity by 89 percent, it is reasonable to consider placing the source of radiation within the tumor to minimize the dose that would be delivered to the surrounding tissue.

Radioactive isotopes produce radiation with a decreasing dose rate as time passes. Every isotope has a half-life and the dose rate will decrease by 50 percent with each half-life. There are situations in which a constant dose of radiation is desired and a long-lived isotope is inserted and removed after a prescribed dose is delivered. In other cases, it may be difficult to remove radioactive sources, and a permanent implant is used. The half-lives of some commonly used isotopes are listed in Table 19-1.

Table 19-1 Characteristics of Commonly Used Clinical Isotopes

ISOTOPE	HALF-LIFE		EFFECTIVE ENERGY	
Radium 226	1622	years	1.1	MeV
Radon 222	3.8	days	1.1	MeV
Gold 198	2.7	days	326	KeV
Iridium 192	74.5	days	670	KeV
Cobalt 60	5.26	years	1.25	MeV
Iodine 125	60	days	27	KeV
Palladium 103	17	days	21	KeV

Percent Depth Doses for Electron and Photon Beams

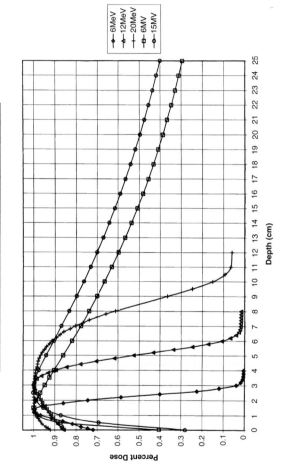

Figure 19-1 Sample depth dose curves for 6 MeV electrons (-◊-), 12 MeV electrons (-△-), 20 MeV electrons (—|—), 6 MV X-rays (—□—), and 15 MV X-rays (—o—).

II. RADIOBIOLOGY

Radiation causes its effects in tissue by producing ionizations within the cell. The target in cells is the DNA molecule, and the ionizations will produce breaks in the DNA strand. Cells can repair this damage if it is confined to a single strand because the opposite strand serves as a template for repair. If two strand breaks occur on opposite chains in close proximity, it is possible that the two ends of the chromosome will drift apart. These fragmented chromosomes may adhere to other chromosomes or they may sort out randomly when the cell divides. These daughter cells may be missing critical segments of DNA or have excess and unregulated copies of other genes, either of which may be fatal to the cell. This is thought to be the reason that cells are observed to die a mitotic death (i.e., the lethal effect of the radiation is not expressed until the cell dies).

Radiobiologic research has been directed at identifying the factors that affect the survival of cells and methods to selectively increase these effects on tumor cells. The easiest method to assay the effect of radiation is to deliver a dose of radiation to a suspension of single cells and then measure the percentage of surviving cells. The technique uses a suspension with a known concentration of cells. A sample is placed on a culture plate and the colonies are counted. At the same time, a similar sized sample is radiated and plated and the number of colonies counted. The ratio of number of colonies developing on the two plates is the surviving fraction. A typical survival curve is shown in Figure 19-2.

Since a rad represents a specific amount of energy transferred to tissue, each rad would have an equal physical effect on the cell. As the survival curve in Figure 19-2 shows, the biologic effect is less for the first rad than it is for the 101st rad. This shows that cells are capable of accumulating a certain amount of damage that is not lethal. The second curve in Figure 19-2 shows what happens if the radiation dose is split up and delivered over several fractions with time between fractions to repair this sublethal damage. The sublethal damage is expressed as a shoulder on the cell survival curve. Once the dose of radiation exceeds this shoulder, then each subsequent increment of radiation will kill a constant fraction of the surviving cells. If the radiation is stopped and the cells are given time to repair the effects of the first dose, a second dose of radiation will have the same effect on the surviving cells as it would have if they had never been radiated. Because normal cells repair this damage much more efficiently than tumor cells, recent studies have delivered two doses of radiation to some tumors each treatment day and shown that it may increase the efficacy of treatment. This is because in vitro studies have shown that normal cells repair this damage more efficiently than tumor cells.

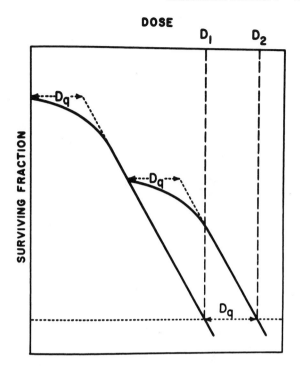

Figure 19-2 A typical survival curve in for a mammalian cell line. D_q describes the extent to which the cell line can accumulate less than lethal damage.

Oxygen is known to enhance the effects of radiation. Cells are more sensitive when radiated under oxygenated conditions than when they are hypoxic. Normal tissues are always oxygenated, but experimental measurements in tumors have shown that these cells will pile up around a capillary and consume the available oxygen, and diffusion into the tissues is limited. This creates a situation in which there are well-oxygenated, relatively sensitive cells adjacent to the capillary and necrotic material at a distance from the capillary. Between these two areas is a region of viable but hypoxic cells that are more resistant to radiation. In vitro studies have shown that all cells are more sensitive to radiation in the presence of oxygen. All in vitro studies thus far show that hypoxic cells require 1.5 to 3.0 times as much radiation to achieve the same cell kill.

Efforts are underway are being made to develop substances that will act like oxygen in cells but are able to diffuse through tissue without being metabolized like oxygen. It is hoped that this will help to deal with the problem of hypoxic tumor cells without affecting the sensitivity of normal cells. In vitro work showed that these compounds sensitized hypoxic tumor cells to the effects of radiation, but clinical trials were limited by the other toxicities of the sensitizer. Similarly, there was an effort to develop drugs that would protect the normal cells from the effects of radiation. These trials have also failed to show in vivo benefit, but efforts continue to develop a new generation of sensitizers and protectors. More importantly, chemotherapy and hormonal therapies have been observed to affect tumor sensitivity in vivo and these agents form the basis of many current combined modality trials.

III. TREATMENT PLANNING

The delivery of radiation to a tumor requires a physician to perform five functions: (1) identify and locate the structures to be treated; (2) identify those adjacent structures that need to be protected; (3) prescribe the appropriate dose of radiation for the tumor based on its size and histology; (4) consider the tolerance of tissue within the target that may be affected by treatment; and (5) consider the tolerance of tissues between the skin and the target (transit volume). In theory, this appears to be a complex but solvable problem, but, in fact, most clinical situations will require some compromise on one or more issues. The clinician must select those compromises that will minimize the effect on the desired outcome of uncomplicated tumor control.

Modern equipment will allow for sophisticated three-dimensional treatment planning. Patients may undergo CT-based treatment planning in which a series of axial images is obtained of the target as well as the adjacent critical structures. The target, the bony structures, and the sensitive normal tissues are defined on each computed tomography slice. When these are loaded into a computer, it is possible to create a reconstruction of the target and the critical structures. Newer and more versatile machines are able to deliver radiation from a much wider range of angles. Radiation oncologists are no longer restricted to one plane for treatment delivery. The system can then calculate the dose to many small volumes within the target and to the adjacent tissues.

The target consists of the prostate and a margin of tissue to account for day-to-day variation in setup, beam edges where the dose is not uniform, and organ motion. Newer techniques of localization allow for tighter margins. New positions allow for better immobilization of the prostate and linear accelerators have sharper edges. Figure 19-3 shows the dose volume histogram for the prostate and the rectum of a patient with prostate cancer. The dose through the prostate is homogeneous, with a minimum dose that is only 4.3 percent less than the maximum dose. Similarly, a small volume of rectum will tolerate a high

DVH-VOI id 1 PROSTATE
Volume (ccm): 55.
Calc. pnts 518/518

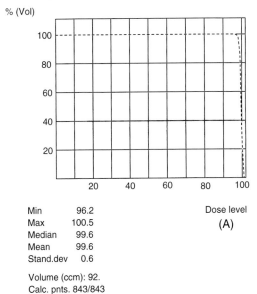

% (Vol)

Min	96.2	Dose level
Max	100.5	(A)
Median	99.6	
Mean	99.6	
Stand.dev	0.6	

Volume (ccm): 92.
Calc. pnts. 843/843

% (Vol)

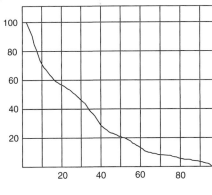

Min	2.1	Dose level
Max	95.6	(B)
Median	27.1	
Mean	30.6	
Stand.dev	24.5	

Figure 19-3 Dose volume histograms for the prostate (A) and the rectum (B) of a patient treated for prostate cancer.

dose of radiation as is shown in the figure, but most of the organ receives a much lower dose. In this histogram, 7 percent of the rectum received more than 80 percent of the tumor dose, but 79 percent received less than 50 percent. Older methods using anterior–posterior and lateral fields delivered at least 60 percent of the dose to the entire rectum and 40 percent of the rectum received more than 80 percent of the dose. These newer techniques allow for higher doses to be delivered to the prostate without increased complications.

Once a plan has been developed by the dosimetrist and approved by the physician, the patient is taken to a simulator. This is a machine that uses the same projection and localization system as the treatment machine but produces a low energy beam to produce diagnostic quality films. These machines are useful because the radiation machine produces a rectangular beam. It is possible to use the diagnostic film to draw blocks. The film is then used to cut a block out of a low-melting-point lead alloy, which can be hung on a plate from the head of the machine. This allows the field to be shaped to conform to the shape of the target. The field is then confirmed with a high-energy low-resolution film that is obtained with the treatment beam. Simulation films for fields shown in Figure 19-4A can be seen in Figure 19-4B and the Port films for those fields are shown in Figure 19-4C.

Fixed fields may be used when blocks are critical, but when they are not needed rotational fields may be used. In this method, the tumor is placed on the central axis of rotation of the machine. Radiation is delivered as the machine rotates around the patients in either a full circle or one or more limited arcs. Because the contour of the target and the patient change as the patient rotates, rotational techniques may not be feasible. An example of the dose distributions in a patient using four-fixed field is shown in Figure 19-5. In treating prostate cancer, the fixed fields treat a smaller volume of normal tissue but deliver a higher dose to that volume, while the rotational technique treats a substantially larger volume of tissue to a substantially lower dose.

One attempt to circumvent the inability to shape rotational fields is the development of multileaf collimation. This is a series of 80 to 120 lead "leaves," each mounted with individual motors so that a computer system can set each leaf's position quickly. With this technique, it is possible to approximate the shape of a customized block and using a "stop and shoot" method with a large number of fields to approximate a rotational treatment with blocks. Prototypes of these computer control systems are currently being tested, and the multileaf collimator is generally available. Because the collimator only approximates an individual customized block, the field edges may not be as sharp as the individual block. Whether the use of additional fields with a slightly fuzzier edge will lead to better results is currently being studied.

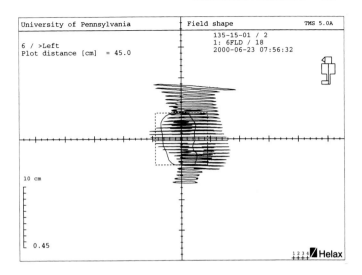

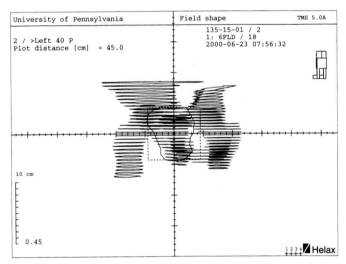

Figure 19-4 (*A*) CT reconstruction of two of the six fields (Left Lateral and Left Posterior Oblique) used to treat the prostate cancer. Shows wire rim outlines of pelvic bones (thin lines), treatment field edges (dashed lines), block edges (irregularly shaped solid lines), and Planning Target Volume (central darker lines). (*B*) Simulation films for fields shown in (A). Lateral and Posterior Oblique. (*C*) Port films for fields shown in (A). Taken with a 15MV beam. PTV is the Planning Target Volume (prostate and margin) defined by treatment planning CT scan.

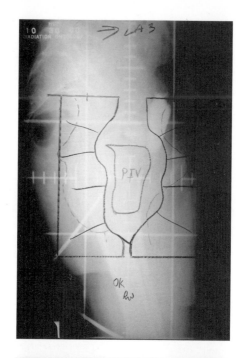

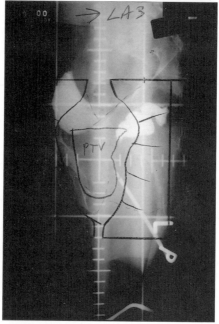

Figure 19-4 (*continued*)

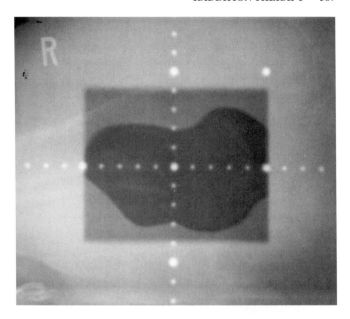

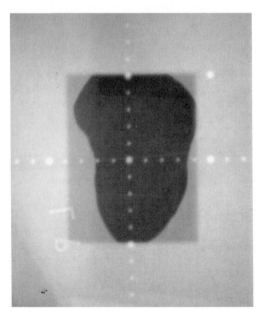

Figure 19-4 (*continued*)

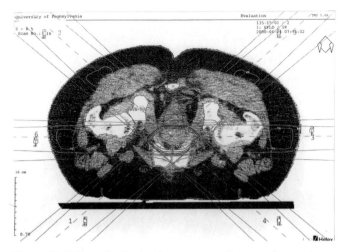

Figure 19-5 Dose distribution for treatment of prostate for a patient treated in the prone position with a six field technique.

An alternative method is to deliver the radiation from within the tumor using interstitial radiation. Permanent implants are usually used to treat the prostate. Figure 19-6A shows a reconstruction of the prostate obtained from a postimplant CT scan demonstrating the seeds within the prostate. Figure 19-6B shows the dose volume histogram for the bladder and the rectum for the implant. It is clear that the implant delivers lower doses to the periprostatic tissues, but substantially higher doses to the interior of the prostate. Although this may appear to be advantageous, it must be remembered that many tumors have some degree of extracapsular extension, and this would not be effectively treated with an implant. There is also an acquired facility with the implant procedure that allowed experienced users to deliver a more homogeneous dose to the prostate while minimizing the dose to adjacent structures. This skill increases with increased experience. Currently, only sophisticated CT and ultrasound planning equipment will allow preplanning of the implant and post-treatment evaluation of the dose distribution.

Other recent developments have improved the staging and treatment planning for prostate cancer. Magnetic resonance imaging has allowed the detection of clinically occult extracapsular extension and seminal vesicle extension. This has reduced the risk of local recurrence in clinical T2 tumors by filtering out the occult T3 tumors that are then sent for radiation and hormones. Similarly, the use of CT-based treatment planning allows

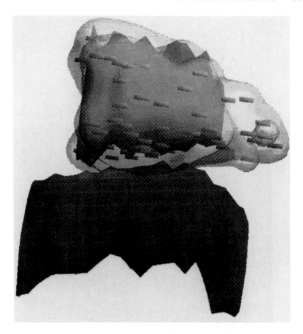

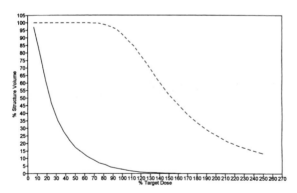

Figure 19-6 (*A*) CT reconstruction of Iodine-125 implant of the prostate showing seeds with the prostate surface (upper dark structure), the rectum (lower dark structure) and the 160 Gy isodose volume (lighter upper structure). Seeds are depicted as small cylinders. (*B*) Dose volume histogram demonstrating the much reduced dose to the rectum compared to the prostate.

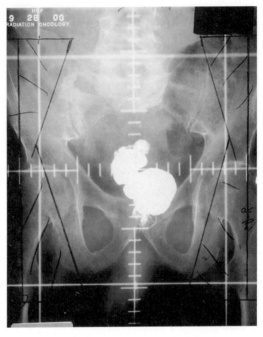

Figure 19-7 Typical field arrangement to treat pelvic lymph nodes in a patient with prostate cancer using opposed anterior and posterior fields (*A*) and opposed lateral fields (*B*).

the clinician to precisely determine the border of the prostate and to treat the necessary volume with tighter margins. Open table tops (the belly board), body casting, and other immobilization techniques allow better immobilization of the prostate and the more accurate treatment setup. This has allowed further tightening of the margins with better definition of the treatment volume, which reduces the dose to the bladder and rectum. More versatile machines and computer systems allow the clinician to use multiple fields in multiple planes to minimize the overlap of entrance and exit beams as they traverse the normal structures. Recently, some investigators have used daily ultrasound to check the location of the prostate. The end result of these modifications is that clinicians have been able to increase the dose delivered to bladder tumors from 50 to 60 Gy to 63 to 67 Gy, and for prostate cancer from 65 to 66 Gy to 77 to 85 Gy. It remains to be determined whether this increase in dose will translate into an improved long-term survival rate.

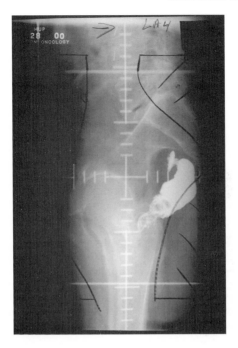

Figure 19-7 (*continued*)

IV. CLINICAL RADIATION ONCOLOGY

There is no role for radiation (alone or with chemotherapy) in the treatment of unresected renal cell carcinoma. The use of radiation in the treatment of patients following resection is somewhat controversial. Among patients with tumor transgressing the renal capsule, the risk of local recurrence is higher and radiation can reduce the risk of local recurrence. Rafla reviewed his experience and found an apparent benefit to the use of adjuvant radiation therapy for patients with involvement of the renal capsule (T3).[1] Among patients receiving adjuvant radiation, the 5-year survival was 57 percent compared to 28 percent for patients treated with surgery alone. It is presumed that the improved survival was related to the reduced incidence of local recurrence, although this could not be documented as these patients were treated in the pre-CT era. Subsequent trials reported by Finney[2] and Kjaer et al[3] found no benefit to treating these patients with adjuvant radiation. The results of the Finney trial are limited by the small number of patients and the 8 percent treatment-related mortality due to liver injury in the radiation arm. The results reported by Kjaer are clouded by the registration of node positive patients where Rafla demonstrated no benefit. This study also was complicated by the fact that 16 percent of the patients randomized to radiation did not receive radiation and those patients that were treated experienced a 44 percent incidence of major toxicity. Kao has reported that this toxicity can be avoided by using CT-based treatment planning.[4] Both Finney and Kjaer used anterior and posterior fields and the toxicity was in patients with right sided tumors where large parts of the liver were treated to 45 Gy, which is well past liver tolerance. Whether there is still benefit is also complicated by the fact that many tumors are found incidentally at the time of diagnostic CT scan for other reasons. It is not clear that these patients have the same prognosis after surgery as patients in these older studies who presented with hematuria, mass, or other more ominous findings.

Radiation can be used for metastatic renal cell carcinoma to palliate bleeding, pain, or neurologic symptoms related to spinal or central nervous system (CNS) involvement. The tumor has traditionally been thought to be radioresistant, and some experts have argued for surgical excision of limited metastatic disease. Onufrey[5] and Halpern[6] reviewed the experience in their institutions and reported that these tumors tended to respond more slowly than other tumors and that unlike other tumors, renal cell carcinomas did seem to respond to higher doses of radiation. They also noted that they achieved good palliation of symptoms in most cases. There are still cases that favor surgical excision as it removes the tumor focus immediately and allows the patient to begin rehabilitation more rapidly than following radiation.[7] The clinician must compare the relative risks and benefits of radiation against the functional deficits and more rapid rehabilitation after surgery in selecting the appropriate treatment for individual patients.

The one area of active radiation research is in the management of CNS metastases. Previous problems with control of the tumor frustrated both radiation oncologist and the neurosurgeon. It is difficult to deliver an adequate dose of radiation to the tumor to produce durable local control because of the toxicity to normal CNS tissues with high doses. Similarly, the neurosurgeon cannot get a margin around the tumor because the residual neurologic effects are related to the manipulation of the normal tissues at the margin of the tumor. Many tumors are not accessible to the neurosurgeon because of the deep location of some metastases. Patients also need whole brain radiation after resection because most patients with a clinically isolated metastasis will have other microscopically occult metastases. The most common site of recurrence of tumor following neurosurgical excision without radiation is the CNS.

Because of the problems managing brain metastases, many patients were managed with combined surgery and postoperative radiation. Recently, the development of stereotactic radiosurgery has allowed the delivery of a single large dose of radiation to a small volume encompassing the tumor without a margin. The purpose of this radiation is to produce areas of necrosis within the gross tumor. This is used for deep-seated lesions or tumor adjacent to critical structures. Whether this will lead to improved local control and improved quality of survival is being studied in prospective trials.

V. RENAL PELVIC AND URETERAL CARCINOMA

There is very limited data on the use of radiation to manage tumors in the renal pelvis and ureter. The rationale that supports the use of radiation is based on the anatomy of the retroperitoneum as it affects the surgical resection. Tumors of the renal pelvis and ureter are resected with wide proximal and distal margins. The resection includes the kidney and a generous bladder cuff because these tumors are frequently multifocal and can spread along the urothelium. The radial margin is more problematic and radiation may be indicated to sterilize any tumor in this region. The thin wall of the ureter is the only barrier to lateral spread of the tumor and the surgeon is limited in the ability to extend the dissection laterally. There are no additional barriers to tumor spread in the retroperitoneum. There have been no recent reports of the use of radiation in the post operative setting but an older report from Anderson[8] described 8 patients out of 58 patients that underwent nephro-ureterectomy for transitional cell carcinoma that were thought to have a high risk for local recurrence. The proximal and distal margins of resection were negative, but because of the thin wall of the ureter and the transmural extension of the tumor, there was concern that the radial margin may not have been adequate. These 8 patients received 40 to 60 Gy of radiation to the ureteral bed, which was delivered without major morbidity, although most of the patients did develop anorexia, nausea, and diarrhea. Four of the 8 patients died with tumor, but only one of these patients had a recurrence of tumor in the retroperitoneum. A similar logic can be applied to the renal pelvis, which would suggest that patients with transitional cell carcinomas lower in the pelvis or extending into perinephric fat may benefit from adjuvant radiation.

The fields that have been used in patients with renal pelvis tumors are the same as those used in the adjuvant radiation of renal cell carcinomas to encompass the renal bed and the renal hilar structures. Although there is no proven benefit to adjunctive radiation in patients with lymph node metastases, these nodes are frequently sampled in conjunction with the nephrectomy so there is concern about possible contamination of the medial structures. Most radiation oncologists will include the pre-aortic, para-aortic, and para-caval lymph nodes. Ureteral tumors are generally treated with fields that extend proximally and distally to encompass the preoperative tumor volume with a 5- to 7-cm margin. The medial and lateral margins are determined by the surgical resection and the gross lateral extent of the tumor although the prevertebral structures are generally not included. The decision regarding the use of radiation must be individualized. An assessment is made of the potential risks of recurrence and benefits of adjunctive radiation so that an appropriate recommendation can be reached.

VI. BLADDER CARCINOMA

The application of radiation in the management of transitional cell carcinoma of the bladder (TCCB) is very controversial. Radiation was initially used prior to cystectomy to increase the probability of successful cystectomy. The group at Memorial Sloan-Kettering Cancer Center (MSKCC) evolved a policy in the treatment of bladder carcinoma that showed possible benefit to radiation as well as the possibility of tumor control with radiation alone.[9,10] A substantial number of patients taken to cystectomy did not complete the procedure because of the presence of extravesicle extension or lymphadenopathy. This was especially true in patients with T3b and T4 tumors and patients with poorly differentiated carcinomas. They initially gave patients a dose of 40 Gy in 4 weeks with a 4-week break prior to resection and found that many patients had substantial regression of tumor with greater probability of complete resection and a reduction in the risk of pelvic recurrence. The surgical procedure was more difficult because of fibrosis, which limited the amount of ureter that could be used in the urinary reconstruction. They also found that many of these patients could have such dramatic responses that they could send these patients to further radiation to a total dose of 60 Gy with the chance for tumor control, although the 4-week break did reduce the efficacy of radiation compared to 60 Gy continuous radiation over 6 weeks.

They subsequently used a dose of 20 Gy in 1 week during the week prior to surgery and found that there was less fibrosis but the complication rate did not change because of the effects of radiation on the normal tissues, which impaired postoperative healing. Subsequent to the MSKCC report, Montie et al,[11] at the Cleveland Clinic, and Skinner and Lieskovsky[12] at the University of Southern California, reviewed their experience and found that survival and pelvic failure in the patients treated with surgery alone had the same survival and pelvic recurrence rates as patients treated with preoperative radiation. Montie did select a significant number of patients who were thought to be marginally resectable or thought to be at high risk for local recurrence to receive radiation and excluded them from the analysis. Many of the patients reported by Skinner received adjuvant chemotherapy, and it is not clear whether the results are due to the fact that there is no benefit from adjuvant radiation or whether a similar effect can be achieved with adjuvant chemotherapy. A large intergroup trial randomized patients to receive adjuvant chemotherapy versus no adjuvant therapy and the results of this trial are pending.

In a large meta-analysis, Parsons showed that there was an apparent survival benefit to preoperative radiation.[13] This analysis has been criticized because the trials that did not meet the criteria for inclusion generally supported the use of surgery alone, although most of them were not randomized or critical parameters were not reported. In the absence of a randomized trial, there is no role for radiation except in unusual circumstances. The reports of neo-adjuvant chemotherapy show a clear benefit to the use of chemotherapy in marginally resectable lesions by increasing the rate of resection, although there is no evidence to support or disprove an effect on survival. The response rates reported with methotrexate, vinblastine, cisplatin, $\pm$ doxirubicin (MCV or MVAC) approach 80 percent. More recent results suggest that taxol and carboplatin have similar efficacy and may have reduced toxicity.

In Europe and Canada, the initial focus for radiation was to deliver high-dose external beam radiation in an attempt to preserve the bladder and sterilize the tumor. A sampling of the reported experience for patients is shown in Figure 19-2.[14–17] These experiences show that the local control rates are only 35 to 45 percent in T2 tumors and even poorer for patients with T3-4 tumors. This compares to the survival rates in patients undergoing cystectomy, which are approximately 75 percent in T2 tumors and 50 to 65 percent for patients with T3 tumors. In an effort to improve these results, some centers have used radiation sensitizers or particles such as neutrons and π^- mesons.[18–21] There was some improvement in the rates of local control and survival, but at the expense of a 15 to 30 percent risk of major complication, which was usually due to small bowel or rectal injury or severe bladder contracture or bleeding. This morbidity precludes the general recommendation for these treatments.

Interstitial radiation has been used by a number of centers to treat bladder tumors and deliver a higher dose to a small portion of the bladder with relative sparing of the rectum and the rest of the bladder. Van der Werf-Messing treated patients with 3 fraction of 3.5 Gy to reduce the risk of intraoperative dissemination and then carried out a cystotomy to perform a radium needle implant under direct vision.[22] The sources were attached to suture material that was brought out through a stab wound adjacent to the incision. The sources were left in place to deliver a dose of 70 Gy in 7 to 8 days, following which they were removed through the stab wound. This reduced the risk of local recurrence in T1 or T2 tumors from 75 percent to 18 percent and reduced the need for cystectomy from 65 percent to 20 percent. A similar reduction was seen in the 10-year risk of metastatic tumor from 50 percent to 18 percent. For more extensive low-grade tumors, including larger T2 tumors and small T3 tumors, she would deliver a preimplant dose of 30 Gy in 3 weeks to the pelvis and then deliver 45 Gy with the implant. This treated any subclinical disease that may have extended beyond the high dose implant volume and also delivered a higher dose to the larger gross tumor.[25] The local control in this group was 92 percent with an actuarial disease free survival of 74 percent.

In the United States, there has been an interest in chemosensitized radiation in treating a number of tumors based on the theories advanced by Steele and Peckham.[26] Chemotherapy can reduce the tumor burden so that radiation can deal more effectively with the residual tumor. Similarly, there can be spatial cooperation allowing the radiation to deal effectively with the bladder tumor while the chemotherapy will treat subclinical metastatic tumor. The response rates to chemotherapy suggest that it may also be active in the adjuvant setting. The final mechanism that may enhance the effect of combined modality therapy is true chemosensitization. Soloway et al[27] evaluated the response of a bladder cell line in vitro and found that a dose of chemotherapy that produced a 1 log cell kill and in vitro without a growth delay in nude mice could be given in conjunction with a dose of radiation that would produce a 3 log cell kill and a 5-week growth delay. The result was a 4 to 5 log cell kill with a 9-week growth delay suggesting a three- to seven-fold enhancement of the individual effects due to a synergistic interaction between the radiation and cisplatin.

The National Bladder Cancer Cooperative Group (NBCCG) in the United States[28] and the group in Innsbruck, Austria[29] sponsored trials delivering cisplatin on days 1, 22, and 43 of radiation following TURBT, with reevaluation after 40 Gy had been delivered. Patients with less than visual complete responses after 40 Gy were sent to cystectomy as there is very small chance of achieving a complete response with an additional 20 to 25 Gy. Among patients with complete responses or only positive cytology, the 2-year relapse-free survival rates were 68 percent and 53 percent in the Innsbruck and NBCCG, respectively. In an effort to improve the results with conservative surgery and chemosensitized radiation, the NBCCG and RTOG began a joint trial delivering 2 cycles of MVC prior to radiation-cisplatin therapy. The 4-year survival rate with bladder conservation was 44 percent and the overall survival rate was 62 percent.[30] A subsequent trial randomized patients to neoadjuvant chemotherapy prior to chemosensitized radiation versus immediate chemosensitized radiation. This study showed no benefit to the neoadjuvant therapy.[31]

The current role for neoadjuvant chemotherapy is restricted to patients who decline cystectomy unless they have no other curative option. In this setting, a trial of chemotherapy may allow the identification of patients with chemoradiation sensitive disease that may be controlled with radiation-cisplatin. Patients with clearly unresectable tumors should proceed directly to radiation-cisplatin. The availability of continent diversions has sharply reduced the utility of bladder conservation because continent diversion has been shown to preserve normal voiding function in men with the chance of preserving potency. Women, and some men, will intermittently catheterize an internal reservoir, which is much easier than maintaining an external appliance. This must be balanced against the risks of radiation including the risk of rectal ulcer (7 percent), bladder contracture (10 percent), impotence in men (more than 50 percent), and bowel injury (3 percent). In centers with the availability of continent diversions, chemosensitized radiation is generally reserved for patients with unresectable tumors or patients unable or unwilling to undergo cystectomy.

VII. PROSTATE CANCER

As controversial as the treatment decisions may appear in patients with bladder cancer, the disagreements surrounding the management of prostate cancer are that much greater. With the advent of prostate specific antigen (PSA) screening the incidence of prostate cancer has skyrocketed from 120,000 new cases annually to more than 270,000 new cases. Many of these tumors are probably not clinically significant as there is a high prevalence of occult prostate cancer found incidentally in autopsy series. It is difficult to distinguish the men with incidental tumors from those with clinically significant tumors. It has also been noted that the annual number of deaths from prostate cancer in the United States has fallen from 44,000 to 36,000 in the last 6 years.

The critical elements in evaluating a man with prostate cancer require that the clinician estimate the annual risk of tumor dissemination and tumor-related mortality as well as the annual nonprostate cancer-related mortality for the individual. Census reports suggest that a 70-year-old male has an average life expectancy of 13 years for whites and 9.5 years for African Americans. At age 75, the median survival rates fall to 9.2 and 7.0 years, respectively. This estimate must be adjusted downward for comorbid conditions such as diabetes, atherosclerotic disease, renal insufficiency, and chronic lung disease, and adjusted upward for men who are in good health with no comorbid conditions. In completing an ad hoc risk–benefit analysis, it is also necessary to factor into the equation any conditions that may increase the risk of radiation-related morbidity including prior abdominal surgeries, any history of peritonitis or pelvic inflammatory conditions including Crohn's disease or ulcerative colitis, or a history of diverticulitis. Less ominous risk factors include renal insufficiency, diabetes, hypertension, and increasing age.

It is necessary to have the proper equipment to deliver radiation for prostate cancer. The Patterns of Care studies were inaugurated in 1976 to identify treatment factors that are associated with better outcomes in radiation oncology. One of the first sites studied was prostate cancer and the factors associated with better control and/or less morbidity are: (1) treatment simulation; (2) customized blocking to shape fields; (3) computerized treatment planning; (4) treatment with machines with beam energies at or higher than 10 million volts (MV); and (5) a dose of or more than 66 Gy for T2 tumors and 70 Gy for T3 tumors to a point 4 cm lateral to the center of the prostate.[32]

Recent developments suggest that newer methods that further improve the results in managing prostate cancer include CT-based treatment planning, three-dimensional conformal radiation therapy (3-DCRT), and escalation of the dose to the prostate past 70 Gy. CT-treatment planning is available in most institutions and has allowed the clinician to treat larger fields with less morbidity. Previously, the clinician used his or her best clinical judgment to set the field location and size based on the diagnostic CT scan as well as bladder and rectal contrast placed at the time of simulation. The volumes from a diagnostic CT cannot be translated directly to a plain film because the CT is done on a curved table top and the patient is treated on a flat table top, so there is some distortion in the anatomy between the two images. There is also the potential for errors in translation that require the clinician to use wider margins to be confident that the tumor is adequately covered.

CT-based treatment planning uses a CT scan directed by the radiation oncologist to define the pelvic anatomy with techniques that are better adapted for translation to a plain film. The diagnostic study is done to maximize the resolution of structures to identify any abnormality, discern the nature of the process and to determine its extent; whereas the treatment planning study is done to define the location of the organs in the region of the tumor. It is possible on the CT scan to outline the prostate, the bladder, and the rectum, as well as the bony structures to locate in three dimensions the edges of each of the organs (see Fig. 4A). This information can then be translated onto a beam's eye view projection of the treatment field, which shows the bony structures, the bladder, and rectum. Bladder and rectal contrast are used in this technique to register the beam's eye view projection onto the simulator film using many different reference points. From the beam's eye view projection, it is possible to draw blocks that will shield areas not at risk for cancer from the radiation. This is done because machines only produce rectangular treatment fields and it is necessary to customize the shape of the field to the shape of the irregularly shaped target.

The plan that is produced is still a two-dimensional plan of a cross-section through the center of the tumor along the common axis of all the beams. This is useful for simple plans, but just as the isodose lines will be more round shaped at the edges of the field, it is most pronounced at the corners of the treatment volume. This can result in a point being technically in the field, but not receiving the full dose. To determine the extent of this inhomogeneity, it is necessary to look at a three-dimensional plan. 3-DCRT can render dose distributions in any plane, and also will produce a dose volume histogram that will visually demonstrate how much of the target is receiving in excess of any specified dose. Sample histograms for a patient with early stage low-grade prostate cancer are shown in Figure 19-3. Figure 19-3A shows that when a dose of 76 Gy is delivered to the point where the beams cross, the target volume receives a minimum dose of 73.1 Gy. The second graph (Fig. 19-3B) shows a similar histogram for the rectum where the maximum dose is 72.6 Gy and the minimum dose is 1.6 Gy. It also shows that only 10 percent of the rectum receives more than 53.2 Gy. A second advantage of 3-DCRT is that it will allow the use of multiple beams that are not coplanar and still calculate the dose throughout the entire target. It is possible to use a tetrahedral or pyramidal field arrangement to minimize the overlap of entrance and exit beams outside of the target volume.

The use of these precise prostate localization techniques allow for the use of tighter margins with adequate coverage of the tumor. This maximum tolerated dose of radiation to the prostate is being defined. Many centers currently use doses of 74 to 81 Gy and others, such as Memorial Sloan Kettering and the University of Michigan, are exploring doses of 84 to 91 Gy. In order to further improve the precision of treatment, these centers and many others will use individualized immobilization devices, such as body casts, as well as specialized techniques to reduce organ motion.

In comparing the results from different series it is necessary to compare the definitions of tumor control and treatment related morbidity. There is no generally accepted definition of biochemical control after radiation as there is after surgery. Following the surgery, the generally accepted definition of biochemical cure is an undetectable PSA. Following radiation there is still residual normal prostate epithelium that will produce PSA. Some investigators have argued that the PSA should be less than 0.5 or 1.0 or 1.5 ng/mL. Others argue that it only needs to be stable and not rise during the follow-up period. The problem with these definitions is that experts who use higher doses of radiation will report that follow-up PSAs are lower. It is not clear whether this reflects a better tumor control, or perhaps just more fibrosis of the normal residual prostate. Similarly, many studies have use concurrent hormones and radiation. Hormones cause the normal prostate to involute, and when hormones are withdrawn, and prostate function may return to normal, the PSA will rise to its baseline level. If the clinician is too sensitive to the results of the serum PSA determination, the risk of recurrence may be overestimated.

Similarly, individuals who have had radiation can develop painless rectal bleeding. When they undergo proctoscopy they are found to have some mucosal atrophy and telangiectasias. Many physicians would score this as a minimal or grade I toxicity. Others would score it as a grade II toxicity because they may have a lower threshold to recommend symptomatic treatment. Some studies have also considered rectal hemorrhage requiring transfusion or laser ablation of the anterior rectal wall as grade II toxicity. Others consider it grade IV (life-threatening) toxicity. Similarly, men who advise their physicians they are able to obtain partial erections may be considered by some physicians to be potent, although they are not able to complete vaginal intromission. Others require that men be able to sustain an erection and reach orgasm.

A controversy in the treatment of prostate cancer is the definition of the target volume. Many centers will deliver a dose of 45 Gy to the obturator, hypogastric, external iliac, and common iliac lymph nodes and boost the prostate to the final total dose. Others will treat the prostate only and this volume may or may not include the seminal vesicles. One of the major contradictions in the literature arises out of retrospective reviews of several hundred men at both Stanford[33] and the Cross Clinic in Alberta.[34] Both centers had an experience that had evolved over the years, initially treating the lymph nodes as well as the prostate and subsequently, only the prostate. Each found that the risk of distant metastases was higher in patients treated to only the prostate when compared to patients who received prophylactic pelvic radiation. The Radiation Therapy Oncology Group (RTOG) carried out a subsequent randomized trial that sampled lymph nodes in men with prostate cancer. Men with negative lymph nodes were randomized to either prostate radiation alone or to prophylactic pelvic radiation plus prostate radiation. There was no difference in the survival of these men following surgical lymph node staging.[35]

In a contemporaneous series of men with involved lymph nodes, Sause[36] and the group at Memorial Sloan Kettering Cancer Center (MSKCC) found that the clinical disease-free survival curves in node positive patients continued to deteriorate for more than 15 years and that there was no evidence of cure. In a review of RTOG studies of men with involved lymph nodes from prostate cancer, only 2 of 90 men were biochemically without evidence of progression at 10 years. The 10-year overall survival rate was 29 percent and the clinical without evidence

Table 19-2 Effect of Treating Lymph Nodes in Patients with Prostate Cancer

INSTITUTION	PATIENT NUMBER	TREATMENT VOLUME	NODAL[e] STATUS	10-YEAR RELAPSE-FREE SURVIVAL (%)
Stanford	51	Prostate	−	95
Stanford	NS[a]	Pelvis + prostate	?	73
Stanford	NS	Prostate	?	50
Stanford	61	Pelvis + prostate	+	18
Cross Clinic[b]	70	Prostate	?	63[c]
Cross Clinic[b]	126	Pelvis + prostate	?	30[c]
MSKCC	84	Prostate	−	92[d]
MSKCC	124	Prostate + PLND[e]	+	46[d]

[a]Not specified.
[b]Stags B2 and C Only.
[c]8-year data.
[d]5-year data.
[e]Pelvic lymph node dissection.
+, positive; −, negative; ?, node dissection not done.

of disease (NED) survival rate was 7 percent[37] (Table 19-3). It appears contradictory but true that men with negative lymph nodes do not benefit from prophylactic nodal irradiation, while men with positive nodes cannot be cured. Yet, when the nodal status is unknown there is a benefit to prophylactic lymph node irradiation. The explanation may lie in the fact that all of the studies were conducted before the general availability of CT scanning. It is possible that the fields used for prostate radiation may not have treated the superior–lateral prostate gland, which was included in the pelvic lymph node field.

A sample of the treatment portals used to treat the pelvic lymph nodes are shown in Figure 19-7 and a typical field to treat only the prostate gland is shown in Figure 19-4A. The large field is designed to include the common, external, and internal iliac lymph nodes as well as the obturator and presacral nodes because these are the most common sites of lymph node metastases. It also includes the entire prostate and the proximal pendulous urethra. To include these structures and nodes, the field extends from the middle of L5 to the bottom of the ischial tuberosity and laterally goes at least 1 cm lateral to the pelvic brim. On the lateral fields, the fields extend 1cm anterior to the symphysis and to at least the S3–S4 interspace.

The prostate field is designed to encompass the prostate as defined by treatment planning CT scan. The CT-rendered images are registered to the simulation film using the bladder, rectum, and boney structures as landmarks. A urethrogram is performed at the time of treatment planning CT scan to identify the proximal prostatic urethra. Some clinicians will include the seminal vesicles in the treatment volume; others will not. Still others will include them in selected patients. The concern in this area is related to the fact that seminal vesicle involvement occurs in 20 to 30 percent of men with stage T2 prostate cancer and in approximately 50 percent to 70 percent of men with T3-4 prostate cancer. If this portion of the tumor is not treated then the tumor cannot be cured, but when the seminal vesicles are included the amount of rectum in the treatment field will sharply increase. Roach has developed an algorithm that allows the clinician to predict the risk of nodal involvement based on the Gleason score and the PSA,[38] and D'Amico has demonstrated that MRI with an endorectal coil is extremely sensitive in detecting actual involvement.[39]

Although node positive prostate cancer has become less frequent in this era of community screening, there is still controversy over the treatment of node positive disease. Because these patients have such a high rate of distant metastases, many oncologists do not recommend local therapy. A review of the results in patients with conservatively treated prostate cancer shows that there is a significant risk of bladder outlet obstruction, bladder invasion, hemorrhage, and pain, which may be

Table 19-3

INSTITUTION	PTS.	TREATMENT	NODAL STATUS	FOLLOW-UP (YEARS)	CLINICAL RFS
Stanford	NS[a]	Pelvis + prostate	?	10	73
Stanford	NS	Prostate only	?	10	50
Stanford	61	Pelvis + prostate	+	10	95
Stanford	51	Prostate only	−	10	18
Cross Clinic	126	Pelvis + prostate	?	8	63
Cross Clinic	70	Prostate only	?	8	63
RTOG	104	Pelvis + prostate or prostate only	−	10	67[b]
RTOG	90	Pelvis + prostate	+	10	2

[a]Not specified.
[b]Reported "no difference" between the two arms, but specific figures not reported.

prevented with radiation. A second consideration is that radiation may offer the opportunity to "debulk" the tumor to leave a smaller tumor burden to be treated by the hormones.

There is a spectrum of androgen sensitivity in prostate tumors at diagnosis, and hormonal therapy will select the androgen independent population to proliferate while the more androgen dependent population involutes entering an extended G_0 state or undergoes apoptosis. In men with locally advanced nonmetastatic prostate cancer treated with deferred therapy and androgen ablation at the time of symptomatic progression, the median time to develop hormone resistant tumor was 48 months. Men treated with immediate androgen ablation did not develop hormone independent tumor until a median of 84 months after diagnosis.[40] The most common sites of progression when androgen resistance develops is at sites of previous disease. We developed a policy of treating these men with concurrent hormones and radiation to address both the pelvic tumor and occult distant metastatic disease. In a series of 80 patients with a median follow-up of 5 years, the 12-year cancer specific survival rate was 90 percent and the biochemical relapse-free survival rate was 57 percent.[39]

For men with earlier stage prostate cancer there are three accepted treatments from which they can choose; radical prostatectomy, external beam radiation, and interstitial therapy. In reviewing large series of men, most physicians divide patients into three groups. The group with a low risk of recurrence within 5 years consists of men with PSA less than or equal to 10.0 ng/mL and a Gleason score less than or equal to 6. The intermediate-risk group has PSAs between 10.0 and 20.0 ng/mL, or a Gleason score of 7. The high-risk group has a PSA greater than or equal to 20.0, or a Gleason score greater than or equal to eight. In one analysis comparing these three treatments in the three risk groups, D'Amico found no difference in the relative risk of recurrence between the treatments in the low-risk population.[41] Among intermediate- and high-risk patients, there was a threefold higher risk of recurrence among men undergoing interstitial therapy when compared to external beam or surgery, although the difference disappeared in the intermediate-risk group when men were treated with 6 months of androgen ablation therapy in addition to the implant. Among men with high-risk cancers the risk of recurrence was greater than 65 percent in all of the treatment groups, but the recurrences occurred earlier after interstitial therapy than with surgery or external radiation. The inference from these results is that new treatment approaches are needed, possibly combining current therapies with androgen ablation or introducing new therapies such as cytotoxic chemotherapy, higher radiation doses, or more extensive surgery.

A number of centers have reported that men in the intermediate-risk group appear to have a longer biochemical disease-free survival with higher doses of radiation, but the follow-up thus far is less than 5 years in these series and further follow-up is necessary to determine whether the difference will translate into a longer overall survival and whether the morbidity is acceptable. Hanks initially reported in a retrospective review that the bNED survival was better with doses greater than 76 Gy than with doses less than 70 Gy.[42] A preliminary report of a randomized trial of 70 Gy versus 78 Gy is being carried out at M.D. Anderson showing that the bNED survival is 47 percent with 70 Gy and 68 percent with 78 Gy, although the median follow-up is only 30 months.[43]

The use of combined hormonal and radiation therapy has been prospectively studied in four studies. The earliest study from M.D. Anderson demonstrated comparable 10-year survival rates among men with T3 tumors treated with radiation including the pelvic lymph nodes with or without lifelong adjuvant diethylstilbesterol (DES) 5 mg/day.[44] In reviewing these results it was found that there was an excess of cardiovascular deaths in the hormone group and an excess of cancer related deaths in the control group. Two subsequent RTOG[45,46] trials randomized men to radiation with or without hormone therapy and found that the hormones prolonged disease-free survival, although they have yet to show a benefit in overall survival. One study treated men with 4 months of androgen deprivation therapy using an LHRH agonist delivering 2 months of therapy before starting radiation and completing treatment with the end of radiation. The second study began radiation concurrently with the LHRH agonist and continued the therapy indefinitely. The median duration of hormone therapy in this group was 24 months. In a recent analysis of the results of these two trials there appeared to be a small advantage favoring the longer course of therapy, although the results are not conclusive since there were slight differences in the eligibility for the two studies. Most of the patients on both studies had T3 N0 tumors, but patients with involved lymph nodes, positive margins following radical prostatectomy, and high-grade tumors were eligible for the study with indefinite hormones. There is currently a randomized trial being conducted by the RTOG to compare these two regimens.

A study was reported by Bolla,[47] who reported a European randomized trial comparing radiation and 3 years of hormonal therapy to radiation alone. His report is the only one thus far to find a clear survival benefit with a 5-year overall survival of 79 percent in the patients receiving radiation and hormones versus 62 percent in men treated with hormones alone. Most of these men had T3 N0 disease based on CT scan, lymphangiogram, or node sampling, although approximately 10 percent of the patients on each arm had T3 WHO Gr. 3 tumors. One concern here is that men treated with radiation alone ended treatment within 2 months after registration, whereas the hormone group had

3 years of treatment after registration, so the follow-up after treatment is significantly shorter in the latter group. There is also the problem that many men will develop permanent hypogonadism after prolonged androgen deprivation although the exact incidence of testicular failure is not known.

There are still challenges remaining in managing a man with prostate cancer. The first is to assess each man as an individual and specifically address the potential of each treatment to render the patient free of tumor and simultaneously to weigh the effects of treatment on quality of life including the effect of and on associated conditions, such as bladder outlet obstruction and bladder and rectal dysfunction, and the effect of comorbid conditions such as diabetes, vascular disease, and intra-abdominal processes. The second is to develop a treatment plan within the abilities of the institution which should include, but is not limited to, CT-based treatment planning and simulation, customized treatment planning and blocks, and development of a treatment plan that allows the delivery of an adequate dose to control the tumor. In high-risk patients with extracapsular disease, PSAs greater than 20.0 ng/mL, Gleason scores higher than or equal to 8, or metastatic lymphadenopathy, consideration should be given to adjuvant hormones with or without higher doses of radiation.

VIII. TESTICULAR CANCER

The role of radiation in managing testicular tumors is limited to the management of seminoma. There are data showing efficacy for radiation in clinical stage I nonseminomatous germ cell tumors, but the necessary dose and the associated toxicity suggest that these patients are better treated with more extensive staging and close observation or chemotherapy if indicated. Radiation is a standard treatment for seminoma because of the unique sensitivity of these germ cell tumors to radiation. Almost all cells need to divide to express the lethal effects of radiation, seminoma cells undergo an intermitotic death because of their inability to accumulate and repair sublethal damage. Because of this characteristic, there is no shoulder on the cell survival curve.

Staging of seminomas requires chest roentgenography, serum α-fetoprotein and β-human chorionic gonadotropin, and abdominal CT scan or lymphangiography. In men who have not completed their family, a semen analysis is in order as 10 percent of newly diagnosed seminoma patients are infertile and an estimate of fertility is needed to counsel a patient concerning the effects of treatment on fertility. The use of chest CT is limited to patients with disease beyond the testicle because the incidence of distant metastases in patients with stage I disease is small, as evidenced by the less than 5 percent relapse rate among patients treated with adjuvant radiation.

The treatment of seminoma has evolved over the last 10 years with the findings that patients followed without adjuvant therapy in reports by Duchesne[48] and Thomas[49] that the risk of recurrence is less than 20 percent. For men willing to undergo close follow-up with CT scanning and chest x-ray every 3 months for 2 years, observation may be an option with the understanding that they may need higher doses of salvage radiation or chemotherapy if they relapse. Younger men are the largest group with this tumor and preservation of fertility is an issue. Many steps are taken to minimize the scattered radiation to the opposite testicle, but many men elect to avoid radiation entirely. In an effort to further reduce the dose to the testicle, Fossa[50] has reported the results of a randomized trial with treatment to the para-aortic nodes and renal hilum versus the same field as well as the common and external iliac nodes as well. Most of the scattered dose to the testicle comes from the pelvic portion of the field. Eliminating this part of the field substantially reduces the dose to the testicle and the risks of treatment-related infertility. Doses between 24 and 30 Gy are used to treat these tumors as that will reduce the risk of retroperitoneal recurrence by more than from 15 percent to less than 1 percent in both groups, whereas the incidence of azospermia was reduced from 30 percent in the group treated to the iliac region to 11 percent in the group treated to the para-aortic nodes only. The 11 percent figure is identical to the risk of primary infertility with no adjuvant therapy in men with a history of seminoma.

Stage II tumors are a heterogeneous group including patients with retroperitoneal nodes between 1 and 20 cm. Patients with nodes smaller than 5 cm are generally treated with radiation portals similar to those used to treat a stage I tumor, although the field will generally include the external and common iliac nodes as well. After a dose of 25 to 30 Gy is delivered, the initially involved nodes are boosted to a dose of 35 to 40 Gy. Relapse-free survival rates are about 90 percent.[51] Some experts argue that this can be further reduced by prophylactic radiation to the mediastinum, although this is a matter of institutional policy and has not been studied in a prospective trial. In general, most centers in the United States will treat the mediastinum to a dose of 25 Gy.

Stage II tumors with lymph nodes larger than 5 cm are rare and more controversial. In the United states, these tumors may be treated with combination chemotherapy, whereas in Canada and Europe many of these patients are treated with radiation. The difficulty in carrying out primary radiation in patients with bulky adenopathy is that the lateral extent of the retroperitoneal lymph node mass is difficult to define without a treatment planning CT scan and CT-based treatment planning. In spite of this limitation, the rate of control of infra-diaphragmatic tumor is high and long-term disease-free survivals are between 50 and 60 percent. The most common site of recurrence is in the mediastinum, so many institutions recommend prophylactic mediastinal radiation. In a review of the major series that provide mediastinal radiation it was found that the 5-year relapse-free survival rate was 76 percent.[52–57] This is not significantly different from the disease-free survival rates reported with chemotherapy.[58] A sample of the reported results with chemotherapy and radiation is listed in Table 19-4.

In making the decision, the choices must be balanced based on acute and long-term toxicity. Abdominal radiation to a dose of 40 Gy will cause some scarring, increasing the risk of peptic ulcer and complicating any future surgery that might be necessary in these relatively young patients. Prophylactic mediastinal radiation will substantially increase the cure rate but would complicate the delivery of any salvage chemotherapy that might be necessary. This must be balanced against the effect of chemotherapy including the pulmonary effects of bleomycin and the higher risk of infertility associated with chemotherapy. There are also reports of an increased risk of Reynaud's phenomena and a possible increased risk of cerebrovascular disease in men treated with cisplatin, vinblastine, and bleomycin, and it remains to be determined whether either of these phenomena are associated with ciplatin, etoposide, and bleomycin. It would appear that neither treatment offers a survival or disease-free survival benefit and therefore treatment should be individualized. There is little modern experience with radiation for stage III and IV seminoma, and the results that are available suggest that these patients are better treated with chemotherapy.

IX. PENILE CANCER

Squamous cell carcinoma of the penis is rare in the United States and is more prevalent in other countries. Most patients are treated with initial surgery, but some patients are not candidates for surgery or refuse surgery. Superficial lesions can be treated with either external radiation or interstitial radiation using radium needles or iridium seeds in catheters. It is frequently necessary to treat the superficial inguinal nodes because 50 percent of men will have palpable adenopathy and the risk of occult involvement of nodes is high in men with poorly differentiated tumors or tumors of the glans. If a patient is treated with external radiation they may most easily be treated with an en face electron beam to treat the penis and the lymph nodes (which can lie at a depth of 5 cm below the skin) within one field. In this situation, a lucite block is placed behind the penis to spare the scrotum. A dose of 45 to 50 Gy is sufficient to treat clinically uninvolved skin and lymph nodes, but the primary tumor needs to be treated to a dose of 65 to 70 Gy. The morbidity of this procedure is the occurrence

Table 19-4

INSTITUTION	NUMBER OF PATIENTS	MEDIASTINAL RADIATION	MEDIASTINAL RECURRENCE (%)	CHEMO SALVAGE	(%)	SURVIVAL (YEARS)
Princess Margaret	16	No	50	87%	94	10
Vancouver	15	No	20	3/3	93	5
Patients without mediastinal radiation	61		36		70	5
Vancouver	8	Yes	0		87	5
Cross Clinic	14	Yes	0		54	5
Royal Marsden	34	Yes	3	Unknown	70	10
Mayo Clinic	16	Yes	0		100	5
M.D. Anderson	11	Yes	0		64	10
University Southern California	17	Yes	0		94	5
All Patients with mediastinal radiation	100		0		83	5
Chemotherapy	14		1		70	10
					100	5

of moist desquamation of the penis and scrotum with accompanying edema that will last for 8 to 12 weeks after radiation. After node dissection, the frequency and severity of edema will increase. For small low-grade tumors (2 cm or smaller) of the shaft of the penis, the risk of nodal involvement is low and these patients may be treated with interstitial radiation.

Most of the series of definitive radiation are small but as a group they suggest that radiation is effective in controlling the tumor, but the morbidity is substantial. Haile and Delclos[59] reported that 8 patients were treated with external radiation and 7 of 8 were controlled, but one patient required surgical amputation due to necrosis, whereas 11 of 12 patients treated with brachytherapy were controlled, with one patient requiring amputation for necrosis. In older series, Knudsen and Brennhovd[60] and Lederman[61] described a lower control rate (38 and 30 percent respectively), and 6 percent of the patients required amputation of the penis for necrosis. Duncan and Jackson[62] reported the experience of the Holt Radium Institute initially with brachytherapy and subsequently with external beam radiation. They found that the control rates improved from 46 percent to 90 percent as they emphasized external radiation because of the ability to treat larger volumes with a more homogeneous dose and adequately cover the tumor. At the same time, these clinicians found that the risk of urethral stricture or penile necrosis rose from 4 to 10 percent. Although radiation can be used to treat this disease, there is significant morbidity and the treatment requires adequate equipment and a commitment on the part of the patient and physician to persist in treatment in the face of the acute reactions. It remains to be determined whether radiation and chemotherapy may be combined to reduce the risk of distant metastases and to allow lower doses of radiation to be used to minimize the morbidity.

X. SUMMARY

There is extensive experience with radiation in the treatment of genitourinary tumors that demonstrates that it is an effective adjuvant treatment for selected patients with renal cell carcinoma, stage I seminoma, and selected patients with biochemical recurrences after radical prostatectomy. External and interstitial radiation, possibly with hormones, may be an effective alternative to radical prostatectomy or to penectomy or emasculation procedures. Radiation with chemotherapy may be an alternative to radical cystectomy in patients with comorbid medical conditions or extensive nonmetastatic tumors.

Treatment decisions must be individualized based on the clinical findings and the experience and capabilities of the center providing treatment. Although the incidence of incontinence following radical prostatectomy may vary from 1 to 30 percent, the incidence of both local and proctitis following radiation can vary from 3 to 20 percent following radiation. In facilities with state of the art equipment and physicians with specialized skills, there may be little to recommend one treatment over another. In other facilities, one department may have special abilities that would suggest that there may be a treatment preference based on the institutional experience.

It is likewise necessary to consider the working relationship between the departments of urology and radiation oncology within the institution. Even though chemosensitized radiation may be equivalent to radical cystectomy, it may not be desirable to pursue a course of bladder conservation if the urologist does not feel that a salvage cystectomy is possible after radiation.

Because there may be alternatives that are similarly effective, it is important to avoid confusing patients with conflicting claims of superior results. Patients can be presented with alternative treatments and select the treatment that will produce the results that are most desirable with morbidity risks they find most acceptable. The current directions of radiation research include exploring combinations of hormones and radiation and higher doses of radiation in the management of prostate cancer. Radiation oncologists are also looking at new radiation and chemotherapy schedules in bladder carcinoma to improve the chances for organ preservation.

BIBLIOGRAPHY

1. Rafla S: Renal cell carcinoma: Natural history and results of treatment. *Cancer* 24:26–40, 1970.
2. Finney R: An evaluation of postoperative radiotherapy in hypernephroma treatment: A clinical trial. *Cancer* 32:1332–1340, 1973.
3. Kjaer M, Frederiksen PL, Engelholm SA: Postoperative radiotherapy in stage II and III renal adenocarcinoma. A randomized trial by the Copenhagen Renal Cancer Study Group. *Int J Radiat Oncol Biol Phys* 13:665–672, 1987.
4. Kao GD, Malkowicz SB, Whittington R, D'Amico A, Wein AJ: Locally advanced renal cell carcinoma: Low complication rate and efficacy with post-nephrectomy irradiation during the computed tomography (CT) - era. *Radiology* 193:725–730, 1994.
5. Onufrey V, Mohiuddin M: Radiation therapy in the treatment of metastatic renal cell carcinoma. *Int J Radiat Oncol Biol Phys* 11:2007–2009, 1985.
6. Halperin EC, Harisiadis L: The role of radiation therapy in the management of metastatic renal cell carcinoma. *Cancer* 51:614–617, 1983.
7. Middleton RG: Surgery for metastatic renal cell carcinoma. *J Urol* 97:973–977, 1967.
8. Babaian RJ, Johnson DE, Chan RC: Combination nephroureterectomy and postoperative radiotherapy for infiltrative ureteral carcinoma. *Int J Radiat Oncol Biol Phys* 6:1229–1232, 1980.

9. Whitmore WF, Grabstald H, Mackenzie AR, Iswariah J, Phillips R: Preoperative irradiation with cystectomy in the management of bladder cancer. *Am J Roentgenol* 102:570–576, 1968.

10. Batata MA, Chu FCH, Hilaris BS, et al: Preoperative whole pelvis versus true pelvis irradiation and/or cystectomy for bladder cancer. *Int J Radiat Oncol Biol Phys* 7:1349–1355, 1981.

11. Montie JE, Straffon RA, Stewart BH: Radical cystectomy without radiation therapy for carcinoma of the bladder. *J Urol* 131:477–482, 1984.

12. Skinner DG, Lieskovsky G: Contemporary cystectomy with pelvic node dissection compared to preoperative radiation therapy plus cystectomy in management of invasive bladder cancer. *J Urol* 131:1069–1072, 1984.

13. Parson JT, Million RR: Planned preoperative irradiation in the management of clinical stage B2-C (T3) bladder carcinoma. *Int J Radiat Oncol Biol Phys* 14:787–810, 1986.

14. Goffinet DR, Schneider MJ, Glatstein EJ, et al: Bladder cancer: Results of radiation therapy in 384 patients. *Radiology* 117:149–153, 1975.

15. Duncan W, Quilty PM: The results of a series of 963 patients with transitional cell carcinoma of the urinary bladder primarily treated by radical megavoltage x-ray therapy. *Radiother Oncol* 7:299–310, 1985.

16. Yu WS, Sagerman RH, Chung CT, Dalal PS, King GA: Bladder carcinoma experience with radical and preoperative radiotherapy in 421 patients. *Cancer* 56:1299, 1985.

17. Goodman GB, Hislop TG, Elwood JM, Balfour J: Conservation of bladder function in patients with invasive bladder cancer treated by definitive irradiation and selective cystectomy. *Int J Radiat Oncol Biol Phys* 7:569–573, 1981.

18. Battermann JJ: Results of d + T fast neutron irradiation on advanced tumors of bladder and rectum. *Int J Radiat Oncol Biol Phys* 8:2159–2164, 1982.

19. Laramore GE, Davis RB, Hussey DH, et al: Radiation Therapy Oncology Group phase I–II study on fast neutron teletherapy for carcinoma of the bladder. *Cancer* 54:432–439, 1984.

20. Abratt RP, Barnes DR, Hammond JA, Sarembok LA, Tucker RD, Williams, AM: Radical irradiation and misonidazole for T2 grade III and T3 bladder cancer: 2 year follow-up. *Int J Radiat Oncol Biol Phys* 10:1719–1720, 1984.

21. Studder UE, Von Essen CF, Enderli JB, Bodendorfer G, Zingg EJ: Preliminary results of a phase I/II study with pi-messon (pion) treatment for bladder cancer. *Cancer* 56:1943–1952, 1985.

22. Van der Werf-Messing B, Hop WCJ: Carcinoma of the urinary bladder (category T1 Nx Mo) treated either by radium implant or by transurethral resection only. *Int J Radiat Oncol Biol Phys* 7:299–303, 1981.

23. Mazeron JJ, Marinello G, Leung S, et al: Treatment of bladder tumors by iridium 192 implantation: The Créteil technique. *Radiother Oncol* 4:111–119, 1985.

24. Strauss KL, Littman P, Wein AJ, Whittington R, Tomaszewski JE: Treatment of bladder cancer with interstitial iridium-192 implantation and external beam radiation. *Int J Radiat Oncol Biol Phys* 14:265–271, 1988.

25. Van der Werf-Messing B, Menon RS, Hop WCJ: Carcinoma of the urinary bladder category T3 Nx Mo treated by the combination of radium implant and external irradiation: Second report. *Int J Radiat Oncol Biol Phys* 9:177–180, 1983.

26. Steel GG, Peckham MJ. Exploitable mechanisms in combined radiotherapy– chemotherapy: The concept of additivity. *Int J Rad Oncol Biol Phys* 5:85–91, 1979.

27. Soloway MS, Morris CR, Sudderth B: Radiation therapy and cis-di-ammine-dichloroplatinum (II) in transplantable and primary murine bladder cancer. *Int J Radiat Oncol Biol Phys* 5:1355–1360, 1979.

28. Shipley WU, Prout GR, Einstein AB, et al: Treatment of invasive bladder cancer by cisplatin and radiation in patients unsuited for surgery. *JAMA* 258:931–935, 1987.

29. Jakse G, Frommhold H, Nedden DZ: Combined radiation and chemotherapy for locally advanced transitional cell carcinoma of the urinary bladder. *Cancer* 55:1659–1664, 1985.

30. Tester W, Caplan R, Heaney J, et al: Neoadjuvant combined modality program with selective organ preservation for invasive bladder cancer: Results of RTOG phase II trial 8802. *J Clin Oncol* 14:119–126, 1996.

31. Shipley WU, Winter KA, Kaufman DS, et al: Phase III trial of neoadjuvant chemotherapy in patients with bladder cancer treated with selective bladder preservation by combined radiation therapy and chemotherapy: Initial results of Radiation Therapy Oncology Group 89-03. *J Clin Oncol* 16:3567–3583, 1998.

32. Leibel SA, Hanks GE, Kramer S: Patterns of care outcome studies: Results of the National Practice in Adenocarcinoma of the Prostate. *Int J Radiat Oncol Biol Phys* 10:401–409, 1984.

33. Bagshaw MA: Potential for radiotherapy alone in prostatic cancer. *Cancer* 55:2079–2085, 1985.

34. McGowan DG: The value of extended field radiation therapy in carcinoma of the prostate. *Int J Radiat Oncol Biol Phys* 7:1333–1339, 1981.

35. Hanks GE, Asbell SO, Krall JM, et al: Ten-year outcome for lymph node dissection negative T1b, 2 (A-2,B) prostate cancer treated with external beam radiation therapy in RTOG 77-06. *Int J Radiat Oncol Biol Phys* (suppl 1) 19:195, 1990.

36. Sause WT, Richards RS, Plenk HP: Prostatic carcinoma: 5-year follow-up of patients with surgically staged disease undergoing extended field radiation. *J Urol* 135:517–519, 1986.

37. Hanks GE, Buzydlowski J, Sause WT, et al: Ten-year outcomes for pathologic node positive patients treated in RTOG 75-06. *Int J Rad Oncol Biol Phys* 40:765–768, 1998.

38. Roach M: The role of PSA in the radiotherapy of prostate cancer. *Oncology* 10:1143–1153, 1998.

39. D'Amico AV, Schultz D, Whittington R, et al: A multivariable analysis of clinical factors predicting for pathologic features associated with local failure after radical prostatectomy for prostate cancer. *Int J Rad Oncol Biol Phys* 30:293–303, 1994

40. The Medical Research Council Prostate Cancer Working Party Investigators Group: Immediate versus deferred treatment for advanced prostatic cancer: Initial results of the Medical Research Council trial. *Brit J Urol* 79:235–246, 1997.

41. D'Amico AV, Whittington R, Malkowicz SB, et al: Biochemical outcome after radical prostatectomy, external beam radiation therapy, or interstitial radiation therapy for clinically localized prostate cancer. *JAMA* 280:969–974, 1998.

42. Hanks GE, Hanlon AL, Horwitz EM, Price RA, Schultheiss T: Dose selection for prostate cancer patients based on dose comparison and dose response studies. *Int J Rad Oncol Biol Phys* 46:823–832, 2000.

43. Pollack A, Zagars GK, Smith LG, Antolak JA, Rosen II: Preliminary results of a randomized dose-escalation study comparing 70 Gy to 78 Gy for the

treatment of prostate cancer. *Int J Rad Oncol Biol Phys* 45(suppl 1): 146–147, 1999.

44. Zagars GK, Johnson DE, von Eschenbach AC, Hussey DH: Adjuvant estrogen following radiation therapy for stage C adenocarcinoma of the prostate: Long-term results of a prospective randomized study. *Int J Rad Oncol Biol Phys* 14:1085–1092, 1988.

45. Pilepich MV, Krall JM, al-Sarraf M, et al: Androgen deprivation with radiation therapy compared with radiation therapy alone for locally advanced prostatic carcinoma: A randomized comparative trial of the Radiation Therapy Oncology Group. *Urology* 45:616–622, 1995.

46. Pilepich MV, Caplan R, Byhardt RW, et al: Phase III study of androgen suppression using goserelin in unfavorable-prognosis carcinoma of the prostate treated with definitive radiotherapy: Report of Radiation Therapy Oncology Group protocol 85-31. *J Clin Oncol* 15:1013–1021, 1997.

47. Bolla M, Gonzalez D, Warde P, et al: Improved survival in patients with locally advanced prostate cancer treated with radiotherapy and goserelin. *N Engl J Med* 337:295–300, 1997.

48. Duchesne GM, Horwich A, Dearnaley DP, et al: Orchidectomy alone for stage I seminoma of the testis. *Cancer* 65:1115–1118, 1990.

49. Thomas GM, Gospodarowicz M, Duncan W, et al: A preliminary report of surveillance of stage I seminoma (SEM) post orchidectomy (PO). *Proc ASCO* 6:427, 1988.

50. Fossa SD, Horwic, JM, Russell JP, Roberts RJ, Stenning S: Optimal field size in adjuvant radiotherapy (XRT) of stage I seminoma-A randomised trial. *Proc Am Soc Clin Oncol* 15:595, 1997.

51. Einhorn LH: Radiotherapy in seminoma: More is not better. *Int J Radiat Oncol Biol Phys* 8:309–310, 1981.

52. Warde P, Gospodarowicz M, Panzarella T, et al: Management of stage II seminoma. *J Clin Oncol* 16:290–294, 1998.

53. Ball D, Barrett A, Peckham MJ: The management of metastatic seminoma testis. *Cancer* 50:2289–2294, 1982.

54. Smalley SR, Evans RG, Richrdson RL, Farrow GM, Earle JD: Radiotherapy as initial treatment for bulky stage II testicular seminomas. *J Clin Oncol* 3:1333–1338, 1985.

55. Zagars GK, Babaian RJ: The role of radiation in stage II testicular seminoma. *Int J Radiat Oncol Biol Phys* 13:163–170, 1987.

56. Green N, Broth E, George FW. et al: Radiation therapy in bulky seminoma. *Urology* 50:467–469, 1983.

57. Willan BD, McGowan DG: Seminoma of the testis: A 22-year experience with radiation therapy. *Int J Radiat Oncol Biol Phys* 11:1769–1775, 1985.

58. Laukkanen E, Olivotto I, Jackson S: Management of seminoma with bulky abdominal disease. *Int J Radiat Oncol Biol Phys* 14:227–233, 1988.

59. Haile K, Delclos L: The place of radiation therapy in the treatment of carcinoma of the distal end of the penis. *Cancer* 45:1980–1984, 1980.

60. Knudsen OS, Brennhovd IO: Radiotherapy in the treatment of the primary tumor in penile cancer. *Acta Chir Scand* 133:69–71, 1966.

61. Lederman M: Radiotherapy of cancer of the penis. *Br J Urol* 25:224–232, 1953.

62. Duncan W, Jackson SM: The treatment of early cancer of the penis with megavoltage x-rays. *Clin Radiol* 23:246–248, 1972.

CHAPTER 20

Male Sexual Dysfunction

Ashok K. Batra
JC Trussell

I. GENERAL CONSIDERATIONS

The new millennium has brought with it a combination of explosion in the scientific study and recently acquired understanding of sexual function and dysfunction. A lot was learned in the last decade of the 20th century. Historically, physicians have always had a concern for the sexual issues of their patients. In fact, Hippocrates believed that "preoccupation with business and lack of attractiveness can cause impotence." Later, Aristotle discussed "engorgement" and recognized some of the physiologic aspects of ejaculation.

Both professional and public interest in sexual dysfunction has been sparked by recent developments in several areas: (1) major advancements in understanding neurovascular mechanisms of sexual response; (2) several new drugs offering a spectrum of treatment options for male erectile disorders; and (3) changes in both cultural attitudes and population demographics. A recent survey (1992) of adults aged 18 to 59 years reported a male sexual dysfunction rate of 31 percent. The female population reported an even greater rate of dysfunction (43 percent). Such figures are indicative of a problem much more common than cancer or heart disease; one that deserves continued serious consideration.

II. PHYSIOLOGY OF SEXUAL FUNCTION
A. Erection

An erection is the result of complex interactions between the physiologic, neuroendocrine, and vascular mechanisms acting on the penile erectile tissue. Erections are the result of relaxed sinusoidal smooth muscles, triggered by various reflexogenic and psychogenic stimuli, which result in the release of modulator neurotransmitters. Recent observations strongly suggest nitric oxide to be a major neurotransmitter.

---

*The views expressed in the chapter are those of authors and do not represent the policies of the FDA.

This is followed by a net increase in the blood flow that engorges the cavernous spaces.

1. *Corporal bodies.* The erectile tissue consists of three corporal bodies: the two corpora cavernosa dorsally and a corpus spongiosum ventrally. The latter encloses the urethra and expands distally to form the glans penis.

   At the root of the penis, the bulbospongiosum and corpora cavernosa are covered by the bulbocaverosus and the ischiocavernosus muscles respectively. Erectile tissues within the covering of the complex fibrous tunic contain cavernous spaces capable of considerable distention.

   Microscopic examination of the flaccid canine corpora demonstrates small sinusoids, constricted arteries/ arterioles, and venules, which drain into emissary veins. During an erect state, the sinusoidal spaces are distended, the arterioles/arteries are dilated, and the venules appear small and compressed between the sinusoidal wall and the tunica albuginea. The tunica albuginea, which surrounds the corpora cavernosa, is bilayered (with multiple sublayers). The outer layer is notably absent between the 5 and 7 o'clock position. (Note: penile prosthetics tend to extrude through the corpora canvernosal ventral groove—where the tunica is most thin).The inner layer surrounds the cavernous tissues and also extends into this tissue in the form of the intracavernosal pillars that augment the septum and provide support. In contrast, the tunica albuginea covering of the spongeosum is a single layer without internal struts—ensuring a low-pressure structure during tumescence. The glans is not covered by the tunica albuginea.

2. *Vasculature* (Fig. 20-1). Internal pudendal arteries arise from the internal iliac arteries and continue as the penile arteries. The penile arteries give off three terminal branches: (1) the cavernosal artery, which gives off helicine arteries and, is responsible for tumescence of the corpus cavernosum; (2) the dorsal artery controls engorgement of the glans; and (3) the bulbourethral artery, which supplies the bulb and corpus spongiosum. Occasionally, the penis is supplied by accessory vessels that achieve added importance in the event of the problem with the main vessels. Venules, which drain the sinusoidal spaces, form emissary veins and pierce the tunica albuginea. Emissary veins ultimately drain into four structures: circumferential veins (which in turn drain to the deep dorsal vein), crural, cavernous, and internal pudendal veins.

3. *Hemodynamics.* The mechanism of penile erection and hemodynamics has become much more clearly understood with recent research and advances.

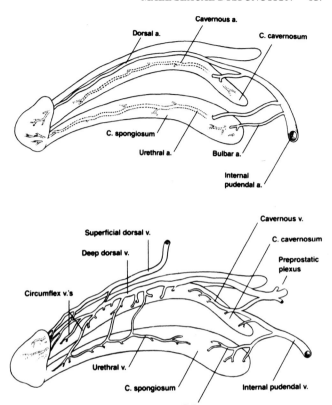

Figure 20-1 Arterial supply (*top*) and venous drainage (*bottom*) of the human penis. (*Reproduced from Orvis BR, Lue TF: New Therapy of Impotence. In: Lytton B (ed): Advances in Urology. Chicago, Year book Medical Publishers, 1988.*)

In the flaccid state (due primarily to tonic sympathetic stimuli), the terminal arterioles and sinusoidal smooth muscle are contracted and a minimal amount of blood flows through the sinusoidal spaces (for nutritional purposes). The flow through cavernous tissue is estimated to be 2.5 to 8 mL/min/100 g of tissue. Following sexual stimuli, the cavernous nerves release neurotransmitters that cause a relaxation of the vascular and sinusoidal smooth muscle. There is a twofold increase in blood flow through the pudendal artery. No changes occur in the systemic blood pressure. This reflects a decrease in the peripheral resistance (due to smooth muscle relaxation) at the level of the terminal arterioles and sinusoids). When full erection is achieved, the flow through the cavernous tissue gradually decreases to its minimum as the intracavernous pressure (ICP) reaches 10 to 20 mg Hg below that of systolic blood pressure. The incoming blood is trapped in the dilated cavernous tissue and the tunic is stretched to its capacity. The draining venules are compressed against the relatively indistensible tunical albuginea, thus preventing the escape of blood. This assures storage of blood during the erection phase.

4. Phases of penile erection

The state of erection can be divided into six phases (Fig. 20-2):

a. *Flaccid phase.* There is minimal arterial and venous flow, and the penile blood gas values are identical to those of venous blood. A minimal amount of blood enters the cavernous tissue for nutritional purposes. High-resolution Doppler studies of the cavernous arteries show an inner diameter of 0.05 cm and a range of flow rates from 15 cm/sec to undetectable.

b. *Latent or filling phase.* There is increased blood flow through the internal pudendal artery during both systolic and diastolic phases. There is penile elongation without change in the ICP. Highest flow occurs in this phase. In a healthy potent man, there is a twofold dilatation of the cavernous artery to 0.1 cm and a peak flow velocity of more than 30 cm/sec.

c. *Tumescence phase.* As the ICP increases, flow starts to decrease. The penis elongates and expands to its maximal capacity. After the ICP rises above the diastolic pressure, the inflow occurs only during the systolic phase.

d. *Full erection phase.* The ICP stabilizes at a value equal to 85 percent of the systolic blood pressure. Blood flow within the pudendal artery is slower than during the tumescence phase, yet greater than during the flaccid phase. All the while, the arterial diameter remains constant. During this phase, penile volume and pressure remains steady and venous flow equals arterial flow (venous flow is greater than in earlier phases). Intracavernous blood gas values resemble those of arterial blood.

e. *Rigid or skeletal erection phase.* Due to the contraction of the ischiocavernosus muscle, the ICP rises well above that of systolic pressure, resulting in a rigid erection. During this phase there is no inflow of blood. Due to muscle fatigue, the duration of this phase is short—preventing ischemia and tissue damage.

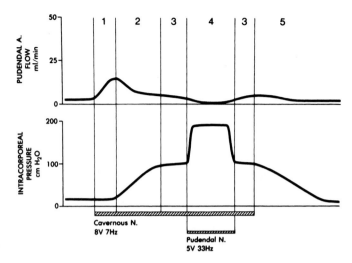

Figure 20-2 Five phases of penil erection: (1) latent phase, (2) tumescence phase, (3) full erection phase, (4) rigid erection phase, (5) detumecene phase. *Upper graph* shows the change in the arterial flow in the internal pudenal artery; *lower graph* demonstrates the change in ICP during these five phases. (*Reproduced from Lue TF: The mechanism of penile erection in the monkey. Semin Urol 136:158, 1986.*)

      f. *Detumescence phase.* After the cessation of erotic stimuli (or ejaculation) tonic sympathetic discharge causes contraction of smooth muscle in the sinusoids and arterioles and diminishes the blood flow to flaccid levels. Sometimes it's further subdivided into a slow and fast phase.

5. *Neuroanatomy and neurophysiology of erection.* The cerebral cortex plays a major role in the erectile process. The oldest part of the brain phylogenetically—the limbic system—appears to contain most of the centers from which stimulation can elicit erection. Medial preoptic area and paraventricular nucleus of hypothalamus are known to be the higher integration centers for sexual drive and erection. Both dopaminergic and adrenergic receptors appear to promote sexual drive. These centers have a close physical relationship with areas associated with such emotional functions as fear, rage, olfaction, and vision. Particularly unknown are the pathways and centers involved in erectile inhibition. It appears that serotonin receptors inhibit sexual drive while prolactin (which inhibits dopaminergic activity) will suppress sexual function. Such centers and

neurotransmitters may be linked to the function of psychogenic impotence.

The spinal center is organized centrally into the autonomic and somatic divisions. The autonomic division is further divided into sympathetic part that originates in the ganglia T11–L2 and the parasympathetic part that originates in S2 through S4. The somatic (sensory and motor) division also originates here in S2–4 and is known as the Onuf's nucleus. The somatic sensory center receives the pain, temperature, and tactile sensations and its motor center is responsible for contraction of ischiocavernosus muscles and ejaculation. The sympathetic and parasympathetic nerves originating from the central and peripheral ganglia merge to form cavernous nerves that are primarily responsible for the erection. Neurally mediated erections can be reflexogenic, psychogenic, or nocturnal.

Psychogenic erections are integrated in the medial preoptic area and paraventricular nucleus of hypothalamus (higher integration centers for sexual drive and erection). These are the result of audiovisual stimuli or fantasies. The impulses from brain modulate the spinal erection centers (T11–L2 and S2–S4) to activate the erection. Reflexogenic erections are the result of local genital stimulation. This sets up a complex process. The impulses go to spinal erection centers and some reach the higher centers through ascending pathways to produce sensations. Others go to the autonomic ganglia and via cavernous nerves to the penis to produce erection. Nocturnal erection occurs during REM sleep and the mechanism is yet unknown.

The neurotransmitters involved in erectile function have been the focus of much research. Norepinephrine (from sympathetic nerve terminals) is accepted as the principal neurotransmitter controlling penile flaccidity and detumescence. Recently, endothelin, a potent vasoconstrictor, has been suggested as the major neurotransmitter responsible for detumescence. Other agents proposed for flaccidity are: thromboxane A2, prostaglandin F2-alpha, and leukotrienes. Nitric oxide (from nonadrenergic–noncholinergic nerves) causes an increase in the production of cGMP, which relaxes the cavernous smooth muscle resulting in tumescence and rigidity. Acetylcholine is another important vascular smooth muscle relaxer. Other putative neurotransmitters are: vasoactive intestinal polypeptide (VIP) (from the parasympathetic pathway), calcitonin gene-related peptide, substance P, and neuropeptide Y. In the central nervous system dopaminergic and adrenergic receptors are known to produce sexual drive and serotonin receptors are thought to be usually inhibitory. The neurotransmittors include dopamine, serotonin, norepinehrine, opiods, oxytonin, and prolactin.

Injury to the sacral segments of the spinal cord, sacral roots, or pelvic/pudendal nerves abolishes reflexogenic erections. Spinal cord injury patients with lesions above the sacral segments may have preserved reflexogenic erections. Psychogenic erections are usually lost in the patients with lesions above T9. Psychogenic erections tend to be of less than optimum rigidity.

6. *Endocrinology.* The role of male hormones with regard to erectile physiology and sexual behavior is unclear. Erectile function in males castrated before puberty is thought to be quite rare. The effects of post-pubertal castration range from complete loss of libido and erectile ability to totally normal activity. Generally, there is an overall decrease in sexual activity and ability following medical or surgical castration. After puberty, testosterone may well have more of an influence on libido than erectile ability. The two may be hard to differentiate in the clinical setting.

B. Emission

Emission refers to deposition of the following glandular secretions into the posterior urethra: periurethral glands, prostate, seminal vesicles, and contents of the distal vas. Emission and ejaculation are two reflexogenic phenomena that are closely related temporally—occuring at the culmination of a sexually exciting situation. Each has the potential, in certain situations, to be independent of the other or even, independent of a penile erection.

Although the exact nature of the afferent stimuli preceding emission is not clear, it appears as though both sensorial stimuli from the genitalia and cerebral stimuli are both involved. Cerebral control is such that emission may be halted voluntarily up to the sensation of "inevitability"—caused by the filling and distention of the posterior urethra. Efferent neural control emanates from the T10 to L2 sympathetic outflow. Sympathectomy and adrenergic blockade can eliminate emission (closure of the bladder neck is under sympathetic control).

C. Ejaculation

Ejaculation is a complex phenomenon involving rhythmic contractions of the pelvic floor musculature with compression of the urethra, such that, under normal conditions, the semen is expelled in an antegrade direction through the urethra and out the penile meatus. The afferent stimulus seems to be the passage of semen from the posterior urethra into the bulbous urethra. Little voluntary control exists after this point. Although the control center for ejaculation appears to be located at the T_{11}–L_2 level, outflow at the time of ejaculation also involves the sacral somatic nervous system (S_{2-3-4}). A coordinated neural output controls both the smooth and striated muscles. The bladder neck remains tightly closed (a sympathetic phenomenon), and rhythmic external sphincter relaxation allows semen to enter the bulbous urethra, where it is expelled by contractions of the bulbocavernousus and ischiocavernous muscles (a somatic phenomenon).

D. Orgasm

Orgasm is a central nervous system (CNS) phenomenon that relates genital experiences to whole-body physiology. It can be described as an intense and profoundly satisfying cerebral sensation that represents the explosive discharge of accumulated neuromuscular tensions.

Following orgasm, detumescence takes place and a refractory period ensues in which the male is unable to achieve full erection or repeat orgasm. Detumescence may be a sympathetic event secondary to vasoconstriction.

III. SEXUAL DYSFUNCTION

A. Definitions

1. *Premature ejaculation.* The inability to control ejaculation to satisfy a partner 50 percent of the time. Generally, this is a functional problem—a type of learned behavior—that responds well to several techniques of behavioral therapy. See bibliography for a list of self-help and Masters and Johnson publications.

2. *Ejaculatory incompetence.* Inability to ejaculate during intercourse. This form of dysfunction can be considered the opposite of premature ejaculation. It is relatively rare and usually psychogenic in nature.

3. *Primary impotence.* Never able to maintain erection to achieve successful coitus. This always demands full diagnostic evaluation to rule out an organic etiology.

4. *Secondary impotence.* Previously potent, but subsequent failure to achieve successful coitus in at least 25 percent of coital opportunities.

5. *Libido quantification.* This is very difficult to define. What is adequate for one person or couple may be inadequate for another. The frequency of intercourse varies. If a patient feels his libido is low, the clinician may either attempt to increase it or modify expectations.

6. *Priapism.* Defined as an abnormally persistent (more than 6 hours) erection without sexual desire. Pain and tender-

ness may be present in the ischemic or low-flow variety. It is classified as primary (idiopathic, 33 to 50 percent of all patients) and secondary. The most common etiologies for secondary priapism are injection with a vasculogenic agent such as Caverject (PGE1), alcohol and drug abuse, sickle cell disease, and trauma including arteriovenous and arteriocavernous bypass surgery. Other causes include neurologic disease, malignancy, and total parentral nutrition. Two hemodynamic types of priapism exist.

a. *Low flow (ischemic).* A veno-occlusive phenomenon that causes tissue ischemia and pain if not treated. First-line treatments include α-adrenergic agonists (epinehrine 10 to 20 μg, pheylephrine 250–500 μg, and ephedrine 50 to 100 mg) and corporal aspiration. In persistant erection a form of cavernosal–spongiosum shunting procedure may be required to resume an alternative drainage system. This can later lead to impotence.

b. *High flow (nonischemic).* An arterial phenomenon that is usually painless. Treatment may require diagnosis by arteriography with embolization of the involved cavernosal or internal pudendal artery.

Treatment must be undertaken expeditously in a low-flow state (preferably within 12 to 24 hours) to avoid damage to the tissues and subsequent impotence. In spite of treatment, its overall impotence rate may be as high as 40 percent. High-flow priapism has a better prognosis, with impotence rates of 20 percent.

B. Etiology and Classification of Erectile Dysfunction

Physiologically, there are three types of erections (nocturnal, psychogenic, and reflexogenic); each of which may be impaired by any of the following etiologies.

1. Psychogenic
2. Vasculogenic
3. Neurogenic
4. Endocrine
5. End-organ failure
6. Iatrogenic and drug-induced

1. *Psychogenic impotence.* Until about a decade ago it was generally thought that 80 to 90 percent of impotence was psychogenic and only 10 percent had an organic basis. Recent studies have demonstrated that organic causes of erectile dysfunction are found in approximately 70 to 80 percent of patients. In less than one third of patients the cause may be purely psychogenic. Normal sexual functioning requires a certain degree of self-confidence, absence of anxiety, presence of arousing mental and/or physical

stimulation, and ability to focus attention on sexual activity. Psychogenic dysfunction can produce exaggerated suprasacral inhibition of spinal erection center and/or there may a presence of excessive sympathetic outflow. Both mechanisms will lead to decreased erection. Lue classfied psychogenic erectile dysfunction into following subtypes.

1. Anxiety and fear of failure
2. Depression (drug or disease induced)
3. Marital conflict strained relationship
4. Ignorance, misinformation, and religious beliefs
5. Psychotic and personality disorder (obsessive-compulsive, anhedonia)

A wide variety of psychologically based problems can interfere with these prerequisites, and determination of such an underlying problem is critical to successful treatment. A careful history and an appropriate selection of diagnostic tests to rule out a primary or concomitant organic problem are essential.

2. *Vasculogenic impotence.* Thromboembolic occlusion at the aortic bifurcation (Leriches' syndrome) will result in pain and claudication of the hips and thighs as well as erectile dysfunction. Furthermore, atherosclerosis may cause narrowing of the aortoiliac and pundendal vessels. Fibrosis, calcification, obliteration, scarring, and aneurysmal dilations decrease the blood flow through the penile arteries and result in arterial erectile dysfunction. Additionally, cavernosal arteries become progressively obliterated by the process of aging. Diabetic vasculopathy causes erectile dysfunction, although some attribute diabetic impotence more to neuropathy. Other risk factors include, hypertension, smoking, hyperlipidemia, and blunt pelvic or perineal trauma. Pelvic steal syndrome is seen in large vessel arteriosclerosis in the pelvis where there is shunting of blood to the pelvic and gluteal muscles resulting in detumescence. Veno-occlusive dysfunction is caused by presence of large and abnormal channels, denegenerative and Peyronie's disease, structural alterations in fibroelastic components, insufficient smooth muscle relaxation, and acquired shunts as seen after the treatment of priapism.

3. *Neurogenic impotence.* Neurogenic impotence is due to peripheral nerve, spinal cord, or cerebral lesions. Diabetes, uremia, and amyloidosis are known to involve the peripheral autonomic nerves and are associated with erectile dysfunction. Spinal cord lesions including spinal

cord trauma, multiple sclerosis, tabes dorsalis, spina bifida, syringomyelia, amyotrophic lateral sclerosis, compression due to herniated disks and tumors, lateral chordotomy for intractable pain, and Shy-Drager syndrome may cause sexual dysfunction. Cerebral lesions that may cause erectile dysfunction include frontal lobotomy, Parkinson's disease, stroke, Huntington's chorea, and electrocortical shock therapy (ECT).

4. *Endocrine and metabolic disorders.* The overall incidence of endocrinopathy in impotent patients is 17.5 percent, with diabetes leading as the single most frequent cause of erectile dysfunction in the United States. In diabetic men, it is notable that impotence is more common than either retinopathy or neuropathy. Half of male diabetic patients (2 to 2.5 million men) complain of sexual dysfunction with 30 to 50 percent of all diabetic men over 50 functionally impotent. Of note, impotence does not correlate with the severity of diabetes or the adequacy of its control. Libido is usually normal. When age is accounted for, as the duration of diabetes increases, there appears to be a greater risk for developing impotence. The mechanism of dysfunction is complex and involves vascular, neurologic, and endocrine pathways.

Libido, erectile, and ejaculatory functions all require adequate levels of androgens. The androgens affect synaptic transmission (including synthesis, storage, uptake, and release of neurotransmitters) as well as receptor sensitivity. Hypergonadotropic hypogonadism (primary testicular failure) is the most common endocrinopathy causing sexual dysfunction. Various causes include congenital defects, Klinefelter's syndrome, chemotherapeutic agents, and, radiation therapy. Hypogonadotropic hypogonadism results from failure of primary luteinizing hormone (LH) secretion by the anterior pituitary.

Congenital hypogonadotropic hypogonadism is associated with Kallmann's, Prader-Willi, and Laurence-Moon-Biedl syndromes. Hyperprolactinemia—drug induced, or from a prolactin-secreting pituitary tumor—is also associated with sexual dysfunction. Thyroid disorders are known to cause erectile dysfunction and are indirectly associated with changes in testosterone levels. Reduced erectile ability exists in 40 to 80 percent of dialysis patients, with as many as half being completely impotent. Remarkably, following transplant, as many as 50 percent regain potency.

5. *End organ factors.* Congenital problems include the exstrophy/epispadias complex, microphallus, fusiform megalourethra, and severe penile chordee.

Peyronie's disease is characterized by the development of a fibrous plaque involving the tunica albuginea that surrounds the erectile tissue of the corpora. The earliest pathologic finding is a vasculitis in the loose areolar tissue beneath the tunica. Although the etiology is unknown, subclinical trauma to the erect penis is suspected to be the cause. It is associated with patients having more generalized fibrotic responses to injury. For instance, such patients have an increased incidence of Dupuytren's contractures and often display fibrous degeneration of cartilage in the external ear. Most cases involve men in the fourth or fifth decades. Symptoms include the presence of a plaque or induration within the penis, penile curvature during erection, and painful intercourse. The inelastic tunica albuginea causes the veno-occlusive dysfunction. The natural history is variable with some patients improving spontaneously. Medical treatments have included steroids (orally or injection into the plaque), vitamin E, *para*-aminobenzoate, and local dimethyl sulfoxide. More recently, improvements have also been seen after plaque iontophoresis with verapamil, dexamethasone, and lidocaine. Surgical operations (generally resorted to after a year or so of watchful waiting) include excision of the plaque with placement of a graft, excision of a diamond-shaped portion of the tunica opposite the plaque to foreshorten but straighten the penis, or placement of a penile prosthesis.

Priapism is the pathologic prolongation of a penile erection most often associated with pain (low-flow type) but not with sexual excitement or desire. It is associated with a 50 percent rate of impotence secondary to corporal scarring (regardless of the modality of treatment).

Finally, prostatitis and seminal vesiculitis can cause pain on arousal or ejaculation and constitute end-organ causes of sexual dysfunction.

6. *Iatrogenic and drug-induced impotence.* Vascular surgical procedures, transplant and radical pelvic surgery, surgery for priapism, pelvic irradiation, and trauma to the lower urinary tract are known to cause erectile dysfunction. Certain procedures performed on the spinal cord and brain may result in erectile dysfunction. The incidence of drug-induced impotence is about 25 percent. Various drugs known to cause erectile dysfunction are alcohol, recreational drugs, antihypertensives, and psychotropics.

Most of the antihypertensive drugs currently in use are associated with some degree of impotence or ejaculatory dysfunction. The frequency of which varies dramatically between the different agents used. Both the diuretics and vasodilators (such as hydralazine and minoxidil) rarely cause impotence. The sympatholytic agents, which include methyldopa, clonidine, and reserpine, are the ones most often associated with sexual dysfunction. Alpha-adrenergic blockers (pehnoxybenzamine, phentolamine, and prazosin) adversely affect emission and ejaculation. Beta-blockers (propranolol and metoprolol) are not infrequent offenders.

Psychotropic agents, anticholinergic drugs, and commonly abused substances—including alcohol, amphetamines, barbituates, cocaine, marijuana, and narcotics—are all potentially detrimental to sexual function. It is incumbent upon the physician to review the pharmaceutical profile of each patient with sexual dysfunction to prevent unnecessary diagnostic, surgical, or psychotherapeutic interventions, in cases in where a simple change in medication may be all that is required.

IV. EVALUATION OF SEXUAL DYSFUNCTION
A. History

1. *Physiologic changes.* To evaluate erectile dysfunction properly, both a careful history and a thorough understanding of normal erectile physiology are required. Male sexual drive and performance peak between the ages of 15 and 25. Following this, there is a progressive decline in function. Whereas after the age of 50, a longer stimulation time is generally required for erection. The pre-ejaculation period is longer with a shorter ejaculation sensation and a decreased volume and expulsion force. In addition, the refractory period is increased.

2. *Psychologic dysfunction.* Psychologic dysfunction typically has an abrupt onset, and a careful history will usually disclose the inciting factors. The patient will usually admit to erections in certain situations (masturbation, extramarital coitus, in the early morning, or when awakening from sleep). Performance anxiety, while often a secondary phenomenon in organic impotence, can be the primary problem in psychologic dysfunction.

3. *Organic deterioration.* Life-style choices may cause a predisposition to erectile dysfunction. For this reason, improvements may be seen with cessation of smoking and moderate alcohol use. A low cholesterol diet is also beneficial. Long distance bicycling is another well-known risk factor for impotence. Regarding organic impotence, the patient generally notices a gradual deterioration in potency. The following deterioration sequence is typical: decreased rigidity, decreased frequency, failure with fatigue, erection achieved but not maintained, success only in morning or after waking with erection from

a dream, success only in very exciting circumstances, loss of nocturnal erections, loss of erection with masturbation, and complete loss of erectile function despite no loss of libido. A good history should address all risk factors and medical and surgical problems discussed in the etiology.

B. Physical Examination

Look for changes compatible with endocrine disease (e.g., gynecomastia). Examine the penis and testes (both size and texture), prostate, and seminal vesicles. Conduct a thorough neurologic examination, including evaluation of anal sphincter tone, bulbocavernosus reflex, and perineal and genital sensation. Vascular examination should include a search for bruits, characterization of peripheral pulses, skin temperature, color, and hair distribution.

C. Laboratory Data, Hormonal Evaluation

Screening blood chemistries are helpful to rule out diabetes and renal failure. In addition, a hormonal evaluation that includes testosterone, prolactin, and LH should be obtained. Because of negative feedback on the pituitary-derived LH-releasing hormone (LHRH), prolactin levels over 22 ng/mL should be corrected. Hyperprolactinemia must be corrected since sexual dysfunction is not alleviated by testosterone supplementation alone. Prolactin not only reduces end-organ responsiveness to LH but also reduces conversion of testosterone to dihydrotestosterone. Since prolactin secretion is inhibited by dopamine, bromocriptine (a dopamine agonist), may correct impotence related to elevated prolactin levels arising from pituitary adenomas.

D. Special Studies to Evaluate Sexual Dysfunction

1. *Psychological testing.* The Beck Depression Inventory can be a valuable aid in diagnosing clinically significant depression, a common cause of decreased libido and erectile dysfunction. This questionnaire can be administered in 15 min and is a useful screening aid. The Minnesota Multiphasic Personality Inventory is perhaps the best known of many psychologic examinations and can be self-administered. Abnormal results serve as a "red flag" and suggest the need for further psychologic evaluation. Patients with depression, marital difficulties, or abnormal personality inventories should be referred for psychiatric evaluation prior to undergoing a complete urologic evaluation.

2. *Nocturnal penile tumescence (NPT).* Ohlmeyer first described NPT in infants in 1940 and later in adults in 1944. NPT usually occurs in conjunction with the rapid eye

movement (REM) sleep. Normally, there are three to five erectile episodes per night. Each lasting 10 to 25 min and associated with an expansion in penile circumference by 15 to 30 mm. The use of this test assumes, among other things, that the mechanism of NPT is identical to that of erotic stimulation and that the patient with psychogenic impotence will have NPT. Nocturnal erections are not affected by recent sexual gratification and the dream content is not necessarily erotic in nature. Overall accuracy of NPT in distinguishing psychogenic from organic impotence (its primary purpose) is questionable. Interpretation of this test has also been questioned on the premise that it only measures tumescence and not the rigidity that is required for the vaginal penetration. NPT is best monitored for 1 to 3 nights at home or in a formal sleep laboratory with the aid of loop strain gauges that are placed around the penis and connected to a transducer and monitor that can give a recording of tumescence at the base and the glans throughout the night. The advantage of formal sleep laboratory testing is that both technician and the awakened patient can evaluate penile rigidity. Of note, sleep apnea and periodic limb movement disorders are strikingly prevalent among men with erectile dysfunction. Devices such as rigiscan, snap gauge, and mercury strain gauge are used to measure penile rigidity. All of these devices have associated controversies. Most urologists do not commonly undertake NPT testing these days.

3. Assessment of penile blood flow
   a. *Doppler studies.* The simplest and most common erectile function test to detect impaired hemodynamic blood flow parameters is the use of Doppler ultrasound techniques to record systolic occlusion pressure in the cavernosal arteries of the penis. A pediatric blood pressure cuff is placed around the base of the penis and inflated to a pressure above the brachial systolic blood pressure. As the cuff is slowly deflated, a Doppler ultrasound probe is used to detect the return of pulsation in the right and left cavernosal arteries. A penile systolic pressure less than 70 percent of the brachial systolic pressure [penile brachial index (PBI): less than 0.7] is considered compatible with arterial vasculogenic impotence. It is important to note that this study is typically inaccurate and difficult to reproduce. A decrease in PBI of more than 0.15 after exercise is suggestive of a "pelvic steal." This test is currently not commonly performed.

   Duplex ultrasound and pulsed Doppler analysis with and without intracavernosal vasoactive agent [papaverine and/or prostaglandin E_1 (PGE$_1$)] are very commonly used in many centers for evaluation of penile vascular insufficiency. After an intracavernosal injection, venogenic impotence is ruled out by obtaining a rigid erection (usually within 10 min) that is sustained for half an hour. Following intracavernosal injection, Doppler wave form analysis is done with a 7.5 to 10 Mhz probe. Arterial insufficiency is diagnosed if the duplex scan shows an arterial diameter increase less than 25 percent and a peak systolic velocity of less than 25 cm/sec. Some people have used a criterion of end diastolic velocities of more than 5 cm/sec to represent venous leak. Duplex studies show reasonable correlation with arteriographic studies for arterial insufficiency.

b. *Dynamic infusion cavernometry and cavernosography (DICC).* Following a papaverine injection, the ICP is measured. A normal erection after injection rules out a venous leak. An abnormal result does not distinguish between arterial, venous, or cavernous pathology. The corpora are then infused with warmed, heparinized saline at a flow rate necessary to achieve an erection. This is followed by infusion of contrast. If the dorsal vein is visualized (not normally seen during erect state) and the flow rate required to maintain erection is high, the patient is considered to have venous insufficiency syndrome of the corporal bodies. This patient may be a candidate for dorsal vein ligation. Results are often flawed because lack of privacy, fear, and anxiety in the test setting can all lead to veno-occlusive dysfunction.

c. *Angiography.* Selective Internal pudendal arteriography (coupled with PGE$_1$ and/or papaverine) is the most sensitive procedure for precise evaluation of the anatomy of the entire hypogastric–pudendal–cavernous arterial bed. It is still considered the gold standard. However arteriography is an expensive, invasive procedure associated with significant risks and should be used only in individuals willing to consider penile revascularization procedures. Best results are seen in young men after traumatic arterial disruption, or, in the rare patient with a pelvic steal syndrome.

d. *Assessment of autonomic pathways (neurologic testing).* Having a high index of suspicion for a neurologic basis for sexual dysfunction, corroborative data may be obtained by neurologic testing. Cystometrography and bethanechol supersensitivity testing evaluates the pelvic parasympathetic nerves at the vesicle parasympathetic plexus. At present there is no reliable test of the corporal parasympathetic plexus, and testing integrity of the more proximal vesical pathway can only make indirect inference as to its integrity. Smooth muscle EMG, sympathetic skin response, and somatosesory evoked potentials are performed in specialized centers.

Perineal electromyography and bulbocavernous reflex latency testing can evaluate the somatic pudendal nerve. The pudendal nerves (S2–S4) supply sensation from the penile skin and provide motor innervation to the bulbocavernousus, ischiocavernosus, and external urethral sphincter muscles. The sensory aspect is important for erections while the motor aspect is necessary for ejaculation. Dorsal penile nerve conduction velocity (n = 21–29 m/sec) can be done to assess its function.

Examination of the suprasacral afferent pathways is possible through testing of the genitocerebral evoked response. The penis is stimulated and cerebral/sacral evoked potentials, at various sites within the CNS, are measured.

4. *Assesment of cavernous tissues.* The cavernous smooth muscle biopsy is controversial and proposed in rare cases prior to undertaking highly reconstructive vascular surgery. Biopsy specimens are utilized for typing of collegen, electronmicroscopy, and ultrastructral studies. Nitric oxide synthase test is also performed.

V. NONSURGICAL TREATMENT
A. Time
Many psychologically based sexual problems will disappear with simple reassurance by the physician and with the passage of time. Most men will experience an episode of erectile failure at some time.

B. Psychotherapy and Sexual Counseling
Psychotherapy can run the gamut from reassurance and education, to formal marriage counseling, sexual therapy, and even psychoanalysis. Generally, performance anxiety is targeted and treated by various desensitization techniques. Sensate focus and noncoital techniques are taught so that the sexual experience is not merely looked upon as one in which vaginal intromission is the ultimate end point. This tends to improve sexuality primarily by allaying performance anxiety.

C. Hormonal Therapy
Hormonal supplementation with adjunctive testosterone is often helpful when testosterone levels are low or in the low

to normal range. In our experience, testosterone seems to have its major effect on libido rather than erectile function. It is only indicated in young hypogonal patients as the risks outweigh the benefits in older patients. It can be given by the intramuscular route since oral absorption is quite variable and has a propensity to cause liver damage. Other delivery systems are (1) testoderm—which is applied solely to scrotal skin; and (2) androderm—which can be applied to any skin surface. Transdermal systems have increased testosterone levels to within the normal range in over 90 percent of treated patients. Overall the results of testosterone treatment of impotence have been disappointing. Naturally, testosterone replacement is contraindicated in patients with prostate cancer. A patient receiving testosterone replacement requires a semiannual PSA, DRE, and hematocrit (checking for polycythemia).

D. Pharmacological Therapy
  1. Oral Agents
     a. *Peripherally acting drugs.* After FDA approval of sildenafil citrate (Viagra) in 1999, patient demand and agent efficacy fueled a record within the pharmaceutical community—the largest number of prescriptions ever written for any newly released agent. Sildenafil is a peripherally acting agent, a selective inhibitor of cyclic guanosine monophosphate (cGMP)-specific phosphodiesterase type 5 (PDE5). PDE5 is the predominant isozyme, which metabolizes cGMP in the corpus cavernosum. Sildenafil has no direct relaxant effect on human corpus cavernosum but enhances the relaxant effect of nitric oxide (NO) by inhibition of PDE5, which is responsible for degradation of cGMP in this tissue, thus making more of NO available to the cavernous tissue (Fig. 20-3). When sexual stimulation causes a local release of NO, increased levels of cGMP are possible since sildenafil inhibits its breakdown. Alternatively, in the absence of sexual stimulation, sildenafil should not alter the sexual function of a patient. The effective response rate is up to 80 percent and has been found to work equally well in patients with psychological and organic (diabetes, spinal injury, and surgical nerve damage) impotence. It is least effective in the patient with extensive damage to the neurovasculature that some times occurs after radical prostatectomy. Use of this agent is contraindicated in men taking organic nitrates since it potentiates the hypotensive effects of nitrates. Furthermore, use with caution in men with heart disease and those in poor

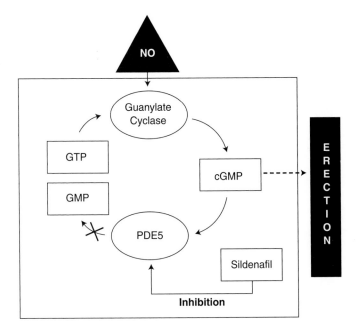

Figure 20-3

physical health due to lack of exercise. Other phosphodiesterase inhibitors like milrinone, rolipram, and zaprinast are being tried intracavernously in conjunction with PGE_1 with some promise. Peripherally acting pentoxifylline is a vasoactive agent used to treat patients with symptoms of claudication. Serendipitously, these patients were noted to have improved erectile function.

b. *Centrally acting drugs.* Centrally acting agents include phentolamine, yohimbine, apomorphine, and trazodone. Yohimbine is an α-adrenergic antagonist oral agent that has been reported to have a beneficial effect on sexual function in humans, and was most commonly used until the arrival of Viagara. Usual response rate is approximately 25 to 30 percent. Recent trials with sublingual apomorhine and oral phentolamine have shown some promise. Trazodone is a commonly prescribed antidepressant and is known to cause penile erection as a side effect.

2. Intraurethral and transdermal agents. PGE_2 placed into the fossa navicularis as a suppository (Muse) has induced full tumescence in 30 percent and partial tumescence in 40 percent of patients. Overall, 50 percent of the patients had erections adequate for coitus. Side effects include penile pain (burning) in 10.9 percent patients, 2.8 percent complained of hypotension, 3.8 percent felt dizzy, and 0.2 percent developed a urinary tract infection. Minioxidil 2 percent solution, yohimbine, and nitroglycerine ointments have been used with some success in the induction of penile erection.

E. Intracavernous Injection Therapy

Neurologic stimulation initiates penile erection by inducing hemodynamic alterations in the corporal erectile tissue. It has been proposed that released postganglionic neurotransmitter substances such as acetylcholine or VIP, and more recently NO, result in the relaxation of smooth muscle in the corporal end arterioles and the surrounding sinusoids. When injected intracorporally, pharmacologic agents that result in vascular and cavernous smooth muscle relaxation may mimic the action of physiologic neurotransmitter substances. As expected, the net effect of increasing cavernosal arterial inflow and decreasing venous drainage, is an accumulation of corporal blood volume and an increase in the ICP. If the ICP exceeds 90 mm Hg, there is sufficient rigidity for vaginal penetration.

It is now possible for patients to administer a combination of papaverine and/or phentolamine or PGE_1 by direct injection into the corpora to initiate an erection. This is an excellent option for patients with neurogenic impotence, refractory psychogenic impotence, and some patients with minimal vascular disease. Intracavernosal pharmacologic erections have proven to be a useful diagnostic tool by giving an indication of the degree of vascular impairment. Sensation, emission, ejaculation, and orgasm are not different after using injection therapy. At present, PGE_1 (alprostadil) is the most commonly used agent and is marketed as Caverject. After injection, 96 percent is metabolized locally without any significant absorption into the peripheral blood stream. In doses of 10 to 20 μg, 70 to 80 percent of patients with erectile dysfunction had full erections. It is an effective agent for diagnosis and treatment of erectile dysfunction. The most common side effects are a burning sensation and localized pain. More recently, an injectable, triple drug combination (papaverine/phentolamine and alprostadil) has yielded 89 percent patient satisfaction with a significantly lower incidence of painful erections. A worrisome side effect of injection therapy is corporal fibrosis, which has been reported after papaverine injections and may occur (although less frequently) after prostaglandin therapy. Priapism occurs occasionally and usually responds to intracorporal pharmacotherapy with α-adrenergic agents such as ephinephrine, norepinephrine, ephedrine, or phenylephrine. Other experimental intracavernosal agents include VIP, moxisylyte, CG-RP, linsidomanine and sodium nitroprusside, and some newer phosphodiestrase inhibitors. Some of these agents are approved in Europe and are being used alone or as a part of the combination with other commonly used agents.

F. Other Therapeutic Options

1. *Neurostimulation.* Eckhard described the innervation of the dog penis in 1869 and was the first to show the electrical stimulation of the nerves from the sacral roots produced erections in this animal model. Habib, in 1967, produced erections after sacral nerve stimulation in man—an event subsequently reproduced on purpose and by accident (as a by-product of attempts to produce bladder emptying). Erections can be produced by electrical stimulation both centrally and peripherally (at the pelvic plexus). Both Lue and associates reported the use of electrostimulation and erection pacemaker in experimental animals. A rigid and sustained erection without side effects has not been consistently possible in humans. It is not being used clinically at present.

2. *Vacuum erection device.* The exact mechanism is poorly understood. Normally the pressure gradients on arterial and venous sides are 120 and 8 mm Hg, respectively. Application of the vacuum creates a negative venous pressure of 100 mm Hg, thus filling the venous spaces. Engorgement of the sinusoidal spaces produces erections. This erection state is preserved by the placement of a rubber ring at the base of the penis. The should not be left in place for over 30 mins. Patient acceptance rate is about 40 to 50 percent. It is not effective in patients with proximal venous leaks, arterial insufficiency, and patients with fibrosis. Reported complications include pain, ecchymosis, swelling, and petechiae of the shaft of the penis. Caution should be used in patients on anticoagulants.

3. *Corporal dilation and gene therapy.* It has been reported that the penile erections inducted by papaverine and sustained at high pressures by infusing heparinized saline for 45 min may improve subsequent potency. Monthly therapy is given for 6 to 12 months. The mechanism of this therapy is not completely understood. More recently researchers have transplanted cultured endothelial cells into corpora in

an effort to induce expression of nitric oxide synthase by transfection. This is a promising area of research.

VI. SURGICAL TREATMENT
A. History
In 1668, de Graaf injected the hypogastric artery in cadavers and concluded that erections were caused by venous stasis induced by perineal muscle contraction. Ebbehoj and Wagner, Vaclav Mikal, and Virag are some of the pioneers of modern revascularization surgery. In 1936, Borgoras used a rib implantation to simulate an erection. The stage was set for modern prosthetic surgical techniques. All that was needed was the technology to develop a nonreactive substance that could be implanted safely. This effort was lead by Pearman and Scott in 1970s. Today, placement of penile prosthesis—comprises the majority of penile surgery and in rare young patients penile revascularizations are undertaken.

B. Indications
Surgery is indicated in cases of organic impotence (not amenable to non-surgical treatments) and in psychogenic impotence where conventional psychotherapy has failed repeatedly.

C. Prosthetic Surgery
Penile prostheses currently available for implantation can be divided into two major categories: malleable or semirigid and the inflatable devices. After a complete discussion of all the alternative forms of treatments and their risks and benefits, the prosthesis is placed according to the patient and the surgeon's choice and taking the cost factor into account.
1. Malleable or semirigid models include:
   a. *Semirigid.* Small Carion (Mentor)
   b. *Hinged.* Flexirod (Surgitek)
   c. *Malleable* (Fig. 20-4).
      i. AMS Malleable 600 (AMS)
      ii. Jonas (Bard)
      iii. Jonas Trimmable Tail (Bard)
      iv. Mentor Malleable (Mentor)
   d. *Positional.* Duraphase (Dacomed)
   e. *Mechanically activated.* Omniphase (Dacomed)
2. Inflatable prosthetic models include:
   a. *One-piece* (Fig. 20-5): AMS Dynaflex (AMS); Flexiflate (Surgitek)
   b. *Two-piece* GFS (Mentor); GFS Mark 2 (Mentor); AMS 2-piece Ambicor; Uniflate 1000 (Surgitek)
   c. *Three-piece* (Fig. 20-6). AMS 700 CX and ultrex plus (AMS); Alpha 1 Inflatable (Mentor)

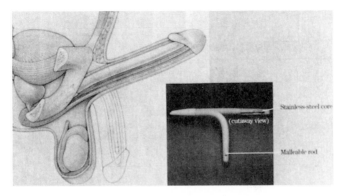

Figure 20-4 AMS Malleable 600 penile prosthesis.

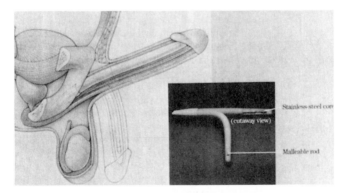

Figure 20-5 AMS Hydroflex self-contained penile prosthesis.

The rigid and semirigid devices are paired flexible or malleable rods composed of medical-grade silicone elastomer or polytetrafluoroethylene or an intertwined central/spiral metalic core. When implanted, they provide the patient with a permanent degree of penile rigidity suitable for vaginal penetration and sexual intercourse. The inflatable penile prosthesis is hydraulically operated. Original models are comprised of four parts: a reservoir placed in the abdomen (extraperitoneally), a pump placed in the scrotum, and paired cylinders placed in the corporal bodies. Newer inflatable models are self-contained and consist only of the

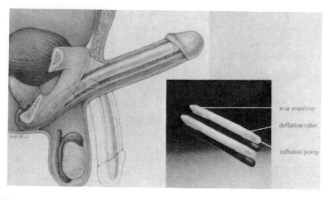

Figure 20-6 AMS 700 CX inflatable penile prosthesis.

corporal cylinders. Inflatable devices provide for both erect and flaccid states.

Patients must understand that to place any prosthesis, the normal erectile tissue must be hollowed out thereby destroyed. If the prosthesis must be removed for any reason, the patient will never be able to attain a normal erection. Because placement of the prosthesis is essentially "burning your bridges," it is not a step to be taken lightly. Nevertheless, when a patient suffers from organic impotence, it is often the best and/or only treatment alternative. The prosthesis does not affect sensation, emission, ejaculation, or orgasm. Regardless of type of device, there is a 1 percent incidence of discomfort—severe enough to require prosthetic removal. Notably, the prosthesis can usually be replaced at another time. The mechanical malfunction rate of the inflatable variety is now somewhere around 3 to 5 percent. The infection rate is usually 0.6 to 8.9 percent. It is more common in patients with spinal cord injury and diabetes.

D. Vascular Procedures

1. *Proximal arterial lesions.* Isolated proximal lesions (aortoiliac occlusive diseases) are rare and small vessel lesions frequently coexist. Occasionally, they are associated with the failure of veno-occlusive mechanisms. Therefore, a complete vascular evaluation is mandatory before any vascular procedure is undertaken. Various techniques to improve blood flow have been described. These include direct iliac to hypogastric artery graft, hypogastric endarterectomy, and transluminal balloon angioplasty.

2. *Distal arterial lesions.* Occlusions of the internal pudendal, common penile, and cavernosal arteries are idiopathic, congenital, atherosclerotic, and traumatic in nature. In general, the revascularization procedures include:
(1) neoartery to cavernosal anastamosis (complications include priapism and corporal fibrosis); and (2) neoarte-rial
anastomosis to the dorsal artery, cavernosal artery, or dorsal vein of the penis. The neoarterial source is either the ar-
terialized saphenous vein or the inferior epigastric artery.
The inferior epigastric artery is considered superior to the
vein. These procedures seem to be most successful in
young patients with trauma-related vascular occlusion.

3. *Venous lesions.* Various procedures to improve veno-occlusive mechanisms have been described. Ligation of the
deep dorsal vein with or without circumflex/crural venous ligation is the most commonly performed procedure. Of course, precise localization of the venous leaks
is an important step in planning therapy. Poor patient selection and the generalized nature of this disease are major causes of therapeutic failure. Relatively younger age
and extremely careful patient selection with advanced diagnostic techniques cannot be overemphasized for the
success of venocorrective surgery. Success rates, previously reported to be in the range of 25 to 74 percent, have
tended to taper off because of late failures. These procedures are rarely performed due to the very high recurrence rates and the generalized nature of this disease.

VII. CONCLUSION

The current treatment costs are as follows; (1) psychosexual
therapy $500 to $2,000, (2) oral therapy $15 to $45/month,
(3) vacuum device $200 to $450, (4) intracavernous injections
$40 to $200/month, (5) prosthesis $5,500 to $14,000, (6) Vascular surgery $8,000 to $17,000. In this day of rising healthcare
cost, one has to make judicious and realistic decisions. The
availability of a safe and effective oral agent to treat most cases
of impotence has revolutionized the field of male sexual dysfunction. Multiple new, possibly synergistic, oral and transmu-
cosal agents are rapidly approaching FDA approval. The scientific study of impotence and its treatment is one of the most
rapidly expanding frontiers of urology. At this point in time, almost any patient presenting to an urologist with sexual dysfunction can be helped.

BIBLIOGRAPHY

Batra AK, Lue TF: Physiology and pathology of penile erection. In: Bancroft J,
ed. *Annual Review of Sex Research.* Iowa, Society for the Scientific Study
of Sex, 1990, vol. 1, pp 251–263.

DeGroat WC, Booth AM: Neurol control of penile erection. In: Maggi CA, ed. *The Autonomic Nervous System*. Nervous control of urogenital system. London, Harwood, 1993, pp 415–513.

Dinsmore W, Evans C: ABC of sexual health: Erectile dysfunction. *Br Med J* 318:387–390, 1999.

Eid JF, Dutta TC: Vacuum constriction devices for erectile dysfunction: A long-term, prospective study of patients with mild, moderate, and severe dysfunction. *Urology* 54:891–893: 1999.

Goldstein I: Current status of surgical correction of vasculogenic impotence. In Lytton B, Catalona WJ, Lipshultz LI, eds. *Advances in Urology,* vol. 7, St. Louis, Mosby, 1994, p 155.

Arterial revascularization procedures. *Semin Urol* 4:252, 1986.

Hashmat AI, Rehman J: In: Hashmat, Das S, eds. *The Penis*. Philadelphia, Lea and Febiger, 1993.

Hellstrom, WJG ed: *The Handbook of Sexual Dysfunction*. San Francisco, The American Society of Andrology, 1999.

Iacono F, Barra S, DeRossa G: Microstructral disorders of tunica albuginea in patients affected by impotence. *Eur Urol* 26:233–239, 1994.

Kirby RS, Carson C, Webster GD, eds: *Diagnosis and Management of Male Erectile Dysfunction*. London, Oxford, Butterworths-Heinneman, 1991.

Krane RJ, Siroky MB, Goldstein I, eds: *Male Sexual Dysfunction*. Boston, Little Brown, 1983.

Laumann E, Paik A, Rosen R: Sexual dysfunction in the United States. *JAMA* 281:537–544, 1999.

Lawless C, Cree J: Oral medications in the management of erectile dysfunction. *J Am Board Fam Pract* 11:307–314, 1998.

Lewis R, Barrett DM, eds: *Problems in Urology, Impotent Man*. Philadelphia, Lippincott, 1991, vol. 5.

Lewis RW; Long term results of penile prosthethesis implantations. *Urol Clin North Am* 7:381–401, 1995.

Lewis RW: Arteriovenous surgeries: Do they make any sense? In: Lue TF, ed. *World Book of Impotence*. London, Smith-Gordan, 1992, pp 199–220.

Lue TF: Intracavernous drug administration: Its role in diagnosis and treatment of impotence. *Semin Urol* 2:100–106, 1990.

Lue TF: Editorial comment. *J Urol* 152:1661, 1994.

Lugg J, Rajfer J: Drug therapy for erectile dysfunction. *A UA Update Series,* vol. 15, lesson 36, 289–296, 1996.

Melman A, Gingell JC: The epidemiology and pathophysiology of erectile dysfunction. *J Urol* 161:5–11, 1999.

Masters WH, Johnson VE: *Human Sexual Inadequacy.* Boston, Little Brown, 1970.

Montague DK: Editorial: Medical therapies for erectile dysfunction. *J Urol* 162:732, 1999.

Montague DK: The current status of penile prosthesis. *A UA Update Series,* vol. 8, lesson 29, 226–231, 1987.

Montague DK, ed: *Disorders of Male Sexual Function*. St. Louis, Mosby, 1987.

Newman HF, Northrup JD: Problems in male organic sexual physiology. *Urology* 21:443–450, 1983.

Padmanathan H, Shabsigh R: Sildenafil citrate (Viagara): A review. *A UA Update Series,* vol. 18, lesson 35, 273–280, 1999.

Reidl CR, Plas E, Engelhardt P, Daha K, Pfluger H: Iontophoresis for the treatment of Peyronie's disease. *J Urol* 163:95–99, 2000.

Shabsigh R, Fishman IJ, Toombs BD, Skolkin M: Venous leaks: Anatomical and physiological observations. *J Urol* 146:1260–1265, 1991.

Steers W: Erectile dysfunction. *AUA News* May/June 25, 1999.

Stief GS, Jonas U: Editorial: After the gold rush: Advancing research based care for patients with erectile dysfunction. *J Urol* 159:120–121, 1998.

Van Arsdalen KN, Wein AJ, Hanno PM, Malloy RT: Erectile failure following pelvic trauma: A review of pathophysiology, evaluation, and management, with particular reference to the penile prosthesis. *J Trauma* 24:579–585, 1984.

Walsh P, Retik A, Vaughan E, et al: *Campbell's Urology,* 7th ed. Philadelphia, Saunders Company, 1998.

Wagner G, Green R: *Impotence.* New York, Plenum, 1981.

Zilbergeld B: *Male Sexuality.* New York, Bantam, 1978.

Zorgniotti AW, Lefleur RS: Auto-injection of the corpus cavernosum with a vasoactive drug combination of vasculogenic impotence. *J Urol* 133:39–41, 1985.

SELF-ASSESSMENT QUESTIONS

1. How prevalant is male sexual dysfunction in the United States?
2. What are the two main erectile cylinders?
3. During erection, is there a contraction or the relaxation of the erectile tissues?
4. What is a major neurotransmitter for the erectile process?
5. What is the major cause of the flaccid state of penis?
6. What is the most common cause of priapism?
7. Is it true that the most common cause of male erectile dysfunction is psychogenic?
8. Other than a history and physical examination, what is the most common diagnostic examination performed in the office?
9. What is the most common drug used in the treatment of erectile dysfunction today?
10. What is the most common surgical treatment for erectile dysfunction?

CHAPTER 21
Male Fertility and Infertility

David M. Nudell
Paul J. Turek

I. BACKGROUND
A. The Problem
1. Approximately 25 percent of women will become pregnant after 1 month of trying to conceive with the same partner. However, only 80 percent of women will be pregnant after 1 year.
2. Approximately 15 to 20 percent of couples will, therefore, have difficulty achieving pregnancy in the woman.
3. During the evaluation of the couple, a male factor alone may be found in approximately 40 percent of couples, and both a male and female factor in an additional 20 percent such that a male factor may be involved in the infertility problem in approximately 60 percent of cases.

B. Chapter Plan: Topics Considered
1. Reproductive anatomy and physiology
2. Evaluation of the infertile male
3. Classification of male infertility problems
4. Treatment modalities

II. REPRODUCTIVE ANATOMY AND PHYSIOLOGY
A. Embryology
1. Genital organs are observed during the 5th gestational week and include an indifferent gonad, a mesonephric duct, and the müllerian ducts.
2. The indifferent gonad forms from a thickening in the urogenital ridge near the mesonephros; germ cells migrate from the yolk sac and populate the urogenital ridge.
3. Sexual differentiation of the embryo stems from the presence or absence of testis determining factor (TDF) located on the Y chromosome. This determines gonadal sex, which then forms the basis for gender-specific phenotypic development (Fig. 21-1).

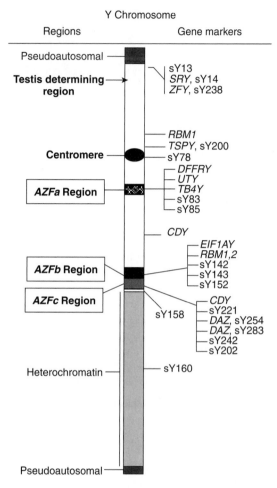

Figure 21-1 Schematic diagram of the human Y chromosome with known regions and gene segments listed. The testis determining region (SRY) is shown on the short arm (Yp) of the chromosome. AZF a,b,c denote the azoospermia regions of the chromosome.

4. Induced to form a testis, the gonad develops clustered cords of germ cells that converge to form the rete testis at the hilum of the testis.

5. During the 8th week of gestation, testosterone is made by differentiating Leydig cells and then declines in produc-

tion after the 12th week, during which, external genital development occurs.

6. The mesonephric duct forms the ureter in both genders and regionally specializes to form the vas deferens and epididymis in the male, joining with the testis in the form of ductuli efferentes testis.

7. The müllerian duct develops into fallopian tubes, the uterus, and the upper portion of the vagina in the female; in the male, this development is inhibited by a müllerian-inhibiting substance produced by the primitive testis. Except for the appendix testis and prostatic utricle, regression is otherwise complete.

8. Late in gestation, the testis descends caudally along the posterior abdominal wall as a result of differential growth and through the gubernaculum testis pulling toward the scrotum under endocrine control. Descent into the scrotum is usually completed by birth, although descent can still occur during the first year of life.

B. Gross Anatomy

1. The male reproductive system includes the following components: the testes and seminiferous tubules, efferent ductules and rete testis, epididymides, vasa deferentia, ejaculatory ducts, seminal vesicles, prostate, penis, and urethra.

2. From the standpoint of infertility, any consideration of anatomy must also include the hypothalamic–pituitary–gonadal axis.

C. Reproductive Hormonal Axis

1. Components (Fig. 21-2)
   a. Extrahypothalamic central nervous system
   b. Hypothalamus
   c. Pituitary
   d. Testes
   e. Steroid sensitive organs

2. Functions
   a. Normal male sexual development
   b. Maintenance of secondary sexual characteristics
   c. Male sexual behavior
   d. Sperm production and maturation

D. Extrahypothalamic Central Nervous System

1. The extrahypothalamic central nervous system is responsible for a variety of stimulatory and inhibitory influences on fertility.

2. The pathways of olfaction and vision are better defined in experimental animals than in humans.

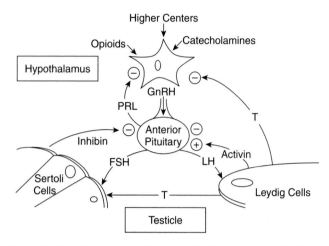

Figure 21-2 Inhibitory and stimulatory feedback loops within the hypothalamic–pituitary–testicular axis. GnRH, gonadotropin releasing hormone; PRL, prolactin; T, testosterone; LH, leutinizing hormone; FSH, follicle stimulating hormone.

3. In humans, the effects of stress of both a physical and/or emotional nature are probably mediated through this system, but again the mechanisms are unknown.

E. Hypothalamus—Gonadotropin Releasing Hormone (GnRH)
1. The hypothalamus is the center of integration for neuronal and humoral messages in the brain. The anterior and ventromedial nuclei are most important for male fertility.
2. The hypothalamus is responsible for production of GnRH, which is the primary releasing substance involved in male sexual function.

F. Pituitary—Leutinizing Hormone (LH) and Follicle-Stimulating Hormone (FSH)
1. The effect of GnRH is the production and release of LH and FSH from the anterior pituitary gland.
2. Both LH and FSH are glycopeptides with two molecular chains. They share a common alpha chain; specificity is determined by a unique beta chain.
3. LH and FSH are both secreted episodically. LH is rapidly metabolized, causing wide swings in its concentration within the bloodstream as determined by radioim-

munoassay techniques. This makes serum determination in patients difficult unless pooled blood samples are assayed. FSH is more slowly metabolized, resulting in a more constant level within the bloodstream.

4. The testes are the primary target for LH and FSH. No other target organs for these hormones have been found.

G. The Testes

1. Microscopic anatomy
   a. Seminiferous tubules comprise the bulk of the testis and are responsible for sperm production.
   b. The interstitium between the seminiferous tubules contains blood vessels, lymphatics, and Leydig cells.
2. Seminiferous tubule structural organization
   a. The tubules consist of long ducts lined by Sertoli cells that engulf and nurture the developing germ cells.
   b. Sertoli cells contain membrane receptors that bind FSH, resulting in increased intracellular cAMP and subsequent cytoskeletal reorganization for protein synthesis.
   c. The primary secretion products from Sertoli cells include müllerian-inhibiting substance in the fetus, androgen binding protein (ABP), transferrin, and inhibin (a nonsteroidal glycoprotein) in the adult.
   d. Sertoli cells appear responsible for regulation of the tubule microenvironment. They govern fluid secretions into the lumen of the seminiferous tubules, phagocytosis, steroid metabolism (in part), sperm production, and sperm movement through their development.
   e. Sertoli cells are also mainly responsible for the blood–testis barrier. This is an anatomic barrier created by the surrounding myoid cells, the basement membrane, and Sertoli cell tight junctions. In addition, a selective physiologic barrier is created by active transport processes across Sertoli cells. Further compartmentalization is established in that Sertoli cells divide the developing cells into two areas, the basal compartment for immature sperm forming cells and the adluminal compartment for germ cells undergoing maturation. This complex blood–testis barrier provides an immunologically privileged site for mature spermatozoa, as these haploid cells harbor unique specific antigens that are not otherwise recognized as "self" by the body's immune system.
3. Seminiferous tubules—spermatogenesis
   a. LH, FSH, and testosterone are all required for normal spermatogenesis.

b. Sertoli cells, lining 250 m of seminiferous tubules in the average testis, regulate the complex process of spermatogenesis.

c. A variety of germ cell types exists, including spermatogonia, primary spermatocytes, secondary spermatocytes, spermatids, and spermatozoa. Actually, 14 germinal cell subtypes are recognized histologically and are associated with six distinct stages of spermatogenesis. Spermatids and spermatozoa have a haploid complement of chromosomes.

d. The process of spermatogenesis takes about 74 days for completion. The average daily output is 125 million spermatozoa, which declines with age. A normal man makes 1200 sperm for every heartbeat.

e. Spermiogenesis is the maturation process of a spermatid to a spermatozoan. This includes nuclear condensation and a programmed repackaging of DNA from histones to protamines, acrosome formation, residual body separation from the sperm, and tail formation. It is one of the most complex series of morphologic changes undertaken by any mammalian cell.

4. Interstitium—Leydig cells

a. Leydig cells contain membrane receptors that bind LH, resulting again in cAMP production, protein kinase activation, and protein phosphorylation.

b. LH stimulation results in the conversion of cholesterol to testosterone in a steroidogenic pathway.

c. Testosterone diffuses into the plasma (endocrine function) or into the seminiferous tubule lumen (paracrine function). In the plasma, testosterone is bound (98 percent) to testosterone-estrogen binding globulin (TEBG) or albumin. Within the seminiferous tubules, testosterone is bound to androgen-binding protein (ABP).

d. Depending on the target tissue, testosterone may be active itself or may be reduced to dihydrotestosterone (DHT) by the enzyme 5-alpha reductase.

e. Testosterone is responsible in part for sexual differentiation, spermatogenesis, gonadotropin regulation, and sexual maturation and behavior.

H. Feedback Mechanisms

1. GnRH, LH, and FSH are generally thought to be responsible for driving the production of testosterone and spermatozoa as noted above. There are also feedback mechanisms, however, that regulate the production and release of these substances (Fig. 21-2).

2. LH regulation

    a. Testosterone and estradiol are the major negative feedback substances that control the formation and release of LH.

    b. Testosterone, therefore, regulates its own production and release by acting on the pituitary and hypothalamus.

    c. Estradiol is produced within the testicle and the liver as it is converted from testosterone (5-alpha reductase). It is found in smaller amounts within the blood stream but is more potent in action. The site of regulation is also at the level of the pituitary and hypothalamus.

3. FSH regulation

    a. Testosterone and estradiol are the major modulators of pituitary FSH secretion.

    b. In man, Sertoli cells produce inhibin, a two subunit hormone in the transforming growth factor family, which has an inhibitory effect on the pituitary FSH output. In contrast, activin, a glycoprotein formed as a homodimer of either inhibin chain, has a stimulatory effect on pituitary FSH. Neither inhibin nor activin affects pituitary LH release.

4. There also appear to be a variety of "short feedback loops" and a variety of other modulating substances that may act to more finely tune this system.

I. Testicular Transport

1. As noted previously, movement of developing germ cells from the basement membrane to the lumen and release into the lumen of the seminiferous tubules appears to be controlled by Sertoli cells. Unlike most mammalian species, the stages of spermatogenesis occur in a patchwork pattern and not in a wave-like manner within the seminiferous tubules.

2. The movement of the spermatozoa from the testis to the epididymis is controlled by four factors.

    a. Fluid pressure generated within the seminiferous tubule.

    b. Myoepithelial contractions of the seminiferous tubules.

    c. Contraction of the tunica albuginea of the testis.

    d. Cilia within and contraction of the wall of the efferent ductules.

3. The spermatozoa enter the epididymis in an immature state.

J. Epididymal Functions

1. Transport and storage

    a. The spermatozoa traverse the length of the epididymis in approximately 12 days. This process is governed by regular slow contractions of the muscular wall in a fashion similar to intestinal peristalsis.

    b. Approximately 700 million sperm are stored within the epididymes and vasa deferentia. Approximately 60 percent of these are stored within the tail (cauda) of the epididymides. Sperm become progressively more motile as they traverse the epididymal tubules, knowledge of which is important in harvesting sperm from the epididymis for *in* vitro fertilization (IVF) with intracytoplasmic sperm injection (ICSI).

    c. At the time of emission, regular coordinated contractions of the tails of the epididymides and the vasa deferentia occur, as mediated by the sympathetic nervous system, propelling sperm into the urethra. During ejaculation, somatic nervous system stimulated rhythmic contractions of periurethral and pelvic floor muscles propel the sperm through the urethra.

2. Sperm maturation

    a. The chemical composition of the intraluminal fluid and spermatozoa changes significantly as it traverses the three anatomic portions of the epididymis.

    b. A variety of membrane changes with regard to permeability and antigenicity also occur.

    c. Motility and fertilizing capacity are gained during transport through the epididymis.

    d. The final process of maturation, sperm capacitation, actually takes place after the sperm have been ejaculated and come in contact with the female reproductive tract. Fertilizing capacity lasts approximately 48 hours within the female internal genitalia, an important finding for counseling patients on the optimum frequency of sexual intercourse around the time of ovulation.

K. Semen Composition

1. The bulk of seminal fluid originates from the accessory ducts, with the spermatozoa adding a negligible amount to the total volume.

2. Prostatic fluid

    a. The prostatic fluid is usually found in the first part of the ejaculate and contributes approximately one third of the total volume.

    b. Specific prostate products include liquefaction factors like prostate specific antigen (PSA), zinc, citric acid, acid, phosphatase, and spermine. The latter substance, when oxidized to aldehydes, produces the characteristic odor of semen.

    c. PSA, a 33kd molecular weight serum protease in the family of glandular kallikreins, serves to liquefy the coagulum of human semen after 5 to 20 min following ejaculation.

3. Seminal vesicle fluid
    a. The seminal vesicle fluid is usually found in the second part of the ejaculate and contributes approximately two thirds of the total volume.
    b. Specific substances secreted by the seminal vesicles include coagulation factors, prostaglandins, and fructose.

III. CLINICAL EVALUATION OF THE SUBFERTILE MALE
A. Fertility History
1. Present relationship history
    a. Duration of infertility.
    b. Contraceptive methods and length of time used.
    c. Length of time trying to conceive.
    d. Number of pregnancies including miscarriages and therapeutic abortions, which gives an indication of the potential to conceive.
2. Previous history and relationships
    a. If the patient has attempted to conceive in the past, the duration and number of pregnancies achieved should be determined.
    b. The duration and number of pregnancies attempted or conceived by the woman or partner should also be determined.
    c. Previous marriages and divorces are common. Potential fertility problems may be suspected if one partner has previously attempted to conceive without success. However, the clinician must remember that the ability to conceive is a phenomenon involving both partners and, therefore, is ultimately determined by the current couple.
3. Sexual history
    a. *Frequency of intercourse and masturbation.* Overly frequent (daily) or infrequent (more than 48 hours apart around the time of ovulation) adversely affects the couple's ability to conceive.
    b. *Libido, potency, and sexual technique.* A normal desire and ability to have intercourse is critical and problems in these areas are often overlooked by clinicians.
    c. *Ejaculation.* One must be certain that ejaculation can occur deep within the vagina. Severe problems with premature ejaculation or severe hypospadias may prevent proper deposition of sperm.
    d. *Dyspareunia and the use of lubrication.* Problems with adequate natural vaginal lubrication can result in painful intercourse for either partner. Most accessory lubricants commonly used are spermicidal. The use of

vegetable oil based substances have been shown to be safe for sperm viability.

e. *Understanding of the ovulatory cycle.* It is important that the couple understand when ovulation occurs.

4. Genitourinary history

a. *Testicular descent.* Bilateral cryptorchidism is associated with impaired spermatogenesis and fertility. With unilateral maldescent, there is only a slight decrease in fertility potential.

b. *Sexual development and onset of puberty.*

c. *Infections.* Venereal, nonvenereal, mumps (at the time of puberty or later), recent febrile illness, or other infectious problems that directly involve the genitalia or urogenital duct system may be associated with a significant amount of scarring and subsequent fertility problems. Viral infections and other febrile illnesses not specifically involving the genitalia can also be related to decreased spermatogenesis and lowered sperm counts.

d. *Trauma or torsion.* Either condition can injure the duct system or result in ischemic damage to the seminiferous tubules.

e. *Exposure to chemicals.* A variety of drugs and industrial compounds may be associated with abnormal semen analyses.

f. *Exposure to heat.* Prolonged exposure to high temperatures can adversely affect spermatogenesis. It is presumed that hot tub baths, saunas, or steam rooms on a regular basis for long periods of time have significance in this regard, although this is not proven at present.

g. *Exposure to radiation.* Even small amounts of ionizing radiation, particularly that used for medical radiation therapy, can destroy sperm forming cells. Spermatogonia are particularly radiosensitive.

5. Previous infertility evaluation

a. *Patient.* A history of previous semen analyses and medical or surgical treatment is certainly important with regard to determining prognosis and additional therapeutic modalities that may be instituted to determine the etiology of infertility.

b. *Woman.* It is always wise to determine the type of fertility evaluation the patient's partner has undergone. Obviously, conception involves two people and if for some physiologic or anatomic reason, an irreversible problem exists in one of the partners, a successful outcome is not likely. The evaluation of each partner should be carried out simultaneously, and the evaluation of the male should be completed prior to performing any invasive procedures on the female partner.

B. General Medical History

1. Although most conditions causing male infertility do not lead to long-term medical consequences, 1 to 2 percent of men undergoing evaluation for infertility will have a significant underlying medical condition (Sigman et al., 1997).

   a. *Medical illnesses.* Medical problems such as diabetes and hypertension or their pharmacologic treatments can adversely affect erectile and ejaculatory function and hence, fertility.

   b. Abnormal metabolism of sex steroids can be associated with various liver and renal diseases and interfere with the regulatory mechanisms of spermatogenesis. Rare medical illnesses such as immotile cilia syndromes and Kartagener syndrome (ciliary defect with situs inversus) can adversely affect fertility.

2. Surgical history

   a. Inguinal herniorrhaphy, particularly when performed on a young child and when performed bilaterally, may be associated with injury to the vas deferens in 1 to 2 percent of patients.

   b. Surgery on the ureter, bladder, bladder neck, or urethra can result in problems with emission and/or ejaculation.

   c. Retroperitoneal surgery and other major pelvic procedures can result in failure of emission and/or problems with retrograde ejaculation. Young males with testis cancer are now being cured with great success. Many with nonseminomatous tumors are treated with retroperitoneal lymphadenectomy and subsequently have fertility problems due to absent ejaculation from either failure of emission or from retrograde ejaculation.

3. Current and past medications

   a. A variety of drugs and chemotherapeutic agents can adversely affect sperm production and/or function. The adverse affects are usually reversible upon discontinuation of the medication (Table 21-1).

4. Occupation and habits

   a. *Occupation and stress.* The effects of daily stress on fertility are poorly quantified. Severe, acute stress has been associated with decreases in ejaculate volume and sperm count. Most patients inquire about stress, but it is unlikely that they would change their job or style of living, making this a difficult problem to treat.

   b. The active ingredients in cigarettes, marijuana, coffee, tea, alcohol, and some naturopathic herbs have all been demonstrated in laboratory studies to be potentially gonadotoxic. The susceptibility of a given patient to these substances is difficult to quantify.

Table 21-1 Drugs and Chemicals with Potential Adverse Fertility Effects

Alcohol
Alkylating agents (e.g., cyclophosphamide)
Arsenic
Aspirin (large doses)
Caffeine
Cimetidine
Colchicine
Dibromochloropropane (pesticide)
DES
Lead
Monoamine oxidase inhibitors
Marijuana
Medoxyprogesterone
Nicotine
Nitrofurantoins
Phenytoin
Spironolactone
Sulfasalazine
Testosterone

5. Family history
   a. Sibling fertility status may help to identify familial conditions like cystic fibrosis and congenital adrenal hyperplasia.
   b. In utero exposure to diethylstilbestrol (DES) can result in testicular, epididymal, and penile anatomic abnormalities. Despite the finding of impaired semen quality in DES-exposed men, proof of decreased fertility has not been shown in extensive follow-up studies.

C. **Physical Examination**
   1. *General examination.* The general physical examination evaluates the patient's body habitus and secondary sexual characteristics. In particular, the pattern of hair distribution and presence or absence of gynecomastia are evidence of general endocrine disorders.
   2. *Examination of the genitalia.* The genitalia are the most important aspect of the examination. This should be performed in a systematic fashion, taking care to palpate and evaluate the areas listed as follows.
      a. *Penis.* The size of the penis and location of the meatus are important in assuring the delivery of spermatozoa deep within the vagina at ejaculation.

b. *Testes.* The location, size, and consistency of the testes should be noted. The testes should be in a dependent part of the scrotum. Testicular size is particularly important; the bulk of the testicle (80 to 90 percent) is composed of seminiferous tubules that are involved in sperm production. The size of each testis can be compared to the other testis as well as to normal values by noting the length and width of the testicle or by attempting to quantify the volume by comparison to plastic models of known volumes. The normal testicle in the adult is greater than 4 cm in length and greater than 2.5 cm in width (20 mL). Each testicle should be of a firm consistency. Ethnic variations in testis size are well described.

c. *Epididymides.* The epididymides should be examined for size and consistency. The obstructed epididymis feels enlarged and firm. The epididymis that is scarred from either trauma or chronic infection may be hard and irregular. Part of the epididymis may be missing in association with congenital absence of the vasa deferentia.

d. *Vasa deferentia.* Each vas deferens should be palpable as a distinct, firm, cord-like structure in the scrotum. In 1 to 2 percent of infertile men, one or both vasa are not palpable in the scrotum, a condition termed congenital absence of the vas deferens (CAVD).

e. *Spermatic cords.* Each spermatic cord should be evaluated for size and consistency with the patient in both the upright and supine positions. The patient should be asked to perform a Valsalva maneuver while standing to accentuate differences in blood volume maintained within the cord, characteristic of a varicocele. The internal spermatic veins fill while standing and this filling may be increased when the Valsalva maneuver is performed. In the supine position, these veins drain more easily and, hence, the varicocele is not as easily palpable. Persistent fullness in the spermatic cord upon reclining is suggestive of cord lipoma and not varicocele. Other abnormalities involving the spermatic cord include hydrocele and spermatocele, which may be detected during this examination.

f. *Inguinal region.* The inguinal canals are palpated looking for evidence of inguinal hernias. In addition, the inguinal regions should be inspected to assess if previous surgery in this area may have injured the vasa deferentia or testicular blood supply.

3. *Rectal examination.* A general rectal examination should be performed to detect lower gastrointestinal pathology.

The rectal examination is useful to examine the prostate and seminal vesicles. The prostate should be small and benign in consistency without tenderness or evidence of inflammation. The seminal vesicles are generally not palpable under normal conditions but may be palpable with obstruction of the ejaculatory ducts.

D. Semen Analyses

1. *Collection.* Generally, at least two semen analyses are needed to establish a baseline for a patient. If a discrepancy exists between the results, a third or, perhaps, even a fourth specimen may be required. Each semen analysis is collected after a 2 to 3 day period of abstinence. The specimen is generally collected by masturbation into a clean, dry, glass container and examined within 2 hours. If the specimen is collected at the patient's home, great care must be taken to keep it near body temperature during transportation to the laboratory (shirt pocket). The patient should avoid lubricants during specimen collection. If needed, silicone condom devices are available.

2. *Minimal standards of adequacy.* There is no absolute measure of fertility on semen analysis. Minimal standards of semen adequacy have been defined by the World Health Organization (Table 21-2).

3. *Additional physical parameters.* Other properties examined at the time of a routine semen analysis include:
   a. *Color.* The semen is generally grayish in color with an opalescent character. It may also appear lumpy.
   b. *Coagulation.* This occurs immediately after ejaculation.
   c. *Liquefaction.* This occurs 5 to 30 min following ejaculation. Prostatic specific antigen (PSA) is the serine protease responsible for this process.

Table 21-2 Semen Analysis: Minimal Standards of Adequacy

Seen on at least two occasions:	
Ejaculate volume	1.5–5.0 mL
Sperm density	> 20 million/mL
Motility	> 60% motile
Forward progression	> 2.0 (scale 0–4)
Morphology (WHO)	> 30% normal morphology
(Strict)	> 14% normal morphology

and

No significant sperm agglutination
No significant pyospermia
No hyperviscosity

    d. *Viscosity.* This parameters refers to the fluid consistency of the semen after coagulation and liquefaction have occurred. Viscosity is normal if it is possible to pour the semen in a drop by drop fashion.

    e. *pH.* The pH of semen is normally in the range of 7.2 to 8.0.

    f. *Fructose.* As noted previously, fructose is produced by the seminal vesicles. It is important to check the semen fructose in cases of azoospermia and when the ejaculate volume is less than 1 mL. Absence of fructose in semen suggests absence of the vasa deferentia and seminal vesicles, ejaculatory duct obstruction, or dysfunction of the seminal vesicles.

E. Other Laboratory Tests

1. *Urinalysis.* This test is useful to rule out infection of the lower genitourinary tract and associated glandular structures.

2. *Endocrine evaluation.* A complete hormonal evaluation includes measurement of serum LH, FSH, testosterone, and prolactin, and 99% of endocrine conditions can be detected through the initial measurement of serum FSH and testosterone only. Hormonal testing can differentiate between hypogonadism due to hypothalamic or pituitary disease and hypogonadism due to primary testicular failure.

3. Other tests regularly recommended in the past now appear to be unnecessary on a routine basis. These include tests of thyroid and adrenal function (less than 0.5 percent of cases). Prolactin levels should be determined if a low testosterone is found or if the patient has gynecomastia, severe headaches, or visual disturbances. Prolactin-secreting pituitary tumors produce high levels of circulating prolactin, and these lesions tend to reduce LH and FSH levels by pituitary compression within the sella tursica.

4. *Genetic testing.* Karyotype analysis is critical for all men with azoospermia and severe oligospermia who are planning IVF/ICSI. In addition, it is now known that specific deletions in the Y chromosome are found in approximately 15 percent of men with azoospermia and 5 to 8 percent of men with severe oligospermia. Several regions of the long arm of the Y chromosome have been classified as azoospermic factor (AZF) regions (Fig. 21-1). Most deletions are found in the AZFc region in a specific gene complex termed *DAZ* (deleted in azoospermia) (Reijo et al, 1996). Deletions in this region appear specific for infertility as they have not been found in fertile men. However, it has been difficult to correlate specific AZF deletions regions with specific histologic findings in the testis.

5. Test of sperm function
   a. *Mucus penetration test.* This test of sperm function determines how spermatozoa move through a mucus medium similar to that found in the cervix. The simplest form of this is the postcoital test in which a specimen of preovulatory, thin cervical mucus is obtained for examination several hours after coitus. Sperm numbers and motility, and cervical mucus quality are assessed to determine whether there is a problem with semen deposition. The most common cause of abnormal mucus penetration is incorrect timing; the cervical mucus is hostile to sperm at all times except during ovulation. Using in vitro variations of this test with standardized mucus media, cross-penetration assays (patient and donor sperm are compared to partner and donor cervical mucus, respectively) are used to better quantify this interaction.
   b. *Hamster egg penetration test.* This is a cross-species assay that assesses the ability of human spermatozoa to penetrate zona pellucida-free hamster eggs. The zone pellucida is digested from the hamster egg, since it is this layer that determines the species-specific penetration ability of sperm. Although not commonly used, this test can assess several steps necessary for sperm capacitation.
6. *Antisperm antibodies.* A link between infertility and antisperm antibodies has been recognized for many years. The effect of these antibodies is to disturb either of two processes: sperm transport through the female reproductive tract or sperm–egg interaction. Enzyme-linked immunosorbent assay (ELISA) and immunobead binding assay are two commonly used tests to detect the presence of antibodies on sperm.
7. *White blood cells.* Reproductive tract infections are a treatable cause of infertility and are often heralded by the presence of excessive white blood cells in the ejaculate. Special stains are needed to distinguish white cells from immature germ cells, the latter of which are not pathologic.

F. Radiologic procedures
1. *Transrectal ultrasound (TRUS).* TRUS is indicated in infertile men with low-volume ejaculates (less than 1.5 mL). Ejaculatory duct obstruction (EDO) may be identified by seminal vesicle dilatation (larger than 1.5 cm in diameter); seminal vesicle hypoplasia or absence is also easily diagnosed. Often the cause EDO, stones, scar, cysts, or a persistent utricle can also be diagnosed by TRUS. Seminal vesicle fluid can be sampled to confirm the presence

of sperm in patients with suspected obstruction or seminal vesiculography can be done to demonstrate obstruction radiographically.

2. *Vasography.* Classically, intraoperative, transcrotal vasography is used to detect abdominal vas deferens and seminal vesicle and ejaculatory duct patency prior to definitive surgery for obstruction.

3. *Scrotal ultrasound.* A scrotal ultrasound is indicated when the testes are not easily palpable due to coexistent hydrocele, to confirm the origin and character (solid versus cystic) of intrascrotal masses, and for confirming the presence of a clinically suspicious varicocele.

IV. CLASSIFICATION OF ABNORMALITIES
A. General Information

1. A variety of classification schemes have been developed to categorize fertility problems. One of the most useful schemes is based on the findings on semen analyses with initial classification of problems into one of four categories: (1) all parameters normal, (2) azoospermia, (3) a single abnormal parameter and (4) multiple abnormal parameters.

2. Distribution of semen abnormalities among infertile men:

Azoospermia	8%
Single abnormal parameter	37%
Multiple abnormal parameters	55%

Among the single abnormal parameters, isolated abnormalities in motility account for the majority of cases.

B. All Parameters Normal

1. When two semen analyses are normal and the history and physical examination are not suggestive of a specific fertility problem in the male, further evaluation of the female partner is recommended.

2. If the evaluation of the female partner is also found to be normal, and the couple still have not conceived, then the tests of sperm function noted previously (i.e., the mucus penetration and hamster egg penetration tests) may be useful. Most couples with unexplained infertility will go on to be treated with intrauterine insemination (IUI) or in vitro fertilization (IVF).

C. Azoospermia

1. When no sperm are found on semen analysis, the specimen should be centrifuged to confirm the absence of any sperm in the specimen (Fig. 21-3). In addition, a collection error and/or retrograde ejaculation must be ruled out as

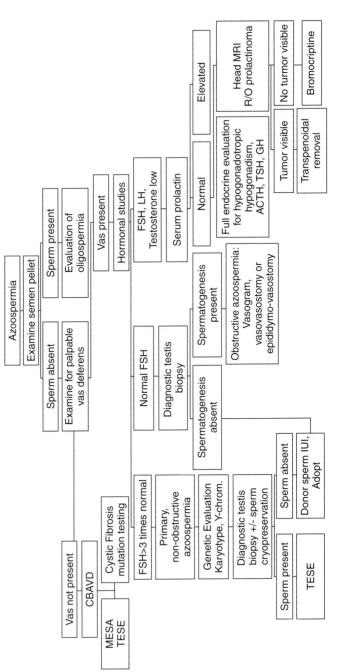

Figure 21-3 Algorithm for the azoospermic patient. CBAVD, congenital bilateral absence of the vas deferens; MESA, microscopic epididymal sperm aspiration; TESE, testicular sperm extraction; FSH, follicle stimulating hormone; LH, leutinizing hormone; ACTH, adrenocorticotropic hormone; TSH, thyroid stimulating hormone; GH, growth hormone.

causes of azoospermia. If retrograde ejaculation is identified by the finding of sperm in the urine (more than 10 to 15 sperm per high-power field), treatment can be initiated with oral alkalization and sympathomimetic agents to promote antegrade ejaculation. Alternatively, sperm can be retrieved from the bladder, processed, and used for IUI.

2. The results of the fructose test and gonadotropin levels determine what additional evaluation and treatment is necessary.

   a. The LH, FSH, and testosterone levels can differentiate primary testicular failure from secondary testicular failure caused by either pituitary or hypothalamic dysfunction.

   b. A serum FSH greater than three times normal along with atrophic testicles on physical examination is essentially equivalent to a "medical biopsy" of the testis and indicates severe testicular failure. This finding obviates the need for a surgical biopsy to rule out obstructive conditions; however, sperm can be found in many of these men for use with IVF/ICSI by testicular sperm extraction techniques (TESE).

3. After ruling out a major endocrine abnormality, the major differential diagnosis is ductal obstruction or testicular failure.

   a. *Negative fructose test.* Three possibilities exist in the azoospermic patient with normal hormone studies and a negative fructose test. These include congenital bilateral absence of the seminal vesicles and vas deferens, bilateral ejaculatory duct obstruction and, rarely, a type of retrograde ejaculation with scant antegrade ejaculation that contains no sperm or fructose. The treatment of CAVD is direct sperm aspiration from the remnant of the head of the epididymis. The sperm are then processed and used in combination with in vitro fertilization (IVF) techniques. Ejaculatory duct obstruction is managed by transurethrally resecting the ejaculatory ducts or unroofing midline cysts.

   b. *Positive fructose test.* A positive fructose test usually rules out complete obstruction of the ejaculatory ducts and severe dysfunction of the seminal vesicles but does not give an indication of the patency of the ductal system from the level of the testis to the ejaculatory ducts. Therefore, a positive fructose test in azoospermia does not differentiate between proximal ductal obstruction and testicular failure.

   c. *Testicular biopsy.* A testicular biopsy is necessary in the azoospermic patient with normal hormones and normal sized testes who has fructose in the ejaculate.

The microscopic examination of the biopsy will indicate whether spermatogenesis is progressing normally. With the advent of IVF/ICSI, sperm found on testicular biopsy can be cryopreserved for future use.

d. If the testicular biopsy indicates active and complete spermatogenesis, scrotal exploration and vasography are indicated. A vasogram is performed by injecting contrast material through one vas deferens to determine its patency. If patency is demonstrated, then exploration of the epididymis is required to determine the site of obstruction. Fluid within the vas deferens lumen should also be examined microscopically to determine if sperm are present or absent. A microscopic vasoepididymostomy is necessary to correct intraepididymal obstruction. If no spermatozoa are detected in the tubules of the epididymis during this exploration, then intratesticular ductal obstruction may be the cause of azoospermia. Since these cases are difficult to correct, IVF and ICSI with testicular sperm is recommended.

D. Multiple Abnormal Parameters on the Semen Analysis
1. Diffuse abnormalities of all or many of the seminal parameters is the most common pathologic pattern identified (55 percent). Determination of the LH, FSH, and testosterone levels are essential to rule out an endocrine abnormality.
2. Stress, infections, and other nonspecific environmental factors such as heat, drugs, and toxin exposures may produce a transient abnormality of all seminal parameters. Therefore, when other specific factors cannot be identified by the history or physical examination, it may be beneficial to follow these patients for an additional 6 to 12 months to determine if there is any self-correction of the abnormality. After this, if spontaneous correction has not occurred, nonspecific therapy can be instituted as discussed below or, more commonly, couples can be offered assisted reproductive technology (IUI, IVF).
3. Varicoceles
   a. A varicocele is defined as dilated, varicose internal spermatic veins producing fullness, dilatation, and poor drainage of the pampiniform plexus. A varicocele is found in 10 to 20 percent of males in the general population but is found in 35 to 40 percent of men presenting with infertility problems and results in abnormal semen parameters. Historically, the repair of varicoceles was based on case reports of oligospermic and azoospermic males who became normospermic and whose wives became pregnant following varicocele ligation.

b. Varicoceles are classified according to size as either large, medium, or small. Large varicoceles can be seen as a "bag of worms" beneath the scrotal skin. Medium varicoceles are readily detected by palpation, especially on standing. Small varicoceles can only be identified by noticing an impulse in the scrotum with the Valsalva maneuver or a difference in the size and fullness of the spermatic cord when the patient moves from the standing to the supine position. The majority of single varicoceles occur on the left side, but bilateral varicoceles are more common than previously believed.

c. The exact mechanism through which the varicocele exerts its detrimental effect is not completely clear; the leading theory is that it leads to increased intrascrotal temperature through retrograde venous blood flow. An increased number of immature and tapered sperm are noted. There may also be decreased sperm motility and varying degrees of oligospermia.

d. Treatment of varicocele involves one of several surgical approaches or transvenous angiographic identification and embolization of the involved internal spermatic veins. The usual surgical approach is retroperitoneal, inguinal, or subinguinal ligation of the internal spermatic and collateral veins. Laparoscopy has also been used and may have a role in bilateral varicocele repair. Newer interventional angiographic techniques and catheters have made it possible to selectively catheterize the internal spermatic veins and introduce a variety of substances, including sclerosing solutions, balloons, and stainless-steel coils to occlude veins.

e. Results of varicocele ligation from a large number of series indicate approximately a 70 percent improvement in semen quality associated with a 40 percent pregnancy rate. With initial sperm counts greater than 10 million sperm per milliliter, the improvement in pregnancy rates is significantly better than if the initial counts are less than 10 million sperm per milliliter. Both surgical and angiographic techniques for occlusion of varicoceles have a small failure rate with persistence and/or recurrence of the varicocele noted during follow-up. Pregnancies, when they occur, generally are noted 6 to 9 months following varico-celectomy.

E. Isolated Abnormal Parameter on Semen Analysis

1. Abnormal semen volume

a. *Large ejaculate volume.* A volume greater than 5.5 mL may result in dilution of the spermatozoa and poor cervical placement of seminal fluid during intercourse (Fig. 21-4). Mechanical concentration of the

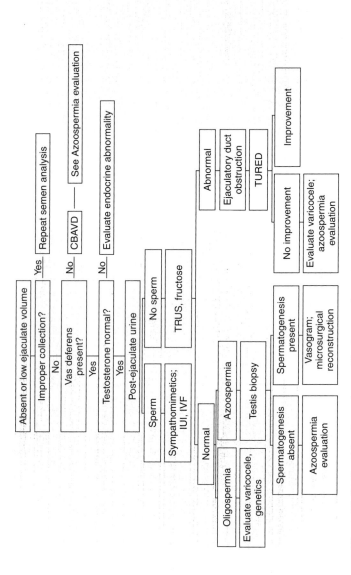

Figure 21-4 Algorithm for patients with absent or low volume (< 1.5 mL) ejaculate. CBAVD, congenital bilateral absence of the vas deferens; IUI, intrauterine insemination; IVF, in vitro fertilization; TRUS, transrectal ultrasound; TURED, transurethral resection of the ejaculatory ducts.

spermatozoa and artificial insemination may be employed if necessary.

   b. *Absent or low ejaculate volume.* Once a collection abnormality has been ruled out, it is essential to consider retrograde ejaculation, infection of the accessory sex glands, or endocrine dysfunction (low testosterone) (Fig. 21-5). The presence of retrograde ejaculation is confirmed by the finding of large quantities of spermatozoa in the postejaculatory urine sample (more than 15 sperm per HPF). Sympathomimetic drugs with α-adrenergic activity may be useful in reversing this problem in some patients. In others, it may be necessary to obtain, wash, and inseminate sperm collected from the postejaculate urine sample. Endocrine abnormalities and infections are treated with the appropriate hormones and antibiotics.

2. *Hyperviscosity.* Problems with hyperviscous semen are rare and may reflect enzymatic imbalance in the semen. A check of the split ejaculate can be useful, as the first portion may be less viscous than the second portion and therefore can be used for artificial insemination. Mechanical disruption of the sample to decrease viscosity, followed by artificial insemination is useful in this situation.

3. Decreased motility and forward progression (asthenospermia)

   a. This is the **most common** isolated abnormality found on analysis of semen and is due to endocrine dysfunction, infection of accessory glands, a varicocele, or epididymal dysfunction. Specific therapy is available for the first three problems. Unfortunately, epididymal dysfunction at the present time is poorly understood and treated.

   b. Sperm motility and forward progression can also be adversely affected by the presence of antisperm antibodies that agglutinate (clump) or immobilize the spermatozoa. Special tests are now available to determine the presence and levels of antisperm antibodies in the semen. Several therapeutic modalities have been tried including sperm washing and short-term treatment with systemic steroids.

4. Oligospermia

   a. Decreased sperm numbers as an isolated problem may be secondary to endocrine dysfunction and genetic or idiopathic conditions. Occasionally the absolute number of sperm is relatively normal, but the number of sperm per milliliter may appear to be low due to the presence of a large ejaculate volume. With sperm densities below 10×10^6/mL, a karyotype analysis and

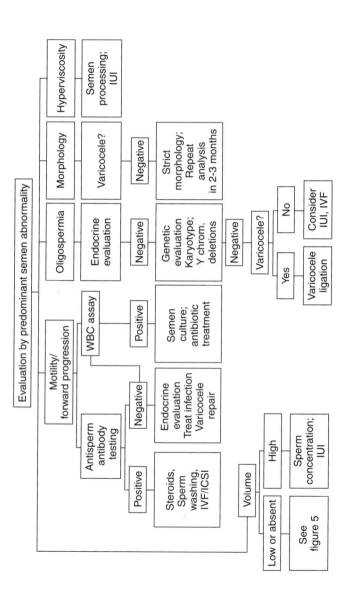

Figure 21-5 Algorithm for the patient with a single predominant abnormality on semen analysis. IUI, intrauterine insemination, WBC, white blood cell; IVF/ICSI, in vitro fertilization with intracytoplasmic sperm injection.

specific deletions in the Y chromosome should be evaluated (Fig. 21-1).

b. In general, there are two treatments for oligospermia. One attempts to stimulate the testes with a variety of drugs to increase the output of spermatozoa (see later section on idiopathic infertility). Alternatively, with advances in assisted reproduction, spermatozoa can be concentrated for use with artificial insemination with IUI. In addition, IVF and ICSI are very powerful methods to produce pregnancies when simpler approaches fail and may be necessary in cases where the above methods fail.

5. *Abnormal morphology.* An isolated problem with morphology is very unusual. It may be a transient abnormality that is self-correcting. There is no known method of treatment.

F. Empirical Treatment of Idiopathic Infertility

1. Second only to the large number of patients who have varicoceles, idiopathic infertility is the next largest group of patients. In fact, nonresponders to varicocele ligation may belong in this category. Essentially, idiopathic infertility refers to men who have an abnormal parameter or parameters on the semen analyses with a normal history, physical examination, and screening hormone analysis. The etiology of the abnormal semen quality is unclear and probably reflects the incomplete knowledge regarding normal spermatogenesis and genetics. Many of these cases are likely to have genetic etiologies that will be evident as knowledge grows.

2. *Nonpharmacologic treatment modalities.* A variety of nonpharmacologic treatment modalities have been suggested, but their efficacy has not been demonstrated. These include the following:

   a. *Vitamins and diet.* Specific vitamins and changes in dietary habits have not been associated with improved semen quality and fertility. Antioxidant therapy has been shown to increase motility during in vitro isolation of sperm (Parinaud et al, 1997), but treatment of men with severe asthenospermia with high dose vitamin E and C did not improve motility in one large, randomized study (Rolf et al, 1999). However, such therapy may be helpful for tobacco smokers to reduce oxidative effects on sperm.

   b. *Changing from jockey shorts to boxer shorts.* Most males have already performed this maneuver prior to being evaluated in the infertility clinic with persistence of their problem. A recent study has refuted the old idiom that a switch from jockey to boxer shorts improves spermatogenesis and semen parameters.

   c. Prostatic massage.

   d. Antibiotics for "occult infection."

   e. Varicocelectomy for the "occult varicocele."

3. Drug therapy for idiopathic infertility

   a. The use of human menopausal gonadotropin (hMG) (Pergonal), essentially FSH; human chorionic gonadotropin (hCG) (APL), essentially LH; or the combination of hMG and hCG has not resulted in significant improvement in sperm counts in idiopathic infertility. They have not been associated with significantly higher pregnancy rates in various studies. GnRH therapy, when given in a pulsatile fashion, has the potential to raise LH and FSH levels, but its administration is complex and costly.

   b. *Testosterone rebound.* This method utilizes complete suppression of spermatogenesis with exogenous testosterone followed by discontinuation of therapy after the patient's sperm counts have been reduced to zero. It is hoped that the recovery of spermatogenesis will be greater than it was prior to therapy. However, there is no physiologic basis for this finding and it has been therapeutically abandoned.

   c. Clomiphene citrate is an antiestrogen that has been used nonspecifically for idiopathic infertility. The scientific rationale for its use is based on its ability to block the negative feedback of estradiol on the hypothalamic–pituitary axis, resulting in increased LH and FSH levels. Overall improvement in the semen analysis is noted in approximately 50 percent of patients and pregnancies occurring in 25 to 30 percent of patients in uncontrolled studies. Men with low-normal testosterone and FSH levels may be the best responders to this therapy.

   d. Tamoxifen is also an antiestrogen that prevents feedback inhibition of GnRH, thus increasing LH and FSH levels. This agent, however, lacks the estrogenic activities of clomiphene and may provide equal efficacy.

   e. Kallikreins may act to increase the blood supply to the testes and may also stimulate prostaglandin synthesis through the production of kinins. Improvement in sperm motility but not overall sperm counts have been seen experimentally with the kallikreins. Presently, the compound is not available in the United States.

   f. L-Carnitine is found in high concentrations in the normal epididymis and is postulated to be important for sperm motility. Oral L-carnitine is currently being evaluated in a multicenter, randomized study to evaluate its possible beneficial effect on sperm motility.

4. Assisted reproductive techniques (ART)

   a. ART attempts to improve the conception by bypassing many or all of the barriers associated with normal fertilization (Fig. 21-6). The simplest techniques involve sperm processing and insemination of the female; the more sophisticated ones involve manipulation of the sperm and ova extracorporeally. Fertilization with these procedures can occur in vitro or in vivo.

   b. Semen processing is used as an isolated procedure or in conjunction with ova processing. Sperm washing, swim-ups, sedimentations, and Percoll gradient centrifugations are commonly employed to remove seminal plasma and leukocytes and to select for and concentrate highly motile sperm. Theoretically, with these procedures, fewer sperm than normal are needed since at least initially, they are placed higher within the female reproductive tract than is an ejaculate during intercourse.

   c. Intrauterine insemination (IUI) can be used to treat male factor infertility. In this technique, a small catheter is used to inject processed sperm through the cervix and into the uterine cavity. By bypassing the cervical mucus, a larger number of motile sperm can progress to the fallopian tubes where normal fertilization occurs. Indications for IUI include male factor and cervical mucus problems, and anatomic abnormalities that may prevent sperm deposition at the cervical os. Usually, greater than 5 million total motile sperm are required for IUI. Pregnancy rates are variable with these techniques, but average 30 to 35 percent in couples who try 3 to 4 times.

   d. IVF, first introduced in 1978, was developed to manage fallopian tube obstruction. It is now important for male factor infertility. Female partners undergo ovarian hyperstimulation to induce the maturation of multiple oocytes, which are harvested ultrasonographically, prior to ovulation. Processed semen and recovered oocytes are mixed in vitro. If fertilization occurs, embryos are placed back into the uterus transcervically. Usually only 20 to 30 percent of replaced embryos survive and become clinical pregnancies. Of those couples who fail the first IVF attempt, 10 to 18 percent will fertilize on the second cycle. Depending on the cause of infertility, and the number of embryos replaced, pregnancy rates can approach 40 to 50 percent per IVF attempt.

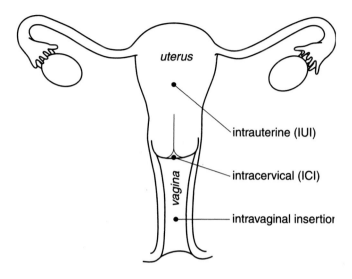

Figure 21-6 A. Available locations for insemination of embryos in the female reproductive tract.

    e. In gamete intrafallopian transfer (GIFT), sperm and ova are placed into the fallopian tubes prior to fertilization. This is done in lieu of uterine placement with the hope that higher pregnancy rates will be achieved if more physiologic placement is used. As this procedure does not improve on the fertilizing capacity of sperm, it has no benefit over IVF in male factor infertility. If zygotes or embryos are transferred to the fallopian tube instead of sperm and ova, the benefits of IVF are added to GIFT. If zygote stage fertilized eggs are transferred, then the technique is called zygote intrafallopian transfer (ZIFT) or pronuclear stage tubal transfer (PROUST). Early embryo stage transfers are labeled tubal embryo transfer (TET) or tubal embryo stage transfer (TEST). Given the recent success of IVF and ICSI, the role of adding tubal transfer to IVF has undergone serious reexamination.

    f. *Micromanipulation.* Sperm and oocyte micromanipulation by intracytoplasmic sperm injection (ICSI) has become the mainstay of addressing the poor fertilizing capacity of sperm often seen in male factor infertility. By injecting a single sperm directly into an oocyte, multiple barriers of fertilization are bypassed and suc-

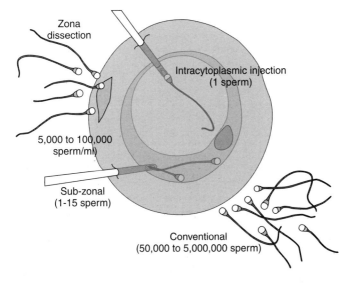

Figure 21-6 (*continued*). **B.** Available methods of in vitro fertilization with micromanipulation of gametes.

cess rates (when compared to standard IVF) are greatly improved. Pregnancy rates of 40 to 50 percent have been obtained using this technique even in the most severe cases of male factor infertility. In addition, not only ejaculated sperm but sperm retrieved from the male reproductive tract are capable of producing pregnancies with ICSI. Vasal, epididymal, and even testicular sperm are now routinely used with this technique.

5. IVF with ICSI should not be performed without karyotype analysis on both partners. Despite great success with ICSI, there remain concerns. Multiple gestations occur in 30 to 40 percent of pregnancies and place a financial and social burden for many. ICSI bypasses many mechanisms of natural selection such that many men would not be able to conceive under normal circumstances are now able to father children. Studies of children born by this technique to date have shown no increase in major or minor birth defects or in developmental milestones. One study showed a significant increase in sex chromosomal abnormalities among ICSI offspring (0.8 percent) that may be attributable to the chromosomal status of the fathers rather than to the technique itself (Bonduelle et al, 1996). As previously

mentioned, from 5 to 8 percent of men with severe oligospermia have deletions in the AZF region of the Y chromosome. It has been shown conclusively that these genetic deletions are passed to the male offspring produced by these fathers through IVF/ICSI (Mulhall et al, 1997). Finally, sperm obtained from some infertile men have been shown recently to have mutations in specific genes that could affect the ability of DNA to repair itself in the offspring. Clearly, children born by ICSI should be followed closely to ensure normal development.

Preimplantation genetic diagnosis is now possible by sampling a single cell from an eight-cell developing embryo in vitro and performing either fluorescent in situ hybridization (FISH) or single-cell polymerase chain reaction (PCR) to examine for aneuploidies, chromosomal translocations, or even specific diseases caused by point mutations. As this technology develops, genetic counseling will become more and more important for these couples.

V. CONCLUSION

The knowledge of the physiology of sperm production, maturation, and transport through the male urogenital system continues to evolve. At this point, fewer male patients evaluated for infertility have an undefined etiology for their condition. Clinicians are beginning to uncover many of the chromosomal and even molecular mechanisms necessary for normal sperm production. Clearly, more genes like those recently found on the Y chromosome in men with infertility will be discovered. At the same time, technology has outstripped the understanding of sperm development, and we are now able to bypass what were in the past natural barriers that prevented the inheritance of genetic defects. As a consequence, the study of human reproduction is in a very exciting and active period at present.

Despite many high-technology advances, the evaluation and treatment of male patients with infertility remains cost effective. The male factor evaluation is centered on a careful history, physical examination, and hormonal and semen analysis. This process helps to define pathologic and otherwise treatable conditions and identifies ways to correct, and not bypass, the infertility problem.

BIBLIOGRAPHY

Bonduelle M, Wilikens A, Buysse A, et al: Prospective follow-up study of 877 children born after intracytoplasmic sperm injection (ICSI), with ejaculated epididymal and testicular spermatozoa and after replacement of cryopreserved embryos obtained after ICSI. *Hum Reprod* (suppl) 4:131–155; discussion 156–159, 1996.

Mulhall JP, Reijo R, Alagappan R, et al: Azoospermic men with deletion of the DAZ gene cluster are capable of completing spermatogenesis: Fertilization, normal embryonic development and pregnancy occur when retrieved testicular spermatozoa are used for intracytoplasmic sperm injection. *Hum Reprod,* 12:503–508, 1997.

Parinaud J, Le Lannou D, Vieitez G, Griveau JF, Milhet P, Richoilley G: Enhancement of motility by treating spermatozoa with an antioxidant solution (Sperm-Fit) following ejaculation. *Hum Reprod* 12:2434–2436, 1997.

Reijo R, Alagappan RK, Patrizio P, Page DC: Severe oligospermia resulting from deletions of azoospermia factor gene on Y chromosome. *Lancet* 347:1290–1293, 1996.

Rolf C, Cooper TG, Yeung CH, Nieschlag E: Antioxidant treatment of patients with asthenozoospermia or moderate oligoasthenozoospermia with high-dose vitamin C and vitamin E: A randomized, placebo-controlled, double-blind study. *Hum Reprod* 14:1028–1033, 1999.

Schlegel PN, Chang TSK: Physiology of male reproduction. In: Walsh PC, Retik A, Vaughan ED Jr., Wein A, eds. *Campbell's Urology,* 7th ed. Philadelphia, Saunders, 1998, pp 1254–1286.

Sigman M, Howards SS: Male infertility. In: Walsh PC, Retik A, Vaughan ED Jr., Wein A, eds. *Campbell's Urology,* 7th ed. Philadelphia, Saunders, 1998, pp 1287–1330.

Sigman M, Jarow JP: Endocrine evaluation of infertile men. *Urology* 50:659–664, 1997.

SELF-ASSESSMENT QUESTIONS

1. Embryologically, the vas deferens and body of the epididymis are derived from what developmental structure?
   a. Müllerian ducts
   b. Wolffian ducts
   c. Urogenital ridge
   d. Gubernaculum testis
2. Within the testicle, which cell type is responsible for testosterone production?
   a. Sertoli cell
   b. Myoid cell
   c. Leydig cell
   d. Spermatozoa
3. In the male infertility evaluation, which of the following findings is the most important to suggest whether or not there is a significant male factor present?
   a. Normal FSH and testosterone levels
   b. Normal testis size
   c. Normal semen analysis
   d. A history of paternity
4. One feature of the semen analysis that may indicate an obstructive condition is:
   a. the presence of white blood cells.
   b. the presence of red blood cells.
   c. the presence of fructose.
   d. a basic seminal pH (> 8.0).
   e. low ejaculate volume.
5. When the sperm density is low (oligospermia), the chance that testing for Y chromosome microdeletions will show a gentic mutation is:
   a. 0%
   b. 5–10%
   c. 15–25%

d. 40–50%

e. > 50%

6. The semen analysis parameter that is most commonly abnormal in male factor infertility is:

   a. sperm density.

   b. sperm motility.

   c. seminal volume.

   d. sperm morphology.

7. The most common and correctable identifiable problem causing male infertility is:

   a. infection.

   b. obstruction.

   c. gonadotoxin exposure.

   d. varicocele.

8. The role of PSA in the ejaculate is:

   a. to coagulate the ejaculate.

   b. to serve as a marker for prostate cancer.

   c. to serve as a liquefaction factor.

   d. to give semen its characteristic odor.

Answers

1. b
2. c
3. d
4. d
5. b
6. b
7. d
8. c

CHAPTER 22

Sexually Transmitted Diseases

Michel A. Pontari

I. **URETHRITIS**

Men with urethritis may be symptomatic or asymptomatic. Symptoms typically include urethral discomfort, dysuria, and/or a purulent or mucoid discharge. The diagnosis of urethritis is made on the basis of either the presence of urethral discharge or the finding of 5 or more PMN per oil immersion field (1000 ×) or a Gram's stain smear of urethral discharge or an intraurethral swab specimen. Gonococcal (GC) urethritis is diagnosed clinically if intracellular gram-negative diplococci are observed. Nongonococcal urethritis (NGU) is more likely if they are not present. NGU is more commonly found as a cause of urethritis in heterosexual men than gonorrhea.

A. **Gonoccal Urethritis (GU)**

1. *Neisseria gonorrhea* is a gram-negative diplococcus. Incubation period is 3 to 10 days. For a man, risk of acquiring GU from a single episode of intercourse with an infected partner is approximately 17 percent. Transmitted via vaginal sex, but also via oral sex in a partner with gonococcal pharyngitis.

2. *Cultures.* Urethral specimens plated on modified Thayer-Martin media.

3. *Treatment.* Ceftriaxone 125 mg IM one dose or cefixime (Supax) 400 mg PO one dose or ciprofloxacin 500 mg PO one dose or ofloxacin 400 mg PO one dose. For patients who cannot tolerate cephalosporins or quinolones, use spectinomycin 2 grams IM single dose.

4. Because coinfection with *Chlamydia* is common in gonococcal urethritis (15 to 35 percent of cases), treatment for **both** gonorrhea and NGU should be initiated.

5. Screen for syphilis by serology if gonorrhea diagnosed.

6. *Long-term sequelae.* Urethral strictures. Disseminated GC occurs in 0.5 percent of patients and produces fever, a pustular rash, and septic arthritis.

B. Non-gonococcal Urethritis (NGU)

1. Incubation period is 7 to 21 days. Most common organisms causing NGU: *Chlamydia trachomatis* (23 to 55 percent), *Ureaplasma urealyticum* (20 to 40 percent), *Trichomonas vaginalis* in up to 11 percent of NGU cases, and others include herpes and *Mycoplasma genitalium* (reported as high as 12 to 25 percent). An infecting organism is not identified in all cases.

2. Cultures are available for *Chlamydia* and should be sent using the intraurethral swab; can also perform ELISA on the swab.

3. Possible complications of NGU in men infected with *Chlamydia* include epididymitis and Reiter's syndrome (urethritis, arthritis, and uveitis). Chlamydial infections transmitted to female sex partners can produce pelvic inflammatory disease (PID), which can cause fallopian tube scarring leading to ectopic pregnancy and infertility, as well as chronic pelvic pain.

4. *Treatment.* Doxycycline 100 mg PO BID × 7 days or azithromycin 1 g in a single dose. *Alternative regimen.* Erythromycin base 500 mg PO × 7 days (or 250 mg × 14 days) or erythromycin ethylsuccinate 800 mg PO QID × 7 days (or 400 mg PO × 14 days) or floxin 300 mg PO BID for 7 days. Sex partners within 60 days of onset of symptoms should also be treated, whether or not they are symptomatic.

5. Patients who return with persistent symptoms or a recurrence after therapy should be restarted with the original regimen if they either failed to comply initially or were reinfected by an untreated sex partner. If this does not apply, do a wet mount of a urethral swab and intraurethral culture for *Trichomonas*. If positive, treat with flagyl 2 g PO in one dose. If negative for *T. vaginalis,* treat with 14 days of erythromycin base 500 mg PO QID to treat possible tetracycline-resistant *Ureaplasma.* Note: Ofloxacin (Floxin) for 7 days will also cover *Chlamydia* and *Ureaplasma.*

6. Urologic evaluation to look for intraurethral anatomic abnormality (stricture, foreign body, condyloma) in patients with chronic urethritis despite multiple courses of antibiotics finds a significant abnormality in only approximately 10 percent of cases. Of these, uroflow will detect the majority of abnormalities.

II. EPIDIDYMITIS

A. Etiology

Epididymitis caused by sexually transmitted disease occurs mainly in men age 15 to 35 years. Common causes include

Neisseria gonorrhea and *Chlamydia trachomatis,* organisms that cause urethritis. In homosexual men, more coliform bacteria, such as *Haemophilus influenzae* are seen. Epididymitis in individuals under 15 and over 35 is more often from common urinary pathogens and commonly associated with urinary tract obstruction. Noninfectious epididymitis can develop with the use of amiodarone for heart disease, as the drug accumulates in the epididymis.

B. Evaluation
1. Gram's stain of urethral smear for gonorrhea and nongonococcal urethritis; culture of urethral swab for GC and *Chlamydia.*
2. Culture of midstream urine for gram-negative bacteria.
3. *Physical examination.* Rule out torsion and testis tumor.

C. Treatment
1. *Age 15 to 35.* Treat as for gonococcal urethritis (e.g., ceftriaxone 250 mg IM plus doxycycline 100 mg PO BID for 10 days to cover *Chlamydia.* Alternative is ofloxacin 300 mg PO BID × 10 days).
2. *Age less than 15 or over 35.* Use broad-spectrum antibiotic to cover gram-negative bacteria and evaluate for underlying urinary tract disease/obstruction, such as meatal stenosis in boys and prostatism or urethral stricture in older men.

III. PELVIC INFLAMMATORY DISEASE
A. Etiology
Pelvic inflammatory disease (PID) is also caused by sexually transmitted diseases, particularly GC, *Chlamydia, Ureaplasma,* and *Mycoplasma.* The risk of acquiring GC for a female from an infected partner approaches 90 percent.

B. Symptoms
1. Abdominal and pelvic pain
2. Vaginal discharge
3. Fever
4. Menorrhagia
5. Dysuria—may mimic a urinary tract infection
6. Infertility caused by untreated asymptomatic disease leading to tubal scarring

C. Evaluation
1. Close examination of labia, perineum, and perirectal areas.
2. Speculum examination with visualization of the cervical os. Take a swab of the os for culture and Gram's stain. Send for both GC and *Chlamydia.*

3. Bimanual examination looking to distinguish unilateral from bilateral pain. Also perform rectal examination looking for trauma, genital warts, or discharge. Palpate for inguinal and systemic adenopathy.

4. The key differential diagnosis to exclude is ectopic pregnancy. Scarring from asymptomatic PID can lead to an ectopic pregnancy. Send a serum pregnancy test.

D. Treatment

1. In *nonpregnant females.* Treat as above for GC and *Chlamydia.*

2. *Pregnant females.* Ceftriaxone 250 mg IM one dose plus erythromycin 500 mg PO QID × 7 days.

IV. GENITAL WARTS: CONDYLOMA ACUMINATA

A. Etiology

Caused by the human papillomavirus (HPV), HPV is a small, nonenveloped virus containing double-stranded DNA. HPV infects basal epithelial cells and multiplies in cell nucleus, causing cell death and perinuclear cavitation, or koilocytosis, a histologic feature specific to HPV.

B. Transmission

Transmission is during sexual contact. Incubation period is 4 to 6 weeks. The male urethra may serve as a reservoir for HPV.

C. HPV and Carcinogenesis

1. HPV has been associated with female genital tract cancer, leading to concerns over sexually transmitted malignancy. HPV types 16, 18, and 31 are found in the majority of cervical malignancies. These types are also found in Bowen's disease (CIS) of the penis and squamous cell carcinoma of the penis.

2. HPV-6 and HPV-11 are more often found in benign condyloma acuminata, but are also sometimes associated with malignancy of genital and respiratory tract.

D. Diagnosis

1. *Clinical infection.* Visible lesions. Fibroepithelial, exophytic, on penis. Urethral lesions occur, and 80 percent are located within the distal 3 cm of urethra. Patients present with dysuria, bloody urethral discharge, changes in urinary stream. Bladder condyloma are rare. If meatal condyloma are identified, urethroscopy should be performed to look for other urethral lesions; urethroscopy should stop at the external sphincter to preventi atrogenic seeding of the prostatic urethra and bladder.

2. *Subclinical infection.* Not apparent to naked eye. Vinegar (3 to 5 percent acetic acid solution) is applied to surface of penis for 10 to 15 mins. Areas that turn acetowhite are suspicious for HPV. Biopsy is required to confirm diagnosis because other benign lesions can stain white. Also see false negative, as unstained areas may contain the virus.

3. Detection of HPV is best by nucleic acid hybridization tests. HPV does not grow in cell culture. Polymerase chain reaction (PCR) is most sensitive, requiring only 10 to 100 copies of viral DNA to detect.

E. Treatment

No treatment has been shown to eradicate HPV. HPV has been found in tissue after laser treatment. There is also evidence of spontaneous resolution of most HPV infections. Goal is to eradicate visible disease and any symptoms caused by the warts. No evidence indicates that treatment of visible warts affects the development of cervical cancer.

1. Small volume disease
   a. Podofilox 0.5% (active ingredient is podophyllotoxin), applied by patient 3 days on, 4 off for up to 4 weeks at a time.
   b. Imiquimod (Aldara) 5% cream, 3 times per week at night, for up to 16 weeks. This is an immune modulator, and success is associated with tissue production of interferon a,b,g and TNF-a.
   c. Cryotherapy with liquid nitrogen.
   d. Intralesional injection of interferon alpha 2b increases success of podofilox but recurrence rate is same.
   e. Trichloroacetic acid (TCA) 50% topically.

2. Larger areas (or when topical therapy fails)
   a. *Laser therapy.* CO_2 laser vaporizes tissue with a shallow depth of penetration. Must use laser mask and vacuum because viral DNA has been demonstrated in the smoke plume. Nd:YAG coagulates tissue and causes less plume. Overall success with laser is 88 to 100 percent. Recurrence occurs in 2 to 3 months.
   b. Surgical excision for very large wart burden.

3. *Intraurethral condyloma.* Fulguration with Nd:YAG via cystoscope. Can use intraurethral 5-FU cream afterward 4 times a week for 6 weeks to prevent recurrence. 5-FU causes severe exfoliative dermatitis so adjacent areas must be protected.

4. *Subclinical disease.* There is no evidence that treatment of male subclinical disease alters the disease course in female contacts. The partner may already be at risk for developing cervical dysplasia and malignancy. Coupled

with the difficulty in eradicating HPV, many clinicians do not advocate treating subclinical disease. In series which have treated subclinical disease, failure rates of up to 70 percent at 4 months follow-up have been reported.

V. GENITAL ULCERS

A. Diagnosis of Genital Ulcers

Diagnosis presents a diagnostic challenge. Even "experts" are wrong in their initial diagnosis over 40 percent of the time. Only three ulcer presentations are pathognomonic:

1. A fixed drug eruption is always triggered by the use of one particular medication.
2. A group of vesicles on an erythematous base that does not follow a neural distribution is pathognomonic for herpes simplex infection.
3. A genital ulcer that develops acutely during sexual activity is diagnostic of trauma. If the clinical picture does not meet these criteria, then the differential diagnosis must include premalignant processes (e.g., erythroplasia of Queyrat), malignant processes such as squamous cell carcinoma of the penis, and nonmalignant processes including syphilis, chancroid, LGV, granuloma inguinale. In the United States, the most common causes are herpes, syphilis, and chancroid. Biopsy of the lesion is most helpful to diagnose malignant or premalignant lesions.

B. Herpes Simplex Virus (HSV)

1. *Etiology.* Herpes virus is a double-stranded DNA virus. Types include HSV-I and HSV-II. Most genital herpes is type II, with 10 to 25 percent type I.
2. *Transmission.* Can be transmitted even if individual is asymptomatic (up to one third of cases). After inoculation in mucocutaneous sites, the virus spreads to neurons to establish latent infection.
3. *Clinical course*
   a. Flu-like symptoms with initial infection are much worse than subsequent episodes, and worse in patients without history of previous oral herpes. Local lesions persist for average of 10 days in initial infection. Tender inguinal adenopathy can develop in 2 to 3 weeks. Dysuria present in 80 percent of females and 40 percent of males with genital herpes.
   b. Minority of patients will have recurrent episodes of genital lesions. Most cases of recurrent herpes are caused by type II.
   c. Late complications include:
      i. CNS: mild meningitis 10 to 30 percent
      ii. Sacral or autonomic dysfunction in 1 percent, and can result in urinary retention

iii. Pneumonitis

iv. Hepatitis

Most serious consequence is neonatal transmission, which carries high rates of morbidity and mortality.

4. *Diagnosis.* Pathognomonic appearance is vesicles grouped on an erythematous base that do not follow a neural distribution. Diagnosis is by viral cultures or other techniques including immunofluorescence with anti HSV-antibodies and DNA hybridization.

5. *Treatment.* No cure for herpes yet.

   a. Acyclovir acts as a guanidine analog, getting selectively phosphorylated by a viral thymidine kinase (therefore selectively active for viral containing cells) and inhibits viral DNA polymerase, terminating the formation of the DNA chain. Acyclovir provides partial control of the current episode of herpes, not a cure. It does not eradicate latent virus or affect subsequent frequency or severity of recurrences after it is stopped. Acts to decrease the duration of viral shedding of the current episode of herpes, reducing time to healing of the lesions and minimizing pain and itching. Most serious side effect is occasional reversible depression of renal function. Valacyclovir is a valine ester of acyclovir with enhanced oral absorption. Famiciclovir also has high bioavailability.

   b. CDC recommendations

      1. First clinical episode of genital herpes: acyclovir 200 mg PO 5 times per day for 7 to 10 days; can also use 400 mg PO TID. Can use famiciclovir 250 mg PO TID or valaciclovir 1g PO BID for 7 to 10 days.

      2. For frequent recurrences (more than 6 episodes per year): acyclovir suppression 400 mg PO BID. Reduces the frequency of HSV recurrences by at least 75 percent in patients with more than 6 recurrences per year. Stop after 1 year and reassess rate of recurrence.

      3. For episodic recurrent infections, patient-instituted therapy at signs of recurrence, use any of the following for 5 days: acyclovir 500 mg PO TID, 200 mg PO 5 times per day or 800 mg PO BID; famiciclovir 125 mg PO BID; valciclovir 500 mg PO BID.

      4. Severe disease or complications requiring hospitalization: IV acyclovir.

C. **Syphilis**

   Caused by *Treponema pallidum,* a spirochete bacteria.

   1. Stages

      a. *Primary.* Ulcer or chancre at site of infection. Most common area on penis is corona. Lesions in primary syphilis are characteristically firm, hard (due to end-arteritis and vascular sclerosis), and painless. Can develop bilateral painless lymph node involvement. Incubation period is 2 to 4 weeks from contact.

b. *Secondary.* Appears 4 to 8 weeks after the primary lesion. Sites include a palmar–plantar rash, mucocutaneous lesions (condyloma lata), adenopathy; this is a highly infectious state of the disease. Resolves if left untreated.

c. *Tertiary.* May develop many years later. *Latent syphilis.* Serologic evidence of syphilis with no clinical findings. Defined as early (less than 1 year) or late (more than 1 year). Characteristic lesions are gummas, which are areas of granulomatous inflammation. Can also include cardiac, with aortic aneurysms or aortic insufficiency; neurologic, which can lead to dementia, tabes dorsalis, and neurogenic bladder; ophthalmic, with Argyll-Robertson pupils that have accomodation but no pupil response; and auditory symptoms.

2. Diagnosis

a. Definitive diagnosis of early syphilis is darkfield examination or direct antibody tests of lesion exudate or tissue.

b. Presumptive diagnosis is based on two types of serologic tests:

1. Non-treponemal: veneral disease research laboratory (VDRL) and rapid plasma reagin (RPR).

2. Treponemal: FTA-ABS (fluorescent treponemal antibody absorption) and MHA-TP (microhemagglutination assay for antibodies to *T. pallidum*).

Need **both** types of tests to make the diagnosis. Non-treponemal antibody titers usually correlate with disease activity and are reported quantitatively. A fourfold change in titers is diagnostic. False positives are seen in pregnant women, IV drug users, and patients with systemic lupus erythematosus (SLE) or systemic viral infections. The treponemal tests correlate poorly with disease activity. Non-treponemal tests should be used to follow disease activity and response to treatment.

3. Treatment. Parenteral penicillin (PCN) G. Preparation, dosage, and length of treatment dependent on stage and clinical manifestations. For primary or secondary disease, or early latent syphilis, use benzathine PCN G, 2.4 million units, IM in single dose. If PCN allergic: use doxycycline 100 mg PO BID × 2 weeks. For late latent or tertiary syphilis, benzathine PCN G, 2.4 million units × 3 weekly doses.

4. *Jarish-Herxheimer reaction.* Acute febrile reaction with headache, myalgia, and other symptoms that may occur within the first 24 hours after any therapy for syphilis. Treat symptomatically with antipyretics.
5. Patients should be re-examined serologically at 3 and 6 months. Failure of VDRL or RPR to decline fourfold should prompt examination of CSF for neurosyphilis.
6. All patients with syphillis should be encouraged to be tested for HIV.

D. Lymphogranuloma Venereum (LGV)

Caused by *Chlamydia trachomatis* serotypes L1, L2, and L3. Incubation period is 2 to 21 days.

1. Presentation. The initial genital lesion typically is painless, nonindurated, and heals quickly. Tender inguinal adenopathy, usually unilateral, appears 1 to 4 weeks later. Suppuration of the nodes can occur along with the spread to involve the rectum. Obstruction of nodes can lead to local elephantiasis of penis and scrotum.
2. Diagnosis. Culture of *C. trachomatis* from aspiration of fluctuant node. Serologic tests used include the microimmunofluorescent antibody test (Frei test no longer used).
3. Treatment. Doxycycline 100 mg PO BID × 3 weeks. *Alternatives.* Erythromycin 500 mg PO QID × 3 weeks, sulfisoxazole 500 mg QID × 3 weeks.

E. Chancroid

Caused by *Haemophilus ducreyi,* a gram-negative rod. Incubation period is 1 to 7 days.

1. Presentation. Painful ulcer, borders are not indurated, frequently covered with pus. One half of patients will have tender inguinal adenopathy, with matting of nodes. Can develop phimosis, even gangrene of glans if untreated.
2. Diagnosis
   a. Gram's stain of base of the lesion.
   b. Selective cultures for *H. ducreyi* using supplemented gonococcal base and Mueller-Hinton agar.
3. Treatment. Azithromycin 1 g PO in single dose or ceftriaxone 250 mg IM in one dose or erythromycin base 500 mg PO QID × 7 days or cipro 500 mg PO BID × 3 days. Healing will be slower in HIV patients—consider using 7 days of erythromycin in this group.

F. Granuloma Inguinale (GI)

Caused by *Calymmatobacterium granulomatosis* (related to *Klebsiella pneumoniae*). Incubation period is 2 to 3 months.

1. Presentation. Ulcers start as nodules that rupture into shallow areas of red velvety granulation tissue. Nodes

usually not involved early in infection. Frequently get secondary infection with cicatricial healing and scarring as late complications.

2. Diagnosis. Crush preparation of area for histology. Giemsa or Wright's stain show characteristic Donovan bodies, which are bipolar staining rods within monocytes. No culture for *C. granulomatosis* available. Must also rule out chancroid as it is commonly mistaken for GI.

3. Treatment. Tetracycline 500 mg PO BID or bactrim DS PO BID or cipro 750 mg PO BID for 3 weeks. IV gentamicin can be used if lesions do not respond to initial oral therapy in several days, or if the patient is HIV positive.

VI. VAGINITIS

The etiologies are distinguished by features found on examination of the pH of the vaginal discharge, the presence of a characteristically fishy odor from the release of amines on the addition of 10% KOH to the discharge, and the examination of a saline wet prep of the vaginal fluid (Table 22-1).

VII. OTHER SEXUALLY TRANSMITTED DISEASES

A. Molluscum Contagiosum

Dermatologic disease caused by the pox virum that has a sexual mode of transmission. Incubation period is 2 to 7 weeks.

1. Presentation. Smooth, dome-shaped lesions, pearly or pink, with a characteristic small dimple impression on top. Often asymptomatic.

2. Diagnosis. Biopsy shows molluscum body, cytoplasmic inclusions containing viral particles.

3. Treatment. Local therapy with cryotherapy or podophyllin. If untreated will regress in 2 to 3 months.

B. Hepatitis B

Six to ten percent of infected persons become hepatitis B carriers and become infectious. Hep B can cause cirrhosis and hepatocellular carcinoma.

VIII. ACQUIRED IMMUNODEFICIENCY SYNDROME (AIDS)

A. Biology of HIV Infection

1. AIDS is caused by infection with the human immunodeficiency virus type I (HIV-I), a retrovirus. Another distantly related virus has been identified in humans from Western Africa and called HIV-2; the two viruses are distinct antigentically and in pathogenicity.

Table 22-1

ORGANISM	pH DISCHARGE	AMINE ODOR ON 10% KOH	WET PREP	TREATMENT
Normal	< 4.5	No	Rare PMN	—
Trichomonas	> 4.5	Yes	Trichomonas many PMNs	Flagyl 2 g once
Yeast	< 4.5	No	pseudomycelia (on KOH)	Miconazole 200 mg suppository (Monistat)
Gardnerella	> 4.5	Yes	Clue cells[a]	Flagyl 500 mg PO BID × 7 days

[a]Clue cells: vaginal epithelium cells covered with bacteria.

2. *Replication of retroviruses.* Retroviruses contain their genetic material as RNA.

HIV-I single strand RNA ⟶ Viral DNA → transcribed by viral DNA polymerase ("reverse transcriptase") integrated into host genome

3. *Characteristics of HIV.* Has spherical shape, an outer envelope composed of glycoproteins, 70 to 80 knob-like surface projections, and a polypeptide shell around the core containing RNA.
4. All retroviruses contain three genes that code for structural proteins

Gene	Product
gag	Viral core proteins
pol	Reverse transcriptase, protease and integrase
env	Envelope proteins

B. Pathogenesis of HIV Infection

1. *Target cells for acute HIV infection.* CD4 molecule, found on CD4+ lymphocytes (T-helper cells), also macrophages, in lymph nodes, and blood. Goes on to infect other cells, such as rectal mucosal cells and cells lining the uterine cavity, and CNS.
2. After entry into host, HIV binds to the CD4 protein on the surface of the T-helper lymphocytes, mediated by the gp120 molecule on the viral envelope.
3. Destruction and depletion of CD4+ T cells results in a profound depression in cell-mediated immune function in the host.
4. Factors leading to HIV protection from normal immune surveillance
   a. Hypervariable regions in the virus envelope genome mutate quickly, leading to selection of variants of the virus that evade the host immune response.
   b. HIV can also induce fusion of host cells with other cells forming large syncitia, a fusion of infected and uninfected cells. This provides a mechanism of transmission from one cell to another without being exposed to the humoral immune system of the host.
   c. Immunosuppression from concurrent syphilis or CMV infection.

C. **Natural History of HIV Infection**
1. Clinical manifestations range from asymptomatic HIV infection to full blown AIDS. Most HIV+ patients are asymptomatic at any given time. AIDS related complex (ARC) is HIV+ patients with a CD4+ count of less than 200/uL and one or two signs or symptoms (e.g., fatigue, weight loss, herpes infection). The functional definition of AIDS is the occurrence of certain systemic infections or malignancies in a patient with no other cause or defective cell-mediated immunity. The case definition of AIDS is made by the CDC.
2. Progression of disease
   a. The rate of progression from asymptomatic infection to AIDS increases with the length of follow-up. The incidence of symptomatic infection is low in the first several years and increases thereafter. More rapid progression in patients age 55 years or older. Predicted time for 50 percent of HIV+ individuals to develop AIDS is 10 to 11 years. Twenty percent of individuals will remain asymptomatic for 10 years.
   b. Poor prognosis is CD4+ lymphocyte count below 200/uL. Over 80 percent of patients with CD4+ counts below this level develop an AIDS-related opportunistic infection or malignancy within 3 years. Patients with CD4+ count above 500 usually are asymptomatic. The median survival in treated AIDS patients is 2 to 3 years.

D. **Transmission of AIDS**
1. Direct sexual contact
   a. *Homosexual contact.* Receptive anal intercourse can produce trauma to the rectal mucosa and provides access for HIV in semen to recipient blood and lymphatic system. HIV can also directly infect rectal epithelial cells.
   b. *Heterosexual contact.* Most commonly from infected males to females. Risk from a single heterosexual contact may be below 0.1 percent. Increased risk of male to female transmission with oral contraceptive use and nonoxyl-9 containing spermicides, both of which may cause irritation of female genital mucosa.
   c. Other risk factors for sexual transmission of HIV
      i. presence of sexually transmitted diseases and/or genital ulcer disease show a three- to fivefold increase in risk of HIV infection. May cause breaks in local genital skin and facilitate infection and also may recruit susceptible WBCs to site of HIV exposure. Chancroid especially

causes more inflammation than other STDs and is more closely linked to HIV transmission.

ii. Lack of circumcision gives a large, moist area of foreskin that can support the virus. Cracks in foreskin from abrasions or inflammation facilitate infection.

iii. Lack of condom use.

2. Bloodborne transmission

a. IV drug use with shared needles.

b. Blood transfusion and organ transplant recipients.

i. Routine screening of blood since 1985. Current risk is estimated at 1 case of HIV transmission for every 83,000 to 122,000 blood transfusions.

ii. Possible for an infected donor to transmit HIV during the "window period" prior to the development of HIV antibodies. The window period is estimated to be 6 months or less, as 95 percent of HIV+ individuals have antibody detectable by 6 months (CDC STD guidelines 1993). Window period may be shorter with improved detection methods, on the order of 25 days.

iii. Seventy percent of patients receiving organs from HIV+ organ donor convert to HIV+ and proceed to clinical AIDS within 2 to 3 years.

c. *Hemophilia.* Typical hemophiliac patients receive approximately 75,000 units of clotting factor concentrate per year. Heat treatment is now used to eliminate HIV from factor concentrates.

d. *Health care workers.* Risk for HIV infection associated with a single needlestick ranges from 0.2 percent to 1 percent. Seroconversion rate after mucous membrane exposure is 0.63 percent. Risk of HIV infection after single cutaneous exposure is 0.04 percent for blood and 0.02 percent for any body fluid that contains HIV.

3. *Perinatal transmission.* Newborn has 40 to 60 percent chance of acquiring HIV from an infected mother.

E. Diagnosis of AIDS

Made by detection of antibodies against the viral antigens by serologic testing.

1. First test is ELISA (enzyme linked immunosorbent assay)

i. Sensitivity: higher than 99 percent

ii. Specificity: 95 to 99 percent

2. A positive ELISA should be confirmed by a second test. Most commonly used is Western blot. Can also use immunofluoresence assays.

3. Window period exists prior to the development of HIV antibodies. The window period is estimated to be 6

months or less. Patient can be infected but antibody negative in this period.

F. Antiviral Therapy
1. Reverse transcriptase inhibitors
   a. Zidovudine (azidodeoxythymidine or AZT) can decrease frequency of opportunistic infections in patients with AIDS or ARC and overall delays progression to advanced disease. Evidence for long-term survival advantage is inconclusive. Usually not started unless the patient is symptomatic or has decreased CD4+ counts. AZT is commonly given after occupational exposure but there is no evidence that it prevents infection.
   b. *Site of action.* Reverse transcription of viral RNA to viral DNA by reverse transcriptase. *Mechanism.* Incorporation into the growing viral DNA chain; since the drug lacks a 3′ hydroxyl group (OH), elongation of the DNA chain is terminated.
   c. Most serious side effect is bone marrow suppression manifested as cytopenia and megaloblastic anemia. Other side effects of AZT include fatigue, nausea, vomiting, headache, pancreatitis, and peripheral neuropathy.
2. Protease inhibitors
   a. These block the late phase of viral replication during assembly of new viral particles. Proteases cleave gag-pol polyproteins into pieces that cannot be successfully assembled into a normal virus. Main problem is the loss of gag protein p24.
   b. Multidrug regimens are used along with the reverse transcriptase inhibitors.
   c. Indinavir (Crixivan) is associated with renal stones in up to 4 percent of cases. Patients usually improve with hydration and discontinuation of the drug. Indinavir crystals are found as part of the stone in 60 percent of cases. The other protease inhibitors have a lower incidence of stone formation.

G. Urologic Manifestations of AIDS
1. *Renal disease.* AIDS associated nephropathy (HIVAN).
   a. *Incidence.* Up to 25 to 35 percent of patients with HIV have proteinuria and develop rapidly progressive, irreversible renal failure. More common in African Americans and IV drug users.
   b. *Pathology.* Affects glomeruli, tubules, and interstitium simultaneously. Most common finding is focal segmental glomerulosclerosis (FSGS). Previously thought

to be similar to heroin nephropathy, but shown to be distinct.

   c. *Progression.* Usually rapid progression to end-stage renal disease in 8 to 16 weeks. Median survival from diagnosis of renal disease to death is 4.5 months.

2. Renal obstruction can result from non-Hodgkins lymphoma causing retroperitoneal lymphadenopathy. Treatment is systemic therapy (chemotherapy) with use of percutaneous nephrostomy tubes or stents as needed in bilateral disease.

3. Malignancies

   a. *Kaposi's sarcoma (KS).* A sarcoma of endothelial origin, which prior to 1981 was seen only in elderly men of Mediterranean descent, affecting the feet and lower extremities, rarely the genitalia, and ran an indolent course (now called "classic" Kaposi's sarcoma). Development of KS in HIV population is from a KS-associated herpes virus that is sexually transmitted.

      i. Twenty percent of patients with HIV-associated KS will develop lesions on the genitalia. Lesions are subcutaneous, nonpruritic nodules. Can be pigmented, sometimes appearing blue. Lymphedema is common.

      ii. *Treatment.* (1) small local solitary lesion: local excision, laser fulguration, or radiation therapy; (2) large multicentric lesions: use radiation therapy for palliation, side effects include urethral strictures and fistulae; and (3) disseminated KS: chemotherapy including vincristine, bleomycin, and doxorubicin. Response rates of up to 88 percent are reported. In patients with CD4 count above 600/uL, IFN-a can be used and results in 18- to 30-month response.

   b. Testicular tumors

      i. Incidence of testicular tumors in AIDS clinic population is up to 0.2 percent, or 50 times that of general population.

      ii. Most series report an increase in nonseminomatous germ cell tumors but one reported an increase in seminomas.

      iii. Testicular lymphoma in HIV+ patients presents in younger men and with higher grade tumor than in non-HIV men. Still overall greater number of germ cell tumors in HIV+ men than testicular lymphomas.

   c. *Urethra.* Primary urethral T- and B-cell lymphomas reported.

4. *Opportunistic infections.* Can see unusual infections found in association with immunosuppression, such as toxoplasmosis, aspergillosis, histoplasmosis CMV, MAI, fungal infections, throughout GU tract including testes and kidneys. Specific infections include the following.

   a. Prostate

      i. Increased incidence of bacterial prostatitis in AIDS (up to 14 percent) versus asymptomatic HIV infections. Treat with minimum of 6 weeks of fluorquinolones; relapses are frequent and require retreatment. Prostatic abscess can develop; abscess must be drained transurethrally or transperineally. Can have abscess despite sterile cultures.

      ii. Fungal prostatitis occurs. Diagnosis on fungal stains or cultures of prostatic tissue. Treatment is with IV amphotericin (total dose 2 g) plus oral flucytosine. Persistent infection or relapses treated with oral fluconazole.

   b. Urethra. There is an unexplained association between AIDS and Reiter's syndrome: urethritis, arthritis, and uveitis. Presents as urethral discharge unresponsive to antibiotic therapy.

   c. Epididymis

      i. Can develop salmonella infection, which is difficult to eradicate. Treatment is 10 days of IV bactrim followed by life-long oral maintenance therapy.

      ii. *Cytomegalovirus (CMV) epididymitis.* Diagnostic histologic appearance for CMV is an inclusion body in the nucleus of the infected cell. Urine culture is positive for CMV. Treatment is gancyclovir or likely epididymectomy.

   d. Higher incidence of tuberculosis infection in HIV + men.

5. *AIDS and semen.* Viral excretion in the semen is independent of clinical stage of the HIV infection; it does correlate with CD8 counts.

   a. Vasectomy does not eliminate HIV in semen, indicating that HIV enters ejaculate through accessory glands or via epithelium of urethra or vas deferens.

   b. Semen analysis in HIV + men shows decreased motility, increased number of round cells, and increased viscosity. Can see maturation arrest of sperm along with interstitial fibrosis. Testicular atrophy occurs from fever, testicular infection, and/or toxic effects of antibiotics and chemotherapy.

6. *Impotence.* Increased incidence of erectile dysfunction from primary and secondary gonadal failure with testicular

atrophy and decreased testosterone levels, psychological depression, AIDS-related dementia, and neurogenic dysfunction including peripheral neuropathy from viral myelitis and myelopathy, which occurs in 30 to 40 percent of AIDS patients.

7. *Voiding dysfunction.* From neurogenic dysfunction as above. Also associated with high incidence of toxoplasmosis opportunistic infection of CNS. Urodynamic findings vary with extent of disease and CNS involvement. Progress from detrusor hyperreflexia from initial involvement of thoracic cord, then to areflexia as sacral cord is involved. Older series note urinary retention and detrusor areflexia as the most common finding (Catanese, 1988). More recent series report detrusor hyperreflexia with dyssynergy as most common urodynamic finding in men with AIDS and associated with HIV-related neurologic disorders, with areflexia much less common.

8. *Fluid and electrolytes.* Increased incidence of hyponatremia. Found in 40 percent of patients in one clinic. Etiology includes hypovolemia from GI fluid loss with hyponatremic replacement and adrenocortical deficiency. Euvolemic hyponatremia from syndrome of inappropriate antidiuretic hormone (SIADH) secondary to pulmonary or CNS infection. Hypervolemic causes include acute renal failure.

9. *Hematuria.* Microscopic hematuria may be present in up to 25 percent of HIV-infected patients. However, genitourinary tumors are uncommon in this group of predominantly young people, especially men, a full evaluation for the hematuria is not routinely warranted.

BIBLIOGRAPHY

Berger RE: Sexually transmitted diseases: The classic diseases. In: Walsh PC, Retik AB, Vaughan ED, Wein AW, eds. *Campbell's Urology.* Philadelphia, Saunders 663–683, 1998.

Busch MP, Lee LLJ, Satten GA, et al: Time course of detection of viral and serologic markers preceding human immunodeficiency virus type I seroconversion: Implications for screening of blood and tissue donors. *Transfusion* 35:91–97, 1995.

Carpiniello VL, Mally TR, Sedlacek TV, et al: Results of carbon dioxide laser therapy and topical 5-fluorouracil treatment for subclinical condyloma found by magnified penile surface scanning. *J Urol* 140:53–54, 1988.

Catanese AJ, Rowan RL, Morales P: *AIDS and the Urologist: PartI. Urologic Manifestations of AIDS.* AUA Update Series, vol VIII, lesson 1, 1988. American Urologic Association, Baltimore, MD.

Centers for Disease Control and Prevention: 1998 Sexually transmitted diseases treatment guidelines. *MMWR* 1998; 47:Jan 23, 1998 (No. RR-1).

Cespedes RD, Peretsman RJ, et al: The significance of hematuria in patients infected with the human immunodeficiency virus. *J Urol* 154:1455–1456, 1995.

Drugs for sexually transmitted diseases. *Med Let* 37:117–122, 1995.

Fife KH: New treatments for genital warts less than ideal. *JAMA* 279:2003–2004, 1998.

Glassock RJ, Cohen AH, Danovitch G, Parsa KP: Human immunodeficiency virus (HIV) infection and the kidney. *Ann Int Med* 112:35–49, 1990.

Kane CJ, Bolton DM, Connolly JA, Tanagho EA: Voiding dysfunction in human immunodeficiency virus infections. *J Urol* 155:523–526, 1996.

Krieger JN: New sexually transmitted disease treatment guidelines. *J Urol* 154:209–213, 1995.

Krieger JN, Hooton TM, Brust PJ, et al: Evaluation of chronic urethritis: Defining the role for endoscopic procedures. *Arch Int Med* 148:703–707, 1988.

Krieger JN: The acquired immunodeficiency syndrome and related conditions. In: Walsh PC, Retik AB, Vaughan ED, Wein AW, eds. *Campbell's Urology.* Philadelphia, Saunders, 1998.

Kwan DJ, Lowe FC: Genitourinary manifestations of the acquired immunodeficiency syndrome. *Urology* 45:13–27, 1995.

Lackritz EM, Satten GA, Aberle-Grasse J, et al. Estimated risk of transmission of the human immunodeficiency virus by screened blood in the United States. *N Engl J Med* 333:1721–1725, 1995.

Levy JA: The transmission of HIV and factors influencing progression to AIDS. *Am J Med* 95:86–100, 1993.

Mellinger BC: *Human Papillomavirus in the Male: An Overview.* AUA Update Series vol XIII, lesson 13, 1994. American Urologic Association, Baltimore, MD.

Phillips AN, Lee CA, Elford J, et al: Serial CD4 lymphocyte counts and development of AIDS. *Lancet* 337:389–392, 1991.

Sande MA, Carpenter CJ, Cobbs G, et al: Antiretroviral therapy for adult HIV-infected patients. *JAMA* 270:2583–2589, 1993.

Schmid GP, Fontanarosa PB. Evolving strategies for management of the nongonococcal urethritis syndrome. *JAMA* 274:577–579, 1995.

Siegel JF, Mellinger BC: Human papillomavirus in the male patient. *Urol Clin N Am* 19:83–91, 1992.

Stamm WE, Hicks CB, Martin DH, et al: Azithromycin for empirical treatment of the nongonococcal urethritis syndrome in men. *JAMA* 274:545–549, 1995.

Stone KM: Human papillomavirus infection and genitalwarts: Update on epidemiology and treatment. *Clin Infect Dis* 20(suppl 1):S91–S97, 1995.

Sutherland SE, Reigle MD, Seftel AD, Resnick MI: Protease inhibitors and urolithiasis. *J Urol* 158:31–33, 1997.

Tyring SK, Arany I, Stanley MA, et al: A randomized, controlled, molecular study of condyloma acuminata clearance during treatment with Imiquimod. *J Infect Dis* 178:551–555, 1998.

Wilkinson M, Carroll PR: Testicular carcinoma in patients positive and at risk for immunodeficiency virus. *J Urol* 144:1157–1159, 1990.

SELF-ASSESSMENT QUESTIONS

1. Men with urethritis refractory to first line medications should be treated with erythromycin to treat which organism that can be resistant to tetracycline?
   a. *Chlamydia*
   b. *Ureaplasma*
   c. *Gonorrhea*
   d. Herpes
   e. *Trichomonas*

2. Which drug can cause noninfectious epididymitis?
   a. Procardia
   b. Dobutamine
   c. Amiodarone
   d. Isordil
   e. Captopril

3. Pelvic inflammatory disease is caused by all of the following except:
   a. *gonorrhea.*
   b. *chlamydia.*
   c. *klebsiella.*
   d. *mycoplasma.*
   e. *ureaplasma.*

4. What is the histologic feature specific to human papillomavirus (HPV) infections?
   a. Koilocytosis
   b. Schiller-Duvall bodies
   c. Michaelis-Guttman bodies
   d. Clue cells
   e. Cowdry A bodies

5. The most common cause of genital ulcers in the USA is:
   a. lymphogranuloma venereum (*Chlamydia*).
   b. herpes virus.
   c. granuloma inguinale.
   d. *Gonorrhea.*
   e. *chancroid.*

6. The venereal disease research laboratory (VDRL) and rapid plasma reagin (RPR) are non-treponemal tests used in the diagnosis of syphillis. They correlate most closely with the:
   a. presence of primary syphillis.
   b. presence of secondary syphillis.
   c. presence of neural syphillis.
   d. length of time from diagnosis.
   e. disease activity.

7. A 35-year-old man presents with tender unilateral inguinal adenopathy. There is some suppuration of the nodes along with the spread to involve the rectum. He does not recall having a genital lesion at any time. The most likely diagnosis is:
   a. lymphogranuloma venereum (LGV).
   b. chancroid.
   c. herpes.
   d. granuloma inguinale.
   e. syphillis.

8. A sexually active 25-year-old female presents with a 3 day history of dysuria and vaginal discharge. The pH of the discharge is > 4.5. There is no amine odor on addition of 10% KOH to the discharge, (i.e., a negative whiff test). On microscopy, there are numerous PMNs and no clue cells. The most likely diagnosis is:
   a. yeast.
   b. *Gardeneralla.*
   c. *Gonorrhea.*
   d. *Trichomonas.*
   e. *Chlamydia.*

9. Which of the following is not a risk factor for the transmission of the HIV virus during sexual contact?
   a. Use of nonoxyl-9 as a spermicide
   b. Being circumcised
   c. Receptive anal intercourse
   d. The presence of other sexually transmitted diseases
   e. Lack of condom use
10. Protease inhibitors block replication of the HIV virus by:
    a. blocking the late phase of viral replication during assembly of new viral proteins.
    b. inhibiting reverse transcriptase.
    c. blocking DNA gyrase.
    d. inhibiting translation of viral proteins.
    e. inhibiting transcription of viral proteins.

Answers

1. b	6. e
2. c	7. a
3. c	8. d
4. a	9. b
5. b	10. a

CHAPTER 23

Nonmalignant Diseases of the Retroperitoneum

E. James Seidmon

I. ANATOMY OF THE RETROPERITONEUM

To evaluate and ultimately treat disease of the retroperitoneum, it would seem reasonable to first address the anatomy of the genitourinary tract and its encompassing structures. The retroperitoneum space is bounded by the following: (1) anteriorly, by the posterior layer of the parietal peritoneum and its contents (stomach, small and large bowel); (2) superiorly, separated from the thorax by the reflection of the diaphragm; (3) inferiorly, by the pelvic diaphragm; and (4) posteriorly, by the body wall muscles (psoas, iliacus quadratus luumborum, and transversalis).

Three distinct spaces can be defined within the retroperitoneum. The anterior paranephric space is located between the parietal peritoneum and Gerota's fascia. The perinephric space is limited by Gerota's fascia and Zuckerkandl's fascia and contains the kidney, adrenal gland, renal collecting system (including the proximal ureter), and the renal vessels; all are surrounded by fatty connective tissue. The posterior paranephric space lies between Zuckerkandl's fascia and the transverse fascia. The division of the retroperitoneal space allows for good correlation of anatomic and radiologic features and its most helpful in the diagnosis of retroperitoneal processes (Table 23-1).

Noncancerous pathologic diseases affecting the retroperitoneal space can be divided into two general categories: diseases of the retroperitoneum and retroperitoneal hemorrhage. Retroperitoneal diseases include ureteropelvic junction obstruction (UPJ), extrinsic ureteral obstruction, retroperitoneal fibrosis (Ormond's disease), retroperitoneal abscess, and pelvic lipomatosis, which is characterized by nonmalignant overgrowth of normal fat in the lower areas of the retroperitoneum (perirectal and perivesical spaces).

Table 23-1 Structures within the Retroperitoneum

UROLOGIC	KIDNEYS, URETERS, ADRENAL GLANDS
Vascular	Great vessels (aorta and inferior vena cava and their branches); portal veins
Gastrointestinal	Pancreas and portions of duodenum and colon; rectosigmoid
Lymphatic	Parietal and visceral lymph nodes and channels; cisterna chyli, thoracic duct
Neural	
Nerve plexuses	Celiac, superoinferior hypogastric, sacral, sympathetic trunks
Nerves	Ilioinguinal, iliohypogastric, lateral cutaneous, femoral, genitofemoral, obturator, sciatic, pudendal

II. URETEROPELVIC JUNCTION OBSTRUCTION

Obstruction of the UPJ, usually unilateral, can be the result of a congenital problem that has been in the past asymptomatic. More commonly, this condition is due to inflammation, ischemia, crossing vessel, polyps, valves, and fibrosis as well as tumor or calculi. The rate of occurrence in men and women is about equal and the incidence has never been established.

The specific cause of obstruction of the ureteropelvic junction is not always clear but there is often found some form of angulation or twist at the junction of the dilated renal pelvis and the proximal ureter. Generally, what is found at the time of surgery is a hypoplastic region that is thin walled. Variations of this condition can also be found with either a high insertion of the ureter into the renal pelvis or UPJ compression by a crossing vessel to the lower pole of the kidney.

Symptoms associated with adult onset UPJ obstruction can vary from increased renal pelvic pressure with vague back pain that often increases with intensity after an increase in fluid intake, to nausea, vomiting, hematuria, urinary tract infection, pyuria, or hypertension. The diagnosis is commonly made by an intravenous urogram or renal ultrasound (US). Alternatively, a diuretic renal scan or antegrade pyelography would be equally helpful.

Once the diagnosis is made, surgical correction of the UPJ obstruction must be entertained. If immediate correction has to be delayed, then drainage and decompression of the renal pelvis must be initiated with a percutaneous nephrostomy tube or a double J catheter. With relief of the obstruction, renal function will gradual improve over the next 6 to 8 weeks. Surgical correction of the UPJ obstruction can include one of the following techniques: excision of the dysfunctional segment and repair (Anderson-Hines dismembered pyeloplasty, most common), antegrade (percutaneous) or retrograde endopyelotomy (incision), or antegrade (percutaneous) or retrograde lateral positioned cutting (electrified) wire using a low-profile (10 F) Acucise balloon cutting device (Applied Urology, Laguna Hills, CA).

III. EXTRINSIC URETERAL OBSTRUCTION

The ureter is normally a well-protected conduit. It can be displaced, compressed, or blocked as a complication from another disease process occurring in the abdomen or the retroperitoneum. For the obstruction to occur, there is generally a long, extensive condition that has progressed and often, the ureteral involvement is secondary and overshadowed by the primary condition (disease process). Extrinsic ureteral obstruction can be the produced by a variety of diseases and ureteral dysfunction is often an incidental finding noted by abdominal diagnostic imaging. Although the treatment of the primary disease process is often effective, urologic intervention may be necessary to resolve the urologic obstruction. Interventions include insertion of a double J stent or retrograde catheter, percutaneous nephrostomy tube, or invasive surgical repair. Tables 23-2 and 23-3 contains lists of the most common nonmalignant causes of extrinsic ureteral obstruction.

IV. RETROPERITONEAL FIBROSIS

Retroperitoneal fibrosis (RPF) is an adult chronic inflammatory process rarely seen in children. It involves the tissues overlying the lower lumber vertebral region, causing unilateral, or more commonly, bilateral ureteral compression. RPF is generally the result of many disease entities: cancer (Hodgkin's lymphoma, breast cancer, colon cancer), drug induced [ergot derivatives; methysergide (Sansert), lysergic acid diethylamide (LSD)], inflammatory bowel disease, an abdominal aortic aneurysm, inflammatory processes of the lower extremities with ascending lymphangitis, multiple abdominal surgical procedures, Henoch-Schonlein purpura with hemorrhage, gonorrhea, biliary tract disease, chronic urinary tract infection, urinary extravasation, tuberculosis, sarcoidosis, radiation-induced, and idiopathic causes referred to as Ormond's disease, (Table 23-4).

Table 23-5 presents a general listing of the symptoms. The range of these symptoms can be mild to severe, with patients presenting with decreasing urine output and ultimately anuria, abdominal pain, lower extremity edema, and ischemic pain from arterial compression. The diagnosis is commonly made by intravenous urogram (IVU), which demonstrates the classic triad of hydronephrosis, medial deviation of the ureters, and extrinsic

Table 23-2 Nononcologic Common Causes of Extrinsic Ureteral Obstruction: Diseases of the Retroperitoneum and Conditions of the Female Reproductive System

CONDITION	CAUSE	EFFECT ON URETER	MEDICAL AND SURGICAL TREATMENT
Retroperitoneal fibrosis	Long-term use of methysergide Retroperitoneal inflammation Radiation therapy Idiopathic	Fibrotic tissue envelopes the ureter with resultant ureteral deviation from the normal anatomic position.	Steroid Treatment with ureteral stenting and ultimately surgical intervention for ureterolysis
Retroperitoneal abscess	Renal calculus Renal carbuncle Appendicitis, diverticulitis, enterocolitis (Crohn's disease) Extravasation of infected urine Perinephric abscess	The larger the abscess, the more displacement of the ureter, kidney, or both, causing a change in the peristaltic movement of the ureter	Percutaneous drainage of the retroperitoneal abscess and intravenous broad-spectrum antibiotics
Retroperitoneal hematoma	Generally due to abdominal trauma	The larger the hematoma, the greater the ureteral displacement	Surgical evacuation
Nonmalignant retroperitoneal masses	Benign primary tumors of the retroperitoneum	Primary tumors often are noted to cause anterior and lateral displacement of the ureter, also renal distortion Partial or complete ureteral obstruction	Surgical excision and/or urinary diversion; temporary or permanent hephrostomy tube

Pregnancy	Gravid uterus causing pressure on the upper urinary tract with increasing dilatation of the upper two-thirds of the ureter, tortuosity and/or kinking at the UPJ, urinary stasis can lead to pyelonephritis, ovarian vein syndrome	In only the severe cases ureteral catheterization or placement of a double J catheter with antibiotic treatment until the fetus is delivered
Benign pelvic masses Fibroid uterus Cystic ovary	— Obstruction of the ureter as it crosses the iliac vessels; the right ureter is more commonly affected	Pelvic laparotomy and excision of the mass
Tubo-ovarian abscess Acute and chronic pelvic inflammatory disease Use of intrauterine device	Blockage occurs at or below the pelvic brim with lateral or medial displacement of the ureter, at least 50% of cases have bilateral ureteral obstruction due to the size of the abscess	In a child-bearing female the surgical procedure would be unilateral salpingo-oophorectomy; the best treatment is a total abdominal hysterectomy with bilateral salpingo-oophorectomy
Endometriosis Growth of normal endometrial tissue in an abnormal location outside of the uterus	Obstruction to the distal third of the ureter with scarring and inflammation by the endometrial adhesions	Total abdominal hysterectomy with oophorectomy and ureterolysis
Severe uterine prolapse Weakness of the levator ani muscle	Obstruction due to stretching and wrapping of the uterine vessels around the ureter as a result of the herniation of the uterus through the levator ani muscle	Vaginal hysterectomy with vaginoplasty; if surgery is contraindicated then use of pessary if an alternative

Table 23-3 Nononcologic Common Causes of Extrinsic Ureteral Obstruction: Diseases of the Gastrointestinal Tract and Vascular Lesion

CONDITION	CAUSE	EFFECT ON URETER	MEDICATION AND SURGICAL TREATMENT
Enterocolitis (Crohn's disease)	Granulomas form on the mucosa of the distal small intestine and colon, causing thickening of intestinal wall and the formation of scar tissue	Fistulas from the ileum and colon develop, allowing for extension of the inflammatory process, causing obstruction to the distal right ureter, a retroperitoneal abscess may result	Surgical resection of granulomatous intestinal tissue
Appendicitis	Inflammatory condition of the appendix	An abscess can develop in the appendiceal wall that expands and causes pressure onto the right ureter at the pelvic brim	Surgical drainage of the abscess and appendectomy if possible
Diverticulitis	Diverticula in the muscular wall of the colon filled with colonic contents and become inflamed	Progression of the inflammatory process leading to perforation and formation of a retroperitoneal abscess	Surgical drainage and bowel resection with or without diverting colostomy
Abdominanal aortic aneurysm (AAA)	Weakness of the abdominal aortic wall that is often below the renal vessels	The AAA may cause unilateral or bilateral obstruction and displacement of the ureters	Ureteral drainage and AAA repair; ureterolysis and even resection may be necessary if scarring of the ureter is noted
Retrocaval ureter	Congenital deformity with the right ureter passing behind the vena cava	Ureteral compression	Conservative treatment in asymptomatic patients but surgery correction when severe hydronephrosis or calculus is found

Table 23-4 Possible Etiologic Factors in Retroperitonneal Fibrosis

Drugs
  Methysergide (Sansert)
  LSD
  Amphetamines
  Ergot alkaloids
  Halperidol
  Reserpine
  Phenacetin
  Methyldopa (Aldomet)

Retroperitoneal malignancy
  Primary tumors
  Metastatic tumors

Radiation therapy

Infections
  Chronic urinary tract infections
  Tuberculosis
  Gonorrhea
  Syphilis

Nonspecific inflammatory conditions
  Collagen-vascular disease and autoimmune diseases
  Periartertis
  Aortic or iliac aneurysm
  Urinoma

Specific inflmmatory conditions
  Inflammatory conditions
  Endometriosis
  Sarcoidosis
  GI tract infections and inflammation

Hemmorhage
  Trauma
  Postsurgical

Table 23-5 Symptoms in Patients with Retroperitoneal Fibrosis

SYMPTOMS	PRECENTAGE OF PATIENTS
Backache	34
Flank pain	34
Abdominal pain	24
Weight loss	13
Nausea, vomiting	4
Lower extermity edema	3
Malaise	3

compression of the ureters with proximal ureteral dilatation and narrowing of the distal ureters at L4 and L5. If the renal function precludes an intravenous study (creatinine higher than 2.0 mg/dL and azotemia), a retrograde ureterogram will be diagnostic and delineate the anatomic length of ureteral involvement. Magnetic resonance imaging (MRI) and computed tomography (CT) scanning are essential in the evaluating the fibrotic process and its affect on the ureters; whereas ultrasound offers a less exact diagnosis, it is very helpful in monitoring the treatment response.

Initial treatment by means of urinary diversion can be initiated with placement of ureteral stents or double J catheters. With failure to gain access via the retrograde approach, percutaneous placement of bilateral nephrostomy tubes or nephroureteral stents may be necessary. If the hydronephrosis is mild and the degree of renal dysfunction does not necessitate ureteral stenting, a course of treatment with corticosteroids may halt the obstructive process and stabilize the ureteral obstruction. Conversely, if the response to the steroid treatment is poor or if the presentation of the disease is severe, surgical intervention is necessary. The surgical management involves an exploratory laparotomy with appropriate biopsies to rule out cancer as the cause of fibrosis. If the frozen sections exclude cancer then ureterolysis should be performed with dissection of the ureter from the plaque and followed by intraperitonealization and omental wrapping of the ureters should be performed. Postoperative treatment with corticosteroids can be considered as part of the management of idiopathic RPF but their efficacy has never been proven.

If ureterolysis must be abandoned, salvage techniques include ureteral-ileo segment interposition, ureteral reimplantation with a psoas hitch or Boari flaps, or autotransplantation. Surgical complications can be avoided by limiting the ureteral dissection. If they occur, they often include vascular injury, ejaculatory dysfunction in males secondary to extensive dissection of the retroperitoneal nerve plexus, and lymphocele. Whatever the treatment remedy involves, life-time follow up is necessary including blood studies to monitor renal function as well as diagnostic imaging studies (renal ultrasound, renal scan, IVU, CT or MRI scanning).

V. RETROPERITONEAL ABSCESS

Retroperitoneal abscess can be related directly to the posterior retroperitoneal space compartment including renal and perinephric infection or to the anterior retroperitoneal space compartment secondary to a gastrointestinal disease. The posterior abscess can be a result of extravasation from a ureteral calculus or ruptured renal caruncle. Perinephric infection can involve urolithiasis, diabetes mellitus, urinary tract infection or obstruction, or polycystic disease. The anterior abscess etiology can be represented by a host of GI tract diseases including: appendicitis, diverticulitis, Crohn's disease, pancreatic abscess, or malignancy. Retroperitoneal abscess can occur with an incompletely resolved retroperitoneal hematoma secondary to some form of blunt abdominal trauma or as the result of a vascular accident such as a renal cancer disruption, percutaneous lithotripsy, gynecologic surgery, anticoagulants, tuberculosis, sarcoidosis, osteomyelitis, epidural abscess, or iatrogenic events.

Patients with a retroperitoneal abscess will present with fever, malaise, diffuse abdominal pain on physical examination, costovertebral tenderness, and a positive "psoas sign" when the psoas muscle is involved. The symptoms will have been present for several weeks and if the retroperitoneal nerves are involved, patients may complain of tenderness in the groin, lower abdomen, flank, and upper thigh. Sepsis is observed in approximately 60 percent of affected patients.

Laboratory testing is nonspecific and leukocytosis being noted in two thirds of patients. Anemia is often present. Sixty percent of the time, pyuria will be observed. Hematuria is present in approximately thirty percent. A routine abdominal x-ray is normal in approximately half the of the patients. Abnormalities can include the following: (1) obliteration of the psoas muscle border on the abscess side, (2) displacement of bowel gas and/or ileus, (3) lumbar scoliosis, (4) paranephric gas, and (5) displacement of the kidney. Abdominal ultrasound may be of some diagnostic help; however, the CT scan will provide definitive diagnostic detail with regard to the size, content, and magnitude of the retroperitoneal abscess.

The treatment involves the combination of antibiotic therapy (broad-spectrum antibiotics until the culture growth sensitivities are available) with early drainage. Traditionally, a surgical incision with irrigation and drainage of the space was the treatment of choice but with the high precision of interventional radiology, percutaneous drainage with one or more tubes has been proven to be highly successful and only in those cases with failed resolution of the infection should open surgical drainage or nephrectomy be performed.

VI. RETROPERITONEAL HEMORRHAGE

A spontaneous retroperitoneal bleed is rare and is most often due to blunt abdominal trauma or rupture of an abdominal aortic aneurysm. Other causes can include bursting of a large renal cell carcinoma, percutaneous lithotripsy or placement of a renal percutaneous drainage tube, extracorporeal shock wave lithotripsy

(ESWL), renal biopsy (open or percutaneous), gynecologic surgery, anticoagulants, gunshot or knife wound, or iatrogenic causes. The physical examination may reveal flank ecchymosis, an adynamic ileus, and hypotension. Blood that accumulates in the retroperitoneum can lead to ureteral deviation or even ureteral obstruction. Radiographic evaluation is helpful and delineation of the exact nature of the retroperitoneal bleed can be made using IVU, US, CT, and/or MRI. These same evaluating parameters should be used to monitor resolution of the bleed hematoma.

VII. BENIGN PRIMARY RETROPERITONEAL TUMORS

Eighty-five percent of primary retroperitoneal tumors are malignant and the remaining fifteen percent are benign; the categorization of the benign lesions includes 4.5 percent neural, 3.3 percent cystic, 2.4 percent lipomas. The majority of the other benign tumors include fibromas, hemangiomas, and leiomyomas. Less often seen lesions consist of xanthogranuloma, pheochromocytoma, teratoma, lymphangioma, hemangioma, mesothelioma, and cystadenoma. The primary goal of treatment is total resection of the lesion with appropriate frozen sections to rule out malignancy. If repetitive frozen sections reveal benign disease, the need for extensive resection of normal adjacent organs can be obviated.

BIBLIOGRAPHY

Baker LRI, Mallinson WJ, Gregory MC, et al: Idiopathic retroperitoneal fibrosis: A retrospective analysis of 60 cases. *Br J Urol* 60:497–503, 1988.

Dalton RR, Donohue JH, Mucha P, et al: Management of retroperitoneal sarcomas. *Surgery* 105:725, 1989.

Felix EL, Wood DK, DasGupta TK: Tumors of the retroperitoneum. *Curr Probl Cancer* 6:3, 1981.

Koep L, Zuidema, GD: The clinical significance of retroperitoneal fibrosis. *Surgery* 82:250–257, 1977.

Sheinfeld J, Eturk E, Spatano RF, et al: Peritoneal abscess:Current concepts. *J Urol* 127:191–194, 1987.

Wagenknect LV, Hardy JC: Value of various treatment for retroperitoneal fibrosis. *Eur Urol* 7:193–200, 1981.

SELF-ASSESSMENT QUESTIONS

1. Which one of the following nerves is not considered to be a structure within the retroperitoneum?
    a. Pudendal
    b. Sciatic
    c. Obturator
    d. Vagus
    e. Femoral

2. Symptoms associated with adult ureteropelvic junction (UPJ) obstruction do not include:
    a. nausea.
    b. hematuria.

   c. vomiting.
   d. diarrhea.
   e. back pain

3. Surgical correction of the UPJ obstruction includes the following except:
   a. excision of the dysfunctional segment and repair.
   b. balloon dilatation.
   c. antegrade (percutaneous) incision.
   d. retrograde incision.

4. Extrinsic ureteral obstruction is caused by many disease entities and one of the answers below should be excluded.
   a. Retroperitoneal fibrosis
   b. Endometriosis
   c. Pregnancy
   d. Appendicitis
   e. Gastroesophageal reflux

5. Retroperitoneal fibrosis is an adult inflammatory process and may be due to all of the following except:
   a. LSD.
   b. inflammatory bowel disease.
   c. tuberculosis.
   d. abdominal aortic aneursym.
   e. Ormond's disease.

6. Which symptom is not considered to be associated with retroperitoneal fibrosis?
   a. Malaise
   b. Weight gain
   c. Abdominal pain
   d. Backache
   e. Nausea and vomiting

7. Which one of the following is not associated with retroperitoneal fibrosis?
   a. Lateral deviation of the ureters
   b. Extrinsic compression of the ureters
   c. Hydronephrosis
   d. Proximal ureteral dilatation
   e. Distal ureteral narrowing

8. Patients with a retroperitoneal abscess will not have:
   a. absent abdominal pain.
   b. fever.
   c. malaise.
   d. sepsis.
   e. costovertebral tenderness.

9. A routine abdominal x-ray in a patient with a retroperitoneal abscess may present with:
   a. obliteration of the psoas muscle border on the abscess side.
   b. displacement of bowel gas and/or ileus.
   c. lumbar scoliosis.
   d. displacement of the kidney.
   e. all of the above.

10. A retroperitoneal hemorrhage may caused by:
   a. blunt abdominal trauma.
   b. rupture of an abdominal aortic aneurysm.
   c. bursting of a large renal cell carcinoma.
   d. renal biopsy.
   e. all of the above.

Answers

1. d	6. b
2. d	7. a
3. b	8. a
4. e	9. e
5. e	10. e

CHAPTER 24

Disorders of the Adrenal Gland

E. Darracott Vaughan, Jr.

Adrenal disorders are rare but easily diagnosed. The pathophysiology of each specific disorder is well known, the diagnostic laboratory tests accurate, and radiographic imaging for localization precise. Unfortunately, the diagnosis is often delayed simply because the disorder is not included in the differential diagnosis by the physician.

I. ADRENAL EMBRYOLOGY
The adrenal cortex develops from mesoderm and the medulla from neuroectoderm. During the 5th week of fetal development, the fetal cortex forms when mesothelial cells invade the mesenchyme near the developing gonad. A second migration forms the definitive cortex. The intimate relationship with the developing gonads and kidneys explains the occasional finding of ectopic or aberrant adrenal tissue in those organs. Neural crest cells migrate at the 7th week to form nodules of neuroblasts within the cortex. By the 20th week there is a primitive medulla but the definitive medulla consisting of chromaffin cells is not present until atrophy of the fetal adrenal cortex. The majority of extra adrenal chromaffin cells atrophy but deposits along the sympathetic chain to the organ of Zuckerkandl persist and can be the site of ectopic ganglioneuromas.

II. ADRENAL ANATOMY
A. General
1. The adrenals are paired retroperitoneal organs that lie within perinephric fat at the anterosuperior and medial aspect of the kidneys.
2. They measure 5 cm in length by 3 cm in width and are 1 cm thick.
3. Gland weight averages 5 g in the adult. The large fetal cortex (5 to 10 g) regresses during the first 6 weeks of life

but is subject to fetal adrenal hemorrhage during traumatic childbirth.

4. Cortical infoldings defined by CT or MRI may be confused for small adenomas.

B. Adjacent Organ Relationships

1. Left adrenal
   a. The kidney is more closely related at the left side and the left renal artery often lies directly beneath the left adrenal vein.
   b. The apical branch of the left renal artery may course adjacent to the inferior surface of the adrenal.
   c. The anterior surface lies behind the body of the pancreas and the splenic vein.

2. Right adrenal
   a. The gland lies posterolateral to the inferior vena cava and is not directly attached to the kidney.
   b. The anterior surface is in direct contact with the peritoneum overlying the inferior posterior surface of the liver.
   c. The posterior surface of both adrenals are in contact with the posterior abdominal musculature and the attachments of the diaphragm.

C. Adrenal Cortex

1. The cortex comprises 80 percent of total adrenal weight.
2. The cortex divides into three zones:
   a. The zona glomerulosa producing aldosterone.
   b. The zona fasciculata producing glucocorticoids.
   c. The inner zona reticularis producing androgens.

D. Adrenal Medulla

1. The medulla consists of chromaffin cells.
2. The medullary cells are rich in catecholamines producing both norepinephrine and epinephrine.

E. Vascular Supply

1. The adrenals have a rich and delicate blood supply. The adrenal blood flow is estimated to be 6 to 7 mL/min.
2. Small arterial vessels enter into the gland in a stellate fashion without a dominant single artery.
3. The source of the adrenal vessels are:
   a. Primarily the interior phrenic artery.
   b. The aorta.
   c. The renal artery.
   d. The gonadal vessels.
4. The venous drainage differs from the two adrenals.
   a. The right adrenal vein lies cephalad and directly enters the posterior aspect of the inferior vena cava (IVC). It

is often short and easily torn during dissection. It may join a right hepatic vein and then enter the IVC.
   b. The left adrenal vein enters the left renal vein. From the medial aspect of the adrenal there is a phrenic vein, which courses cephalad into the diaphragmatic fibers.

III. ADRENAL PHYSIOLOGY

The adrenal can be thought of as two different organs: the cortex and medulla. Each has its own unique physiology and hormonally active secretory products.

A. Adrenal Cortex

1. From a common precursor pregnenolone, the zones of the adrenal cortex produce an array of steroid hormones with specific actions including salt retention, metabolic homeostasis, and adrenarche development (Fig. 24-1).
   a. The zona glomerulosa is the only source of the major mineralocorticoid, aldosterone, which stimulates sodium reabsorption in the kidney, gut, and salivary and sweat glands with reciprocal potassium and hydrogen ion loss.
   b. The zone fasciculata and reticularis produce cortisol, the major glucocorticoid in humans, and the principal androgens, dehydroepiandrosterone (DHEA), dehydro-epiandrosterone sulfate (DHEA-S), and androstenedione.
   c. The deficiency of one of the five enzymes necessary to convert cholesterol to cortisol leads to a family of diseases termed congenital adrenal hyperplasia.
2. The regulation of corticosteroid release involves the hypothalamic release of corticotropin-releasing hormone (CRH), which in turn stimulates release of corticotropin (ACTH) from the pituitary.
   a. Corticotropin (ACTH) secretion is reciprocally related to the circulating cortisol level.
3. Adrenal androgen production is under the influence of corticotrophin, although other mechanisms are involved.
4. Aldosterone production, in contrast to other adrenal steroids, is primarily under the control of angiotensin II (Fig. 24-2).
   a. Other stimuli for aldosterone are potassium and corticotrophin.

B. Adrenal Medulla

1. The large chromaffin cells synthesize and secrete both epinephrine and norepinephrine as well as dopamine (Fig. 24-3).

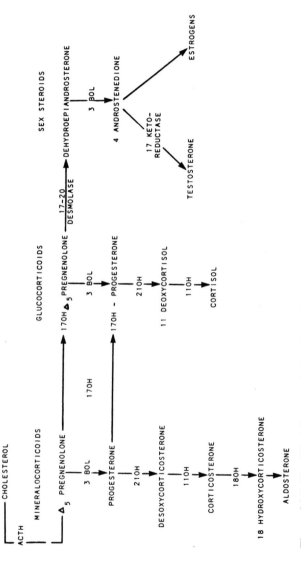

Figure 24-1 Simplified diagram of adrenal steroid synthesis. (*Reproduced from Kroovand RL: Diagnosis and management of adrenogenital syndrome caused by congenital adrenal hyperplasia. AUA Update Series, vol. 5, lesson 36, 1–7, 1985.*)

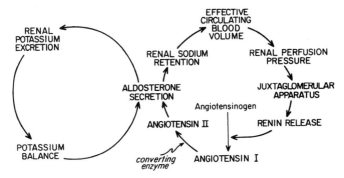

Figure 24-2 Control of aldosterone secretion by means of interrelationships between the potassium and renin–angiotensin feedback loop. (*From Campbell's Urology, 7th Ed, Chapt. 96, p. 2921*)

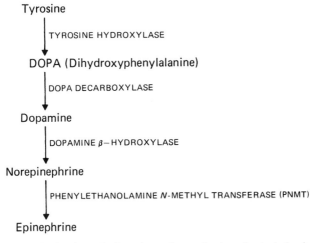

Figure 24-3 Biosynthetic pathway for production of catecholamines in the adrenal medulla.

2. Catecholamines are stored in separate vesicles and released through activation of the preganglionic sympathetic nerves by various stimuli including stress, cold, pain, heat, asphyxia, hypotension, hypoglycemia, and sodium depletion.

3. Catecholamines are rapidly removed from the circulation. Degradation is by the action of catechol-o-methyl transferase (COMT) and monoamine oxidase (MAO).

4. The main urinary metabolite is vanillylmandelic acid (VMA) with metanephrine, normetanephrine, and their derivatives contributing to total metabolic products, which are often measured while evaluating patients for pheochromocytoma.

IV. ADRENAL DISORDERS: INCREASED, DECREASED, AND NORMAL FUNCTION

A. Increased Function
1. Adrenal cortex
   a. Hyperaldosteronism (Conn's syndrome)
   b. Cushing's syndrome
   c. Adrenogenital syndromes
2. Adrenal medulla
   a. Pheochromocytoma

B. Decreased Function
1. Primary adrenal insufficiency (Addison's disease)
   a. Idiopathic adrenal atrophy
   b. Granulomatous disease
   c. Infarction and hemorrhage
   d. Metastatic tumor
   e. Infiltration lesions (i.e., amyloidosis)

C. Normal Function
1. Adenoma and carcinoma
2. Myelolipoma
3. Adrenal cysts

D. Pseudotumors
1. Exophytic renal mass
2. Hepatic mass
3. Interposition of colon into hepatorenal recess
4. Dilated IVC

V. CUSHING'S SYNDROME

Cushing's syndrome is the term used to describe the symptom complex caused by excess circulating glucocorticoids. The first case of Cushing's syndrome was presented in 1912 by Dr. Harvey Cushing.

A. Pituitary hypersecretion of corticotrophin (ACTH)
Pituitary hypersecretion of ACTH, Cushing's disease, accounts for 75 to 85 percent of patients with endogenous Cushing's disease.
1. About 10 to 20 percent of patients with ACTH-dependent Cushing's disease have ectopic secretion of ACTH or CRH from neoplasms, the most common is lung carci-

noma. Patients with adrenal adenoma or carcinoma and suppression of ACTH accounts for the remaining 15 to 25 percent.

B. Source

An exogenous source of Cushing's syndrome should first always be excluded in a patient with clinical signs of steroid excess.

C. Clinical Manifestations

The clinical manifestations of Cushing's syndrome are manifold because of the numerous actions of cortisol (Table 24-1).

1. The physical examination is extremely important in the evaluation looking for the stigmata of Cushing's syndrome.
2. Pseudo-Cushing's is a term utilized to describe patients with clinical manifestations of the syndrome and mild elevations of cortisol.

Table 24-1 Clinical Manifestations of Cushing's Syndrome

	ALL[a] (%)	DISEASE[b] (%)	ADENOMA/ CARCINOMA[c] (%)
Obesity	90	91	93
Hypertension	80	63	93
Diabetes	80	32	79
Centripetal obesity	80	—	—
Weakness	80	25	82
Muscle atrophy	70	34	—
Hirsutism	70	59	79
Menstrual abnormalities/ sexual dysfunction	70	46	75
Purple striae	70	46	36
Moon facies	60	—	—
Osteoporosis	50	29	54
Early bruising	50	54	57
Acne/pigmentation	50	32	—
Mental changes	50	47	57
Edema	50	15	—
Headache	40	21	46
Poor healing	40	—	—

[a]Hunt and Tyrrell, 1978.
[b]Wilson, 1984.
[c]Scott, 1973.

From Scott HW Jr: In Scott HW, ed. *Surgery of the Adrenal Glands*, Philadelphia, J.B. Lippincott, 1990.

a. Causes include depression and excessive alcohol ingestion.

b. Low dose dexamethasone 1 mg at night suppresses plasma cortisol to normal.

D. Laboratory Diagnosis

1. The clinical diagnosis of Cushing's syndrome is confirmed by the demonstration of cortisol hypersecretion (Fig. 24-4).

2. The determination of 24-hour urinary excretion of cortisol is the most direct and reliable index of cortisol secretion.

3. The ideal way to determine whether a patient has ACTH-dependent or ACTH-independent hypercortisolism is the concurrent measurement of both plasma ACTH (corticotrophin) and plasma cortisol.

a. If the plasma ACTH is greater than 50 pg/mL, the cortisol secretion is ACTH-dependent (the patient

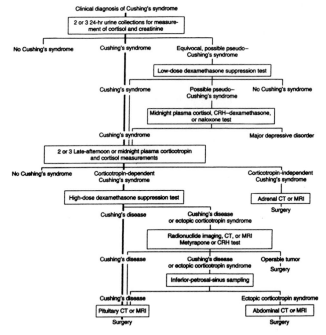

Figure 24-4 Identifying Cushing's syndrome and its causes. (*From Orth DN: N Engl J Med 1995;332:791. Reprinted by permission of the New England Journal of Medicine. Copyright 1995, Massachusetts Medical Society.*)

has Cushing's disease or ectopic ACTH or CRH secretion).

   b. If the ACTH is low, the patient has adrenal disease, adenoma, or carcinoma.

4. If corticotrophin/cortisol assay is not available, the dexamethasone suppression test is utilized.

   a. Low-dose dexamethasone 0.5 mg QID causes plasma cortisol suppression to normal in patients with pseudo-Cushing's and normal patients.

   b. High-dose dexamethasone 2.0 mg QID causes plasma cortisol suppression in patients with pituitary Cushing's (Cushing's disease).

   c. Patients with adrenal adenoma and carcinoma do not suppress plasma cortisol with high-dose dexamethasone.

   d. Patients with ectopic ACTH are often also resistant to high-dose dexamethasone.

   e. The most direct way to demonstrate pituitary ACTH hypersecretion is with petrosal venous sinus sampling.

E. Radiographic Localization

1. In patients with Cushing's disease, CT or MRI of the sella turcica often identifies pituitary adenoma.

2. Adrenal lesions are defined by adrenal CT.

   a. Patients with bilateral hyperplasia show diffuse thickening and elongation of the adrenal rami.

   b. Adrenal adenomas are usually larger than 2 cm and solitary with atrophy of the opposite gland.

   c. Adrenal carcinomas are characteristically greater than 5 cm, irregular, and nonhomogeneous with necrosis and calcification. However, they may be indistinguishable from adenomas.

3. Adrenal MRI may be useful.

   a. Adenomas have low signal intensity.

   b. Adrenal carcinomas may show high signal intensity.

   c. Metastatic tumors to the adrenal show high signal intensity.

   d. Medullary tumors show high signal intensity.

F. Treatment

1. Cushing's disease
   a. Trans-sphenoidal pituitary adenomectomy
   b. Pituitary radiation

2. Ectopic CRH/ACTH secretion
   a. Removal of the primary tumor

3. Adrenal adenoma/carcinoma
   a. Unilateral adrenalectomy
      i. Small—laparoscopic removal

　　　　　ii. Carcinoma or size greater than 6–cm open surgical removal
　　　b. Mitotane (OP-DDD) is utilized for patients with metastatic adrenal carcinoma.
　　4. Preoperative/postoperative management
　　　a. Preoperative steroid suppression with metyrapone to reduce symptoms.
　　　b. Intraoperative glucocorticoid administration.
　　　c. Postoperative steroid replacement with dexamethasone.
　　　d. Patients are at increased risk for infection, hemorrhage, and fractures.

VI. ADRENAL CARCINOMA

A rare tumor, 1 case per 1.7 million with poor prognosis.

A. Classification

Classified by hormonal secretion.
1. Cushing's syndrome
2. Virilization in females
　　a. Increased DHEA, 17-ketosteroid, increased testosterone
3. Feminizing syndrome in men
4. Hyperaldosteronism
5. Mixed secretion (common)
6. Nonfunctional 30 percent

B. Signs and Symptoms

Clinically apparent signs of defeminization or masculinization are typical of carcinoma. Elevated DHEA, androstenedione, or urinary 17 ketosteroids makes carcinoma likely.

C. Treatment

Treatment is excision but the cure rate is less than 50 percent, even in patients with localized disease.

VII. INCIDENTALLY DISCOVERED ADRENAL MASSES

Many adrenal lesions are now accidentally identified with CT or MRI performed for some other reason and 1 to 2 percent of imaging studies show adrenal lesions.

A. Evaluation

Evaluation can be limited.
1. Careful history and physical examination to look for evidence suggesting Cushing's syndrome, hyperaldosteronism, carcinoma, or pheochromocytoma.

2. All patients should have urinary catecholamine studies to diagnose pheochromocytoma.
3. Renin and aldosterone determinations only if hypertension and hypokalemia are present.
4. Cortisol studies only if there is a suggestion of Cushing's syndrome on history and physical examination.

B. Management

The management of patients with an incidentally found adrenal mass is shown in Figure 24-5.

1. All solid lesions greater than 5 cm are removed.
2. All functional lesions are removed.
3. All cystic lesions are observed and only removed when increased size is found.
4. Nonfunctional lesions less than 5 cm are studied with MRI and removed by a laparoscopic technique if the MRI is not hypointense with homogeneous findings typical of an adenoma.

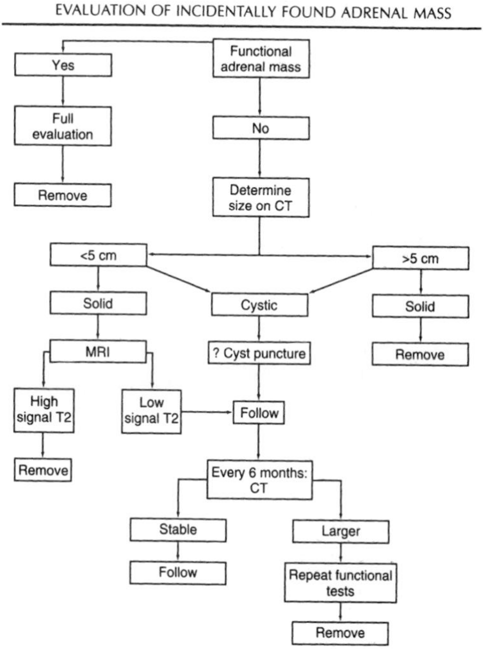

EVALUATION OF INCIDENTALLY FOUND ADRENAL MASS

Figure 24-5 Evaluation of incidentally found adrenal mass. (*From Campbell's Urology, 7th Ed, Chapt. 96, p. 2933*)

VIII. HYPERALDOSTERONISM (CONN'S SYNDROME)

First described by Dr. Jerome Conn in 1955. The clinical triad is hypertension, hypokalemia, and alkalosis. The biochemical triad is hypokalemia, low plasma renin activity (PRA), and high plasma or urinary aldosterone.

A. Pathology
1. Solitary adenoma
2. Bilateral hyperplasia
3. Adrenal carcinoma (rare)

B. Signs and Symptoms
1. Mild hypertension
2. Muscular weakness due to low potassium
3. Polyuria and polydipsia
4. Absence of edema
5. Minimal retinal vascular changes

C. Laboratory Diagnosis
1. Unprovoked hypokalemia is the hallmark of primary hypoaldosteronism (Fig. 24-6).
   a. Monitoring of the potassium after salt loading with 10 g of sodium/day minimizes the false-negative normokalemic finding.
   b. Elevated 24-hour urine potassium excretions verifies renal potassium loss.
2. Low PRA following sodium restriction distinguishes primary hyperaldosteronism from secondary hyperaldosteronism due to renal disease and elevated renin secretions (high PRA).
3. Elevated plasma or urinary aldosterone level indexed against urinary sodium excretion after potassium repletion and sodium loading taken together with a low PRA verifies the diagnosis.

D. Tests to Delineate Adenoma and Hyperplasia
1. With posture, both PRA and plasma aldosterone rise in patients with hyperplasia. Aldosterone does not rise in patients with an adenoma.
2. C-18 Cortisol methyl oxygenated metabolites are only elevated in patients with an adenoma.
3. Adrenal vein aldosterone–Cortisol ratio is unilaterally elevated in patients with an adenoma, bilaterally elevated in patients with hyperplasia.

E. Adrenal Imaging
1. Adrenal thin cut pre- and post-contrast CT
   a. Adenoma: unilateral hypodense usually small, 0.5 to 2 cm.
   b. Hyperplasia bilateral nodular thickening.

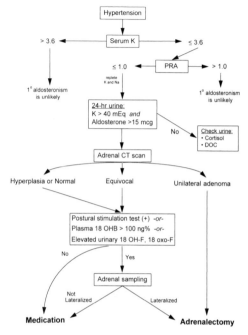

Figure 24-6 Algorithm for the diagnosis and treatment of primary aldosteronism. Abbreviation: 18 − OHB = 18-hydroxycorticosterone; 18 − OH-F = 18-hydroxycortisol; 18 − oxo-F = 18-oxocortisol; CT = computed tomography; DOC = deoxycorticosterone; PRA = plasma renin activity. (*From Blumenfeld JD, Schlussel Y, Sealey JE, et al: Ann Intern Med 121:877–885, 1994.*)

F. Treatment
1. Adenoma: pre-treat with spironolactone to normalize potassium, then laparoscopic adrenalectomy.
2. Hyperplasia: medical management with spironolactone 50 to 200 mg/day (also calcium channel blockers are useful).
   a. With asymmetric aldosterone secretion by sampling, unilateral adrenalectomy may be necessary if medical treatment fails.

IX. OTHER ADRENAL LESIONS
A. Adrenal Cysts
1. Endothelial
2. Lymphangiomatous

   3. Nonfunctional
   4. Usually observe

B. Myelolipoma
   1. Benign tumors containing hematopoietic and fatty elements
   2. Characteristic picture on CT
   3. Usually observed

C. Metastatic Tumors
   1. Common in patients with carcinomatosis (9 percent)
   2. Most common primary site is the lung
   3. Nonfunctional.
   4. Bright on T2-MRI
   5. Irregular in appearance
   6. Treatment depends on the primary tumor

D. Adrenal Hemorrhage
   1. Found in neonates following traumatic delivery
   2. Associated with generalized sepsis
   3. Bright on T2-MRI
   4. Spontaneous resolution
   5. May lead to hypoadrenalism (Addison's disease)

X. ADRENAL INSUFFICIENCY

Adrenal insufficiency is rare, 0.3 per 100,000, with the most common causes being tuberculosis or adrenal atrophy. However, because it is potentially fatal, recognition is critical.

A. Signs and Symptoms (percent)
   1. Addison's disease
      a. Weakness and fatigue (94)
      b. Weight loss (90)
      c. Anorexia (80)
      d. Nausea and vomiting (66)
      e. GI symptoms (61)
   2. Acute adrenal insufficiency
      a. Severe clinical deterioration (100)
      b. Fevers (70)
      c. Nausea and vomiting (64)
      d. Abdominal pain (46)

B. Laboratory
   1. Hyponatremia
   2. Hyperkalemia
   3. Azotemia

C. Diagnosis
   1. Low plasma cortisol.

2. Failure to increase plasma or urinary corticosteroid levels to the normal range with ACTH infusion; 0.25 cosyntropin given IV: measure plasma cortisol before and 60 min later (normal cortisol responses is a rise above 18 μg/dL).

D. Treatment
1. Stress level steroids (8 to 10 mg dexamethasone)
2. Saline
3. Correct hyperkalemia

XI. PHEOCHROMOCYTOMA
A. General
A rare tumor less than 1% of the hypertensive population, which arises from chromaffin cells may cause severe malignant hypertension and sudden death.

B. Clinical Manifestations
1. Sustained hypertension
2. Paroxysmal hypertension with dramatic attacks
3. Sustained hypertension with superimposed paroxysms (50 to 66 percent)
4. Normal blood pressure (10 percent)
5. Other manifestations:

	Paroxysmal (percent)	Persistent (percent)
Headaches	90	72
Sweating	65	69
Palpitations	73	51
Anxiety	60	28
Tremulousness	51	26
Chest pain	48	28

C. Associated Diseases and Syndromes
1. Cholelithiasis
2. Medullary thyroid carcinoma
3. Hyperparathyroidism
4. Neurofibromatosis
5. Von-Hippel-Lindau disease
6. Catecholamine-induced myocardiopathy

D. Localization
1. Adrenal (90 percent)
2. Extra-adrenal (10 percent)
3. Multiple (10 percent)
   a. Children
   b. Familial

    c. Von-Hippel-Landau

    d. Multiple endocrine adenomas.

E. Pathology
1. Greater than 90 percent benign.
2. Less than 10 percent malignant.

F. Diagnosis
1. It is recommended that all hypertensive patients be screened for pheochromocytoma because of the potentially fatal consequence of undiagnosed disease (Fig. 24-7).
2. Five percent of all cases will have normal catecholamines.

G. Radiologic Diagnosis
1. The MRI is the imaging study of choice to localize pheochromocytoma.
   a. The site of the lesion is localized.
   b. Multiple lesions can be localized.
   c. The T2-weighted image of the characteristic bright "light bulb" appearance.
   d. Adjacent structures and venous drainage can be identified.

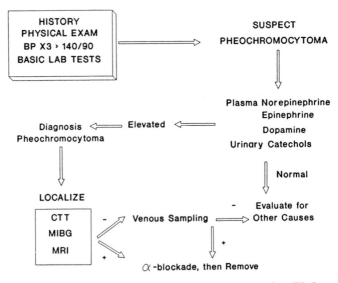

Figure 24-7 Identifying pheochromocytoma (*From Vaughan ED Jr.: Diagnosis of adrenal disorders in hypertension. World J Urology, 1989; 7:111–116.*)

2. Metaiodobenzylguanidine (MIBG) scanning localizes to catechol-secreting tissue and is especially useful in patients with multiple or recurrent lesions.

H. Treatment
  1. Preoperative
     a. Alpha-adrenergic blockade with phenoxybenzamine to a dose to normalize blood pressure.
     b. Beta-adrenergic blockade if cardiac arrhythmias persist.
     c. Alpha-methylparatyrosine-a tyrosine hydroxylase inhibitor (Fig. 24-3) to reduce catecholamine production.
  2. Surgical
     a. Laparoscopic removal for tumors less than 5 cm.
     b. Open removal for tumors greater than 5 cm.
  3. Postoperative
     a. Observe closely for hypotension and arrhythmias.

BIBLIOGRAPHY

Blumenfeld JD, Schlusse, Sealey JE, et al: Diagnosis and treatment of primary hyperaldosteronism. *Ann Intern Med,* 121:877–885, 1994.

Blumenfeld JD, Vaughan ED Jr.: The adrenals. In: *Campbell's Urology.* 7th Ed. Philadelphia, Saunders, 1998, pp. 2915–2971.

Manger WM, Gifford RW Jr.: Pheochromocytoma. A clinical review. In: *Hypertension Pathophysiology, Diagnosis, and Management.* Laragh JH, Brenner BM, eds. 1995, pp. 2225–2246.

Orth DN: Cushing syndrome. *N Eng J Med* 332:791–795, 1995.

Ulchaker JC, Goldfarb DA, Bravo EL, Novick AC: Successful outcomes in pheochromocytoma surgery in the modern era. *J Urol* 161:764–767, 1999.

Vaughan ED Jr.: Adrenal surgery. F. F. Marshall, Ed. In: *Textbook of Operative Surgery.* Philadelphia, Saunders, 1996, p 220–230.

Vaughan ED Jr., (ed): Diagnosis and treatments of adrenal disorders. *World J Urol* 17:1064, 1999.

CHAPTER 25

Renal Transplantation

Ali Naji
Tanmay Lal

Renal transplantation is the treatment of choice for patients with end-stage renal failure. In 1998, 12,232 renal transplants were performed in the United States. Because renal transplantation is economically advantageous and improves quality of life as compared to dialysis therapy, the application of this modality is limited primarily by organ availability. Technical failures claim an estimated 5 percent of grafts, but immunologic rejection, infections, and cardiovascular disease are the major causes of morbidity and mortality. Outcomes reported by the United Network for Organ Sharing (UNOS) in 1998 showed 1-year primary renal allograft and patient survival rates of 88 percent and 93 percent, respectively. The chance of success is optimized by a careful approach that begins with patient selection and proceeds through surgery, perioperative care, and long-term follow-up.

I. PRIMARY ETIOLOGY OF RENAL FAILURE

Patients with irreversible (or approaching) end-stage renal failure who require dialysis are candidates for renal transplantation. Although there is no "age cutoff" for transplantation, only a small number of transplants are performed in recipients over 70 years. The principal etiology of end-stage renal failure in the adult population includes diabetes mellitus, hypertension, and chronic glomerulonephritis. In children, congenital abnormalities of the urinary tract or renal dysplasia constitute the greater majority of patients with renal failure that receive kidney transplantation.

The principal contraindications to renal transplantation are the presence of active infection, substance abuse, and a recent history of malignancy. Although advanced coronary artery occlusive disease constitutes a relative contraindication, a careful cardiac evaluation and a definitive treatment minimizes the risk for the potential candidates of renal transplantation.

II. DONOR CONSIDERATIONS AND HISTOCOMPATABILITY

The majority of the renal grafts are recovered from cadaveric donor sources. However, the organ donor shortage and the improved outcome of kidney transplantation has led to an increased the utility of kidney transplantation from living donors, including genetically unrelated but "emotionally related" donors, such as a spouse or close friend. The genetically unrelated donors (especially spouses) are now considered acceptable by many centers, and in 1991 through 1997 accounted for 1,900 kidney transplants in the United States (almost 10 percent of living donor transplants or 2.7 percent of total transplants). The living unrelated renal transplants have demonstrated surprisingly good graft function (92 percent at 1 year and 72 percent at 5 years) reported to UNOS, which is significantly better than the survival of cadaveric grafts. For the prospective recipients, major advantages of living renal transplantation is the elimination of the discomfort, expense, and risks of prolonged dialysis while waiting for a cadaver kidney. Post-transplant morbidity is also minimized by the reduction of the delayed graft function or early rejection crisis. Moreover, because of the improved histocompatibility, long-term results of related donor transplantation remains superior to cadaveric grafts. In the United States, approximately 30 percent of the kidney transplants are from living donors.

The human leukocyte antigens (HLA) are gene products of alleles at a number of closely linked loci on the short arm of chromosome 6 in humans. The gene products of HLA-A, B, and C loci are referred to as class I major histocompatibility complex (MHC) antigens, and the products of the D region are class II MHC antigens. HLA antigens are inherited as co-dominant alleles and, because of the relatively low recombinant frequency, the HLA genes are usually inherited en bloc from each parent. The long-term renal allograft survival is largely dependent upon the histocompatibility match between the donor and recipient. In immediate families, inheritance of the HLA antigens can be determined serologically and falls into four different combinations of haplotype. Any two siblings have a 25 percent of being HLA identical, that is, having inherited the same chromosome 6 (haplotype) from each parent; a 50 percent chance of sharing one haplotype; and a 25 percent chance of sharing neither haplotype. Parent to child donation always involves a one haplotype identity. The importance of matching HLA antigen in the selection of living related donors for renal transplantation is well established and excellent long-term graft survival (greater than 95 percent) can be expected when a related donor and recipient are HLA identical.

Selection of living donors requires a thorough medical evaluation to assure that the donor will not suffer undue risk. Initial evaluation of potential donors consists of ABO blood group determination and HLA typing (ABO incompatible donors are excluded). All blood group compatible donors are then tested with a T-lymphocyte lymphocytotoxicity assay (cross match). All donors, living or cadaver, are screened for communicable diseases, with particular attention to the HIV and hepatitis B and C viruses. The evaluation of a living donor requires diagnostic studies such as urinalysis, 24-hour urine collection for creatinine clearance and protein excretion, and intravenous pyelogram and aortogram to visualize the anatomy of the collecting system and renal vasculature. Magnetic resonance angiography is now substituted for contrast arteriography at many centers to minimize the risk to the donor.

If the anatomic features of both kidneys are compatible, the recovery of the left kidney is preferred because of the longer renal vein, which technically facilitates the recipient operation. However, if the imaging shows multiple renal arteries, the kidney with a single artery is usually selected to facilitate vascular anastomosis. In an effort to make the procedure more acceptable to prospective living donors by reducing morbidity, several groups have evaluated minimally invasive kidney recovery. The development of laparoscopic nephrectomy has led to a significant increase in the number of living donors. The potential advantage of this procedure includes shortened hospital stay, a quicker postoperative recovery, and earlier return to work. Complications of donor nephrectomy include infection, bleeding, ileus, pneumothorax, and death (0.03 percent); the most common cause of death has been pulmonary embolism.

Cadaver Donors
In 1998, the donation rate was 27.5 per million population of the United States. Due to a failure to identify suitable donors, obtain consent, and retrieve organs, less than 20 percent of suitable donors become available. The optimal cadaveric donors are previously healthy subjects between 3 to 65 years of age, who have sustained fatal head injuries or cerebral vascular accidents. Careful history, physical examination, and laboratory surveys should be carried out to uncover factors that are contraindications to organ donations, such as the presence of generalized infections (including occult ones, such as HIV or hepatitis B and C or a higher risk of these such as the use of intravenous drugs), malignancy (other than non-metastasizing brain tumors), and known renal disease, hypertension, or advanced arteriosclerosis.

In most instances, procurement of cadaveric kidneys are carried out as a component of the multiorgan recovery of thoracic and abdominal organs. The approach utilizes the technique of in situ perfusion and en bloc dissection of the solid visceral organs (liver, pancreas, and kidneys). Kidneys can be preserved by simple cold storage for as long as 48 hours, but the delayed graft function rate (primarily due to acute tubular necrosis) increases markedly with cold storage of greater than 30 hours.

III. RECIPIENT OPERATION

The renal allograft is implanted in the extraperitoneal iliac fossa through a curved oblique incision either in the right or left lower abdominal quadrant. The sequence of vascular anastomosis involves end-to-side anastomosis of the renal vein to the external iliac vein. This is followed by the arterial anastomosis that joins the end of the renal transplant artery (often with a Carrel patch of cadaver donor aorta) to the side of the external iliac artery. The internal iliac artery can be used, but there are frequently extensive arteriosclerotic changes in diabetic recipients. Distal ligation of the internal iliac artery may also contribute to impotence.

The genitourinary tract continuity is established with an extravesical ureteroneocystostomy (modified Lich technique). With this extravesical approach, the spatulated end of the transplant ureter is sewn to the bladder mucosa after incision of the detrusor muscle. The detrusor muscle is then reunited to buttress the anastomosis and create an antireflux valve. Nephroureteric internal stents are usually not utilized. Older techniques for GU continuity include the Leadbetter-Politano and ureteropyelostomy using the native ureter.

If the patient has been anuric or oliguric for several years, the bladder may be contracted and noncompliant. Bladder augmentation using a segment of intestine is then warranted, a procedure which is uniformly completed prior to transplantation. An alternative to augmentation is "stretching" the bladder with a regimen of bladder filling using incrementally larger volumes over time. If the bladder urodynamics are markedly abnormal, the bladder may be used as a reservoir and intermittent self-catheterization instituted after transplantation. This meets with better patient satisfaction and fewer complications than diversion.

IV. IMMUNOSUPPRESSION AND REJECTION

Currently, one of the two immunosuppressive protocols is utilized to control the immune response to the foreign renal graft. These include: 1) cyclosporin (Neoral), prednisone, mycophenolate mofetil (Cell Cept); or 2) FK506 (Prograf, Tacrolimus) and prednisone. Most renal transplant centers monitor the therapeutic trough level of cyclosporin or Prograf to provide effective immunosuppression and reduce the side effects (primarily nephrotoxicity) of these powerful immunosuppressants. In instances of cadaver renal transplantation where the recipient is experiencing delayed graft function, cyclosporin and FK506 may be initially withheld, because of their nephrotoxicity, until a trend in the resolution of acute tubular necrosis (ATN) is observed. In some transplant programs, an immune induction strategy based on the use of polyclonal (thymoglobulin or ATGAM) or monoclonal (OKT3) anti-T lymphocyte antibody has been utilized to maximize the protection of the renal graft from rejection when cyclosporin or FK506 are being withheld to prevent nephrotoxicity.

There has been a marked reduction of the occurrence of the renal allograft rejection with the utility of cyclosporin or FK506 based immunosuppression. Renal allograft rejection is generally manifested by a rise in serum creatinine, which must be differentiated from cyclosporin or FK506 nephrotoxicity. The differential could be aided by a renal biopsy to confirm the diagnosis before initiation of a high dose of steroids. If there is no improvement in the renal function, the refractory nature of the rejection process mandates the use of a monoclonal or polyclonal antibody preparation as a strategy to rescue the renal allograft from irreversible immune destruction.

V. COMPLICATIONS

Complications occurring in the first few hours or days after renal transplantation are commonly related to technical problems in establishing vascular and urinary tract continuity or the damage which occurs during donor nephrectomy or preservation. Because renal allograft rejection may also be an early event, its differentiation from other causes of poor function may be difficult. Arterial thrombosis occurs in less than 1 percent and venous thrombosis is even less common. Other causes of early arterial thrombosis include hyperacute or accelerated rejection, postoperative hypotension, hypercoagulable state, atherosclerosis of the donor or recipient vessels, trauma to the donor artery during recovery or subsequent preservation, disparity in vessels size during anastomosis, or dissection of a distal intimal flap. Acute anuria is suggestive of diagnosis and emergency exploration and thrombectomy are the only chance for salvage of the renal allograft.

Urinary Tract Complications

The most common cause of sudden cessation of urinary output in the immediate postoperative period is presence of a blood clot in the bladder or urethral catheter. More serious causes of fall in urine output (2 to 5 percent in most series) should be investigated simultaneously with consideration of vascular occlusion, ATN, and rejection.

Devascularization of the ureter during donor nephrectomy is a serious problem and may cause ureteral necrosis and urinary fistula within the first few days or weeks following surgery. Analyses of fluid obtained from wound drains or needle aspirations, ultrasound, nuclear scans, cystograms, and antegrade pyelography are other helpful studies to confirm the anatomic diagnosis. Treatment consists of revision of the ureteroneocystostomy or ureteropyelostomy using the patient's own ureter.

Acute Tubular Necrosis

In the absence of vascular or ureteric problem, initial nonfunction of cadaver kidneys may be attributed to ATN (incidence of 5 to 30 percent). Oliguria in the early transplant period should be treated with boluses of fluid for exclusion of hypovolemia. Although mild ATN per se does not significantly worsen the prognosis for eventual transplant success, the overall impact of ATN is an adverse one, primarily because it may interfere with the early diagnosis of rejection and delay antirejection therapy.

Infectious Complications

Infection is the most common complication of immunosuppression and occurs in 30 to 60 percent of patients during the first post-transplant year. Despite more cautious use of immunosuppression over the last decade, it is the major cause of death in the 5 to 10 percent of patients who die during the first year. Bacterial infections are the most common infections during the first month after transplantation, and the urinary tract, respiratory tract, and wound are the most prevalent sites. These infections usually respond to prompt antibiotic therapy and it is important to exclude the possibility of infection before antirejection therapy, since immunosuppression should be decreased rather than intensified in this situation.

The period between the first and 6th month after transplantation, usually the time of most intense immunosuppression, is the most common time for opportunistic infections. Cytomegalovirus (CMV), a member of the Herpes family, is an ubiquitous agent that infects most individuals sometime in their lives. Its causes clinically silent or mild infection in healthy individuals, and the latent virus and seropositivity persist for life. The majority of seronegative recipients who receive a kidney from a seropositive donor develop symptomatic illness, which varies in severity from mild fever and malaise to a debilitating syndrome marked by leucopenia, hepatitis, interstitial pneumonia, arthritis, central nervous system changes, gastrointestinal ulceration and bleeding, renal insufficiency, bacterial or fungal infection, and even death. The incidence of opportunistic infection such as *Pneumocystis carinii* pneumonia has been markedly reduced following routine prophylaxis with bactrim. Bacterial urinary tract infection (UTI) is the most common infectious problem in renal transplant recipients; 50 to 70 percent of patients will suffer a UTI after transplantation. Graft pyelonephritis is often accompanied by fever, chills, serum creatinine elevation, and a tender and swollen renal allograft. Because the renal allograft is denervated, the tenderness is most likely attributed to the inflammation of the renal parenchyma and compression of the peritoneum.

VI. RESULTS

The results of both cadaver and living donor transplantation have steadily improved throughout the years. The development of newer immunosuppressive agents and insights into the immunologic, technical, and medical aspects of renal transplantation have led to the current outstanding results. The benefit of renal transplantation have usually been described in terms of a better quality of life and reduced medical expenses, rather than the prolongation of life. However, analysis of the United States renal data system and transplant scientific registry of UNOS have provided convincing evidence that patients with end-stage renal disease placed on a waiting list for transplantation have a 68 percent reduction in the long-term risk of death once they have received a renal transplant, as compared with those who remain on the waiting list. This finding clearly focuses attention on kidney transplantation as a life-saving, rather than just a life-enhancing procedure.

BIBLIOGRAPHY

Hariharan S, Johnson CP, Bresnahan BA, Taranto BA, McIntosh MJ, Stablein D: Improved graft survival after renal transplantation in the United States, 1988 to 1996. *N Engl J Med,* 342:605–612, 2000.

Makowicz SB, Perloff LJ: Urologic considerations in renal transplantation. *Surg Gynecol Obstet* 160:579–587, 1985.

Terasaki PI, ed: *Clinical Transplants 1998.* Los Angeles, UCLA Tissue Typing Laboratory, 1998.

Wolfe RA, Ashby MA, Milford EL, et al: Comparison of mortality in all patients on dialysis, patients on dialysis awaiting transplantation, and recipients of a first cadaveric transplant. *N Engl J Med* 341:1725–1730, 1999.

CHAPTER 26

Renovascular Disease

Jeffrey P. Carpenter
Ali Naji

I. INCIDENCE

It is estimated that 25 million hypertensive patients are currently being treated in the United States; between 3 and 5 percent have a surgically correctable etiology. Renovascular hypertension (RVH) is present in 2 percent of all patients with high blood pressure. It is the most common cause of surgically treatable high blood pressure and is produced by a critical stenosis of the renal artery.

II. HISTORICAL OVERVIEW

In 1836, Bright was the first to associate hypertension and renal disease. The classic experiments of Goldblatt in 1934 clearly demonstrated that ischemia localized to the kidneys was sufficient to elevate blood pressure, which, in its early stages, was unaccompanied by decreased renal function. In 1937, Butler cured high blood pressure through nephrectomy in a 7-year-old boy with pyelonephritis. Clinical evidence of the validity of Goldblatt's experiment came in 1938 when Leadbetter and Burkland cured sustained diastolic hypertension in a 5-year-old boy by nephrectomy. Pathologic examination of the renal artery from this kidney revealed a lumen severely occluded by a mass of smooth muscle outlined by an elastic lamella representing fibromuscular hyperplasia (FMH). Evidence linking atherosclerotic obstruction of the renal arteries to hypertension was described in 1937 by Moritz and Oldt, who described severe vessel obstruction in an autopsy series of chronic hypertensives. Ultimately, it was the development of translumbar arteriography in the 1950s that opened the door to large-scale investigation and clinical correction of RVH.

III. PATHOLOGY
A. General
1. Significant stenosis of the renal artery, as demonstrated by Goldblatt, is necessary to produce RVH.

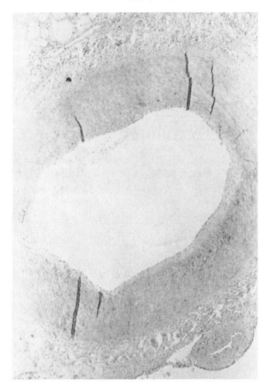

Figure 26-1 Photomicrographs of histologic cross sections of two renal arteries. **A:** Histologic appearance of an unobstructed renal artery. (*Figure continues.*)

2. The specific etiology of the narrowing may be related to atherosclerosis, renal artery fibrodysplasia, developmental renal artery stenosis, renal artery thrombosis or embolism, dissecting aortic, aneurysm, arteriovenous fistula, trauma, Takayasu's arteritis, or renal artery aneurysm.

3. More than 90 percent of all lesions can be classified in two groups, however, atherosclerotic and renal artery fibrodysplasia.

B. Etiology

1. Atherosclerotic renovascular disease is by far the most common etiology of renovascular disease (Fig. 26-1). Men are affected twice as often as women, reflecting the prevalence of arteriosclerosis in the male population. The sex difference is less apparent in the elderly. The fre-

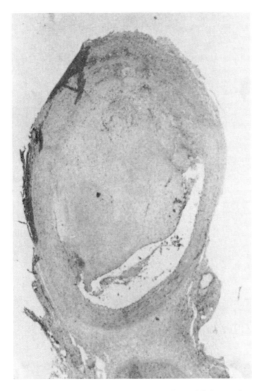

Figure 26-1 (*continued*) **B:** Renal artery with a high-grade obstruction secondary to atherosclerosis.

quency of renovascular arteriosclerosis is more common in elderly patients than atherosclerosis in general. In autopsy series, moderate to severe renal artery atherosclerosis is found in 50 percent of normotensive patients and in 75 percent of hypertensive patients. Most renovascular atherosclerotic lesions occur at the renal artery ostium of the aorta or within the first few centimeters of the main renal artery. These lesions often represent "aortic spillover" lesions and are a continuation of the atherosclerotic disease in the aorta as it enters the renal artery ostium. Distal renal artery arteriosclerotic lesions affect less than 5 percent of patients. Fifty percent of patients have bilateral renal artery disease.

2. Fibrodysplastic lesions affect less than 0.5 percent of the general population. Although uncommon, it is second

only to atherosclerosis as the most frequent cause of RVH. These lesions are found in the distal two thirds of the renal artery and may involve segmental branches. Fibrodysplastic disease is subdivided into the parts of the vessel involved being affected by the dysplastic process: intimal, medial, or perimedial dysplasia.

a. *Intintal dysplasia.* This process accounts for only 5 percent of renal artery fibrodysplastic lesions. It is seen more commonly in infants and young adults than in older patients. It is seen with equal frequency in both genders. It appears angiographically as a smooth focal stenonis of the main renal artery, rarely affecting the segmental vessels. The etiology of this lesion is unknown, but it may represent a proliferation of fetal arterial remnants within the vessel. The intima is hyperplastic. The media and adventitia are usually normal. Intimal fibroplasia can also be an acquired lesion after trauma or intraluminal injury to the vessel.

b. *Medial fibroplasia.* This lesion accounts for 85 percent of renal artery fibrodysplasia. Nearly all of these patients are women. It is often part of a systemic arterial process involving the renal, carotid, and iliac arteries. Although the lesion may be solitary, it is more commonly a series of stenoses with intervening aneurysmal dilatations appearing as a string of beads on arteriography. It is bilateral in 55 percent of patients. The lesions often extend into the segmental branches of the renal artery (Fig. 26-2).

c. *Perimedial dysplasia.* This lesion accounts for 10 percent of renal artery fibrodysplasia. Almost all of these patients are women. These lesions affect the main renal artery as focal stenoses or multiple constrictions without mural aneurysms.

3. *Developmental renal artery stenoses.* These failures of complete development of the renal artery account for approximately 40 percet of childhood RVH.

4. *Renal artery aneurysm.* The most common clinical presentation of renal artery aneurysm is hypertension. The etiology of this hypertension may be associated arterial stenosis, dissection of the artery, arteriovenous fistula formation, thromboembolism, or compression of arterial branches by the aneurysm.

5. *Renal artery dissection.* These lesions may be iatrogenic from catheter injuries or associated with trauma. They may occur spontaneously as a complication of underlying atherosclerotic or fibrodysplastic renovascular disease. All of these patients develop severe hypertension as the kidney becomes ischemic.

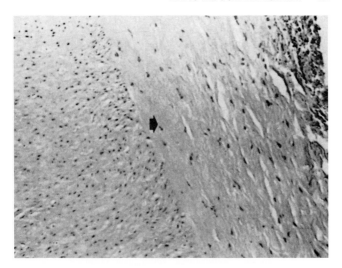

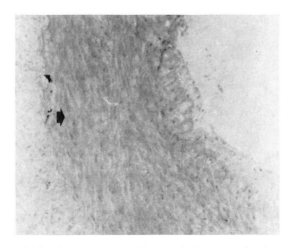

Figure 26-2 High-power photomicrographs demonstrating the appearance of a normal renal artery and tunica media *(arrow)* (*A*). **B:** Vessel with fibromuscular hyperplasia of the tunica media demonstrates overgrowth of the fibrous tissue and smooth muscle of that layer *(arrow)*.

6. *Renal* artery *embolism.* Embolic occlusion of the renal artery is rare. The most common etiology is embolism from the left heart. These patients present with flank pain, hypertension, and hematuria.

C. Age

1. *Atherosclerotic lesions.* These generally occur between the fifth and seventh decades of life.
2. *Fibrodysplastic lesions*
   a. Most frequently identified in younger patients in the second and third decades of life.
   b. Although infrequent in childhood, muscular lesions are the most common cause of RVH in the first decade of life.

IV. PATHOPHYSIOLOGY OF RVH

A. General

1. The renin–angiotensin–aldosterone system is important in maintaining blood volume, blood pressure, and total body sodium.
2. Hemorrhage, sympathetic tone, posture, and renal artery sodium are known factors that alter renin release.

B. Function of the Renin–Angiotensin System

1. Renin is a proteolytic enzyme that is released from the granules of the juxtaglomerular apparatus (JGA) in response to changes in the pressure of the afferent arteriole.
2. Renin is not a vasoconstrictor.
3. Renin acts on a protein in the plasma, angiotensinogen, to produce angiotensin I, which is then proteolytically converted by a plasma enzyme to angiotensin II, an extremely potent vasopressor.
4. Angiotensin II also effects the release of aldosterone from the adrenal cortex, which potentiates sodium reabsorption and potassium excretion in the distal renal tubule.
5. Therefore, in the face of decreasing afferent arteriolar pressure, the compensatory mechanisms cause immediate vasoconstriction and enhance sodium reabsorption to expand the plasma volume.

C. Mechanisms of RVH

1. There appear to be at least two mechanisms producing hypertension in the setting of renal artery stenosis.
   a. Renin-dependent hypertension is documented in 90 percent of patients with high blood pressure and renal artery stenosis.
   b. It is well known that some individuals can become normotensive after surgical therapy even in the ab-

sence of elevated or lateralizing renin values. Current research is focusing on the role of prostaglandins as possible mediators of RVH in this small group of patients.

2. Renin activity is increased in the renal vein when the kidney is perfused through a stenotic renal artery. Moreover, in most patients peripheral blood renin levels are also increased.

3. Experiments reducing renal blood flow, but maintaining perfusion pressure, suggest that decreased renal flow per se will not elicit renin release.

4. Of greater significance is a large pressure gradient across the renal artery lesion or a low diastolic blood pressure, both of which correlate well with renin release.

5. Pharmacologic therapy designed to lower the blood pressure in patients with RVH interferes with this compensatory system designed to increase kidney perfusion pressure. This stimulates even more renin release and occasionally the hypertension cannot be controlled.

6. In patients who respond to antihypertensive agents, the affected kidney may be inadequately perfused. This may explain the higher rate of renal failure and loss of renal mass in patients who are treated by medical therapy alone.

V. HISTORY AND CLINICAL PRESENTATION

There are no distinctive clinical features that enable the clinician to make the diagnosis of RVH. Nevertheless there are suggestive findings in both the history and physical examination that might lead one to suspect RVH.

- Hypertension in young women and children.
- Sudden onset of hypertension.
- Severe hypertension after age 55.
- Sudden difficulty controlling previously well-controlled hypertension.
- Development of renal failure while on angiotensin converting enzyme inhibitors.
- An abdominal bruit. This is audible in 40 to 50 percent of all patients with RVH.

VI. DIAGNOSTIC STUDIES
A. General

1. It is customary to screen hypertensive patients who have unusual presentations or are refractory to medical regimens in order to identify those with surgically correctable causes. Renovascular disease is accurately identified by angiography. However, the demonstration of renovascular disease by angiography does not indicate whether the

patient's hypertension is of renovascular origin. Therefore, the focus of evaluation of these patients is on the functional significance of a stenosis before interventional therapy can be recommended.

B. Specific Tests

1. Laboratory tests
   a. Serum blood urea nitrogen (BUN), creatinine, sodium, potassium, bicarbonate, chloride.
   b. Urinalysis with electrolytes.
   c. Peripheral plasma renin activity. Although often measured, it is not particularly reliable for identifying renovascular hypertension. It is frequently normal in these patients and can be elevated in a large number of patients with essential hypertension. However, when plasma renin activity is measured under strictly controlled conditions (salt and volume restriction, antihypertensive medications withdrawn), most patients who are known to have RVH will demonstrate an elevated secretion of renin.

2. Radiologic evaluation
   a. Rapid sequence intravenous pyelography (IVP)
      (1) Approximately 70 percent of patients with documented RVH will have a positive intravenous pyelogram by the following criteria.
         (a) A difference in length between kidneys of more than 1 cm.
         (b) Delayed pyelocalycele appearance time (which reflects glomerular filtration).
         (c) Decreased concentration or prolongation in the early nephrogram (10 to 30 sec) on the involved side.
         (d)   Underfilling of the collecting systems.
         (e) Segmental renal atrophy.
         (f) Notching of the upper ureter or renal pelvis by enlarged collateral vessels.
      (2) The rapid sequence IVP may appear to be normal in the presence of bilateral stenosis of the segmental renal arteries.
      (3) The utility of the IVP is lessened because of a high false-negative rate. It is specifically for this reason that many clinicians advocate renal arteriography to identify patients with RVH. They believe that all patients with positive IVPs will need angiograms prior to surgery. Furthermore they argue that no patient should be denied the benefit of cure based on a test with a poor specificity.

b. Radionuclide scanning
   (1) This study measures both renal perfusion and excretory function based on renal excretion of hippuran labeled with iodine 131. The addition of technetium 99m dimercaptosuccinic acid and technetium 99m diethylenetriamine penta–acetic acid to the study allows calculation of differential renal excretory function for each kidney. In a patient with unilateral renal artery stenosis, the renogram demonstrates a decreased slope of isotope uptake in the ischemic kidney with delayed excretion, indicating impaired renal perfusion. This test is not ideal for the diagnosis of renovascular disease when bilateral renal artery lesions are present since it depends on comparative assessment between two kidneys. Furthermore, any lesion that decreases renal inflow will give the renographic appearance of renal artery stenosis; thus, it is not a specific test. It has a 25 to 30 percent incidence of false positive and false negative results when used as a screening test for RVH. Its main use is as a noninvasive means of following renal function and identifying deterioration in renal function.
   (2) Radiologic Evaluation
      (a) Rapid sequence intravenous pyelography (IVP)— *this is as stated*
      (b) Radionuclide scanning—*this is stated*
c. *Duplex ultrasonography.* Duplex ultrasound is the cominatin of B-mode ultrasound with pulsed Doppler ultrasound. This allows for imaging of anatomic details along with quantitative measurement of flow. As a screening test for renal artery stenosis, recent series have demonstrated a sensitivity of 84 percent, specificity of 97 percent, and overall accuracy of 93 percent. This test is highly operator dependent and not all centers can duplicate these excellent results.
d. *Captopril renal scintigraphy.* Split renal function studies have shown a reversible decrease in renal function in renal artery stenosis patients, induced by the administration of captopril. The loss of glomerular filtration rate due to captopril administration provides a provocative test for hemodynamically significant renal artery stenosis. If a captopril-induced change in the renogram is noted, revascularization of the affected kidney may be expected to significantly improve the patient's renal perfusion.

e. *Magnetic resonance angiography (MRA).* Arteriographic images generated by the noninvasive modality of magnetic resonance imaging is termed MRA. Magnetic resonance arteriograms of the renal arteries, enhanced with the non-nephrotoxic contrast agent gadolinium, yield highly accurate images of the renal arteries when compared with contrast arteriography. The technique is noninvasive and non-nephrotoxic. Recent series report sensitivities and accuracies in the high 90 percent range. It is rapidly becoming the anatomic imaging modality of choice for screening of patients with suspected renal artery stenosis. Its noninvasive and non-nephrotoxic nature is highly desirable in this patient population.

f. *Computed tomography angiograpy (CTA).* Spiral CT employs contrast agents to form three-dimensional arteriograms. These yield high quality iimages of the abdominal aorta and its branch arteries. Early studies with this technique show high sensitivity and accuracy when compared to contrast arteriography. However, the technique is very dependent on sophisticated image processing and requires contrast doses equivalent to that used for conventional arteriography.

g. Arteriography

  (1) Renovascular lesions are defined by arteriography.

    (a) Intravenous digital subtraction angiography, which allows visualization of the arterial system with intravenous injection of contrast material, has not been able to generate the high-resolution arteriogram necessary to make the diagnosis of renal artery lesions and has not gained wide acceptance.

    (b) Intra-arterial digital subtraction arteriography provides high-resolution arteriograms with less contrast material than either intravenous digital subtraction angiography or standard arteriography.

  (2) The value of arteriography, properly performed, is to evaluate the anatomy of the renal artery.

    (a) Multiple arteries to both kidneys are frequent.

    (b) Atherosclerotic stenosis can be differentiated from fibrodysplastic lesions.

    (c) Although other tests alluded to may indicate the presence of a unilateral abnormality, they cannot specify the site or type of lesion present.

  (3) Atherosclerotic lesions are identified as stenotic areas in the proximal third of the artery (Fig. 26-3).

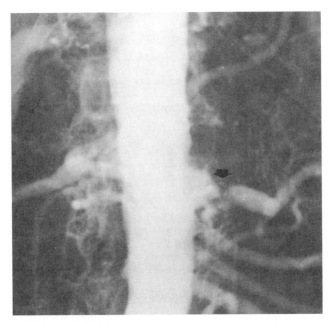

Figure 26-3 Aortogram of a 57-year-old female with severe hypertension that displays a significant proximal left renal artery stenosis consistent with atherosclerotic disease (*arrow*).

    (4) Fibromuscular lesions occur in the distal two-thirds of the vessel and may produce the "string of beads" sign (Fig. 26-4).

    (5) The low morbidity and rare mortality of this test have led to its current widespread use.

VII. FUNCTIONAL RENAL STUDIES
A. General
    1. Although angiography permits the diagnosis of renal artery disease in the presence of hypertension, it does not confirm the diagnosis of RVH. Widespread use of angio-graphy has shown that renal artety stenosis may be present in the absence of hypertension. For this reason, functional assessment of the impact of the stenosis on the kidney must he performed. Two tests are currently available.

B. Differential Renal Function Studies
    1. Originally proposed by Howard with modifications by Stamey. These tests are only infrequently used today but

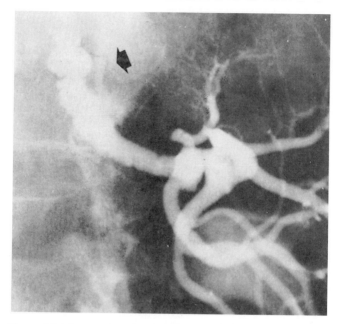

Figure 26-4 Renal arteriogram of a 60-year-old female with hypertension and postprandial pain who was found to have fibromuscular disease of both renal arteries as well as the superior mesenteric artery. The classic "string of beads sign" is demonstrated in the arteriogram.

may be of value, especially in evaluating the viability of severely ischemic kidneys and the likelihood of salvaging them.

2. This test requires catheterization of both ureters, prolonged collection of urine volumes, and multiple sample analysis of specimens for volume, sodium concentration, osmolality, and reabsorption of filtered sodium and water.

3. The test is based on the finding that tubular reabsorption of water is greater in the ischemic kidney than in the normal contralateral kidney. Thus, data can be affected greatly by changes in blood flow, perfusion pressure, and glomerular filtration rate.

4. A test result is considered positive if there are a reduction in urine flow rate and an increase in creatinine as well as an increase in *para*-aminohippuric acid concentration in the urine from the affected kidney when compared with the contralateral kidney.

5. Although this test may be positive in 80 percent of patients with unilateral main renal artery stenosis, it is negative in patients with RVH secondary to a segmental renal artery lesion.

6. It has been found that 73 percent of patients with positive tests were improved after surgical treatment, but 50 percent of patients with negative tests also improved after surgical treatment.

7. The combination of the test's low sensitivity and the relatively high rate of urologic complications (3–5 percent) has caused most clinicians to reserve this study for special situations.

C. Renal Vein Renin Assays

1. Most centers rely on the renal vein renin assay to select patients with hypertension and renovascular disease for corrective treatment.

2. Renin samples are collected from the inferior vena cava and both renal veins by a catheter placed percutaneously in a retrograde fashion via a femoral vein.

3. The renal venous renin ratio is calculated by dividing the renin level of the ischemic kidney by the renin level of the contralateral kidney. A ratio of 1.5 to 1 is considered abnormal by most authors. This test is based on the notion that a unilateral stenosis opposite a normal contralateral kidney will result in unilateral hypersecretion of renin and contralateral suppression of renin secretion. Greater than 90 percent of patients meeting these criteria will respond to corrective interventions.

4. It is interesting that in the small group of patients with severe hypertension and angiographically proven renal artery stenosis but normal renin values, approximately 50 to 80 percent will respond to surgical intervention. Speculation on the reason for this finding centers on the improper preparation of patients for the test. The lingering effects of the antihypertensive agents, inaccurately placed catheters, and failure to restrict sodium intake have all been described. Alternatively the possibility of a nonrenin-dependent mechanism for RVH remain consistent with current data.

5. When bilateral stenoses or contralateral parenchymal disease are present, the normal compensatory mechanisms are not active and hypertension may be multifactorial rather than renin-mediated.

6. The renal vein renin ratio cannot be used as the sole criterion of selection for intervention due to the considerable number of false-negative results and the large number of these patients that benefit from interventions.

7. Confounding factors that may interfere with validity of assay include:

      a. Interference of antihypertensive medication with renin release.

      b. Suppression of renin release by volume expansion and salt loading.

      c. Variability of renin release from the kidney.

      d. Catheter placement error (lumbar vein, left renal vein proximal to gonadal or lumbar vein).

   8. Some have stressed the importance of expressing the renal vein renin assay in relation to systemic renin activity rather than as a ratio of activities between the two renal veins. This renal:systemic renin index has been shown to reliably predict those patients who will be cured of RVH with intervention compared with those whose condition would only be improved.

D. Percutaneous Transluminal Angioplasty (PTA)

   1. Recently it has been proposed that PTA should be performed routinely if angiography demonstrates a significant renovascular lesion amenable to angioplasty. This is based on the observation that a significant number of patients with RVH do not have demonstrable involvement of the renin-angiotensin system and that no tests or combination of tests yield a reliable diagnosis of RVH.

   2. If the patient responds after a first dilatation, this is taken as teleologic evidence that the patient's hypertension was attributable to the angioplastied lesion.

VIII. MEDICAL THERAPY

A. Goal

   1. The goal of medical therapy is good hypertension control without deterioration of renal function.

B. Patient Indications

   1. Considerations that favor a decision of medical therapy include:

      a. Mild hypertension.

      b. Old age with severe associated cardiac, cerebrovascular, or aortic disease.

      c. The presence of adequate blood pressure control with good renal function that remains stable.

C. Methods of Medical Control

   1. Control of dietary sodium and weight loss are important parts of hypertension control.

   2. Diuretics are generally the first medications added.

   3. Other antihypertensive agents are added if the diastolic blood pressure remains above 100 mm Hg.

4. Multiple drug regimens including beta-blockers, calcium-channel blockers, vasodilators, and, rarely, ganglionic blocking agents are often necessary to achieve blood pressure control. (The use of ganglionic blocking agents, although sometimes effective, usually prompts therapeutic intervention in the absence of extreme contraindications.)

5. The use of captopril, an angiotensin inhibitor, helps to control the blood pressure of patients who are otherwise resistant to standard medical therapy.

IX. SURGICAL THERAPY
A. General
1. The goals of surgical intervention include the cure of hypertension and the preservation of functional renal tissue. Innovative surgical techniques, preoperative correction of cardiac and stroke risk factors, and improved anesthesia delivery and monitoring have significantly lowered present-day risks.

B. Surgical Indications
1. Clearly, young patients should undergo surgery to avoid medical treatment of long duration.
2. Failure of medical therapy.
3. Failure to tolerate medical regimens.
4. Deterioration of renal function in the presence of adequate blood pressure control.
5. Renal artery lesions not amenable to angioplasty (orificial stenosis, multiple branch lesions.

C. Preoperative Care and Evaluation
1. Surgical therapy consists of preoperative evaluation to identify patients with a high risk of a myocardial event or stroke. Selective arteriography and revascularization of these areas should be carried out in high-risk patients prior to renal revascularization.
2. One third of patients with RVH have significant intravascular volume deficits that should be slowly replaced preoperatively.
3. Invasive monitoring of blood pressure and volume status should be used routinely.

D. Surgical Procedures
1. Aortorenal bypass
   a. Reversed or nonreversed vein grafts from the infrarenal or supraceliac aorta may be used to bypass a region of renal artery stenosis (Fig.26-5). The distal anastomosis is done in an end-to-end fashion, since end-to-side anastomoses have the potential for

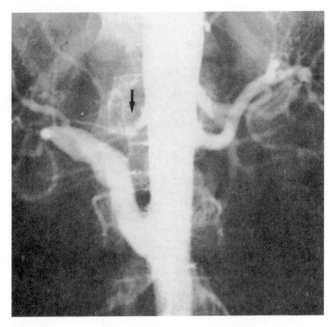

Figure 26-5 Arteriogram of a 40-year-old female, 10 years after revascularization with a right aortorenal bypass for RVH. The origin of the stenotic right renal artery is still visible *(arrow)*.

competitive flow as well as propagation of thrombus into the renal artery.

    b. Prosthetic grafts are reserved for patients who have no suitable autogenous vein, as these grafts have decreased patency rates compared with autogenous material.

    c. The supraceliac aorta, which is usually relatively spared of diffuse atherosclerotic disease, may be used for the proximal anastomosis if the infrarenal aorta is unsuitable.

2. Alternative renal artery reconstructive techniques may be used in specific clinical situations to avoid a diseased or otherwise unsuitable aorta as an inflow vessel.

    a. Hepatorenal bypass.

    b. Splenorenal bypass.

    c. Iliorenal bypass.

    d. Mesorenal bypass.

3. Aortorenal endarterectomy may be performed through an aortic incision. This technique is suited to treatment of ostial lesions, directly removing the diseased intima and plaque.

4. Heterotopic autotransplantation of the kidney to the iliac artery and vein relocating the kidney to the iliac fossa is an effective alternative method of renal revascularization.
5. Ex vivo arterial repair in which the kidney is removed from the patient allowing precise reconstruction of the renal vessels under ex vivo conditions of exposure, illumination, and magnification. This allows for precise reconstruction of complex lesions. The kidney may be replaced back into the renal fossa or autotransplanted to the iliac fossa.

E. Results
1. Most centers now achieve mortality statistics of less than 1 percent for fibrodysplastic lesions and less than 2 percent for atherosclerotic RVH.
2. Surgical cure of RVH is achieved in approximately 40 percent of atherosclerosis patients and 60 percent of fibrodysplasia patients.
3. Improvement in blood pressure is noted in an additional 45 percent of atherosclerosis patients and 30 percent of fibrodysplasia patients, allowing adequate medical control of blood pressure in these previously uncontrollable patients.
4. Overall, a beneficial blood pressure response rate as high as 95 percent can be expected in surgically treated patients with RVH.

F. Preservation of Renal Function
1. Untreated renal artery occlusive disease in patients with progressive renal deterioration has a poor prognosis.
2. Drug therapy of RVH, particularly in patients on angiotensin converting enzyme inhibitors, has resulted in control of hypertension, but often there is progressive loss of renal function.
3. Medical therapy of RVH in no way inhibits the progression of renovascular disease.
4. Renal revascularization is being performed with increasing frequency to prevent or reverse chronic renal failure secondary to renovascular disease.
5. Ninety percent of patients can expect stabilization or improvement of renal function after revascularization. Additionally, there is some evidence that survival in these revascularized patients is significantly improved compared with a comparable age-matched population.
6. Criteria that predict salvageability of renal function in a compromised kidney include:
   a. Renal length greater than 8 cm.
   b. Biopsy findings of greater than 80 percent viable glomeruli.

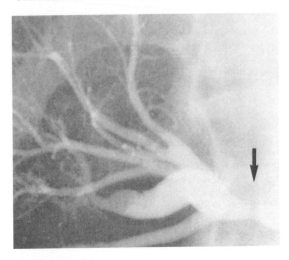

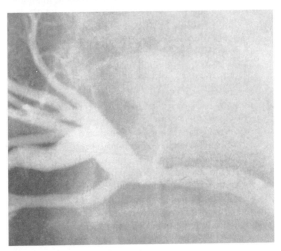

Figure 26-6 A: Arteriogram of a web-like lesion *(arrow)* in the right renal artery of a 17-year-old male with hypertension for 7 months. **B:** The lesion was subsequently treated with successful PTA.

    c. Angiographic evidence of a rich collateral circulation, a distal renal artery that reconstitutes via collaterals, and absence of severe intrarenal arterial disease.

    d. Renal scan findings indicating more than 20 percent of total glomerular filtration rate attributable to the ischemic kidney.

X. PTA

A. General

1. Historically, balloon dilatation of vascular lesions was first performed in 1964. Since that time, renal angioplasties have been performed for RVH using a coaxial catheter system. The first treatment of renovascular lesions by PTA was performed in 1978.

B. Patient Selection

1. Patients with both arteriosclerotic and fibrodysplastic lesions can be treated by PTA.

C. Results

1. Mortality rate is about 1 percent. The major complication rate is between 5 and 10 percent. Thus it is important that angioplasty be done with surgical stand-by available. The most common complications include acute renal failure, peripheral embolization, and vessel damage at the femoral artery catheterization site (Fig. 26-7).

2. For atherosclerotic lesions improvement of blood pressure control can be expected in 70 to 90 percent of patients.

3. For fibrodysplastic lesions a beneficial blood pressure response can be expected in 85 to 100 percent of patients. These particularly good results make it the therapy of choice for fibrodysplastic lesions in the view of most clinicians (Fig. 26-7).

4. Patients who have both aortic and renovascular disease respond poorly to PTA. Lesions at the aortic ostium of the renal artery representing "spillover" atherosclerotic lesions as well as branch fibrodysplastic lesions and congenital stenoses also respond poorly to PTA and should have primary surgical therapy. Recently, stenting of ostial renal artery stenoses has been reported to improve the results with angioplasty of these lesions. Long-term results of this therapy are not yet available.

5. There has never been a prospective randomized comparison of PTA and reconstructive procedures. However, all retrospective comparisons have found surgical results to be superior to PTA for patients with atherosclerotic lesions, whereas those with fibrodysplastic lesions responded well to either therapy.

6. The recurrence rate after PTA has been reported to be between 12 and 23 percent. The rate is higher for atherosclerotic lesions than other types of stenoses.

XI. MEDICAL VERSUS SURGICAL THERAPY

A. Prospective Medical Series

During the late 1970s controversy over the selection of medical or surgical therapy for patients with RVH began to abate

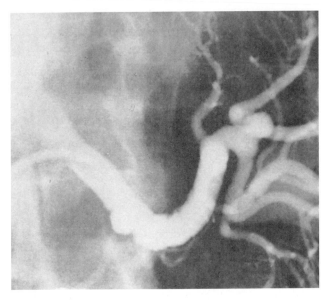

Figure 26-7 Angiogram showing the successful result of dilatation of a stenosis caused by fibromuscular disease. The predilatation film is shown in Fig. 26-4.

as surgical morbidity, mortality, and results improved. Prospective medical studies have contributed to the preference for surgical intervention during the past decade. A series from the Mayo Clinic in 1973 prospectively followed 214 medically managed cases of combined atheromatous and fibromuscular renal artery stenosis. One hundred patients were referred to surgical therapy after the first 3 months because of a failure of medical management (82 percent) or because of exceedingly severe hypertension (18 percent). In spite of this, although the death rate at 7- to 14-year follow-up was 16 percent among surgical patients, it was 40 percent for those who continued on medical treatment. Moreover, 50 percent of surgically treated patients were normotensive without any medication. Mortality was most commonly caused by myocardial infarction, stroke, or renal failure—all known sequelae of poorly controlled hypertension. A prospective study from Vanderbilt University in 1981 confirmed these data in patients that were randomly selected and medically treated for RVH. Forty-five percent of patients had greater than a 25 percent increase in the serum creatinine and a greater than 25 percent decrease in glomerular filtration rate.

Twelve percent went on to a total arterial occlusion. These results occurred despite good blood pressure control in 90 percent of patients with deteriorating renal function.

B. Conclusions

Overall, surgical therapy can cure or lower the need for antihypertensive medication in 90 percent of patients. PTA provides success rates somewhat inferior to these results for atherosclerotic lesions, but is the treatment of choice for RVH secondary to fibrodysplastic lesions. These statistics together with evidence suggesting a genuine prolongation of life due to better hypertension control and preservation of renal function argue effectively for the interventional approach to patients with renovascular disease.

BIBLIOGRAPHY

Calligaro P, *Modern Management of Renovascular Hypertension and Renal Salvage,* Williams & Wilkins, 1996.

Dean RH, Krueger TC, Whiteneck JM, et al: Operative management of renovascular hypertension: Results after a follow-up of fifteen to twenty-three years. *J Vasc Surg* 1:234–422, 1984.

Galanski M, Prokop M, Chavan A, et al: Renal artery stenosis: Sprial CT angiography. *Radiology* 189:185–192, 1993.

Martin LG, Price RB, Casarella WJ, et al: Percutaneous angioplasty in the clinical management of renovascular hypertension: Initial and long term results. *Radiology* 155:629, 1985.

Meier GH, Sumpio B, Black HR, Gusberg RJ; Captopril renal scintography. An advance in the detection and treatment of renovascular hypertension. *J Vasc Surg* 11:770–777, 1990.

Prince MR, Narasimham DL, Stanley JC, et al: Breath-hold gadolinium-enhanced MR angiography of the abdominal aorta and its major branches. *Radiology* 197:785, 1995.

Raynaud AC, Beyssen BM, Turmel-Rodrigues LE, et al. Renal artery stent placement: Immediate and midterm technical and clinical results. JVIR 5:849, 1994.

Strandnesss DE. Duplex scanning in diagnosis of renovascular hypertension. *Surg Clin North Am* 70:109–117, 1990.

CHAPTER 27

Disorders of Sexual Differentiation

Stephen A. Zderic
Howard M. Snyder III

I. NORMAL SEXUAL DIFFERENTIATION
  A. **Genotypic Sex**
   1. Defined at time of conception by a specific combination of the sex chromosomes. Clinically, this is determined by the karyotype: XX female, XY male.
   2. The testes determining factor (TDF) loci have been localized to the Y chromosome. This locus of some 35,000 kB contains a series of highly conserved genes that cause the undifferentiated embryonic gonads to develop into testes.
   3. Other autosomal genes are involved including Wilms' tumor 1 (WT1), which is localized to 11p13 and is abnormal in the Denys-Drash syndrome (genital ambiguity and Wilms' tumor). Other such genes include DAX1 (mutations noted in XY gonadal dysgenesis) and SF1 (mutations noted in murine gonadal and adrenal agenesis). Such autosomal genes may also play a role in gender-specific central nervous system changes.

  B. **Gonadal Sex**
   1. Defined histologically by biopsy-proven presence of testicular, ovarian, or both tissues (ovotestes).
   2. Dysgenetic gonads = histologically resemble neither testis nor ovary.

  C. **Phenotypic Sex**
   1. Defined by the presence of recognizable external genitalia.
   2. Least helpful diagnostic feature.
   3. Often most important factor to parents and child.

4. The findings on examination of the external genitalia may be taken into account in terms of the decision as to which gender to assign.

D. Endocrine Factors

1. Endocrine state is usually determined by gonadal sex and determines phenotypic sex.
2. Testis produces:
   a. Testosterone is produced by the Leydig cells and in the genital tubercle, is reduced by 5α-reductase to create 5-dihydrotestosterone (5-DHT). 5-DHT binds with its cytosolic receptor and crosses the nuclear membrane, binds to a specific genomic site, and initiates transcription. Internally, testosterone causes active wolffian duct development to produce the epididymis, seminal vesicles, and prostate.
   b. Müllerian inhibitory substance (MIS) is produced by the Sertoli cells of the testes and supresses development of internal müllerian structures: fallopian tubes, uterus, and upper vagina.
3. In the absence of the effect of the testis, the external genitalia passively differentiate into the female phenotype, and internal müllerian structures develop.
4. The intersex states can be thought in three broad categories:
   i. Abnormalities of gonadal differentiation.
   ii. Inadequate masculinization of a gonadal male.
   iii. Excessive masculinization of a gonadal female.

E. Sexual and Emotional Identity (Gender)

1. Psychological considerations
   a. Past studies suggested that sexual identity was not fixed until about 18 months of age. Experimental and clinical findings support the concept of fetal gender-specific imprinting in hypothalamic paraventricular nuclei.
   b. Parental uncertainty about their child's gender may be communicated to the child, making the emotional situation more difficult.
   c. In some cases sexual identity can develop independent of chromosomal or gonadal sex. The factors that predict the ability of a child to accept his or her gender are not yet fully understood.
   d. Careful attention must be paid to questions and doubts of parents and children throughout childhood, with preparation for the events of puberty that may be perceived as an illness when brought on by exogenous hormones.

2. Anatomic considerations
   a. In the past, phallic structure status was the major concern with regard to gender assignment in the newborn period. Today, the concepts of fetal hypothalamic imprinting are beginning to sway physicians away from basing their decision only on phallic potential.
   b. In the past, gender reassignment was performed for patients with micropenis; this is no longer the case for long-term studies show that these males have shorter but adequate phalluses in adulthood.
   c. A prominent phallus associated with congenital adrenal hyperplasia should be reduced early on with nerve-sparing techniques if a female sex of rearing is chosen. Milder forms of clitoromegally may dramatically resolve with the institution of cortisol replacement therapy.

II. EVALUATION OF AMBIGUOUS GENITALIA
A. History

1. *Prenatal history.* This is increasingly important as most disorders of sexual differentiation may be detected in utero. For some, such as congenital adrenal hyperplasia, this offers a chance to initiate therapy in utero. In France nearly 80 percent of all intersex cases are detected prenatally allowing for family education and counseling to begin at an early stage.
   a. *Discrepany between karyotype and ultrasound.* This may be seen in congenital adrenal hyperplasia where the virilization results in phallic structures despite a 46XX karyotype. In androgen resistance syndromes a 46XY karyotype will be associated with a lack of virilization.
   b. Discrepancy between the karyotype and the phenotype observed at birth.
2. Family history of:
   a. Abnormal sexual development; unusual changes at puberty
   b. Unexplained infant deaths
   c. Sterility
   d. Amenorrhea
   e. Hirsutism
3. Genetics
   a. Consanguinity facilitates expression of autosomal recessive traits in siblings, which is especially important in cases of congenital adrenal hyperplasia or 5α-reductase deficiency.
4. Maternal virilization during pregnancy or ingestion of any androgenic drugs.

5. In older patients, carefully note growth and development and especially the menstrual history. Patients with androgen resistance syndromes may present with amenorrhea.

B. Physical Examination

Even in cases that are diagnosed or suspected prenatally, a careful physical examination is essential for proper management.

1. Check for the presence of a gonad in the scrotum or labioscrotal fold; this indicates a testes is present. It is extremely rare that an ovotestes might descend.
   a. This finding excludes female pseudohermaphrodite, Turner's syndrome, and pure gonadal dysgenesis.

2. Areolar and labioscrotal hyperpigmentation is common in adrenogenital syndrome.

3. Palpation of uterus or cervix on rectal examination in newborn indicates presence of internal müllerian structures and rules out male pseudohermaphrodites but not bilateral dysgenetic testis syndrome.
   a. Patients with hernia uteri inguinalis do not have external genital ambiguity.

4. Pubertal feminization, virilization, or infantilism is often diagnostic in older child.

5. Careful assessment of the clitoris or phallus and location of urethral and vaginal openings offer little diagnostic help. These are important factors in gender assignment decisions and planning for surgical reconstruction of the genitalia.

6. Note other anomalies, particularly Turner's stigmata.

7. Undescended testes and hypospadias (usually very severe posterior) indicate a possibility that an intersex state may exist. As many as one third will have an abnormal karyotype, usually a mosaic. Sterility is more frequent in this group of patients. Gonadal impalpability increases the chances an intersex state is present. The chances of discovering an intersex state in a patient with a hypospadias and an undescended testes is shown as follows.

Midahsaft and anterior hypospadias and UDT	8%
Posterior hypospadias and UDT	65%

C. Radiographic Evaluation

1. *Pelvic ultrasonography.* Is a rapid means of assessing the newborn to see if any müllerian structures are present (i.e., look for the uterus behind the bladder). This is especially helpful in assessing the newborn male with bilateral impalpable testes.

2. The upper urinary tract should also be assessed by ultrasound examination.

   a. Renal abnormalities of fusion are common in Turner's syndrome.
3. A retrograde flush genitogram is performed by wedging a blunt needle or syringe tip in the urogenital sinus and infusing contrast under fluoroscopy to demonstrate urogenital sinus, urethra, bladder, vagina and cervix, or uterus.
   a. Helps in diagnosis as well as planning the reconstruction.

D. Laboratory Studies
1. Genetic
   a. Karyotyping is readily available with rapid turnovers in 24 hours. Furthermore, the karytotype should be performed in multiple clones; in some instances, the mosaicism will be detected only by assessing the karyotype in up to 100 clones of white blood cells.
   b. In some cases, the presence of mosaicism may only be demonstrated by examining multiple tissues (e.g., white blood cells, gonadal tissue, genital skin).
   c. FISH (fluorescence in situ hybridization) studies may be needed to identify any regions of chromatin containing TDF. This study is indicated in patients with a male phenotype and an XX karyotype.
2. Biochemical
   a. In the past, urinary steroid metabolites offered the clues as to the diagnosis. Today this approach has been supplanted by radioimmunoassay of serum metabolites.
   b. In congenital adrenal hyperplasia, the assay of 17 hydroxy-progesterone is the test that will be positive and establish the diagnosis in 90 percent of these patients (who represent the most common intersex disorder). Assay for deoxycorticosterone (DOC) will be positive for a remaining 9 percent. Other enzymatic blocks producing CAH are far more rare, and must be tested for on an individual basis.
   c. Specific tests to confirm each block as outlined in Figure 27-1 should be ordered selectively and used to confirm a diagnosis made on other grounds. Many of these tests for steroid biosynthesis cannot be performed in routine laboratories, and require genital skin biopsies.

E. Endoscopy and Exploratory Laparotomy
1. A cystovaginoscopy augments findings of a genitogram and is important for diagnosis and treatment.
   a. Distance between the bladder neck and vaginal entry into the urogenital sinus is important in determining which type of vaginoplasty will be required.

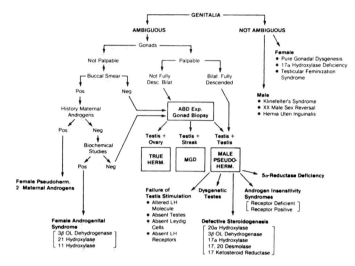

Figure 27-1 An overall approach to the workup of a patient with genital ambiguity or disorders of sexual differentiation. (*Reproduced with permission from Allen TD: Disorders of sexual differentiation. In: Kelalis PP, King LR, Berlman AB, eds. Clinical Pediatric Urology, 2nd ed. Philadelphia, Saunders, 1984, p 914.*)

      b. The endoscopic visualization of a cervix indicates that internal müllerian sexual structures have developed.

      c. Degree of virilization of posterior urethra can be assessed.

  2. Exploratory laparotomy and biopsy of gonads

      a. Necessary in cases where the exact diagnosis is in doubt such as mixed gonadal dysgenesis and true hermaphroditism.

      b. May be omitted in the following four conditions: congenital adrenal hyperplasia, exogenous virilization, Turner's syndrome, and male pseudohermaphrodites with defects in androgen biosynthesis if the specific biochemical assays are available.

III. CLASSIFICATION OF DISORDERS

The major classification scheme used is based on gonadal histology.

A. Female Pseudohermaphrodite (Genetic and Gonadal Female with Masculinized Phenotype)

  1. This is the most common intersex problem and is most often due to the adrenogenital syndrome. Rarely endogenous

Table 27-1 Summary of the Intersex States as Adapted with Modifications

DIAGNOSIS	KARYOTYPE	GONAD	INTERNAL DUCTS	EXTERNAL DUCTS	PUBERTAL CHANGE	FERTILITY	GONADAL MALIGNANCY	SEX ASSIGNMENT	COMMENT
Female									
Pseudohermaphrodite									
3β-OL- dehydrogenase deficiency	XX	Ovary	Müllerian	Mildly ambiguous	Feminization (if treated)	Yes (if treated)	No	Female	Severe salt wasting
11B-Hydroxylase deficiency	XX	Ovary	Müllerian	Ambiguous	Feminization (if treated)	Yes (if treated)	No	Female	Hypertension
21-Hydroxylase deficiency	XX	Ovary	Müllerian	Ambiguous	Feminization (if treated)	Yes (if treated)	No	Female	Frequent salt wasting
Secondary to maternal androgens	XX	Ovary	Müllerian	Ambiguous	Feminization	Yes	No	Female	
True hermaphrodite	XX, XY, XX/XY, etc.	Ovary Testis	Müllerian and wolffian	Ambiguous	Tendency to virilization; gynecomastia	No	Rare	Variable	

(continued)

763

Table 27-1 Summary of the Intersex States as Adapted with Modifications—(*continued*)

DIAGNOSIS	KARYOTYPE	GONAD	INTERNAL DUCTS	EXTERNAL DUCTS	PUBERTAL CHANGE	FERTILITY	GONADAL MALIGNANCY	SEX ASSIGNMENT	COMMENT
Male									
Pseudohermaphrodite									
Hernia uteri inguinalis	XY	Testis	Müllerian and wolffian	Cryptorchid male	Virilization	Rare	Rare	Male	
20α-Hydroxylase deficiency	XY	Testis	Wolffian	Female	Unknown	No	No	Female	Severe salt wasting
3β-OL-dehydrogenase deficiency	XY	Testis	Wolffian	Hypospadiac male	Partial virilization with gynecomastia	No	No	Usually male	Severe salt wasting
17α-Hydroxylase deficiency	XY	Testis	Wolffian	Female	Usually eunuchoid	No	No	Female	Hypertension
17,20-Desmolase deficiency	XY	Testis	Wolffian	Ambiguous	Unknown	No	No	Uncertain	←
17-Ketosteroid reductase deficiency	XY	Testis	Wolffian	Female	Partial virilization with gynecomastia	No	No	Female	
Lubs' syndrome	XY	Testis	Wolffian	Ambiguous (female)	Feminization	No	No	Female	Elevated testosterone and luteinizing hormone
Gilbert-Dreyfus syndrome	XY	Testis	Wolffian	Ambiguous	Partial virilization with gynecomastia	No	No	Variable	

	Chromosomes	Gonad	Ducts	External genitalia					
Reifenstein's syndrome	XY	Testis	Wolffian	Hypospadiac male	Virilization with gynecomastia	No	No	Usually male	
Testicular feminization syndrome	XY	Testis	Wolffian	Female	Feminization	No	Yes	Female	
Pseudovaginal perineoscrotal hypospadias	XY	Testis	Wolffian	Female	Virilization	No	No	Female	
Dysgenetic testes	XO/XY, etc.	Testis	Wolffian and müllerian	Ambiguous	Virilization	No	Yes	Variable	
	XXY, XX. etc.	Testis	Wolffian	Variable	Partial virilization	No	No	Variable	
Mixed gonadal dysgenesis	XO/XY, etc.	Testis and streak	Wolffian and müllerian	Ambiguous	Usually virilization	No	Yes	Variable	
Gonadal dysgenesis Turner's syndrome	XO, etc.	Streak	Immature, müllerian	Female	Eunuchoid	No (one exception)	Usually no	Female	Webbed neck shield chest, etc.
Pure gonadal dysgenesis—XX type	XX	Streak	Immature, müllerian	Female	Eunuchoid	No	Usually no	Female	

T.D.: Disorders of sexual differentiation. *Urology* 7 (suppl 4):4,1976.

androgens secondary to a maternal tumor or exogenous androgens may produce a similar phenotype.

a. *Pathophysiology.* An enzymatic deficiency in any one of several cytochrome P450 type hydroxylase enzymes that lead to the production of cortisol by the adrenal cortex. Mutations in the CYP genes are highly variable; if near the active site, the block may be complete and the child will be severely virilized. If the mutation is farther away from the active site, enzymatic activity will be preserved and the virilization will be mild. Virilization is secondary to an abnormal feedback loop between the adrenal and pituitary. The pituitary senses a loss of cortisol and compensates by overproduction of ACTH, which drives the early stages of steroid biosynthesis. Since the steps leading to cortisol production are blocked, the resulting steroid precursors are shunted into the androgenic pathways culminating in testosterone biosynthesis (Fig. 27-2).

b. 21-Hydroxylase deficiency is most common enzyme defect (90 percent), producing clinical salt wasting and dehydration (in approximately one half) and variable masculinization.

c. II-β-Hydroxylase deficiency is much less common and leads to accumulation of deoxycorticosterone (DOC), a mineralocorticoid, thus producing hypertension as well as a masculinized phenotype.

d. 3β-OL-dehydrogenase deficiency is also rare and produces ambiguity in both sexes, although males are more severely affected; the adrenal insufficiency may be lethal in the newborn period.

2. Exogenous androgens are a rare cause.

a. Exposure to androgenic progestational agents during gestation

b. Arrhenoblastoma

3. Clinical features (quite variable)

a. Enlarged clitoris, sometimes equaling that of a normal newborn male. This diagnosis must be suspected no matter how normal the penis appears if the gonads are bilaterally impalpable.

b. Fusion and rugation of labioscrotal folds, sometimes with increased pigmentation

c. A uterus and vagina are always present. The vagina may enter urogenital sinus at any level, most commonly low near the perineal opening (which determines the type of vaginoplasty).

d. Autosomal recessive pattern of inheritance

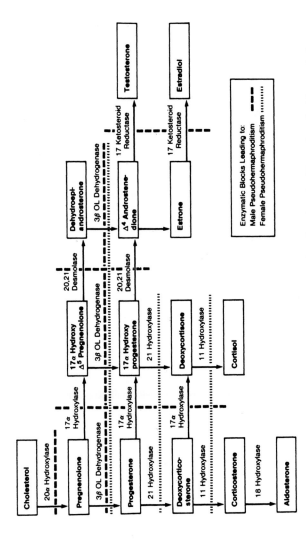

Figure 27-2 Androgenic steroids produced in both adrenal and testis. (*Reproduced with permission from Allen TD: Disorders of sexual differentiation. In: Kelalis PP, King LR, Bertman AB, eds. Clinical Pediatric Urology, 2nd ed. Philadelphia, Saunders, 1984, p 908.*)

4. Management
   a. *Medical management.* It is crucial to institute replacement of cortisol and mineralcorticoid. This is usually done with hydrocortisone and fluorinef.
   b. For male patients with CAH, medical replenishment will be effective at preventing a preventing 2 major complications: (1) premature closure of the epiphyses and short stature and (2) precocious puberty.
   c. For female patients, medical replenishment is essential and may obviate the need for any clitoral reduction surgery in many mild cases. A feminizing genitoplasty is considered the preferred form of management in the neonatal period. In delayed presentations over 6 months of age with massive virilization, strong consideration should be given to maintaining a male gender and removing the uterus and ovaries.

B. **True Hermaphrodite (Testicular and Ovarian Tissue Present with Some Degree of Virilization)**
   1. Defined histologically by the presence of both testicular and ovarian tissue.
      a. Each gonad may be all ovary, all testis, or a combination of ovary and testis (ovotestis).
      b. Ovotestis may be arranged in a linear fashion or one gonadal type tissue may be contained within the other.
      c. A deep linear biopsy of each gonad is required to establish the diagnosis.
   2. Rare; approximately 300 cases reported; more common in blacks.
   3. Clinical features—external phenotype
      a. Severe hypospadias associated with one undescended testis.
      b. Most of these patients are sufficiently masculinized and can be raised as males, but 80 percent of these have severe hypospadias.
      c. Gonads can be present at any level but generally only a testis will descend into the scrotum (a rare ovotestis might be palpable in the scrotum).
      d. Eighty percent develop gynecomastia at puberty, 50 percent menstruate; fertility has been reported in both sexes, but is rare.
   4. Clinical features—internal phenotype
      a. Nearly all have a urogenital sinus, and most have a uterus, albeit atretic.
      b. Internal sexual duct differentiation lateralizes according to the gonad on that side; those with ovotestis may have both an epididymis and a fallopian tube, but only 15 percent have a vas deferens.

5. Genetics
    a. Some familial cases (autosomal recessive); 51 percent
       are 46XX, 19 percent 46XY, and 30 percent mosaics
       or chimeras. The presence of an XX karyotpye in a vir-
       ilized patient with hermaphroditism means that some-
       where in the genome there exists some segment of the
       TDF locus. This may not be present in the lympho-
       cytes for karyotypes done on peripheral blood. Alter-
       natively, there may be mosaicism, which means that
       many clones will need to be screened to identify the 1
       to 10 percent that may carry the TDF locus. To iden-
       tify the TDF locus under these conditions, it will be
       necessary to carry out a FISH (fluorescence in situ hy-
       bridization) study.
4. Management considerations
    a. Making this diagnosis requires bilateral gonadal biopsy.
    b. In the absence of a phallus, female sex of rearing is
       considered. Most patients (75 percent) however will
       be moderately virilized, and male gender assignment
       is recommended. This decision will mandate a major
       hypospadias correction in most cases.
    c. Once sex of rearing is established, inconsistent go-
       nadal tissue and internal sexual ductal tissue are re-
       moved, and reconstruction as indicated is carried out.
    d. Gonadal malignancy is not common except in unde-
       scended testicular tissue.

C. **Male Pseudohermaphrodite (Genetic and Gonadal
   Male with Inadequately Masculinized Phenotype)**
   Three very broad categories exist including inadequate androgen production, inadequate androgen conversion, and androgen receptor deficiency (androgen resistance).
1. Inadequate androgen production.
    a. Five possible enzymatic blocks lead to inadequate an-
       drogen production (Fig. 27-2).
    b. Diagnosis is usually made only after gonadal biopsy,
       as endocrine assays to permit establishment of diag-
       nosis are not clinically available in most centers.
    c. *External phenotype.* Varies from male with hypospa-
       dias to normal female.
    d. *Internal phenotype.* Absent upper vagina, uterus, or
       fallopian tubes. This is on the basis of normal MIF
       production.
    e. Management depends on the degree of external geni-
       tal development.
2. *Inadequate androgen conversion.* Inadequate testosterone to dihydrotestosterone conversion (5α-reductase
   deficiency, pseudovaginal perineoscrotal hypospadias,

incomplete male pseudohermaphroditism type 11). It is also known as the sex reversal syndrome.

a. *Pathophysiology.* Deficiency of 5x-reductase leads to inadequate conversion of testosterone to 5-DHT and therefore failure of masculinization of external genitalia, and in later life, a failure of the prostate to hypertrophy. These observations were the basis for the development of finastride. This is an autosomal recessive trait.

b. *Clinical features.* Female phenotype in infancy with mild phallic enlargement, large utricle (pseudovagina), normal internal wolffian structures with vas terminating in the utricle.

c. If testes left in place at puberty, severe virilization (probably due to direct action of testosterone) occurs with sexual function as male possible. High incidence of this syndrome in Dominica. In Dominica, it is socially accepted to raise infants and children in a female gender role. At puberty, when virilization takes place, the adolescents change over to a male gender role.

d. Diagnosis requires gonadal biopsy.

e. Past recommendations in most countries called for a female sexual assignment with early orchiectomy due to long-term concerns about inadequate genitalia. Certainly, the Dominican experience has provided a basis for raising these children without any medical intervention, but an optimization of social acceptance. However, other cultures are not so adaptable, and a child would have to tolerate inadequate male genitalia until puberty and probably into adulthood. Opponents of gender reassignment see this as a far better alternative than gender reassignment.

3. Androgen resistance syndromes—incomplete androgen resistance

a. Incomplete male pseudohermaphroditism type 1; a spectrum of X-linked recessive disorders with variable degrees of genital ambiguity.

b. *Pathophysiology.* Incomplete effect of 5-DHT to produce normal masculinization of the external genitalia.

c. Reifenstein's syndrome describes a family with nearly adequately masculinized males; Lub's syndrome describes a family with very poorly masculinized males. All grades in between (such as Gilbert-Dreyfus syndrome) are also possible.

d. Cryptorchid small testes with maturation arrest and sterility are common.

e. Except in very virilized cases, male sexual assignment is inappropriate and feminizing genitoplasty, orchiectomy, and female gender assignment produce a more functionally satisfactory individual.

4. Androgen resistance syndrome—complete androgen resistance

   a. *Pathophysiology.* T and 5-DHT production is normal but is not bound in cells of external genitalia secondary to absence or malfunction of the cytosol binding protein. Thus external genitalia passively develop into the female phenotype. As testicular production of MRF is normal, there is suppression of fallopian tube, uterus, and upper vaginal development.

   b. *Clinical features.* Phenotypic females with short, blind-ending vagina.

   c. *Present with amenorrhea or hernia.* One to 2 percent of inguinal hernias in phenotypic females. Identifying müllerian structures (rectal examination or on vaginoscopy) will rule out testicular feminization.

   d. Incidence is 1 in 20,000 to 1 in 64,000; less than gonadal dysgenesis and equal to congenitally absent vagina as cause of primary amenorrhea.

   e. Diagnosis requires gonadal biopsy.

   f. Removal of testes is mandatory due to high incidence of malignancy; pubertal feminization will occur with testis in place.

5. Hernia uteri inguinalis

   This rare syndrome is also classified as male pseudohermaphroditism. It reflects a testis that is capable of normal testosterone secretion; what is lacking is müllerian inhibition substance (MIS).

   a. May be X-linked or autosomal recessive.

   b. *Clinical features.* Phenotypic male with unilateral cryptorchidism and contralateral inguinal hernia containing fully developed müllerian structures.

   c. Fowler-Stephens orchidopexy may be required; uterus and vagina usually should be left as the vas may run in the broad ligament. Fertility in these patients has been reported.

D. Mixed Gonadal Dysgenesis

1. Second most common intersex disorder.

2. Very similar to dysgenetic male pseudohermaphroditism (bilateral dysgenetic gonads in XY infant).

3. Usually a mosaic 45XO/46XY in karyotype; testis on one side lacking germ cell elements and streak gonad opposite (resembling ovarian stroma histologically).

4. *Clinical findings.* Severe hypospadias and unilateral cryptorchidism. Internal phenotype—atrophic hemi

uterus, vagina, and one fallopian tube (on the side of the streak gonad reflecting the absence of MIS).

5. One third exhibit Turner's stigmata.
6. Incidence of seminoma and gonadoblastoma is 2 percent in mixed gonadal dysgenesis and 15 percent in dysgenetic male pseudohermaphroditism; tumor occurs prior to puberty in one half of cases.
7. Early bilateral gonadectomy and female rearing have been recommended in the past. However, male gender assignment is appropriate with virilized phenotype and a scrotal testis.

E. Gonadal Dysgenesis (Turner's Syndrome)

1. Distinguish from Noonan's syndrome (autosomal dominant affecting males and females with normal gonads and karyotype), mixed and pure gonadal dysgenesis by XO or XO/XX genotype, absence of testis/virilization, and presence of stigmata (shield chest, low hairline, webbed neck, cubitus valgus, short stature, sexual infantilism, and renal malformations in 50 percent of cases).
   a. Suspect in short female with horseshoe, ectopic, or absent kidney.
2. Variable expression depending on exact chromosome content.
   a. Loss of part or all of one X or Y chromosome before first cleavage division, resulting in isochromosome formation or translocation.
3. All should be raised as female.
   a. Gonadectomy is indicated in those with a Y chromosome or virilization.

F. Pure Gonadal Dysgenesis

1. Phenotypic females with bilateral streak gonads, infantile uterus and tubes, sexual infantilism, normal height, no other anomalies, and 46XX or 46XY karyotype.
2. Clinical features are indistinguishable from gonadal dysgenesis or mixed gonadal dyspenesis, but X-linked and autosomal recessive inheritance has been demonstrated, providing compelling evidence that autosomal genes influence gonadal development and that at least one X gene is required for testicular differentiation.
3. Severe estrogen deficiency may be accompanied by osteoporosis.
4. Those with Y chromosome in karyotype develop dysgerminoma or gonadoblastoma in one third of cases, which may produce secondary virilization.
5. Management
   a. All are raised as females.

    b. Gonadectomy is required when there is a Y chromosome present.

    c. Exogenous estrogen maintenance from puberty balanced with progestational hormones is required. The combination reduces risk of endometrial malignancy that can result from estrogen therapy alone.

G. Miscellaneous Disorders

  1. A group of 46XY patients with predominantly female phenotype and no functioning gonads has been classified as testicular regression, gonadal agenesis, dysgenetic testes, or vanishing testis syndrome. Variations in internal and external development indicate that testosterone influence was lost very early in some (50-mm crown–rump length) and later in others.

  2. Micropenis results from loss of androgen influence after complete differentiation (12 weeks); if of central etiology (hypogonadotropic hypogonadism), micropenis will enlarge with human chorionic gonadotropin (HCG). In the past, gender reassignment was considered for patients with micropenis. Today, it is accepted that most of these patients will respond well enough to medical management to produce a phallus that is adequate. Long-term follow-up studies from England suggest patient and partner satisfaction with the long-term genital outcome.

IV. MANAGEMENT

A. Gender Assignment

  1. The family should be dissuaded from the belief that the child has no proper gender.

    a. The initial statement should be that development *is incomplete* and further tests will reveal the appropriate gender.

    b. A family should never be told that their child is male but *will* be made female or vice versa. It is important to have a lengthy meeting with the family, and explain the process of normal sexual differentiation and how this process may on occasion vary. An honest and forthright discussion with the family upfront is essential for short-term and long-term management.

    c. This meeting should be multidisciplinary with representatives from the neonatology, endocrinology, urology, and psychiatry services. Even more critical is the presence of the nursing staff, for it is they who will be spending the most time with the family and neonate. For some families inclusion of the clergy is a valuable resource. The input of an ethicist should also be sought whenever possible.

d. In years past, there was a tendency to skirt around the long-term issues of gender assignment in hopes that the family might be "spared" any uncertainty and that this would improve the long-term outlook for child and family.

e. We now believe it best to discuss with families the current state of the literature including the notion of behavioral imprinting by exposure of the fetal brain to androgens. While there is always a tendency to want to put difficult information in the best possible light, families will ultimately learn everything there is to know. When families gain access to such critical information from the Internet or medical texts, faith in their physicians is undermined.

f. Families should be told that there is a movement advocating that nothing be done for these children surgically in the newborn period. The child may be assigned a gender, but any definitive surgery will be delayed until the child can make their own informed decision. Some have even advocated the notion of a third sex. Diamond has called for a moratorium on any surgical reconstruction until long-term follow-up studies are completed. Clearly such approaches to so a complex problem are not without their own long-term psychological risks. Furthermore, other long-term data from patients with intersex states has suggested that 50 percent of these patients are happy that their surgery was completed prior to the age of recall. Much more long-term clinical outcomes research is being conducted so that patients may better guide the profession and their families through these difficult decisions.

g. It must be expected that the literature surrounding this controversial topic will expand greatly over the next decade. The American Academy of Pediatrics and the Societies for Fetal and Pediatric Urology have established a task force to look at long-term outcomes in older patients.

h. Families opting for a surgical reconstructive procedure must understand that the surgery is cosmetic and possibly functional. It is not a panacea, and cannot alter the patient's long-term gender identity no matter how successful it might appear.

2. In the past, the overriding consideration for male gender assignment was the adequacy of a phallic structure.

a. Patients with a large phallus and bilateral undescended testes must be evaluated thoroughly as many will have female adrenogenital syndrome. Others may present with true hermaphroditism or mixed gonadal dysgenesis. In the past many such patients were raised in a female gender; yet as more evidence supports the notion of androgen imprinting on the central nervous system, an overiding concern may become what the patient's future sexual identity will become. As of this time, there is no predictive test that can help the clinicians and family answer this question in advance.

b. Fertility is a consideration in gender assignment. Only patients with the adrenogenital syndrome, some with hernia uteri inguinalis, and rarely true hermaphrodites can be expected to be fertile. However, the potential for fertility that may be preserved is of little benefit if the patient is left with a poor sexual identity. For example, long-term follow-up data suggests that although fertility is preserved in female patients with congenital adrenal hyperplasia, many (20 to 30 percent) of these patients never develop a female gender identity.

3. The traditional view was that definitive gender assignment (a poor term) must be made prior to age 18 months because sexual identity is established by that time. Today this is no longer accepted. There is no question that androgen imprinting of the central nervous system occurs in utero, and for many patients, this is a dominant factor developing their sexual identity.

B. Reconstruction

1. Male reconstruction

   a. May require hypospadias repair, usually carried out between 6 months and 1 year of age, orchidopexy, removal of inappropriate gonads as well as internal müllerian structures.

   b. Total phallic reconstruction is a possible option for patients, but expertise is limited to a few centers. The radial forearm flap, which commits the patient to a penile prosthesis, and the osteocutaneous fibula flap are two such techniques.

2. Gonadectomy is considered when gonadal tissue inappropriate to the assigned gender has been identified or the risk of malignancy exists.

3. Female reconstruction—feminizing genitoplasty

   a. Clitoral reduction is carried out as early in life as possible, as it is the presence of a large phallus that is most disturbing to parents who have been told they have a little girl. This can be done in a nerve-sparing fashion so as to preserve sensation and allow for orgasm. Minor clitoromegally should be left alone such that involution will take place once the source of androgen is shut down.

b. Vaginoplasty is required either to widen the introitus (minor) and separate it from the urethra or to create an entire vagina de novo (major). The type of vaginoplasty that will be required may be predicted from the genitogram and confirmed by endoscopic evaluation.

   i. A perineal flap vaginoplasty for a low entry vagina into the urogenital sinus can usually be carried out at the time of clitoral reduction in first 2 months of life.

   ii. If needed, a substitution vaginoplasty (bowel or skin graft—Mcindoe) is usually carried out when the patient is ready to become active sexually.

4. Psychological and metabolic support

   a. Requires a team approach involving primary care physicians, geneticists, endocrinologists, and psychiatrists. Long-term psychological counseling should be provided for the patient and family.

   b. Long-term metabolic care and follow-up are essential for patients with CAH to ensure adequate steroid supplementation.

5. Future pregnancies

   a. The likelihood of sibling involvement should be assessed and discussed with the family.

   b. Should be closely followed, and maternal treatment with dexamethasone may diminish the degree of virilization allowing for in utero therapy of future siblings.

BIBLIOGRAPHY

Aaronson IA: Sexual differentiation and intersexualiy. In: Kelalis, PP, King LR, Belman AB, eds. *Clinical Pediatric Urology,* 3rd ed. Philadelphia, Saunders, 1992, vol. 11, p 977.

Aaronson IA: Micropenis: Medical and surgical implications. *J Urol* 152:4, 1994.

Allen TD: Disorders of sexual differentiation. *Urology* 7:4, 1976.

Allen TD: Disorders of sexual differentiation. In: Kelalis PP, King LR, Belman AB, eds. *Clinical Pediatric Urology.* Philadelphia, Saunders, 1985, vol. 11, pp 904–921.

Baskin L, Erol A, et al: Anatomical studies of the human clitoris. *J Urol* 162:1015, 1999.

Blyth B, Duckett JW: Gonadal differentiation: A review on the physiologic process and influencing factors based on recent experimental evidence. *J Urol* 145:689–694, 1991.

Diamond M: Pediatric management of ambiguous genitalia and traumatized genitalia. *J Urol* 162:1021,1999.

Diamond M, Sigmundson HK: Sex reassignment at birth. Long term review and clinical implications. *Arch Ped Adols Med* 151:298, 1997.

Duckett JW: Hypospadias. In: Walsh PC, Retik AB, Vaughan ED Jr, Wein AJ, eds. *Campbell's Urology,* 7th ed. Philadelphia, Saunders, 1997, 2093.

Gustafson ML, Donohoe P: Male sex determination: Current concepts of male sexual differentiation. *Ann Rev Med* 45:505, 1994.

Kaefer M, Diamond D, Hendren WH, et al: The incidence of intersexuality in children with cyryptorchidism and hypospadias: Stratification based on gonadal palpability and meatal position. *J Urol* 162:1003, 1999.

LeVay S: *The Sexual Brain.* Cambridge, MIT Press, 1993.

Reilly JM, Woodhouse CRJ: Small penis and the male sexual role. *J Urol* 142:569, 1989.

Reiner W: To be male or female—That is the question. *Arch Ped Adols Med* 151:224, 1997.

Snyder HM: Management of ambiguous genitalia in the neonate and young infant. In: King LR, ed. *Urologic Surgery in the Neonate,* 2nd ed. Philadelphia, Saunders, 1988, pp 346–385.

Snyder HS, Retik AB, Bauer SB, Colodny AH: Feminizing genitoplasty: A synthesis. *J Urol* 129:1024, 1983.

SELF-ASSESSMENT QUESTIONS

1. A normal male newborn is noted to have bilaterally impalpable testes with a flat but rugated scrotum. Appropriate initial management is:
   a. arrange for urologic consultation at 6 months of age.
   b. administer HCG and measure LH, FSH, and testosterone levels.
   c. rule out the presence of a uterus by a rectal examination and pelvic ultrasound.
   d. carry out an immediate orchiopexy.
   e. order a karyotype.

2. In working up a suspected diagnosis of congenital adrenal hyperplasia, which one laboratory test has the best chances of establishing the diagnosis?
   a. Karyotype
   b. Urine ketosteroids
   c. Serum testosterone
   d. Serum müllerian inhibitory substance
   e. 17 Hydroxy-progesterone

3. An 8-year-old boy is explored for an impalpable left undescended testis and a right hernia. At exploration, müllerian structures are found in the hernia sac. The most likely diagnosis is:
   a. true hermaphrodite.
   b. hernia uterii inguinalis.
   c. androgen resistance syndrome.
   d. congenital adrenal hyperlasia.
   e. 5 α-reductase deficiency.

4. A newborn male presents with a severe penoscrotal hypospadias and a unilateral undescenced and impalpable testes. Possible diagnoses include:
   a. congenital adrenal hyperaplasia.
   b. androgen resistance.
   c. true hermaphrodite.
   d. true hermaphrodite or mixed gonadal dysgenesis.
   e. mixed gonadal dysgenesis.

5. The distinction between mixed gonadal dysgensis and hermaphroditism is best made by:
   a. serum testosterone.
   b. serum MIS levels.
   c. a well-performed genitogram.
   d. pelvic MRI.
   e. laparotomy and gonadal biopsy.

6. Which hormone and receptor combination function normally in patients with an androgen resistance syndrome?
    a. MIS
    b. Testosterone
    c. Dihydrotestosterone
    d. Testosterone receptor
    e. Dihydrotestosterone receptor

Answers

1. c	4. d
2. e	5. e
3. b	6. a

CHAPTER 28

Pediatric Oncology

Michael C. Carr
Howard M. Snyder III

I. WILMS' TUMOR
  A. General
  1. Characterized by Wilms in 1899, first described by Rance in 1814.
  2. Seven new cases per million children per year in the North America (450 cases per year).
     a. Eighty percent of all childhood solid tumors.
     b. Eighty percent of all genitourinary (GU) cancers in children under 15 years of age.
     c. Seventy-five percent in children between 1 and 5 years of age; peak incidence 3 to 4 years of age; 90 percent before 7 years of age.
     d. Male:female ratio equal, 1 percent familial; slightly higher rates in black population and lower in Asian children.

  B. Pathology—Embryology
  1. Gross pathologic features
     a. Sharply demarcated, encapsulated
     b. Usually solitary
     c. Frequently hemorrhagic or necrotic
     d. True cyst formation rare
     e. Pelvis invasion rare; venous invasion 20 percent
     f. Extrarenal sites (retroperitoneum, inguinal, mediastinal, sacrococcygeal) rare
  2. Microscopic features—wide spectrum
     a. Triphasic: metanephric blastema, epithelium (glomerulotubular), and stroma (mixoid, occasionally differentiated into striated muscle, cartilage, or fat).
     b. Unfavorable histology (UH) in 10 percent of cases; two types:
        i. Anaplasia: threefold variation in nuclear size with hyperchromism and mitoses. Monomorphic sarcomatous-appearing tumors.

      ii. Rhabdoid: uniform large cells with large nuclei, prominent nucleoli, and eosinophilic cytoplasmic inclusions (fibrils), metastasize to brain, is probably not metanephric. Rhabdoid tumor of the kidney and clear cell sarcoma of the kidney have been reclassified and are now considered distinct entities from Wilms' tumors sarcoma.

      iii. Clear cell sarcoma, "bone metastasizing tumors of childhood:" vasocentric spindle cell pattern, may be malignant version of congenital mesoblastic nephroma (pure blastemal origin) and not a true form of Wilms' tumor.

  c. Favorable histology (FH) consists of all other types, tubular predominance being perhaps most favorable of all.

  d. Cystic nephroma (CN) and cystic, partially differentiated nephroblastoma (CPDN) are benign neoplasms currently considered by many experts to be part of the spectrum of nephroblastoma; tumors occur in both adults and children, are generally asymptomatic, but may cause hematuria. Cystic nephromas are all cystic, without solid component, with septa purely stromal without blastemal elements. CPDN are also cystic, but septae contain blastemal elements (or nephrogenic rests). It is important to note that nephroblastomas, clear cell sarcomas, and mesoblastic nephromas may also be predominantly cystic.

  e. Congenital mesoblastic nephroma occurs in early infancy. It is associated with polyhydramnios, resembles leiomyoma grossly, and histologically exhibits sheets of spindle-shape uniform cells that appear to be fibroblasts. There is no capsule but when completely excised, it follows benign course; it may be a hamartoma. The spindle cell variant may behave with a more malignant potential.

3. Genetics and associated anomalies

  a. 11p chromosomal deletion and sporadic, not congenital aniridia associated with a 20 percent incidence of Wilms' tumor.

  b. 11p deletion common in tumor genotype; 12q also reported.

  c. Trisomy 8 and 18, 45 X0 (Turner's) and XX/XY mosaicism associated.

  d. Loss of heterozygosity for portion of chromosome 16q may portend poorer outcome.

  e. Sporadic (nonfamilial) aniridia associated; full syndrome includes early tumor (less than 3 years), other GU anomalies. External ear deformities, retardation, facial dysmorphism, hernias, and hypotonia.

    f. Hemihypertrophy (1 in 14,000 general population, 1 in 32 in Wilms' patients) along with other malignancies (i.e., adrenal carcinoma, hepatoblastoma), as well as pigmented nevi and hemangiomas.

    g. Beckwith-Wiedemann syndrome: visceromegaly involving adrenal, kidney, liver, pancreas, often with hypoglycemia; gonads, with omphalocele, hemihypertrophy, microcephaly, retardation, macroglossia; 10 percent develop a neoplasm to liver, adrenal, or kidney.

    h. Musculoskeletal deformities exhibited in 2.9 percent, with 30-fold increase in neurofibromatosis incidence.

    i. GU anomalies exhibited in 4.4 percent including renal hypoplasia, ectopia or fusion, duplications, cystic disease, hypospadias, cryptorchidism, pseudohermaphroditism.

4. The nephroblastomatosis complex appears to be a precursor of Wilms' tumor and consists of persistent primitive metanephric elements beyond 36 weeks of gestation; occurs in three forms.

    a. Superficial infantile form in which entire kidney is replaced by blastema; infant presents with massive nephromegaly and dies shortly after birth; rarest form.

    b. Multifocal juvenile form or nodular renal blastema (NRB) consists of gross or microscopic NRB nodules that may be sclerotic or glomerulocystic and papillary, usually in the subcapsular region or along the columns of Bertin.

    c. Wilms' tumorlet exhibits triphasic histology in nodules between 1 and 3.5 cm.

    d. Some component of nephroblastomatosis is present in 100 percent of bilateral Wilms' patients, at least 40 percent of unilateral cases.

    e. May represent Wilms' tumor precursor in the "two-hit" theory of oncogenesis of Knudson and Strong.

    f. NRB should be sought, mobilizing and inspecting the contralateral kidney carefully. Any area of abnormal color or a cleft should be biopsied; it does respond to chemotherapy, but the best program and full therapeutic implications remain to be demonstrated.

C. Management of Wilms' Tumor

1. Diagnosis and management

    a. Three-fourths present with palpable abdominal mass, usually smooth and rarely crossing midline (in contrast to neuroblastoma).

    b. One-third present with abdominal pain, often associated with minor trauma and hemorrhage within tumor.

    c. Hypertension accompanies 25 to 60 percent of cases.

    d. Differential diagnosis includes other tumors and hydronephrosis or cystic disease (Table 28-1).

    e. Abdominal ultrasound will diagnose most Wilms' tumors, as well as evaluate the retroperitoneum, liver, and vena cava for extension of disease.

    f. Four-view chest x-ray completes the metastatic work-up.

    g. Angiography and cavography are rarely indicated; computed tomography (CT) may be helpful with very extensive lesions, detecting bilateral disease and providing functional assessment of contralateral kidney.

    h. Complete blood count, urinalysis, serum creatinine, and urea nitrogen levels complete the preoperative testing; urine catecholamines help to rule out neuroblastoma.

2. Surgical treatment

    a. Exploration is carried out as soon as the child is stable, the above studies are completed, and the situation is no longer considered an emergency.

    b. Transverse abdominal incision provides adequate exposure in most cases; from the tip of the 12th rib on the involved side to the lateral rectus border on the opposite side.

    c. Exploration of the contralateral kidney with biopsy as needed should be carried out first; reflection of colon and complete mobilization of kidney are required for adequate visualization and manual inspection of front and back surfaces of the kidney.

    d. Resectability depends largely on the degree of attachment to the liver, duodenum, pancreas, spleen, diaphragm, abdominal wall, or major vascular invasion

Table 28-1 Childhood Tumors

Malignant abdominal tumors
  Renal: Wilms' tumor, renal cell carcinoma
  Neuroblastoma
  Rhabdomyosarcoma
  Hepatoblastoma
  Lymphoma, lymphosarcoma
Benign abdominal masses
  Renal: renal abscess, multicystic dysplastic kidney, hydronephrosis, polycystic kidney, congenital mesoblastic nephroma
  Mesenteric cysts
  Choledochal cysts
  Intestinal duplication cysts
  Splenomegaly

into the vena cava. Heroic extirpation involving major resection of these organs or cardiopulmonary bypass to remove high caval or atrial tumors is not warranted.

e. Unresectable lesions should be treated with chemotherapy and reexplored; usually the tumor may then be removed. Pretreatment of large tumors reduces the rate of intraoperative rupture but does not influence survival and may alter histology (FH versus UH distinction). As the preoperative diagnostic error rate has been 5 percent in the United States, routine pretreatment has not been recommended.

f. Beginning the dissection along the posterior abdominal wall inferiorly and the great vessels medially, with early ureteral ligation, allows early exposure and ligation of renal vessels prior to mobilization of the mass.

g. Biopsy of the tumor or localized operative spill does not upstage the tumor unless it is massive, in which case, whole abdomen irradiation is needed to avoid an increased incidence of abdominal recurrence. Largest relative risk for local recurrence in NWTS-4 observed in patients with stage III disease, those with unfavorable histology (especially diffuse anaplasia), and those reported to have major tumor spillage during surgery.

h. The adrenal is taken if the tumor involves the upper pole.

i. Gross assessment of nodes has a 40 percent false-positive and 0 percent false-negative rate, and thus routine biopsy of hilar and periaortic nodes is warranted; radical node dissection does not influence survival but does improve staging. The absence of lymph node biopsy is associated with an increased relative risk of recurrence, which was largest in children with presumed stage I disease due to understaging.

j. Remaining tumor in nodes or other organs should be marked with surgical clips to facilitate direction of radiation therapy.

k. NWTS investigators found a 20 percent incidence of surgical complications, with the most common being intestinal obstruction and hemorrhage.

3. Staging (Table 28-2)

a. Histopathology and tumor stage are the most important predictors of survival in Wilms' tumor patients. The staging system has undergone refinement over the years as data has been examined with each NWTS study.

b. In NWTS-3, the distribution by stage of favorable histology tumors was stage I, 47 percent; stage II, 22 percent; stage III, 22 percent; and stage IV, 9 percent.

Table 28-2 Staging System of the NWTS

STAGE	DESCRIPTION
I	Tumor limited to the kidney and completely excised. The renal capsule is intact and the tumor was not ruptured prior to removal. There is no residual tumor. The vessels of the renal sinus are not involved.
II	Tumor extends beyond the kidney but is completely excised. There is regional extension of tumor (i.e., penetration of the renal capsule, extensive invasion of the renal sinus). The tumor may have been biopsied or there may be local spillage of tumor confined to the flank. Extrarenal vessels may contain tumor thrombus or be infiltrated by tumor.
III	Residual nonhematogenous tumor confined to the abdomen; lymph node involvement, diffuse peritoneal spillage either before or during surgery, peritoneal implants, tumor beyond surgical margin either grossly or microscopically, or tumor not completely removed.
IV	Hematogenous metastases (lung, liver, bone, brain, etc.) or lymph node metastases outside the abdominopelvic region are present.
V	Bilateral renal involvement at diagnosis.

Both the surgeon and pathologist have responsibility for determining local tumor stage.

4. Chemotherapy and radiation therapy are given in NWTS-5 according to Table 28-3.

   a. NWTS-4 demonstrated that a short administration schedule (6 months) of vincristine and dactinomycin is equally as effective as longer duration therapy (15 months) with respect to 4-year relapse-free survival (RFS).

   b. The use of single-dose (pulse-intensive) treatment with dactinomycin have equivalent 2-year RFS to those treated with standard 5-day regimen. Pulse-intensive drug administration provides for equal efficacy, greater administration dose intensity, and less severe hematologic toxicity.

   c. Patients with bilateral Wilms' tumor and/or nephrogenic rests should be managed with nephron-sparing approach following primary chemotherapy. Those patients with anaplasia are at much greater risk for recurrence, so that a renal sparing approach is not beneficial.

Table 28-3 Protocol for NWTS-5

	RADIOTHERAPY	CHEMOTHERAPY REGIMEN
Stage I, FH < 24 mo and < 550 g tumor weight	None	None (surgery only for this group)
Stage I, FH > 24 mo and/or > 550 g tumor weight	None	EE-4A (AMD plus VCR; 18 wk)
Stage II, FH		
Stage I, anaplasia		
Stage III-IV, FH	Yes[a]	DD-4A (AMD, VCR, and DOX; 24 wk)
Stage II-IV, focal anaplasia	Yes[a]	I (VCR + CPM + E; 24 wk)
Stage II-IV, diffuse anaplasia	Yes[a]	I as above
Stage I-IV CCSK	Yes[a]	RTK (Carbo + E + CPM; 24 wk)
Stage I-IV RTK	Yes[a]	
Stage V, bilateral: biopsy or limited surgery, both kidneys		
Stage I or II, FH		EE-4A as above
Stage III or IV, FH		DD-4A as above
Stage I-IV, anaplasia		I as above

[a]Consult protocol for details regarding radiation therapy.

Abbreviations: FH, favorable histology; AMD, dactinomycin; VCR, vincristine; DOX, doxorubicin; CPM, cyclophosphamide; E, etoposide; carbo, carboplatin.

5. Treatment of relapses
   a. Variable prognosis based upon initial stage, site of relapse, time from initial diagnosis to relapse and prior therapy.
   b. Risk of tumor relapse in NWTS-3 at 3 years was 9.6, 11.8, 22, and 22 percent, respectively, for stages I through IV. Relapses occurred in 36 percent of stage I through III and 45 percent of stage IV patients with unfavorable histology.
   c. Adriamycin, dacarbazine, cis-platinum, or higher doses of vincristine and/or Cytoxan are used to treat relapses.
6. Complications of therapy
   a. Bone marrow suppression, early or delayed radiation enteritis, bowel obstruction, hepatic dysfunction, scoliosis, radiation nephritis, interstitial pneumonitis, cardiomyopathy with congestive heart failure, and sterility.
   b. Secondary neoplasms are reported in 3 to 17 percent in 20- to 25-year survivors, especially in radiation fields.
7. Cooperative group trials
   a. Prospective randomized trials have been necessary to answer questions about optimal treatment. The Children's Cancer Study Group and the Pediatric Oncology Group collaborated within the National Wilms' Tumor Study Group.
   b. Results of NWTS-3 summarized in Table 28-4.

Table 28-4 Results of the National Wilms' Tumor Study 3

STAGE	HISTOLOGY	FOUR-YEAR POST-NEPHRECTOMY SURVIVAL (%)
I	Favorable	97
II	Favorable	92
III	Favorable	84
IV	Favorable	83
I-III	Unfavorable	68
IV	Unfavorable	55
All patients		
Unfavorable		89
Clear cell sarcoma		75
Rhabdoid sarcoma		26

Adapted from D'Angio GJ, et al: *Cancer* 64:349–360. 1989.

(*Reproduced from Snyder HM, D'Angio GJ, Evans AE, Raney RB: Pediatric Oncology. In: Walsh PC, Retik AB, Stamey TA. Vaughan ED, eds. Campbell's Urology, 6th ed. Philadelphia, Saunders, 1992, chap 54, p 1981.*)

c. NWTS-5 is focusing on correlating biologic parameters with the outcome of treatment of Wilms' tumor. Genes on chromosome 11 may be responsible for induction of Wilms' tumor. Loss of heterozygosity for a portion of chromosome 16q in 20 percent of patients with Wilms' tumor has been noted.

II. NEUROBLASTOMA

A. Incidence

Represents eight to ten percent of all childhood malignancies and is the most common malignant tumor of infancy. Following brain tumors, it is the most common malignant solid tumor of childhood. One third of cases are diagnosed in first year of life and additional quarter between 1 and 2 years of age.

B. Etiology

1. Arise from primitive, pleuripotential sympathetic cells (sympathogonia) derived from neural crest.
2. Ganglioneuromas and ganglioneuroblastomas also arise from neural crest cells.
3. Characterized cytogenetically by deletion of the short arm of chromosome 1.

C. Pathology

Gross tumors are lobular, tend to be infiltrative, often associated with stippled calcification. Histologically, one of "small, round blue-cell tumors" of childhood. May form rosettes and exhibit neurofibrils if differentiation is good. Ultrastructure shows characteristic peripheral dendritic processes. Gradual degree of malignancy from neuroblastoma (most malignant) to ganglioneuroblastoma (intermediate) to ganglioneuroma (benign).

D. Location and Presentation

Can arise anywhere along the sympathetic chain from the head to pelvis. More than half arise in the abdomen and two thirds of these in the adrenal. Presents as an irregular, firm, nontender fixed mass often extending beyond the midline. Abdominal paravertebral sympathetic ganglion origin has an increased incidence of dumbbell-shaped intraspinal extension, which may produce signs of cord compression. Presacral tumors may result in urinary frequency, retention, or constipation. Cervical sympathetic tumors can cause Horner's syndrome. Thoracic tumors may be asymptomatic or produce cough, dyspnea, or infection from airway compression. As many as 70 percent of patients have metastasis (liver is most common in younger children, bone in older children) at presentation. Unexplained fever, malaise, anorexia, weight loss, and irritability are common.

E. Diagnosis

Anemic if disease has disseminated. Bone marrow aspirate is indicated in all suspected cases: 50 to 70 percent positive. Ninety-five percent of patients have elevation of urinary catecholamines produced by tumor (vanillylmandelic acid and/or homovanillic acid). Can be checked on spot urine sample. Appropriate radiographic imaging will depend on site. For abdominal tumors, intravenous pyelography, ultrasound, computed axial tomography (CT), and magnetic resonance (MR) contribute to staging tumor and determining resectability. Chest x-rays, skeletal survey, and often, bone scan are routine. Table 28-5 depicts minimum recommended tests for determining extent of disease.

F. Staging and Prognosis

1. The current, favored staging system is based on clinical, radiographic, and surgical evaluation of children with neuroblastoma. The International Neuroblastoma Staging System (INSS or Evans classification) provides for

Table 28-5 Minimum Recommended Tests for Determining Extent of Disease

TUMOR SITE	TESTS
Primary	Three dimensional measurement of tumor by CT scan or MR or ultrasound
Metastases	Bilateral posterior iliac bone marrow aspirates and core biopsies (4 adequate specimens necessary to exclude tumor)
	Bone radiographs and either scintigraphy (^{99m}Tc-diphosphonate or ^{131}I- (or ^{123}I-) meta-iodobenzylguanidine (MIBG) or
	Abdominal and liver imaging by CT scan or MR or ultrasound
	Chest radiograph (AP and lateral) and chest CT scan
Markers	Quantitative urinary catecholamine metabolites (VMA and HVA)

For evaluation of bone metastases, ^{99m}Tc-diphosphonate scintigraphy is recommended for all patients and is essential if MIBG scintigraphy is negative in bone.

(From Brodeur GM, Castleberry RP: Neuroblastoma. In: Pizzo PA, Poplack DG, eds. Principles and Practice of Pediatric Oncology, 2nd ed. Philadelphia, Lippincott C.; 1993, p 750.)

uniformity in staging of patients, facilitating clinical trials and biologic studies around the world (Table 28-6).

2. A histologic-based prognostic classification (Shimada) is formulated around patient age and the following histologic features.
   a. Presence of absence of schwannian stroma
   b. Degree of differentiation
   c. Mitosis-karyorrhexis index (MKI)
3. Retrospective evaluation of the Shimada method demonstrated that histologic patterns were independently predictive of outcome, whereas stage was prognostically less important.
4. A simplified system has been devised, which predicts a favorable outlook based upon presence of calcification and a low mitotic rate (less than 10 mitoses/10 high power field). Grading system developed for finding tumors with both features (grade 1), with the presence of only one of these features (grade 2), or absence of both features (grade 3). Combining grade with age (less than 1 or older

Table 28-6 International Neuroblastoma Staging System

STAGE	DESCRIPTION
1	Localized tumor confined to the area of origin; complete gross excision, with or without microscopic residual disease; identifiable ipsilateral and contralateral lymph nodes negative microscopically
2A	Unilateral tumor with incomplete gross excision; identifiable ipsilateral and contralateral lymph nodes; identifiable contralateral lymph nodes negative microscopically
2B	Unilateral tumor with complete or incomplete gross excision; with positive ipsilateral regional lymph nodes; identifiable contralateral lymph nodes negative microscopically
3	Tumor infiltrating across the midline with or without regional lymph node involvement; or, unilateral tumor with contralateral regional lymph node involvement; or, midline tumor with bilateral lymph node involvement
4	Dissemination of tumor to distant lymph nodes, bone, bone marrow, liver, and/or other organs (except as defined in stage 4S)
4S	Localized primary tumor as defined for stage 1 or 2 with dissemination limited to liver, skin, and/or bone marrow

than 1 year) and surgicopathologic staging, low- and high-risk groups emerge. Further evaluation will take into account histologic modifiers, such as level of serum ferritin, *N-myc* copy number and tumor DNA content. *N-myc* amplification occurs in 25 to 30 percent of primary neuroblastomas from untreated patients and amplification is associated primarily with advanced stages of disease.

G. Treatment

1. *Treatment of low-risk disease.* Those patients with localized and resected tumors, or infants with regional disease and infants with INSS stage 4S disease will fare better. Radiation therapy is reserved for those patients who fail to respond to either primary or secondary chemotherapy.

2. *Treatment of intermediate-risk disease.* Children with metastatic disease to regional lymph nodes and infants with INSS stage 4 tumors comprise this group. Moderately aggressive chemotherapy and radiation have led to improvement in disease-free survival.

3. *Treatment of high-risk disease.* Patients with disseminated disease require intensive treatment with multi-agent therapy of various combinations, but overall survival has remained disappointingly low (below 15 percent). The use of high-dose chemotherapy, surgery, intraoperative radiation, and bone marrow transplantation has resulted in improved 3-year survival rates (Table 28-7).

III. GU RHABDOMYOSARCOMA

Rhabdomyosarcoma arise from primitive totipotential embryonal mesenchyme. Genitourinary involvement occurs with the second greatest frequency besides head and neck tumors. Sites include bladder, prostate, vagina, and cervix or paratesticular tissue. They comprise approximately 20 percent of all rhabdomyosarcomas. The incidence of GU rhabdosarcomas is 0.5 to 0.7 cases per million children less than 15 years of age.

A. Pathology

1. Tumor arises from any site that develops from embryonic mesenchyme.
   a. Rhabdomyoblasts are the progenitor cell.
   b. Tumor subtypes differ based on extent of differentiation from mesenchymal progenitor.
   c. Classification system of Horn and Enterline based upon primary histologic subtype: embryonal (60 percent); botyroid; alveolar (20 percent); spindle cell; and pleomorphic.
   d. New international classification system proposed by IRS (Table 28-8).

Table 28-7 Disease-Free Survival (Two-Year) Based on Risk Category and Age

RISK CATEGORY	PATIENT AGE (YEAR)	INSS STAGE	TWO-YEAR DISEASE-FREE SURVIVAL (%)
	All	1	> 90
	All	2A	85
Low	< 1	2B/3	87/89
	< 1	4S	57–90
Intermediate	> 1	2B/3	59
	< 1	4	75
High	> 1	4	40/15[a]

[a]Difference relates to complete versus partial surgical resection, respectively.

Table 28-8 IRS-IV Staging

STAGE	TUMOR LOCATION	T	SIZE	N	M
TNM CLASSIFICATION					
1	Favorable sites	T1 or T2	a or b	N0 or N1	M0
2	Unfavorable site	T1 or T2	a	N0	M0
3	Unfavorable site	T1 or T2	a	N1	M0
		T1 or T2	b	N0 or N1	M0
4	Metastatic disease	T1 or T2	a or b	N0 or N1	M1

T1, confined to anatomic site of origin; T2 extension and/or fixation to surrounding tissue; Ta, tumor less than 5 cm in greatest diameter; Tb, tumor is 5 cm or larger; N0, regional lymph nodes are not clinically involved; N1, regional nodes are clinically involved by tumor; M0, no distant metastases; and M1, metastases are present. GU tumors considered to be favorable sites include the vulva and vagina. GU tumors considered to be unfavorable sites include the bladder, prostate, and uterus.

B. Presentation

1. Signs and symptoms dependent on organ of involvement and size of the primary at initial assessment.
   a. Bladder or prostate-irritative voiding symptoms, urinary retention, incontinence, or infection. Trigonal involvement leads to hydronephrosis and progressive obstruction. Hematuria and constipation are also seen.
   b. Vagina-visible mass, hemorrhage, vaginal discharge.

C. Evaluation

1. Thorough assessment of both local and metastatic sites.
   a. Computed tomography and ultrasound scan abdomen and pelvis.
   b. Lobulated soft tissue mass with homogeneous echogenicity seen on ultrasound.
   c. Transrectal ultrasonography can document involvement of prostate and facilitate biopsies.
2. Computed tomography most widely used modality for GU rhabdomyosarcomas—employ oral, rectal, and intravenous contrast.
3. Magnetic resonance imaging with gadolinium-DTPA facilitates intravesical imaging and invasion into adjacent pelvic structures.
4. Accurate diagnosis based on histologic examination. Many GU tumors are amenable to endoscopic biopsy, either percutaneously, transvaginally, or transrectally.
5. Liver, lung, bone, bone marrow, and retroperitoneal nodes are most common sites for metastatic spread. Serum chemistries, including CBC and liver function tests, x-ray or CT of chest, bone scan, and bone marrow biopsy are needed to complete evaluation.

D. Staging

1. Intergroup Rhabdomyosarcoma Study (IRS) represents collaborative efforts from multiple institutions. IRS staging is dependent on resectability of primary tumor and status of draining lymph nodes.
2. Group 1: local disease (without lymph node involvement) that has been completely removed both grossly and microscopically.
3. Group 2: tumors grossly removed but residual microscopic disease (2A), regional nodal involvement with no microscopic residual disease (2B), or both nodal involvement and residual disease (2C).
4. Group 3: incomplete removal of gross disseminated disease.
5. Group 4: distant metastatic involvement present.

This system is dependent on the extent of surgical resection. The IRS-IV staging system (TMN) has been designed to overcome some of these shortcomings. The most important change is the inclusion of pretreatment stage (Table 28-8), rather than surgical staging alone.

E. Intergroup Rhabdomyosarcoma Studies

1. The collective experience of a number of institutions was needed to assess a growing number of treatment options. IRS-I determined that:

   a. Postoperative radiation therapy of the tumor bed was helpful in group I patients.

   b. Chemotherapy with vincristine, actinomycin D, and cyclophosphamide (VAC) was superior to vincristine and actinomycin D alone (VA) in group 2 patients.

   c. Pulse VAC following initial irradiation in groups 3 and 4 was beneficial.

   d. Adriamycin provided additional benefit in those with advance disease (groups 3 and 4).

2. With the favorable results achieved in IRS-I, IRS-II (1978 to 1984) determined the feasibility of primary chemotherapy. Following biopsy-proven rhabdomyosarcoma, VAC therapy was initiated, response documented, and chemotherapy continued for 16 weeks. The residual mass was resected and chemotherapy continued for 2 years. Radiation therapy was added for gross or microscopic disease following resection.

3. IRS-III (1984 to 1988) addressed five specific issues regarding chemotherapeutic protocols and response to therapy. More aggressive chemotherapeutic protocols were used in patients with unfavorable histology (alveolar, anaplastic, and monomorphous types). The use of second- and third-look surgery to assess response in groups 3 and 4 would lead to improved local control.

The results of IRS-III proved superior to IRS-I and II. There was a 60 percent salvage rate of functioning bladder at 4 years from diagnosis compared to only 22 percent and 25 percent in prior studies. Mortality in patients with disseminated disease (groups 1 through 3) declined to less than 10 percent.

F. Treatment

IRS-IV results are demonstrating the continued refinement in the management of patients with greater success using chemotherapy along with more limited operative resection (less exenterative surgery).

1. Prostatic and bladder RMS is best managed with delayed surgery following intensive chemotherapy. Subsequent radiotherapy used following removal of all gross disease.

2. Localized vaginal RMS is best managed by primary chemotherapy after initial biopsy. Local resection may be appropriate, but complete vaginectomy / hysterectomy is needed only with refractory disease.

3. Previous studies have suggested that patients with uterine RMS present at an older age, are less responsive to treatment and have a poorer prognosis than patients with vaginal RMS. More effective chemotherapy protocols are showing that less vigorous surgical resection may be possible in combination with primary chemotherapy.

4. Paratesticular rhabdomyosarcoma are associated with good prognosis and are considered separately from pelvic primaries because of differences in treatment. The majority of tumors are embryonal with lymphatic spread noted in 28%.

   a. Presents with scrotal or inguinal mass that requires exploration to establish tissue diagnosis: radical inguinal orchiectomy is performed.

   b. Evaluation for metastatic disease should include chest x-ray and retroperitoneal node imaging by CT or MRI.

   c. Retroperitoneal lymph node dissection previously recommended for all patients, but now *not* recommended for those children with localized, completely resected tumors, whose retroperitoneal node imaging study results are grossly negative. Chemotherapy cures microscopic retroperitoneal disease.

   d. Staging and treatment—see Table 28-9.

   e. Most favorable prognosis of all RMS:

   Five-year Event-free Survival Rate (percent)

Groups I and II	93
Group III	55.5
Group IV	37.5

G. Complications

1. Hematologic complications similar to those seen with the same drugs in Wilms' tumor therapy occur.

2. The high radiation dose required to control this tumor often produces severe proctitis and fibrosing cystitis, which may destroy normal bladder function and complicate any subsequent surgery such as reconstruction.

Table 28-9 IRS-IV Staging and Treatment Paratesticular Rhabdomyosarcoma

CLINICAL GROUP	TUMOR STATUS	THERAPY
1	Tumor completely excised[a] (not alveolar subtype)	Vincristine and actinomycin D for 1 year[b]
2	Tumor excised with microscopic residual disease at margin and/or positive lymph nodes involving ipsilateral hilar-para-aortic chain	Vincristineplus actinomycin D plus cyclophosphamide versus vincristine plus actinomycin D plus ifosfamide for 1–2 years plus radiation therapy to involved region[c]
3	Gross residual local and/or regional disease (retroperitoneal nodes) that is not surgically removable	Three-to-7 drug regimen plus radiation therapy to involved region[d]
4	Distant metastasis	Same as group 3

[a]If there has been scrotal contamination, hemiscrotectomy and relocation of the contralateral testis into the thigh are advised to avoid the effects of local radiation on the remaining gonad.
[b]No radiation for group 1 patients.
[c]Conventional radiation.
[d]Conventional or hyperfractionated radiation.

IV. TESTIS TUMORS

Testis tumors are uncommon in children, accounting for approximately 1 to 2 percent of all pediatric solid tumors. Incidence in children is 1/100,000. Peak age incidence is 2 years of age; more benign tumors and fewer germinal testis tumors than in adults.

A. Classification

1. Classification has been debated (Table 28-10).
2. Germinal tumors constitute only approximately 77 percent, compared with 95 percent of testis tumors in adults.
   a. Yolk sac carcinoma (embryonal carcinoma, endodermal sinus tumor, orchioblastoma) comprises approximately 39 to 62 percent of all testis tumors in children. Rarely (4 percent) spreads to retroperitoneal nodes; more frequently (20 percent) spreads to lungs,

Table 28-10 Classification of Prepubertal Testis Tumors

I	Germ cell tumors	Yolk sac tumor
		Teratoma
		Mixed germ cell
		Seminoma
II	Gonadal stromal tumors	Leydig cell
		Sertoli cell
		Juvenile granulosa cell
		Mixed
III	Gonadoblastoma	
IV	Tumors of supporting tissues	Fibroma
		Leiomyoma
		Hemangioma
V	Lymphomas and leukemias	
VI	Tumor-like lesions	Epidermoid cyst
		Hyperplastic nodule attributable to congenital adrenal hyperplasia
VII	Secondary tumors	
VIII	Tumors of the adnexa	

especially if child is older than 1 year of age. Alphafetoprotein elevated 90 percent of time. Average age of presentation is 3 years.

   b. Teratoma constitutes approximately 14 percent; uniformly benign tumor in children under 2 years of age, even when histology appears malignant.

   c. Seminoma is extremely rare before puberty and in essence, should be considered a postpubertal tumor.

3. Nongerminal tumors (stromal tumors); peak age of presentation is 4 to 5 years.

   a. Interstitial cell (Leydig cell) tumors are approximately 18 percent of all testis tumors, usually virilizing or virilizing with gynecomastia (rarely malignant). Must be differentiated from hyperplasia; nodules that develop in testes of boys with poorly controlled congenital adrenal hyperplasia. Leydig tumors are unresponsive to ACTH and dexamethasone and gonadotropin stimulation.

   b. Gonadal stromal (Sertoli cell) tumors: approximately 8 percent of all prepubertal testis tumors; usually present as painless mass and are rarely malignant.

   c. Paratesticular rhabdomyosarcoma constitutes approximately 4 percent of testis tumors in children.

Reticuloendothelial malignancy, primarily lymphomas and leukemias, may present with testicular secondary tumor in 2 to 3 percent. Patients with leukemias rarely present with a testicular mass and no evidence of systemic disease.

B. Examination

Although all boys with a testis mass will come to surgical exploration through the groin, a careful preoperative evaluation should be carried out. If it suggests a tumor is benign, the tumor may be removed with preservation of the gonad.

1. Scrotal ultrasound should be done in most cases; it helps to establish that the testis is abnormal with or without presence of a hydrocele. If calcium and cysts are present, a benign teratoma is suggested. A hypoechoic pattern is characteristic of leukemia or lymphoma.
2. Four-view chest radiographs should be done; chest CT to follow any suspicious area.
3. CT is a mainstay of retroperitoneal evaluation, although ultrasound can also be useful.
4. All children should have alpha-fetoprotein (AFP) determined because it is a marker of yolk sac tumor.

C. Endocrine Evaluation

1. In cases of Leydig cell tumor, urinary 17-ketosteroids are elevated. Chorionic gonadotropins, follicle-stimulating hormone (FSH), and leutinizing hormone (LH) are normal or low. Height, weight, bone age, and pubertal changes are advanced.
2. Sertoli cell tumors exhibit normal or elevated estrogens and androgens in urine and serum; 17-ketosteroids are normal, as are gonadotropins.

D. Management

1. Radical inguinal orchiectomy is standard unless preoperative evaluation suggests benign tumor when testis-sparing local resection may be carried out.
2. Staging is similar to that of adult testis tumors (Table 28-11).
3. Yolk sac tumor.
   a. For those patients with organ-confined yolk sac tumor, AFP will fall rapidly to normal. If the CT scan is negative, close surveillance is the treatment of choice. Monitoring should include monthly AFP and chest x-ray for the first year, then bimonthly during the second year. CT scan of the chest and abdomen may also obtained every 3 months for the first year and every 6 months for the second year (varies by institution).
   b. Approximately 15 percent of children will present with metastatic disease. For those with stage II disease, both retroperitoneal lymph node dissection

Table 28-11 Intergroup Staging System for Testicular Germ Cell Tumors

STAGE	EXTENT OF DISEASE
I	Limited to testis (testes), completely resected by high inguinal orchiectomy: no clinical, radiographic, or histologic evidence of disease beyond the testes; tumor markers normal after appropriate half-life decline (AFP, 5 days; β-hCG, 16 hours); patients with normal or unknown tumor markers at diagnosis must have a negative ipsilateral retroperitoneal node sampling to confirm stage I disease
II	Transcrotal orchiectomy: microscopic disease in scrotum or high in spermatic cord (≤ 5 cm from proximal end); retroperitoneal lymph node involvement (≤ 2 cm) or persistently elevated increased tumor markers
III	Retroperitoneal lymph node involvement (≤ 2 cm), but no visceral or extra-abdominal involvement
IV	Distant metastases, including liver

    (RPLND) and chemotherapy have been used alone and in combination. There is no clear concensus as to what is the optimal treatment because the number of cases are too few to draw valid conclusions.

  c. Metastatic disease has been treated with vincristine, actinomycin D and cyclophosphamide or cisplatin, bleomycin and vinblastine. Children with hematogenous metastatic disease have been treated with combination regimens, with salvage rates approaching 100 percent.

  d. RPLND should be reserved for patients with nonbulky tumor mass confined to the retroperitoneum, or for persistently elevated AFP levels anytime following orchiectomy without evidence of disease elsewhere.

4. Teratoma is treated with orchiectomy alone, but if the diagnosis is suspected preoperatively, the cord can be cross-clamped and the tumor shelled out for frozen section examination with testicular preservation.

5. Gonadal stromal tumors (Leydig, Sertoli) are thought to be benign in almost all cases and are treated with orchiectomy alone. Tumors have ultrasound appearance of an intraparenchymal homogeneous, hypoechoic lesion. Enucleation of the tumor is a possible alternative to radical orchiectomy. Regression of virilizing signs is unpredictable.

6. Reticuloendothelial tumors are managed by biopsy and systemic therapy.

E. Prognosis
1. More pediatric than adult testis tumors are benign.
2. Yolk sac tumors in children under 2 years of age have approximately a 90 percent chance of survival. The prognosis is worse in older child.
3. Tumor registry for pediatric testis tumor has been developed by the Urologic Section of the American Academy of Pediatrics. Therapy continues to evolve.

BIBLIOGRAPHY

Andrassy RJ, Wiener ES, Raney RB, et al: Progress in the surgical management of vaginal rhabdomyosarcoma: A 25-year review from the Intergroup Rhabdomyosarcoma Study Group. *J Pediatr Surg* 34:731–734, 1999.

Batata MS, Whitmore WF Jr, Chu FCH, et al: Cryptorchidism and testicular cancer. *J Urol* 124:382, 1980.

Beckwith JB, Kiviat NB, Bonadio JF: Nephrogenic rests, nephroblastomatosis and the pathogenesis of Wilms' tumor. *Pediatr Pathol* 10:1–36, 1990.

Bowman LC, Hancock ML, Santana VM, et al: Impact of intensified therapy on clinical outcome in infants and children with neuroblastoma: The St. Jude Children's Research Hospital Experience, 1962–1988. *J Clin Oncol* 9:1599–1608, 1991.

Brodeur GM, Castleberry RP. Neuroblastoma: In: Pizzo PA, Poplack DG, eds. *Principles and Practice of Pediatric Oncology*, 2nd ed. Philadelphia, J Lippincott 1993, p 750.

Brosman SA: Testicular tumors in prepubertal children. *Urology* 18:581, 1979.

Carr MC, Mitchell M: Neuroblastoma. In: Oesterling JE, Ritchey JP, eds. *Urologic Oncology*. Philadelphia, Saunders, 1997, pp 637–647.

D'Angio G, Sinniah D, Meadows AT, Evans AE, Pritchard J, eds. *Practical Pediatric Oncology*. New York, Edward Arnold, 1992.

Evans AE, D'Angio GJ, Koop CE: The role of multimodal therapy in patients with local and regional neuroblastoma. *J Pediatr Surg* 19:77, 1984.

Evans AE: Neuroblastoma: Diagnosis and treatment. *Curr Concepts Oncol* 4:10, 1982.

Evans AE: Staging and treatment of neuroblastoma. *Cancer* 65:1799, 1980.

Ferrari A, Casanova M, Massimino M, et al: The management of paratesticular rhabdomyosarcoma: A single institutional experience with 44 consecutive children. *J Urol* 159:1031–1034, 1998.

Hays DM, Raney RH Jr, Lawrence W Jr, et al: Primary chemotherapy in the treatment of children with bladder-prostate tumors in the Intergroup Rhabdomyosarcoma Study (IRS-II). *J Pediatr Surg* 17:812, 1982.

Kaefer M, Retik AB. Rhabdomyosarcoma of the pelvis and paratesticular structures. In: Oesterling JE, Ritchey JP, eds. *Urologic Oncology*. Philadelphia, Saunders, 1997, 666–678.

Kaplan GW: Testicular tumors in children. *AUA Update Series,* vol. 2, lesson 12, 1983.

Lobe TE, Wiener E, Andrassy RJ, et al. The argument for conservative, delayed surgery in the management of prostatic rhabdomyosarcoma. *J Pediatr Surg* 31:1084–1087, 1996.

National Wilms' Tumor Study Committee: Wilms' tumor: Status report 1990. *J Clin Oncol* 9:877–887, 1991.

Ritchey ML, Coppes MJ: Wilms' Tumor. Oesterling JE, Ritchey JP, eds. *Urologic Oncology*. Philadelphia, Saunders, 1997, 648–665.

Schneck FX, Peters CA: Pediatric testicular tumors. Oesterling JE, Ritchey JP, eds. *Urologic Oncology.* Philadelphia, Saunders, 1997, 679–694.

Silber JH, Evans AE, Friedman M: Models to predict outcome from childhood neuroblastoma: The role of serum ferritin and tumor histology. *Cancer Res* 51:1426–1433, 1991.

Snyder HM, D'Angio GJ, Evans AE, Raney RB. Pediatric oncology. Walsh PC, Retik AB, Stamey TA, Vaughan ED Jr, eds. *Campbell's Urology,* 7th ed. Philadelphia, Saunders, 1998, 2210–2256.

SELF-ASSESSMENT QUESTIONS

1. Describe the approach taken for a 2-year-old child who presents with bilateral Wilms' tumors.
2. Neuroblastoma involving the cervical ganglia can cause Horners syndrome. How else can neuroblastomas present?
3. Prostatic rhabdomyosarcoma (RMS) can cause urinary retention or constipation. How would a 4-year-old child who is found to have a prostatic RMS be evaluated and managed?
4. Vaginal RMS can present in toddlers as blood noted in the diapers. What would you tell the family of a 2-year-old girl who is discovered to have sarcoma botyroides that is confined to her vagina?
5. What is your evaluation of an 8-month-old boy who presents with a scrotal mass that does not transilluminate? If a yolk sac tumor is diagnosed and there is no evidence of retroperitoneal involvement, what is recommended for treatment and follow-up?

CHAPTER 29

Enuresis and Voiding Dysfunction in Children

Gregory E. Dean

I. NEURAL ANATOMY OF LOWER URINARY SYSTEM
A. Autonomic Control
1. Parasympathetic
   - S2–S4
   - Acetylcholine primary neurotransmitter
   - Efferent stimulation with resultant detrusor contraction

2. Sympathetic
   - T10–L1
   - Norepinephrine primary neurotransmitter. Alpha receptor stimulation in bladder neck and posterior urethra mediate contraction at these sites and Beta receptor stimulation results in bladder relaxation.

B. Somatic Control
1. Pudendal nerve. Efferent stimulation with increased activity of external sphincter.

II. ONTOGENY OF CONTINENCE
1. Requirements. Increase in bladder capacity.
2. Bladder capacity (oz) = Age (yrs) + 2 (Koff)
3. Twenty voids/day during first year
4. During first 3 years of life, number of daily voids decreases to 11 and mean voided volume increases approximately four-fold. At ages 1 to 3 years, development of voluntary control of striated sphincter occurs and uninhibited bladder contractions continue until adult pattern of control. At ages 3 to 5 years, development of voluntary control of spinal micturition reflex occurs as does cortical inhibition of involuntary detrusor contractions.

III. HISTORY

1. Age at toilet training
2. Enuresis primary or secondary?
3. Diurnal, nocturnal, or both?
4. Frequency of voiding?
5. Is initial AM voiding skipped?
6. Frequency of wetting?
7. Quality of urinary stream?
8. Associated urinary tract infections (UTIs)?
9. History of urgency/hesitancy/ staccato voiding pattern?
10. Frequency of bowel movements?
11. Hard bowel movements or encopresis?
12. Social factors/stress

IV. PHYSICAL EXAMINATION

1. External genitalia: rash, labial adhesions, and underwear/introital dampness.
2. Lower back
   a. Evidence of hair tuft or dimple—MRI examination for tethered cord mandatory.
   b. Absent gluteal cleft—found with sacral agenesis.
3. Evidence of fecal soiling
4. Rectal tone
5. Gross assessment of gait
6. Gross lower extremity motor function including strength
7. Deep tendon reflexes
8. Perineal/lower extremity sensation
9. Urinalysis
   a. Glucose—screen for diabetes mellitus.
   b. Specific gravity—screen for concentrating defect.
   c. Leukocytes—screen for infection.

V. RADIOGRAPHIC IMAGING

Not indicated with isolated nocturnal enuresis

A. Renal Bladder Ultrasound

1. Indicated when daytime wetting or other symptoms of dysfunctional voiding present.
2. Thickened bladder commonly seen.
3. Hydroureteronephrosis may be seen with Hinman syndrome.

B. VCUG

1. Indicated with history of urinary tract infection (UTI).
2. Indicated in males if poor stream reported.
3. Trabeculation of bladder may be present.
4. Incomplete voiding common.

     5. *Spinning-top urethra.* Dilated posterior urethra secondary to voiding against dysynergic external sphincter.

C. Lumbar/Sacral MRI
1. Rule out tethered cord. Obtain if lower back examination abnormal or if lower extremity findings present. Consider if dysfunctional voiding refractory to therapy although yield low.

VI. DYSFUNCTIONAL VOIDING
A. Common Symptoms
1. Urinary frequency
2. *Urinary urgency (urge syndrome).* Associated holding maneuvers include crossed legs, squatting with heal in perineum, and genital holding.
3. *Diurnal enuresis.* Nocturnal enuresis may also be present.
4. Staccato voiding pattern
5. *Incomplete voiding (lazy bladder syndrome).* High post-void residual associated with UTIs.
6. Encopresis and constipation

B. Functional Etiology
1. Characterized by dysynergy between external sphincter and detrusor. Failure of normal synchronous relaxation of external sphincter with detrusor contraction.
2. Results in detrusor contracting against closed bladder neck. Manifested by staccato voiding pattern.
3. May result in bladder hypertrophy and detrusor instability such as diminished bladder capacity and results in urge incontinence.

C. Precipitating event
1. Emotional. Family issues, school stress, and sexual abuse.
2. Dysuria. UTI and pool chlorine and soaps.
3. Idiopathic

D. Fecal Symptoms
1. Constipation
2. Encopresis
3. History often difficult to elicit. Parents often unaware of child's bowel habits. Ask children directly. Look for evidence of fecal soiling on examination.
4. Failure to isolate and relax pelvic floor during voiding/defecating.
5. Vicious cycle whereby hard, painful stools result in child's fear of voluntary pelvic floor relaxation during defecation.

E. Urodynamics

May be helpful in making diagnosis although this can usually be achieved on the basis of history and review of a voiding diary. Common findings include involuntary detrusor contractions, staccato uroflow associated with sphincteric dysynergy, and poorly contractile detrusor (lazy bladder).

F. Therapy

1. Stool softeners if constipation present.
   a. High fiber diet
   b. Colace
   c. Mineral oil. Chilled or mixed with honey increases compliance.
2. Timed voiding q 2 to 3 hours regardless of desire.
3. Double voiding to assist with incomplete voiding.
4. Voiding diary
   a. Assists in diagnosis.
   b. Increases child's self-awareness of voiding patterns. Can focus on initial awareness of bladder fullness.
5. Anticholinergic therapy (if urgency or frequency present)
   a. Ditropan × 8 weeks if initially responsive.
   b. Longer therapy periods if necessary but periodically withdraw to ascertain role of continued therapy.
   c. Side effects include dry mouth and decreased perspiration.
6. Alpha blockers
   a. Preliminary reports suggest may enhance emptying.
7. Comfortable seating position on toilet.
   a. Stepstool to support feet.
8. Observation of parents voiding can be helpful to correct staccato pattern.
   a. Enhances ability of child to relax pelvic floor.
9. Antibiotic prophylaxis
   a. Indicated in the presence of VUR.
   b. Consider with absence of VUR if UTIs recurrent.
10. Biofeedback therapy
    a. Appropriate when above measures fail to elicit a satisfactory response.
    b. Highly effective with 80 percent success with 6 month follow-up.
    c. Uroflow. Staccato voiding easily demonstrated. Attempt to achieve continuous flow without interference from a dyscoordinated sphincter.
    d. Pelvic floor EMG. Additional modality to demonstrate normal pelvic floor relaxation during voiding. Assists in teaching awareness and control of these muscles.

G. Lazy Bladder Syndrome

1. Variant of dysfunctional voiding.
2. Characterized by infrequent (more than a 4 hour interval) voiding.
3. Children preoccupied by friends and activities.
4. Wetting results from overflow incontinence.
5. Elevated post-void residuals increase risk of UTIs.
6. Easily identified. Voiding diary completed with assistance of parents. "Voiding hat" useful in documenting volumes.

Treatment is to enforce a strict timed voiding regimen. Double voiding may be useful.

H. Vesicoureteral Reflux (VUR) and Disfunctional Voiding (DV)

1. Of children with VUR 43 percent have DV.
2. Refluxing children with DV more likely to have breakthrough infections and resultant ureteral reimplantation than those with normal voiding patterns (82 percent versus 18 percent).
3. Persistence of reflux associated with recurrent UTIs.
4. Surgical success less in VUR associated with DV.

VII. NON-NEUROGENIC NEUROGENIC BLADDER (HINMAN-ALLEN SYNDROME)

1. Severe form of dysfunctional voiding.
2. Seen in the older child.
3. Upper tract findings consistent with neurogenic etiology although neurologically intact. They include a severely trabeculated bladder, high-grade VUR is common, and potential renal insufficiency.
4. Respond to same therapies as dysfunctional voiders although more likely to be refractory to therapy.
   a. Course of clean intermittent catheterization and anticholinergic therapy may be necessary.
   b. Biofeedback helpful.
   c. Severe cases can result in renal failure if untreated.
   d. Temporary diversion (vesicostomy) option for cases refractory to therapy.

VIII. OCHOA SYNDROME (UROFACIAL SYNDROME)

1. Variant of non-neurogenic neurogenic bladder with inherited component.
2. Associated with inversion of facial expression when laughing.
3. Autosomal recessive expression mapped to chromosome region 10q23-q24.

IX. MISCELLANEOUS ENTITIES

A. Interstitial Cystitis
1. Although controversial, may exist in children.
2. Sensory urgency, frequency, and bladder pain.
3. In small series, majority responded to hydrodistension
   a. Diffuse glomerulations and hematuria post hydrodistension.
   b. No evidence of involuntary contractions on urodynamics.

B. Giggle Incontinence
1. Wetting associated with laughter or emotion.
2. Part of narcolepsy/catoplexy complex.
3. Treated with methylphenidate.

C. Vaginal Voiding
1. Post-void dampness seen in girls
2. Common
3. Responds to positional changes in voiding

X. NOCTURNAL ENURESIS

A. Etiology
1. Developmental factors
   a. Associated with delayed onset of verbal skills and walking.
   b. Associated with attention deficit disorder (ADD). Children with ADD three times more likely to have nocturnal enuresis.
   c. Associated with delayed bone age.
   d. Higher incidence of EEG abnormalities.
2. Functional factors
   a. Reduction in functional bladder capacity common.
   b. Normalization of capacity with anticholinergics suggest that this functional rather than a reduction in total bladder capacity.
   c. Uninhibited bladder contractions common (50 to 80 percent) in contrast to normal children. Forty-five percent of children with detrusor contractions able to awaken with voluntary voiding. Remaining 65 percent wet with failure to contract external sphincter during contractions.
3. Sleep factors
   a. Families report that enuretic children are "deep sleepers," however, sleep studies have been inconclusive.
   b. Enuretic episodes occur throughout the night through all levels of sleep.
   c. Some enuretics wet during very light sleep or when awakening.

      d. Incidence of nightmares less in enuretics, suggesting that they may sleep better.

      e. Signal from subcortical centers controlling inhibition of micturition may not be registering.

  4. Social factors

      a. Children in families with stress are three times more likely to have enuresis.

      b. More common in lower socioeconomic groups. Twice as common in unskilled workers compared to professionals.

  5. Genetic factors

      a. Both parents enuretic: 77 percent offspring enuretic.

      b. One parent enuretic: 44 percent offspring enuretic.

      c. No parental history enuresis: 15 percent offspring enuretic.

  6. Antidiuretic hormone (ADH) and nocturnal enuresis

      a. Some enuretics fail to demonstrate normal rise in antidiuretic hormone during sleep. Resultant increased nocturnal urine volume.

      b. Some studies also suggest a receptor level defect in some enuretics demonstrated by high ADH levels with fluid restriction.

  7. Other associated factors

      a. Food allergies: chocolate/dairy products, caffeine may elicit effect through diuretic-related increase in urine volume rather than allergy.

      b. Obstructive sleep apnea: associated with enlarged adenoids in children, responds to adenoid surgery.

      c. *Entorobius vermicularis* (pinworm): associated with enuresis in females, diagnosis with recovery of eggs from feces and skin, and excellent response to antihelminthic therapy.

B. Incidence

  1. Fifteen percent of children wet at age 5 years.

  2. Resolution rate of 15 percent per year thereafter.

C. Secondary Enuresis

  1. Twenty-five percent of patients with control by age 12 will relapse.

  2. May be associated with social/family stress issues.

D. Association with Dysfunctional Voiding

      a. Encopresis in 10 to 25 percent.

E. Therapy

  1. Dry-bed training

      a. Awakening of children with alarm clock or by parents.

      b. Cure rate of 50 percent at 6 months.

2. Bell-pad alarm
   a. Circuit completed by voided urine contacting pad with resultant sounding of alarm. Child arises and completes voiding in bathroom. May need parental assistance initially but should be responsible for changing own linens. Recommend single training cycle per night to avoid sleep deprivation.
   b. High cure rate: 60 to 100 percent.
   c. Explained by classical conditioned theory. Nocturnal bladder distension associated with alarm stimulated inhibition of micturition and subsequent volitional voiding. Recent evidence also demonstrates improvement in functional bladder capacity.
   d. Requires parental involvement with treatment times extending for several weeks or months.
3. Desmopressin (DDAVP)
   a. Analog of vasopressin without pressor properties.
   b. Available as nasal spray or as tablets.
   c. Mechanism of action: Can overcome blunted ADH response in enuretics
   d. Reduction in wet nights up to 30 to 60 percent.
   e. Up to 50 percent with complete response.

Two-thirds of complete responders with wetting recurrence once DDAVP discontinued. Children with very low or very high native vasopressin levels less responsive to therapy. Responding children tend to have high nocturnal urine volumes. *Same group of children also demonstrate increase in fractional excretion of sodium suggesting abnormal tubular handling of sodium.* Responding children tend to void during early or late portion of sleep in contrast to non-responders who void throughout night.

   f. Safety profile excellent with short-term use. Limited long-term trials suggest excellent safety. Periodic monitoring of serum sodium recommended. Rare instances of hyponatremic seizures with overdose.

4. Imipramine
   a. Tricyclic antidepressant
   b. Enuresis suppressed in more than 50 percent. Relapse rate is 60 percent once discontinued. Acts as an anticholinergic as well as on the sympathetic control of the bladder with a 35 percent increase in average bladder capacity. Decreases time spent during REM sleep, *this action not involved with antienuresis effect.*

F. Nocturnal Enuresis in Adults
1. Respond to DDAVP, wetting alarm, or imipramine: 83 percent.
2. Dry after completing therapy: 38 percent.
3. Refractory to all modalities: 17 percent.

BIBLIOGRAPHY

Caldamone AA, Schulman S, Rabinowitz R: Outpatient pediatric urology. In: Gillenwater JY, Grayhack JT, Howards SS, Duckett JW, eds. Adult and Pediatric Urology, 3rd ed. St. Louis, Mosby, 1996.

Close CE, Carr MC, Burns MW, et al: Interstitial cystitis in children. *J Urol* 156:860–862, 1996.

Combs AJ, Glassberg AD, Gerdes D, Horowitz M: Biofeedback therapy for children with dysfunctional voiding. *Urology* 52:312–315, 1998.

Hunsballe JM, Hansen TK, Rittig S, Pedersen EB, Djurhuus JC: The efficacy of DDAVP is related to the circadian rhythm of urine output in patients with persisting nocturnal enuresis. *Clin Endocrinol* 49:793–801, 1998.

Koff SA, Wagner TT, Jayanthi VR: The relationship among dysfunctional elimination syndromes, primary vesicoureteral reflux and urinary tract infections in children. *J Urol* 160:1019–1022, 1998.

Neveus T, Stenberg A, Lackgren G, Tuvemo T, Hetta J: Sleep of children with enuresis: A polysomnographic study. *Pediatrics* 1193–1197, 1999.

Ochoa B, Gorlin RJ: Urofacial (ochoa) syndrome. *Am J Med Genet* 27:661–667, 1987.

Oredsson AF, Jorgenson TM: Changes in nocturnal bladder capacity during treatment with the bell and pad for monosymptomatic nocturnal enuresis. *J Urol* 160:166–169, 1998.

Van Gool JD, Hjalmas K, Tamminen-Mobius T, Olbing H: Historical clues to the complex of dysfunctional voiding, urinary tract infection and vesicoureteral reflux. The International Reflux Study in Children. *J Urol* 148:1699–1702, 1992.

SELF-ASSESSMENT QUESTIONS
True/False
1. Imipramine is effective in the treatment of nocturnal enuresis through its effect on altering the level of sleep.
2. Renal-bladder USG is indicated in the evaluation of nocturnal enuresis.
3. Control of the striated urinary sphincter occurs from ages 1 to 3 years.
4. Ochoa syndrome is an autosomal dominant disorder.
5. Children with nocturnal enuresis who respond to DDAVP have high nocturnal urine volumes.

Multiple Choice
6. How likely is a child (percent) with a family history notable for the presence of resolved nocturnal enuresis in both parents to have nocturnal enuresis?
   a. 100
   b. 75
   c. 40
   d. 25
   e. 15

7. What percent of 5-year-old bed-wetters will resolve by the following year?
   a. 10
   b. 15
   c. 20
   d. 25
   e. 40
8. Which of the following are not routinely recommended in the treatment of dysfunctional voiding?
   a. Colace
   b. Oxybutinin
   c. Mineral oil
   d. DDAVP
   e. Timed-voiding
9. Which of the following is a complication of DDAVP therapy?
   a. Metabolic ketosis
   b. Hyperkalemia
   c. Hypernatremia
   d. Hyponatremia
   e. Hypomagnasemia
10. The presence of a sacral hair-tuft on examination mandates:
    a. an MRI.
    b. urodynamics.
    c. evoked potential measurements.
    d. voiding diary.
    e. all of the above.

Answers

1. False	6. b
2. False	7. b
3. True	8. d
4. False	9. d
5. True	10. a

CHAPTER 30

Congenital Anomalies

Douglas A. Canning
William F. Tarry
Howard M. Snyder III

I. **UPPER URINARY TRACT**
  A. **Abnormalities of the Kidney Position and Number**
    1. Simple ectopia
      a. Incidence is approximately 1 per 900 (autopsy) (pelvic, 1 per 3000; solitary, 1 per 22,000; bilateral, 10 percent). Left side favored.
      b. Associated findings include small size with persistent fetal lobulations, anterior or horizontal pelvis, anomalous vasculature, contralateral agenesis, vesicoureteral reflux, müllerian anomalies in 20 to 60 percent of females; undescended testes, hypospadias, urethral duplication in 10 to 20 percent males; skeletal and cardiac anomalies in 20 percent.
      c. Only work-up, voiding cystourethrography.
    2. Thoracic ectopia
      a. Comprises less than 5 percent of ectopic kidneys.
      b. Origin is delayed closure of diaphragmatic anlage versus "overshoot" of renal ascent.
      c. Adrenal may or may not be thoracic.
    3. Crossed ectopia and fusion (Bauer)
      a. Incidence is 1 per 1000 to 1 per 2000, 90 percent crossed with fusion, 2:1 male, 3:1 left crossed; 24 cases solitary, five cases bilateral reported.
      b. Origin is presumed abnormal migration of ureteral bud or rotation of caudal end of fetus at time of bud formation (Stephens, 1983).
      c. Associated findings include multiple or anomalous vessels arising from the ipsilateral side of the aorta and vesicoureteral reflux; with solitary crossed kidney only; genital, skeletal, and hindgut anomalies in 20 to 50 percent.

4. Horseshoe kidney
   a. Incidence is 1 per 400 or 0.25 percent; 2:1 males.
   b. Origin is fusion of lower poles before or during rotation (4½ to 6 weeks of gestation).
   c. Associated findings include anomalous vessels; isthmus between or behind great vessels; skeletal, cardiovascular, and CNS anomalies (33 percent); hypospadias and cryptorchidism (4 percent), bicornuate uterus (7 percent), urinary tract infection (UTI) (13 percent); duplex ureters (10 percent), stones (17 percent); 20 percent of trisomy 18 and 60 percent of Turner's patients have horseshoe kidney.
   d. Excluding other anomalies, survival is not affected.
   e. Stones; infection may result from stasis; rarely is true obstruction present [see "Ureteropelvic Junction Obstruction (UPJO)"].

5. Bilateral renal agenesis
   a. Incidence is 1 per 4800 births or 1 per 400 newborn autopsies (75 percent are male).
   b. Origin is thought to be either ureteral bud failure or absence of the nephrogenic ridge.
   c. Associated findings include absent renal arteries, complete ureteral atresia in 50 percent, bladder atresia in 50 percent, Potter's syndrome (Potter, 1972). Also: low birth weight, oligohydramnios, pulmonary hypoplasia, bowed limbs.

6. Unilateral renal agenesis
   a. Incidence is 1 per 1100 in autopsy series, 1 per 1500 in radiographic series, 2:1 male, left kidney is more often involved than right kidney.
   b. Origin is probably ureteral bud failure; there is a familial trend.
   c. Associated findings include absent ureter with hemitrigone (50 percent); adrenal agenesis (10 percent) genital anomalies (20 to 40 percent in both sexes).
      (1) Müllerian anomalies in females include uterovaginal atresia (Rokitansky syndrome), uterus didelphys, and vaginal agenesis.
      (2) In males, the vas and seminal vesicle are absent or atretic.
   d. If the single kidney is normal, no special precautions need to be taken and survival is not affected; management of the genital abnormalities is covered in section III.

7. Supernumerary kidney
   a. Incidence is unknown.

    b. Origin is presumed to be a combined defect of ureteral bud and metanephros.

    c. Associated findings are hydronephrosis (50 percent), common ureter (40 percent), duplex ureter (40 percent), and ectopic ureter or one ending in the pelvis of the ipsilateral kidney (20 percent).

B. Cystic Abnormalities of the Kidney (Glassberg)

  1. Autosomal dominant polycystic kidney disease (Tables 30-1 and 30-2)

    a. 2 gives chromosome 16 and chromosome 4.

    b. Autosomal dominant transmission.

    c. Adult type is the most common cystic disease in humans, with an incidence of 1 per 1250 live births, and accounts for 10 percent of all end-stage renal disease.

    d. Usually presents between ages 30 and 50 years with pain, hematuria, progressive renal insufficiency, but can occur in children. Has been noted in newborns.

    e. Intravenous urography (IVU) reveals irregular renal enlargement with calyceal distortion; ultrasound shows multiple cysts of variable sizes.

    f. Associated findings are liver cysts without functional impairment in one third of patients and berry aneurysms in 10 to 40 percent.

Table 30-1 Cystic Diseases of the Kidney

Genetic
  Autosomal recessive (infantile) polycystic kidney disease
  Autosomal dominant (adult) polycystic kidney disease
  Juvenile nephronophthisis-medullary cystic disease complex
    Juvenile nephronophthisis (autosomal recessive)
    Medullary cystic disease (autosomal dominant)
  Congenital nephrosis (familial nephrotic syndrome)(autosomal recessive)
  Familial hypoplastic glomerulocystic disease (autosomal dominant)
  Multiple malformation syndromes with renal cysts (e.g., tuberous sclerosis, von Hippel-Lindau disease)
Nongenetic
  Multicystic kidney (multicystic dysplastic kidney)
  Benign multilocular cyst (cystic nephroma)
  Simple cysts
  Medullary sponge kidney
  Sporadic glomerulocystic kidney disease
  Acquired renal cystic disease
  Calyceal diverticulum (pyelogenic cyst)

Table 30-2 Comparison of Autosomal Recessive and Autosomal Dominant Polycystic Kidney Disease

	AUTOSOMAL RECESSIVE POLYCYSTIC KIDNEY DISEASE (RPK)	AUTOSOMAL DOMINANT POLYCYSTIC KIDNEY DISEASE (DPK)
Gene defect	Chromosome 6	Chromosomes 4, 16
Incidence	1:5000 to 1:40,000	1:500 to 1:1000
Usual age of clinical presentation	Perinatal	Third to fifth decades
Typical sonographic appearance of kidneys	Symmetrically enlarged homogeneous, hyperchogenic kidneys	Large cystic kidneys sometimes asymmetrical
Histology	Colleting duct ectasia; cysts derived principally from collecting duct	Micro- and macrocysts derived from entire nephron
Liver	Always congenital hepatic fibrosis but of varying severity	Cysts, mostly in adults (on very rare occasions, a newborn may have congenital hepatic fibrosis)
Other system involvement	None	Intracranial aneurysms; colonic diverticuli; mitral valve regurgitation; cysts of other organs

    g. Complications include uremia, hypertension, myocardial infarction, and intracranial hemorrhage (9 percent).

    h. Management involves control of blood pressure and urinary infection, relief of cardiac failure, and eventually dialysis or transplantation.

    i. *Pathology.* Rounded or irregular cysts located in all parts of the nephron.

2. Autosomal recessive polycystic kidney disease

    a. Chromosome 6.

    b. *Infantile type.* Rare (1 per 10,000 live births), usually presents with bilateral flank masses in infancy, but can present in childhood with renal or hepatic insufficiency.

    c. IVU shows huge (12 to 16 times normal) kidneys with very delayed nephrogram and characteristic streaked appearance ("sunburst" pattern).

    d. May be distinguished from hydronephrosis, renal tumor, and renal vein thrombosis by IVU and ultrasound. (Bright echoes on ultrasound.)

    e. Associated findings are congenital hepatic (periportal) fibrosis and dilation of bile ducts with the degree of hepatic insufficiency varying inversely with the severity of renal disease and directly with the age of presentation; cysts elsewhere are uncommon.

    f. Complications are renal and hepatic failure, hypertension and respiratory compromise in the newborn; patients usually die within the first 2 months of life.

    g. Although respiratory support, blood pressure control, and dialysis can improve survival, the longer the survival is, the greater the chance the patient will suffer from the complications of cirrhosis.

    h. Pathology is fusiform dilation of collecting ducts and tubules resulting in small subcapsular cysts.

3. Medullary sponge kidney (tubular ectasia) is an adult disease pathologically characterized by enlarged tortuous collecting ducts and occasional tiny cysts in the pyramids (75 percent bilateral; incidence, 1 per 20,000)

    a. *Diagnosis.* IVU shows collections of contract adjacent to the calyces ("bristles on a brush") often with calcifications in the medulla.

    b. *Complications.* Infection, stones, distal renal tubular acidosis, and hematuria.

    c. Medical management of calculi and infections is often required.

    d. One third of patients with hypercalcemia.

4. Medullary cystic disease (juvenile nephronophthisis) refers to a group of disorders with various genetic patterns characterized pathologically by bilateral small kidneys,

attenuated cortex, atrophic and dilated tubules, medullary cysts, and some interstitial fibrosis.

a. Patients progress to end-stage renal disease by about age 20; juvenile form is said to be responsible for 20 percent of childhood renal failure deaths.

b. Medical management of renal failure can delay need for transplant.

c. Polydipsia and polyuria in 80 percent, retinitis pigmentosa in 16 percent.

5. Unilateral multicystic dysplastic kidney is the most common cystic disease of the newborn and the second most common abdominal mass in infants after hydronephrosis.

a. The left kidney is more commonly involved, but there is no sex predilection or familial tendency.

b. Origin is thought to be either ischemic, from failure of the normal shift of vasculature as the kidney migrates, producing also the associated atretic ureter (Stephens, 1983), or failure of ureteral bud to stimulate metanephric blastoma.

c. Contralateral renal abnormalities are most common when the multicystic kidney is small and/or the ureteral atresia is low. Vesicoureteral reflux may be present (20 percent).

d. Ultrasound is most diagnostic study (multiple sonolucent areas of various sizes without connections or dominant medial cyst and without identifiable parenchyma, as IVU or renal scan demonstrates ipsilateral nonfunction; IVU and voiding cystourethrography (VCU) are done to evaluate the remainder of the urinary tract.

e. Pathology includes atretic artery, cysts, some solid central stroma, low cuboidal epithelium, and some primitive nephrogenic structures, immature glomeruli occasionally.

f. Although the cystic kidney usually does not enlarge as the child grows and thus becomes relatively less conspicuous, a few adults have had problems related to multicystic kidneys (tumor, infection, pain) and it is not unreasonable to recommend removal of the multicystic kidney, although the risk of tumor is no greater than in normal kidneys.

C. **Collecting System Abnormalities (Bauer)**

1. Calyceal diverticulum occurs in 4.5 per 1000 urograms.

a. Origin is failure of degeneration of third- and fourth-order branches of ureteral bud, leaving a pocket lined with transitional epithelium connected to the collecting system near the calyceal fornix.

    b. In approximately one third of patients, stones will form; some will become sites of persistent infection due to stasis; the rest remain asymptomatic.

    c. Treatment involves removal of stones, drainage of pus, and marsupialization to the renal surface with closure of the collecting system and cauterization of the epithelium.

2. Hydrocalycosis is a rare lesion involving vascular compression, cicatrization, or achalasia of the infundibulum; it rarely requires any intervention.

3. Megacalycosis is a rare lesion involving all of one or both kidneys and defined as dilated unobstructed calyces usually numbering more than 25 per kidney (normally 8 to 10). May be confused radiographically with obstructive uropathy.

    a. Results from combination of faulty uretral bud division, hypoplasia of juxtamedullary glomeruli, and maldevelopment of calyceal musculature.

    b. Males 6:1 over females, only in Caucasians. X-linked recessive gene.

    c. May be associated with stones or infection but in itself causes no deterioration of renal function.

4. Infundibulopelvic stenosis may involve part or all of one or both kidneys.

    a. The calyces become quite large but usually no progressive functional deterioration occurs.

    b. May be associated with dysplasia and lower tract anomalies (e.g., urethral valves).

    c. Commonly associated with vesicoureteral reflux.

5. Ureteropelvic junction obstruction (UPJO) is the usual cause of the most common abdominal mass in children (hydronephrosis).

    a. There are a 2:1 male predominance in children and left-sided predominance in all ages.

    b. Several etiologies have been postulated, including segmental muscular attenuation or malorientation, true stenosis, angulation, and extrinsic compression. Crossing vessels are implicated in approximately 20 to 30 percent of cases, but an intrinsic lesion of some sort (either noncompliant or nonconducting) is most often found.

    c. Associated findings include reflux (5 to 10 percent), contralateral agenesis (5 percent), and contralateral UPJO (10 percent); dysplasia, multicystic kidney, or other urologic anomaly is occasionally seen.

    d. Symptoms and signs include episodic flank pain, flank mass, hematuria, infection, nausea and vomiting, and sometimes uremia. In infants, the flank mass may be the only sign, whereas the older child will exhibit any of the others; very often gastrointestinal distress or poorly localized upper abdominal pain are the only symptoms.

e. Radiologic findings are delayed excretion on the affected side with variable dilation of pelvis and calyces or even nonvisualization on intravenous pyelography (IVP); on ultrasound, multiple interconnected lucencies with dominant medial lucency and identifiable cortical rim; usually some measurable function on renal scan. When function is fairly good, the drainage will be delayed even in the face of furosemide (Lasix) administration beyond 20 min.

f. Prompt surgical repair by excision of the narrow segment and spatulated reanastomosis of the ureter to the tailored renal pelvis is indicated in all symptomatic cases. Most cases now present antenatally and can be followed with serial renal scan and ultrasound.

g. Follow-up consists of ultrasound at 1 month and renal scan at 3 months and ultrasound at 1 year postoperatively in most cases.

D. Ureteral Anomalies

1. Duplication of ureter occurs in 1 per 125 autopsies; 1.6:1 female, 85 percent unilateral.

   a. Autosomal dominant with incomplete penetrance.

   b. Seems to arise from two ureteral buds meeting the metanephros in most cases, but may also be caused by a bud that bifurcates immediately after arising, before meeting the metanephros.

   c. Associated with reflux (42 percent), renal scarring and dilation (29 percent), ectopic insertion (3 percent), large kidneys with excess calyces, dysplasia/hypoplasia, infection, and ureteroceles.

   d. Duplication per se is of no clinical significance but the associated anomalies may require intervention (see ureterocele, ectopia, etc.).

2. Atresia is usually associate with a multicystic dysplastic kidney; distal segment atresia is often associated with contralateral hydronephrosis or dysplasia (50 percent) (Table 30-3).

3. Mega-ureter carries a 3:1 male and 3:1 left-sided predominance; the term has been used rather loosely to describe any dilated ureter, but there are three distinct types that should be distinguished.

   a. Refluxing type may originate because of the reflux, although some cases have an abnormal distal segment and some element of obstruction.

Mega-ureter (Wide) Examples

Reflux mega-ureter		Obstructed mega-ureter		Nonreflux–nonobstructed megaureter	
Primary	Secondary	Primary	Secondary	Primary	Secondary
			E X A M P L E S		
Primary reflux mega-ureter [a]Prune-belly	Urethral obstruction Neuropathic bladder	Intrinsic obstruction stenosis adynamic segment	Urethral obstruction Neuropathic bladder Extrinsic obstruction Retroperitoneal tumor	[b]Nonreflux-nonobstructed mega-ureter	Polyuria infection · Remaining wide after reflief of distal obstruction

[a]Some conditions (eg., prune-belly, ureteroceles, ectopic ureters) may appear under several other columns.
[b]As proved not to be obstructed.

An occasional mega-ureter may show reflux and apparent obstruction.

Adapted from Report of Working Party to Establish an International Nomenclature for the Large Ureter. In: Bergsma D, Duckett JW Jr, eds. *Urinary System Malformations in Children: Birth Defects: Original Article Series.* vol 13, No 5. New York, Alan R. Liss, 1977.

    b. A widened ureteral bud gives rise to a ureter dilated down to the orifice, which is in the normal position, and there is no obstruction (nonreflux, nonobstructed type).

    c. The primary obstructed type is the most common and results from a stenotic or aperistaltic distal short segment; the orifice is in the normal position.

    d. The refluxing type, with its laterally ectopic orifice, may be associated with a dysplastic kidney, one scarred by infection, or both; the other types drain normal or hydronephrotic kidneys.

    e. The ultrasound will show moderate-to-severe hydronephrosis and proportionately greater ureteral dilation; VCU diagnoses the reflux type; a Lasix renogram may be needed to distinguish obstructed from nonobstructed types.

    f. There are mild primary obstructed megaureters with only a spindle-shape dilation of the distal ureter and normal (sharp) calyces; these require no treatment.

    g. Surgical correction is needed for some obstructed and refluxing mega-ureters. Refluxing ones more commonly require tailoring than obstructed ones, which tend to decrease in caliber after excision of the aperistaltic distal segment.

    h. Follow-up includes ultrasound at 1 month and renal scan at 3 months. An ultrasound is done 1 year postoperatively.

4. Vesicoureteral reflux (VUR) occurs in approximately 1 per 1000 in the general population, but is 8 to 40 times more frequent in affected families; it will be found in 50 percent of infants and 30 percent of children with a UTI.

    a. It may occur because the ureteral bud arises ectopically leading to a laterally placed orifice and short submucosal tunnel or because the development of the intrinsic smooth muscle of the distal ureteral segment is delayed or incomplete. High intravesical pressures may cause a marginally competent ureterovesical junction to reflux, and evidence is growing that voiding dysfunction in the child may cause or exacerbate reflux.

    b. Duplicated ureters and renal hypodysplasia may be associated with refluxing ureters with laterally ectopic orifices. Infection and renal scarring are prominent findings with all types of refluxing ureters regardless of grade. Voiding dysfunction and urethral obstruction by valves are associated with an acquired form of reflux.

    c. Reflux is best graded I to V by the International Reflux Study system (see Fig. 30-1).

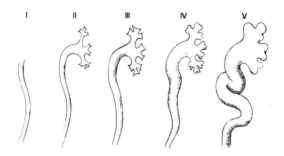

Figure 30-1 International classification of vesicoureteral reflux. Grade I: Ureter only. Grade II: Ureter, pelvis, and calyces; no dilatation, normal calyceal fornices. Grade III: Mild or moderate dilatation and/or tortuosity of ureter and mild or moderate dilatation of renal pelvis *but no or slight blunting of fornices.* Grade IV: Moderate dilatation and/or tortuosity of ureter and moderate dilatation of renal pelvis and calyces; complete obliteration of sharp angle of fornices *but* maintenance of papillary impressions in majority of calyces. Grade V: Gross dilatation and tortuosity of ureter; gross dilatation of renal pelvis and calyces; papillary impressions are no longer visible in majority of calyces. (*Reproduced from Duckett JW, Levitt S: Medical versus surgical treatment of vesicoureteral reflux: An international collaborative prospective study. J Urol 125:277, 1981.*)

    d. All children with reflux should be placed on prophylactic antibiotics at one-fourth the therapeutic dose given once a day. Trimethoprim-sulfamethoxazole and nitrofurantoin are the most commonly used drugs. Children require periodic upper tract radiographic assessment usually with ultrasound and reevaluation of the reflux by VCU or nuclear VCU. We prefer annual follow-up with ultrasound (US) and biannual nuclear VCU. Some centers use dimercaptosuccinic acid (DMSA) to screen for scarring in patients monitored with VUR.

    e. Grades I to III (minimally dilated) are usually treated medically initially; Grade IV–V usually require surgical correction. At our center, low volume (VUR Grades I–III) resolved at a rate of 17 percent per patient-year. Grade IV VUR resolved at a rate of 4 percent per patient-year.

    f. Reimplantation of the refluxing unit by the Cohen technique is the standard surgical management, with nearly complete success; duplicated ureters are reimplanted in their common distal muscular sheath.

g. Breakthrough infections, failure to comply with the antibiotic prophylaxis regimen, persistent reflux into puberty in females, progressive scarring, and worsening renal function are all considerations which favor surgical intervention, but there are no absolute indications for surgery for reflux.

5. The incidence of ureteral ectopia is approximately 1 per 1900; ectopic ureters are duplex in 80 percent of females, more often single in males; there is a 3:1 female predominance, and approximately 10 percent are bilateral.

a. The etiology is a failure of the ureteral bud to separate from the mesonephric duct, probably due to its ectopic origin on the duct.

b. Locations are shown in Table 30-4.

c. Associated findings

1. Renal dysplasia correlates with the degree of ectopy.

2. Single ectopic ureter is accompanied by contralateral duplication in 80 percent.

3. Incontinence and ureteral obstruction are variable findings; incontinence may be due to an orifice located below the sphincter in females or to failure of bladder neck development.

4. Bilateral single ectopic ureters where the orifice is distal to the bladder neck lead to poorly developed bladder and incontinence due to outlet incompetence and failure of bladder cycling.

d. Management is most often removal of the renal segment and ectopic ureter; rarely the segment may be salvageable by ureteroureterostomy or reimplantation.

6. Ureterocele occurs with a frequency between 1 per 500 and 1 per 4000 in autopsies, accounting for approximately 1 percent of pediatric urologic admissions, and is bilateral in 10 to 15 percent of cases. Females 4:1 over males.

a. The embryologic origin is thought to be a combination of an abnormal ureteral bud with either a stenotic orifice or involvement of the distal ureter in the expansion of the vesicourethral canal. The ureter is usually duplicated in children (80 percent), with the ureterocele affecting the upper pole ureter; simple ureterocele subtending a single ureter is less common in children.

b. Associated anomalies include contralateral ureteral duplication in 50 percent; renal segmental dysplasia; renal fusion, and ectopia; reflux (50 percent); and, rarely, incontinence.

c. Classification has recently been simplified (Table 30-4).

Table 30-4 Ureterocele Classification

Simple: intravesical with single ureter

Intravesical: entire ureterocele, including the usually stenotic orifice contained within the bladder, duplicated ureter

Ectopic: part of ureterocele, including orifice, extends into urethra

Adapted from *Report of the Committee on Terminology, Nomenclature and Classification, Section on Urology.* American Academy of Pediatrics, Glassberg, KI, Baren V, Duckett JW, et al.

    d. Cecoureterocele, a subclassification of ectopic ureterocele, differs in that a "cecum" extends beyond the orifice down the urethra; it may be associated with poor bladder neck development and incontinence.

    e. Management is controversial.

       1. Puncture of the ureterocele as newborn.

       2. Upper pole nephrectomy with decompression of the ureterocele.

       3. Intervention as in 2, with lower excision of the ureterocele with common sheath reimplantation and bladder neck reconstruction.

       4. Intervention as in 1, with delayed excision of ureterocele plus reimplant with bladder neck reconstruction if vesicoureteral reflux persists or occurs following step 1. Because we believe that the distortion of the trigone by the ureterocele and not the method of initial management determines the development and persistence of VUR, we favor intervention 1, followed in 50 percent of cases by step 4. This allows those patients who *do not* develop persistent VUR to escape with minimal surgery.

II. LOWER URINARY TRACT (GEARHART)

A. Extrophy and Epispadia—Spectrum of Anomalies

    1. Origin is failure of the cloacal membrane to migrate toward the perineum at 4 weeks gestation, preventing ingrowth of lateral mesoderm and coalescence of genital tubercles.

       a. The most consistent finding is some degree of separation of symphysis pubis.

       b. Epispadias (30 percent) may be penopubic with incontinence in males (55 percent), penile (20 percent) with or without incontinence, balanitic (5 percent), or may occur in females with incontinence (20 percent). It consists of a dorsal meatus with a distal mucosal groove, flattened glans, or bifid clitoris; in males, there is a variable dorsal chordee with shortening of the corporal bodies in severe forms (penopubic).

c. Nearly all cases of epispadias are best managed with the complete disassembly (Mitchell) technique.

d. Classic exstrophy (60 percent) occurs in 1 per 50,000 births with 3:1 male predominance; the bladder and the urethra are open dorsally, and the penis is short or the clitoris is bifid.

e. Cloacal exstrophy (10 percent) results from the condition of failure of the urorectal septum to descend and occurs approximately 1 per 200,000 births, about equally in males and females.

2. Associated findings

a. In classic exstrophy, undescended testes and inguinal hernias are common; often the infraumbilical rectus fails to develop; vaginal stenosis and/or bifid uterus may be present; the upper urinary tract is usually normal, or may be duplex.

b. In cloacal exstrophy, there are a vesicointestinal fissure opening into the center of the exstrophied bladder, short blind distal colon, absent or duplicated appendix, and often omphalocele. Two thirds of females have an absent or duplex and stenotic vagina; nearly all have a tethered spinal cord with 50 percent having myelomeningocele. The penis or clitoris is bifid or may be absent.

3. Exstrophy may be managed in stages, beginning with bladder closure in the newborn period (Fig. 30-2A–D).

a. Penile lengthening by freeing corpora from pubic bone attachments and dividing the urethral plate is accomplished at the same sitting.

b. In cloacal exstrophy, the omphalocele and vesicoenteric fissure must be dealt with by lateral closure of the bowel end colostomy, and omphalocele repair.

4. Second stage is now epispadias repair, in most cases at approximately 1 to 2 years of age.

5. The third stage in those with functioning, sufficiently large bladders is achieving continence by bladder neck tubularization (60 percent success).

a. Those who fail this are candidates for augmentation plus intermittent catheterization.

b. Most cloacal exstrophy patients have undergone early ileal loop diversion, but a few may be reconstructed along the same principles.

6. A second option is complete penile disassembly with bladder closure and bladder neck and epispadias repair all done at a single stage.

7. All patients require careful follow-up throughout life with survey of the upper tracts by IVU or ultrasound,

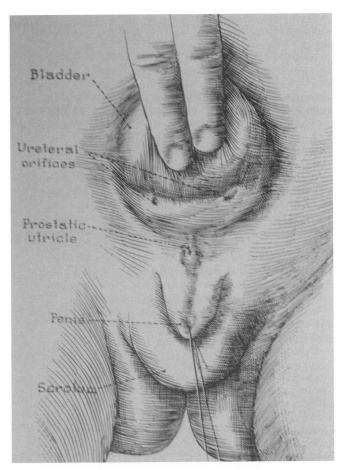

A

Figure 30-2 A. Bladder exstrophy before closure.

monitoring of acid–base balance with USO, renal function tests, and supportive counseling. Each case must be largely individualized within this general outline.

B. Urachus

Patent urachus and persistence of portions of the urachus as cysts result from failure of fibrosis of the cranial embryonic bladder segment; they are treated by excision

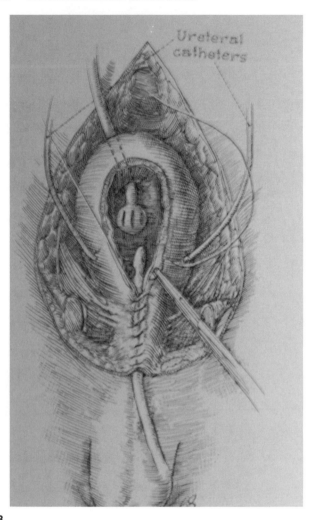

B

Figure 30-2 (*continued*)   **B.** After full mobilization and tubes are placed for a staged repair. In the complete dissassembly repair (not shown), the penis is split into its components two corpora cavernosa and the spongiosal tissue. This maneuver helps provide exposure to the bladder base and prostatic urethra which allows better mobilization and suspension of the bladder neck deep within the pelvis. (*Reprinted with permission from Gearhart JP, Jeffs RD: Exstrophy epispadias complex and bladder anomalies. In: Walsh PC, Retik AB, Vaughn ED, Wein AJ, eds. Campbell's Urology, 7th ed. Philadelphia, Saunders, 1998,*

when symptomatic. In a few cases, they may undergo malignant transformation (adenocarcinoma).

C. Posterior Urethral Valves (Type I)

1. *Incidence.* In boys, 1 per 5000 to 8000; more than 50 percent are diagnosed in the first year of life, generally with more severe obstructions.

2. Proposed etiology is failure of regression of the terminal segment of the mesonephric duct, which is normally represented by the plicae colliculi. Type II valves are nonobstructing normal folds in the prostatic urethra; Type III valves represent either more marked anterior fusion of the valve leaflets or congenital urethral membrane (a separate embryologic entity). Recent data suggest that types II and III are rariations of type I valves.

3. Associated findings
   a. Vesicoureteral reflux (40 percent, approximately one-half bilateral) resolves in approximately one third of cases generally within 2 years. Persistent unilateral reflux is usually associated with a nonfunctioning kidney, most commonly the left one.
   b. Severe renal dysplasia is common in those with severe obstruction.
   c. Severe hydroureteronephrosis.
   d. Acute renal failure and acidosis in the newborn are an obstructive phenomenon; chronic renal insufficiency may be related to dysplasia or may occur when obstruction is not recognized early.

4. Diagnosis
   a. Antenatal diagnosis.
   b. UTI or poor stream in an infant or older child; incontinence occasionally in an older child.
   c. A newborn with palpable bladder and kidneys and urinary ascites.
   d. VCU is *the* diagnostic study; ultrasonography, and renal scan are employed to assess the extent of upper tract damage and postoperative recovery.

5. Management
   a. In the sick infant, bladder drainage by small feeding tube (6 F) per the urethra is maintained while acidosis and sepsis are treated; VCU may be done with this catheter in place.
   b. The healthy infant or older child may undergo transurethral fulguration of valves initially; the sick infant when creatinine stabilizes and sepsis resolves.
   c. Cutaneous vesicostomy can be employed as a temporizing measure in a very small infant, but is rarely required with today's endoscopic equipment.

  d. Nonfunctioning kidneys with refluxing ureters should be preserved to be used as tissue for augmentation of the bladder if needed at the time of renal transplant.

  e. Ureteral tailoring and reimplantation are almost never indicated and are often fraught with failure.

  f. Antibiotic prophylaxis is maintained as long as reflux persists or upper tract emptying is slow (usually through adulthood).

 6. Results

  a. Children whose creatinine levels stabilize below 0.7 mg/dL after relief of obstruction generally do well, whereas those with creatinine levels above 1.0 often "outgrow" their renal function by puberty and require transplantation.

  b. Continence is eventually achieved in virtually all following valve incision.

D. Megalourethra

 1. This rare lesion is seen most often in association with prune belly syndrome.

 2. Occurs in two types

  a. Scaphoid type is a deficiency of corpus spongiosum allowing ballooning of the urethra during voiding; it can be repaired with hypospadias techniques.

  b. Fusiform type involves deficiency of corpora cavernosa as well as corpus spongiosum, resulting in elongated flaccid penis with redundant skin. This form is seen usually in stillborn infants with other cloacal anomalies.

E. Miscellaneous

 1. Anterior urethral valve or diverticulum is a rare obstructing lesion with a large saccular outpouching and obstructing distal lip of mucosa; the diverticulum is excised with careful attention to the obstructing flap distally.

 2. Enlarged utriculus masculinus is a dilated müllerian remnant, usually asymptomatic, associated with hypospadias or an intersex state; it can be excised retrovesically or transvesically if stasis leads to UTI or the full utricle interferes with bladder emptying. These rarely require surgical intervention.

 3. Aphallia and diphallia are exceedingly rare failure of fusion of the genital tubercles or failure of differentiation of the phallic mesenchyme.

 4. Micropenis is often associated with CNS lesions or an intersex state; gender conversion may be considered in severe cases.

III. EXTERNAL GENITAL MALFORMATIONS
A. Hypospadias
Hypospadias occurs in 1 per 300 live male births; there is a 14 percent incidence in siblings and an 8 percent incidence in offspring.

1. *Origin.* Failure of mesodermal urethral folds to converge in midline; chordee results from failure of urethral plate disintegration or fibrosis of inner genital folds (which form the spongiosum and dartos fascia).

2. Associated findings
   a. Variable endocrine findings such as blunted human chorionic gonadotropin response and low androgen receptor levels in a few cases.
   b. Undescended testes in 9.3 percent (30 percent with penoscrotal or more proximal meatus); as many as one third of patients with hypospadias and undescended testes have an intersex state, usually genetic mosaicism.
   c. Inguinal hernia in 9 percent.
   d. Upper tract anomalies in 46 percent when associated with imperforate anus, 33 percent when meningomyelocele is present, 12 to 50 percent when one other system anomaly is present, 5 percent with isolated hypospadias (screening IVP not needed for simple hypospadias).

3. Classification (simplified) (Fig. 30-3)
   a. Hypospadias without chordee (straight erections, meatus between midshaft and corona)
   b. Hypospadias with chordee
      1. Meatus penile or penoscrotal after release of chordee
      2. Meatus scrotal or perineal
   c. Chordee with hypospadias
      1. With normal urethra
      2. With short or hypoplastic urethra

4. Management
   a. One-stage correction between 4 and 12 months of age is preferred.
   b. Glanular hypospadias may be corrected by meatal advancement and glanuloplasty (MAGPI) (Fig. 30-4), Snodgrass (TIP), or onlay island flap (Fig. 30-5) procedure, depending on meatal position.
   c. Penile shaft or more proximal hypospadias may be managed by inner preputial transverse island flap (Fig. 30-6).
   d. Severe penoscrotal hypospadias may require combined island flap and primary (Duplay) closure of the

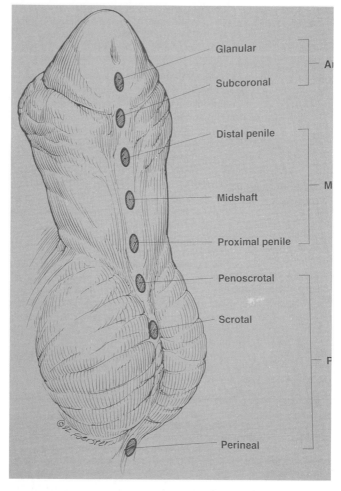

Figure 30-3 Classification scheme for hypospadias. The location of the urethral meatus is described as well as the severity of chordee. (*Reproduced from Duckett JW: Hypospadias. In: Walsh PC, Retik AB, Vaughan ED, Wein AJ, eds. Campbell's Urology, 7th ed. Philadelphia, Saunders, 1998, p 2094.*)

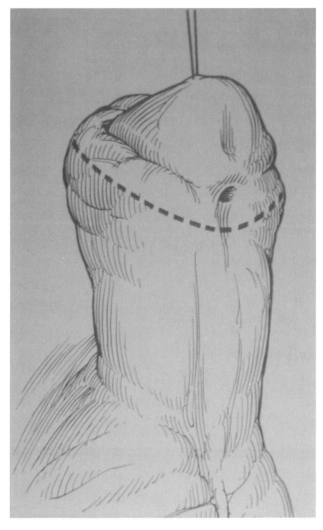

Figure 30-4 Meatal advancement and glanuloplasty incorporated (MAGPI) repair (Duckett). **A.** Line of incision.

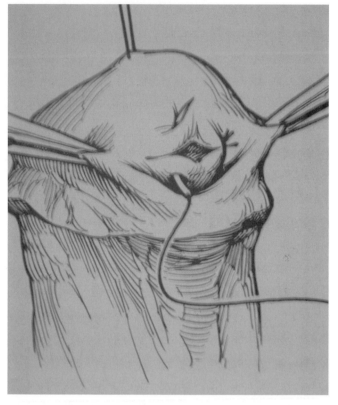

Figure 30-4 (*continued*)   **B.** Meatal incision from urethral meatus to glanular dimple.

       proximal urethra and also may need secondary scroto-
plasty to improve the cosmetic result.

  e. Skin chordee without urethral involvement may be treated by degloving the penis and mobilizing the urethra.

  f. Chordee with hypoplastic urethra requires island flap urethroplasty after chordee release due to bowstring effect of short urethra.

  g. Urinary diversion is used for 2 weeks in all but very distal repairs, with a small silastic urethral stent.

  h. Compressive dressing for 2 to 3 days is commonly used.

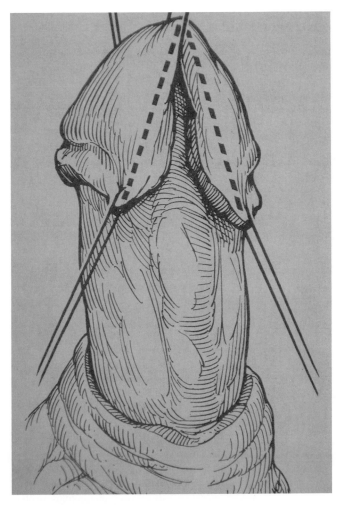

Figure 30-4 (*continued*)   **C.** Advancement suture.

5. Results and complications
    a. Small urethrocutaneous fistulae are the most common complication and can be closed in layers without diversion with 90 percent success.
    b. Postoperative bleeding can usually be stopped by compression.
    c. UTI occurs in less than 10 percent of cases and can be treated with the usual oral agents.

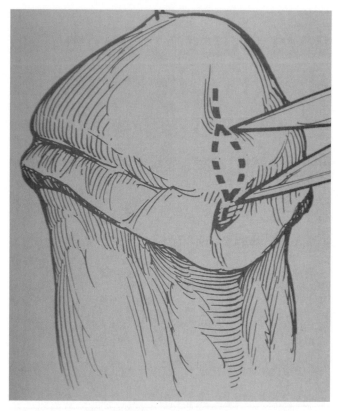

Figure 30-4 (*continued*)   **D.** Glanular cuff is advanced distally.

    d. Strictures are rare and usually occur at the meatus or the proximal end of the island flap and are treated by Y-V meatoplasty; direct vision urethrotomy is often successful for usual short proximal stricture.

    e. When carefully done, the procedures outlined provide functional and cosmetically nearly normal penis and meatus, even in the most severe hypospadias cases.

B. Cryptorchidism

    1. Incidence is 1 percent of live male births.

    2. *Origin.* Aberrant testicular descent; possible failure of pituitary–gonadal axis in late gestation (i.e., absent luteinizing hormone (LH) surge or blunted testicular response).

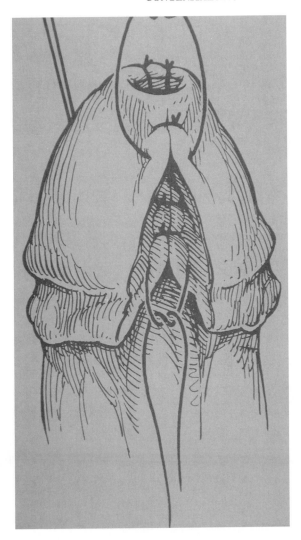

Figure 30-4 (*continued*)   **E.** Glans is closed in two layers.

3. Associated findings
    a. Patent processus vaginalis 90 percent; symptomatic hernia rarely
    b. Infertility approaches 50 percent in untreated unilateral undescended testis; surgery before age 2 and treatment

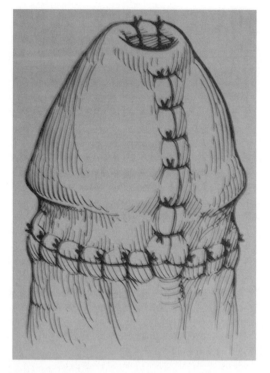

Figure 30-4 (*continued*)   **F.** Final appearance. (*Reproduced from Duckett JW: Hypospadias. In: Walsh PC, Retik AB, Vaughan ED, Wein AJ, eds. Campbell's Urology, 7th ed. Philadelphia, Saunders, 1998, p 2102.*)

        with an analogue of luteinizing hormone releasing hormone may improve fertility. Ectopic testis is normal histologically and not usually associated with infertility.

    c. Testicular malignancy is 20 to 35 times more common than in the general population (inguinal, 1 percent; abdominal testes, 5 percent).

    d. Undescended testis is part of many syndromes, for example, prune belly, exstrophy, genetic disorders, and intersex states (when associated with even mild hypospadias).

  4. Diagnosis

    a. Must discriminate retractile from truly undescended testis by careful examination. A testis that can be manipulated into the scrotum with stretch of the cremaster by gentle traction and does not retract into the canal is retractile and requires no surgery.

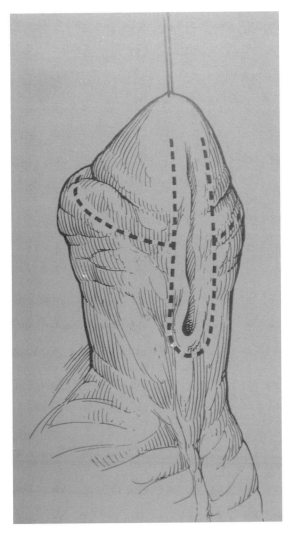

Figure 30-5 Island onlay repair (Duckett). **A.** Line of incision.

5. Management
   a. Inguinal exploration at 6 months of age (spontaneous descent is rare after 3 months).
   b. Most undescended testes are palpable; 85 percent are canalicular even if impalpable and can be brought down with conventional orchiopexy.

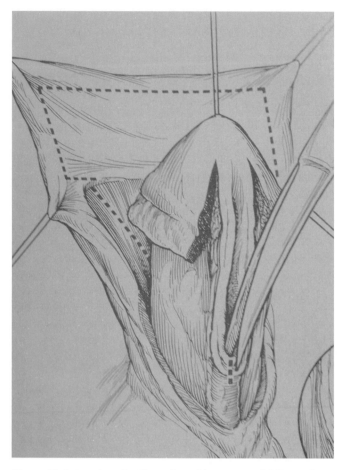

Figure 30-5 (*continued*)   **B.** outline of inner prepucial flap and incision of urethral plate to good spongiosal tissue.

    c. If the canal is empty, the peritoneum is opened; either a testis or blind ending vas deferens and gonadal vessels are found overlying the psoas above the internal inguinal ring. Only identification of the vessels proves testicular absence and constitutes sufficient exploration as the vas may embryologically be separate from the testis.

    d. An intra-abdominal testis may be brought down by Fowler-Stephens orchidopexy dividing the spermatic vessels and relying on collateral flow to the testis via the artery to the vas.

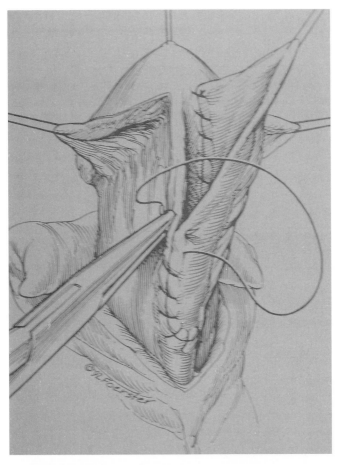

Figure 30-5 (*continued*)   **C.** Flap is sewn to urethral plate.

     e. A testis that cannot be brought into the scrotum should be removed if the contralateral one is normally descended.

6. Results

     a. The Fowler-Stephen's procedure in our experience has been 70 percent sucessful, as judged by palpation of a normal-feeling testis in the scrotum.

     b. Results of conventional orchidopexy are better in terms of viability.

     c. Fertility seems to be improved by earlier orchidopexy but is not guaranteed.

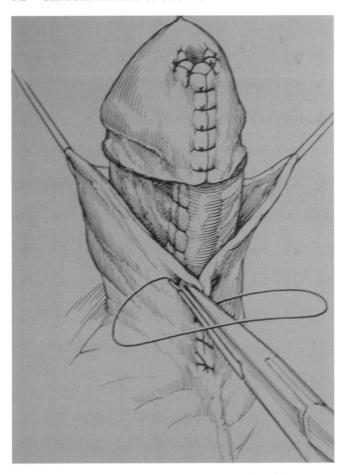

Figure 30-5 (*continued*)   **D.** Skin closure. (*Reproduced from Duckett JW: Hypospadias. In: Walsh PC, Retik AB, Vaughan ED, Wein AJ (eds): Campbell's Urology, 7th ed. Philadelphia, Saunders, 1998, p 2106.*)

C. Hernia and Communicating Hydrocele
1. Incidence is 1 to 4 percent of mature infants and 13 percent of premature infants.
2. Origin is failed closure of processus vaginalis after testicular descent or may be associated with incomplete descent.
3. Only associated findings may be frank hernia (sac containing bowel or other organ) or undescended testis.

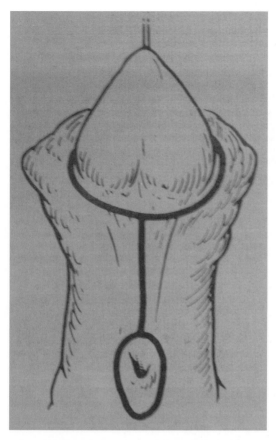

Figure 30-6 Transverse prepucial island flap (TPIF) (Duckett).
A. Line of incision

4. Principal differential diagnosis is with a stable hydrocele associated with a closed processus vaginalis. Stable hydroceles are often seen in infants and will usually be reabsorbed by 12 to 15 months of age. No surgery is required. A communicating hydrocele is suggested by a waxing and waning in the amount of fluid around the testicle. It is important not to confuse contraction of the dartos muscle of the scrotal wall with a change in hydrocele size.

5. Unlike a true hernia, which must be repaired promptly in infants due to frequency of incarceration, a communicating hydrocele may be fixed electively.

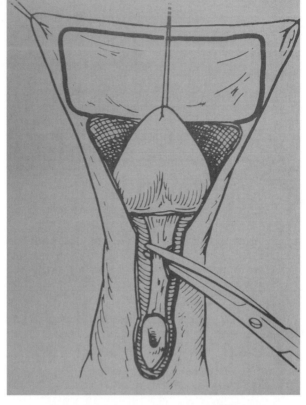

Figure 30-6 (*continued*)   **B.** Incision of ventral chordee tissue. If additional bend persists, dorsal tucks may be taken to straighten the penis further.

D. Appendages
1. Testicular and epididymal appendages are present usually at the upper pole of the testis or epididymis, represent müllerian or wolffian duct remnants, and are only significant when torsion of the appendage occurs.
2. Torsion of the appendix can sometimes be differentiated from testicular torsion by point tenderness and swelling at the upper pole or the "blue dot" sign, in which the infarcted tissue is apparent beneath the scrotal skin as a dark spot.
3. When doubt exists, exploration is essential; when the diagnosis is certain, treatment is symptomatic; pain will usually resolve in 3 to 5 days. If pain persists, excision transscrotally is needed.

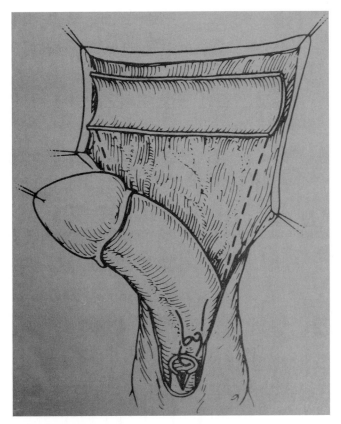

Figure 30-6 (*continued*)   **C.** Flap is harvested and

IV. CLOACAL DYSGENESIS

A. Cloaca Anomaly

A cloaca anomaly represents failure of the urorectal septum to descend, resulting in a single perineal opening or sinus into which the rectum, vagina, and urethra enter.

1. Upper urinary tract is usually normal but should be visualized.
2. Sinography, VCU, if possible, and cystovaginoscopy are necessary to assess the anatomy; diverting colostomy is usually done early, as in an imperforate anus, and this assessment can be performed under the same anesthetic.
3. Reconstruction via a midline posterior approach (Pena-DeVries) is carried out at age 4 to 12 months and consists of the following.

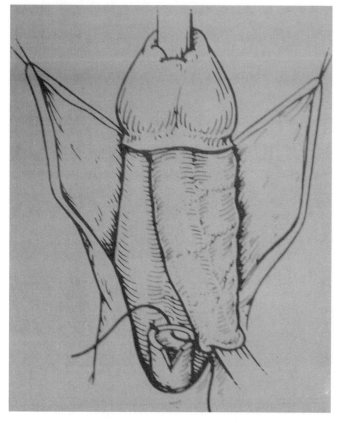

Figure 30-6 (*continued*)   **D.** rotated to

    a. Rectal tapering and pull through.
    b. Combined mobilization of the vagina and urethra as a unit with longitudinal separation of the urogenital sinus.
    c. Spinal anomalies and neurogenic bladders are common.

  B. Vaginal Atresia and Mayer–Rokitansky–Küster–Hauser Syndrome
    1. Primary vaginal atresia can be distinguished from a short vagina seen with testicular feminization by normal LH and follicle-stimulating hormone (FSH) levels and low testosterone levels with primary vaginal atresia.
      a. Failure of müllerian duct to penetrate urogenital sinus or a vascular accident.

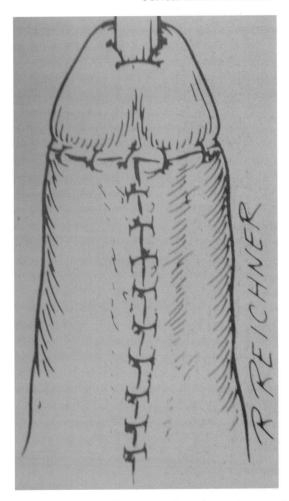

Figure 30-6 (*continued*)   **E.** anastomosis to glans and proximal urethra. **F.** Final appearance. (*Reproduced from Duckett JW: Hypospadias. In: Walsh PC, Retik AB, Vaughan ED, Wein AJ (eds): Campbell's Urology, 7th ed. Philadelphia, Saunders, 1998, p 2107.*)

       b. Isolated anomaly.
       c. Often presents at puberty with amenorrhea.
       d. Usually atretic or agenetic uterus.
       e. Vaginoplasty usually performed using a 10 cm loop of colon, which is reversed and brought to the perineum at the introitus.

2. Rokitansky syndrome
   a. Combination of müllerian duct abnormality, often duplication with vaginal atresia with ipsilateral renal agenesis.
   b. Abnormality of the müllerian ducts may be associated with mesonephric duct absence as both structures are closely associated in early embryonic differentiation.
   c. May present in newborn period with hydrocolpos but commonly presents with amenorrhea or hematocolpos at puberty; some discovered during investigation of a solitary kidney.
   d. Those with complete uterovaginal agenesis are managed as primary vaginal atresia; some have normal or septate uteri above obstruction requiring vaginoplasty.
   e. A special case is the patient with complete uterovaginal duplication and unilateral vaginal atresia. Presents with normal menstrual periods, cyclic abdominal pain, and pelvic mass. Manage by making obstructed vagina into a normal one by transvaginal marsupialization.
   f. Ultrasound is the study of choice for the evaluation of these genital anomalies; VCU is done to rule out reflux and cystovaginoscopy helps to delineate the introital anatomy.

BIBLIOGRAPHY

Bauer, SB: Anomalies of the kidney and ureteropelvic junction. In: Walsh PC, Retik AB, Vaughn ED, Wein AJ, eds. *Campbell's Urology,* 7th ed. Philadelphia, Saunders, 1998, pp 1708–1756.

Canning DA, Koo HP, Duckett JW: Anomalies of the bladder and cloaca. In: Gillenwater, JY, Grayhack JT, Howards SS, Duckett JW, eds. *Adult and Pediatric Urology,* 3rd ed. St. Louis, Mosby Year Book, 1996, pp 2445–2488.

Duckett JW: Hypospadias. In: Walsh PC, Retik AB, Vaughan ED, Wein AJ, eds. *Campbell's Urology,* 7th ed. Philadelphia, Saunders, 1998, pp 2093–2119.

Gearhart JP, Jeffs RD: Exstrophy-epispadias complex and bladder anomalies. In: Walsh PC, Retik AB, Vaughn ED, Wein AJ, eds. *Campbell's Urology,* 7th ed. Philadelphia, Saunders, 1998, pp 1939–1990.

Glassberg KI: Renal dysplasia and cystic disease of the kidney. In: Walsh PC, Retik AB, Vaughn ED, Wein AJ, eds. *Campbell's Urology,* 7th ed. Philadelphia, Saunders, 1998, pp 1757.

Grady RW, Mitchell ME: Complete primary repair of exstrophy. *J. Urol* 162:1415–1420, 1999.

Hagg MJ, Mourachov PV, Snyder HM, et al: The modern endoscopic approach to ureterocele. *J. Urol* 163:940–943, 2000.

Maizels M: Normal and anomalous development of the urinary tract. In: Walsh PC, Retik AB, Vaughn ED, Wein AJ, eds. *Campbell's Urology,* 7th ed. Philadelphia, Saunders, 1998, pp 1543–1600.

Snyder HM: Anomalies of the ureter. In: Gillenwater JY, Grayhack JT, Howards SS, Duckett JW, eds. *Adult and Pediatric Urology,* 3rd ed. Chicago, Mosby Year Book, 1996, pp 2197–2231.

Stephens FD: *Congenital Malformations of the Urinary Tract.* New York, Praeger, 1983, p 195.

CHAPTER 31

Specific Infections of the Genitourinary Tract

Ashok K. Batra

I. **GENITOURINARY TUBERCULOSIS**
  A. **General Considerations**
    1. Tuberculosis is a prehistoric disease, known to occur in humans as far back as 7000 years. In 18th-century Europe, it reached epidemic proportions and wiped out one fourth of the population of England. The cause of this disease remained shrouded in mystery until the 19th century. Robert Koch first discovered the cause of tuberculosis (TB) in 1882, and Medlar was first to describe its renal involvement in 1926. He demonstrated the renal lesions that occurred bilaterally and almost always in the renal cortex. *Mycobacterium tuberculosis* and *M. bovis* are the two most common human pathogens.
    2. The incidence of TB in the developed countries is 13 per 100,000, whereas in the developing countries it reaches as high as 400 per 100,000. About 10 million new cases occur worldwide each year, claiming 3 million lives. Of these, about 40,000 cases occur in the United States and a majority of them arise from reactivation of previously healed loci. A recent resurgence of TB is seen with the growing numbers of acquired immunodeficiency cases in certain areas. In the developed countries, there has been decrease in the incidence of this disease at a rate of about 12 percent annually. However, this decline is not been observed in the developing nations.
    3. Worldwide genitourinary TB accounts for 14 percent of nonpulmonary manifestations. Approximately 9 percent of patients with pulmonary TB and 26 percent of those with miliary disease have associated infection of the kidney, ureter, or genital organs.

The views expressed in the chapter are those of the author and do not represent the policies of FDA.

4. The genitourinary (GU) tract is the leading secondary site of involvement among the extrapulmonary organs, primarily involving young adults. Male cases predominate over female in a ratio of 2:1.

B. Pathogenesis

1. TB of the kidney is a secondary manifestation and is carried by bloodborne TB bacilli following tuberculous infection of the lungs or pulmonary hilar lymph nodes.

2. Involved sites may be dormant for many years, but given favourable conditions, these reactivate and eventually begin to spread and develop caseation and cavitation.

3. The causes of the reactivation of these dormant bacilli are debilitating disease, trauma, steroid therapy, diabetes, anemia, immunosuppression, and acquired immunodeficiency syndrome (AIDS).

4. The characteristic granulomatous lesion, with central giant cell of Langhans surrounded by chronic inflammatory cells, is known as tubercle. Tubercles in the glomeruli may heal or spill into the nephrons and may be caught in the narrow loop of Henle, where they form more tubercles.

5. Tubercles caseate and slough into the calyceal fornix. Bacilli are spilled down the ureters with potential for ureteral stricture formation, bladder inflammation, and contracture.

6. Approximately 4 percent of initial tubercles result in destructive TB. When caseation is progressive, the disease may involve the entire renal pelvis leading to a calcified mass of caseous material called a "putty kidney."

7. If early renal lesions do not heal (the response of each kidney is independent of the other), passage of infected urine through the urogenital tract can lead to involvement of the ureters, bladder, prostate, seminal vesicles, vas deferens, epididymis, and testis. Rarely, the primary hematogenous lesion in the urinary tract may settle in the prostate.

8. Bacillus calmette-guerin (BCG) therapy is commonly employed for the treatment of superficial bladder cancer. Sometimes, this results in TB infection in bladder, prostate, and occasionally, in the kidney. Even miliary TB has been reported after BCG treatment.

C. Clinical Features and Diagnosis

1. Renal involvement is largely silent (Table 31-1). It often presents with vague urinary symptoms. Therefore history taking and high index of suspicion is very important particularly a history of "contact" and/or a previous history of pulmonary TB, as well as a history of recurrent urinary tract infections that are nonresponsive to common antibiotics. In the male the earliest indication may be tubercu-

Table 31-1 Clinical Findings in Genitourinary Tuberculosis

Sterile pyuria
Nocturnal painless frequency of micturition
History of present or past TB elsewhere in the body
Unexplained hematuria
Chronic cystitis unresponsive to antibiotics
Chronic epididymitis with epididymal nodularity and/or thickened or
  beaded vas deferens
Nodularity of prostate, shrunken "bean bag" prostate
Induration of seminal vesicles
Dull flank pain and renal colic
Chronic draining scrotal sinus
Hemospermia (rare)

---

lous epididymitis or cystitis. Females may present with bladder pain and dysuria. Back pain and hematuria are not uncommon. A recurrent *Escherichia coli* infection should serve as a warning sign for the urologist.

2. The severity of symptoms does not correlate with the degree of urinary tract involvement.
3. The diagnosis is made by finding *M. tuberculosis* in the urine or semen.
   a. Three to five consecutive early morning urines are cultured: repeat if results are negative.
   b. Acid-fast stains on concentrated urinary sediment from 24-hour specimen may be positive in 50 to 60 percent of cases, but culture corroboration is essential. Once the cultures are positive, the antibiotic sensitivities are performed. Fluorescence microsopy and other modern diagnostic techniques have enhanced the yields. DNA probes have allowed clinicians to differentiate between various mycobacterial species and strains.
   c. A negative tuberculin skin test makes the diagnosis unlikely, but a conversion of previously negative test to positive should raise the index of suspicion.
   d. Radiographs alone are not sufficient for diagnosis. However, an intravenous urogram may reveal various features of TB and helps rule out obstruction and non functioning unit.
   e. Drug-sensitivity testing is essential.
4. Differential diagnosis
   a. Chronic nonspecific cystitis or pyelonephritis
   b. Acute or chronic nonspecific epididymitis
   c. "Urethral syndrome," interstitial cystitis
   d. Necrotizing papillitis of one or both kidneys
   e. Schistosomiasis

D. Therapy

1. General considerations (Table 31-2)
   a. The aim of antituberculous therapy is to treat the active disease promptly and render the patient noninfective in the shortest period of time.
   b. The size of the bacillary population is related to the extent of the disease.
   c. Multiple drugs work synergistically against resistant organisms in early treatment.
   d. Close follow-up of upper tracts is essential during therapy, as asymptomatic uretetal strictures (especially in the lower third) may occur during the healing phase Tuberculous strictures lend themselves to percutaneous or transurethral dilatation techniques. Steroids may be beneficial.
   e. Surgical intervention may play an increasing role with trends toward shorter duration of chemotherapy.

D. Medical and Surgical Therapy Subject to Sensitivity Results

1. Primary agents are rifampicin, isoniazid, pyrazinamide, and streptomycin. Currently, a combination therapy is employed, usually for 4 to 6 months.

   Combination therapy popularized by Gow includes: pyrazinamide, 25 mg/kg daily plus INH, 300 mg daily and rifampin, 450 mg daily for 2 months followed by isoniazid 600 mg and rifampin 900 mg three times weekly for a further 2 months.

2. Secondary agents include ethambutol, ethionamide, cycloserine, para aminosalycic acid, and capreomicin. (See Table 31-2 for dose and side effects.)

3. Surgical therapy
   a. Surgery, when indicated, is performed 4 to 6 weeks after chemotherapy has begun.
   b. Surgical procedures are undertaken to drain perinephric abcess, remove nonfunctioning renal tissue, bypass ureteral strictures, and to augment severely contracted bladders.
   c. Nephrectomy is done for grossly diseased nonfunctioning kidney or diseased kidney with severe secondary hypertension.
   d. Partial nephrectomy is some times undertaken for calcified polar lesion increasing in size.
   e. Reconstructive surgery is performed as necessary.

E. Follow-up

1. Patients should be seen at 3, 6, and 12 months after completion of therapy and their urines cultured for acid-fast

Table 31-2 Common Antituberculous Chemotherapeutic Agents

DRUG	DOSES	SIDE EFFECTS	REMARKS
Isoniazid (INH)	5–10 mg/kg per day, max 300 mg/day	Peripheral neuritis, hepatitis	Bactericidal, pyridoxin for neuritis
Rifampicin	10–20 mg/kg per day, to maximum 600 mg/day	Hepatotoxicity, hypersensitivity, transient leukopenia, thrombocytopenia	Bactricidal, orange discoloration of urine
Ethambutol	15 mg/kg per day	Retrobulbar neuritis, color vision changes	Tuberculostatic baseline visual acuity tests
Streptomycin	750–1000 mg/day IM for 1 month, then 95 mg/kg twice per week	Nephrotoxicity, ototoxicity	
Pyrazinamide	15–30 mg/kg to max 2000 mg/day	Hepatotoxicity, elevates serum uric acid	Monitor Liver function and serum uric acid
Para-aminosalicylic acid	150 mg/kg to max 12 g/day	Hypersensitivity, GI irritation, hepatotoxicity	Tuberculostatic
Cycloserine	10–20 mg/kg per day to maximum 500 mg/day	Psychosis	Contraindicated in epileptics
Capreomycin	500–1000mg/day once per day for 3 months, then twice per week	Nephrotoxicity ototuxicity	Use with caution in elderly

bacillus (AFB). Patients can discharged following a year of disease-free follow up.

2. Kidney, ureter, and bladder (KUB) x-rays and intravenous urography (IVU) are required to follow the status of calyceal deformities and renal calcifications.

II. GENITOURINARY SCHISTOSOMIASIS
A. General Considerations
1. Caused by a blood fluke, this disease was first recognized by Egyptian physicians of the 12th Dynasty (1900 B.C.). Theodore Bilharz first described the worms in the human mesenteric venous plexus and linked it to the disease. Contrary to the other common infections, its incidence is on the increase.

2. Approximately 300 million humans are infested with schistosomes namely, *Schistosama mansoni, S. japonicum,* or *S. haematohium,* an estimated 500,000 living in the United States. Incidence of urinary involvement is 40 to 60 percent.

3. GU schistosomiasis is caused primarily by *S. haematohium.* It is endemic mainly in Africa and certain areas in the Middle East.

4. *S. mansoni* and *S. japonicum* cause intestinal schistosomiasis.

B. Etiology and Life Cycle
1. Adult schistosomes are delicate cylindrical worms, 1 to 2 cm in length, that are adapted for existence in venules and have a mean life span of 3.4 years. A single pair spawns about half a million eggs in their life time.

2. Humans are infected through contact with infested fresh water in small canals, ditches, or drains. The infective larval stage, free swimming cercariae, penetrates the skin or mucous membranes.

3. Cercariae (shed by the snails in fresh water source) penetrate through the human skin and reach the general circulation and are pumped by the heart throughout the body. Only worms that reach the portal circulation live.

4. Adult worms reaching their definitive destinations in the venous plexi, mature and mate. Females lay eggs (200 to 500/day) in the subumcosa of the involved tissues—the bladder, lower ureters, and seminal vesicles in the case of GU schistosomiasis. Eggs are quite antigenic and produce intense inflammatory reactions in the tissues they are deposited. About 20 percent erode through the viscera of deposition (intestine, bladder) and are eliminated.

5. Ova are eliminated in human feces and urine. If they reach freshwater, they start their asexual cycle (snail) resulting in the production of sporocyst. They hatch, and

the contained larvae, ciliated miracidia, find a specific freshwater snail that they penetrate. There, they form sporocysts that ultimately form the cercariae that leave the snail and pass into the freshwater to begin their sexual cycle (human) after reaching their human host.

C. Pathogenesis of Genitourinary Manifestations

1. Stage 1: generalization or incubation period.
   a. A young schistosome rapidly acquires host derived antigenic materials on its body surface and is immunologically camouflaged.
   b. Secretions and excretions of the worms may engender hypersensitivity and general manifestations of illness.
   c. Allergic skin reactions, cough, fever, malaise, body and bone aches, and gastrointestinal (GI) symptoms may be present.
2. Stage 2: deposition of ova by mature worms in the target area.
   a. Because female worms may lay eggs for years, the disease is slowly progressive.
   b. Toxic and antigenic products of a viable miracidium pass through the shell of the egg and elicit a granulomatous inflammatory response around the egg, forming pseudotubercles.
   c. General symptoms include "swimmers itch" and Katayama fever.
   d. GU symptoms include painful terminal hematuria, dysuria and pyuria, hemospermia, and vesical irritability.
3. Stage 3 : late complications.
   a. End result of repeated, chronic infection.
   b. Infection of urinary tract—usually coliform organisms (*E. coli, Klebsiella, Pseudomonus*). Definite association with *Salmonella typhi* infections.
   c. Schistosomal bladder polyps, secondary infection, stones, urinary tract calcification.
   d. Fibrosis is the ultimate result of infection and involves the bladder, urethra, and ureters, leading to hydronephrotic renal atrophy and bladder contraction.
   e. Relationship to bladder malignancy—usually squamous cell carcinoma.

D. Diagnosis

1. Diagnosis of infection
   a. Urine sediment reveals terminally spined eggs of *S. haematobium* (midday urine sample is most diagnostic).
   b. Rectal or bladder mucosal biopsy to look for eggs.
   c. Serologic tests are not yet completely reliable. However, the new and developing DNA probes may become useful in the future for the diagnosis.

    2. Diagnosis of sequelae and complications
       a. Plain x-ray of abdomen classically reveals bladder calcification. Seminal vesical, urethral, and distal ureteral calcification may be seen.
       b. IVU is essential to look for obstructive uropathy. More recently, CT scanning and ultrasound have been employed for the detection of obstructive and destructive lesions.
       c. Cystoscopic appearance.

E. Treatment
    1. Medical management
       a. *S. haematobium* is sensitive to metrifonate (Bilharcil), praziquantel (Biltricide), hycanthone mesylate (Etrenol), niridazole (Ambilhar), and Oltipraz.
       b. Praziquantel, a heterocycline prazinoisoquinoline, is the drug of choice for treatment of all species. Dosage for *S. haematobium* is 40 mg/kg by mouth in single dose.
       c. Metrifonate (7.5 to 10 mg/kg) is given in three oral doses at 14-day intervals. It is the drug of choice for endemic infections caused by *S. hematobium.*
       d. Niridazole (Ambilhar) is a nitrofuran given orally in two divided daily doses of 25 mg/kg per day for 5 to 7 days.

         These drugs may have many side effects, and in edemic areas the clinician must be cognizant of risk–benefit ratios, as low-level infection is well tolerated by many persons and generally will not produce symptomatic chronic disease or chronic obstructive uropathy.

    2. Surgical management
       a. Surgical procedures are reserved for complications of infection such as ureteral stenosis, bladder fibrosis, and bladder carcinoma. Procedures include ureteral dilatation, ureteral reimplantation, partial cystectomy, bladder augmentation, and cystectomy with urinary diversion.

III. GENITAL FILARIASIS (BANCROFTIAN FILARIASIS)
  A. General Considerations
    1. Approximately 300 million people are infected with filarial diseases.
    2. Filarial infection is widespread in tropical countries. Although numerous filarial species cause human disease, urologic problems are most common with *Wuchereria bancrofti* (90 percent). *Onchocerca volvulus,* the agent of African river blindness, can also cause scrotal elephantiasis, also known as hanging groin. *Brugia malayi* infections are rare in this country.

3. *W. bancrofti* is a human parasite without a known animal reservoir and with a cycle that proceeds from human to mosquito and back to human. Mosquito bites transmit the filarial larvae into the human host.

4. Periodic bancroftian filariasis is found throughout tropical Africa, North Africa, tropical coastal borders of Asia, southern parts of Indian subcontinent and Queensland, the West Indies, Puerto Rico, and northern South America.

B. Etiology

1. Adult filarial *W. bancrofti* are 4- to 10-cm worms approximately 0.2 mm in diameter; they reside in the lymphatic system and live for decades.

2. The female worm is viviparous, producing microfilariae that are found in the peripheral blood at night (nocturnal periodicity) and in the lungs during the day. Microfilariae live 3 to 6 months.

3. If ingested by suitable mosquitoes, microfilariae develop in the thoracic muscles of the insect and move to the mouth parts in 2 weeks.

4. They enter the skin of a human through the puncture wounds of a mosquito bite and move to the lymphatics where males and females meet, mate, and mature; 1 year later, microfilariae appear in the blood.

C. Pathogenesis and Clinical Manifestations

1. Host reaction to microfilariae is different from that to adult forms. Various features of occult and overt infections have been described. The clinician will see a range of pathology from circulating eosinophilia to eosinophylic granulomas in the lymph nodes and spleen.

2. Severity of lesions is related to
   a. Load of adult worms
   b. Site of infection
   c. Host susceptibility

3. Maturing adults in the lymphatics cause fibrotic and inflammatory changes, producing lymphatic obstruction.

4. Filarial fever involves fever, headache, lymphadenopathy, and urticarial rash.
   a. It occurs in acute phase.
   b. Often, no history of this can be obtained.

5. Chronic phase: lymphatics of inguinal region, upper arm, and spermatic cord are affected. Funiculoepididymitis and orchitis is known to occur.
   a. Chronic lymphadenopathy
   b. Retrograde lymphangitis
   c. Lymphatic obstruction and resulting edema (elephantiasis), especially in lower limbs and scrotum, hydrocele formation.

    d. Bacterial and mycotic superinfection

    e. Chyluria from renal lymphaticourinary fistula formation.

  6. Tropical pulmonary eosinophilia

    a. This due to hyperergic reaction to filariae.

    b. It is characterized by peripheral eosinophilia, lymphadenopathy, and pulmonary infiltrates. There is very little to no urologic involvement.

D. Diagnosis

  1. In early stages, microfilariae are usually present in smears of blood obtained at night.

  2. In long-standing, chronic disease, blood smears are usually negative.

    a. Look for eosinophilia.

    b. Look for microfilariae in hydrocele fluid or chylous urine.

    c. Filarial complement fixation tests are useful for the detection of disease. Currently, specific serodiagnostic tests for *W. bancrofti* are available. ELISA test for IgG_4 antibody against recombinent filarial antigen is also useful.

  3. Differential diagnosis includes nonfilarial congenital lymphatic defects and obstructions, tuberculous, inguinal lymphadenitis, schistosomiasis, and lymphatic obstruction from malignancy.

E. Treatment

  1. Even though chemotherapy is effective in eliminating *W. bancrofti,* structural changes may not be reversible. Treatment goals are the elimination of adult worms and microfilarae.

  2. Diethylcarbamazine (Hetrazan)

    a. Mainstay of the treatment. It is known to be effective against adult worms and microfilarae.

    b. Mechanism of action unknown.

    c. Dose: 6 mg/kg per day. Total course: 72 mg/kg. Some recommend lower doses initially; 3 mg/kg/day and increasing gradually. Repeat at 3- to 6-month intervals.

    d. Toxicity (anorexia, nausea, vomiting, pruritis) may be due to dying microfilaria.

  3. Ivermectin

    a. It is effective against microfilarae, but has no effect on the adult worms.

    b. Single dose of 20 to 25 μg/kg. It is usually well-tolerated with fewer side effects. Like Hetrazan, it needs to be repeated to prevent recurrent filaremia.

  4. Suramin (Antrypol, Moranyl)

    a. Complex derivative of urea.

      b. Intrapelvic instillations of silver nitrate 1 to 2 percent solutions.
      c. Rarely, surgical interruption of renal pedicle lymphatics.
    5. Desideratum
      It is a new anti-adult filarial drug that has shown promise.

IV. RARE PARASITIC GENITOURINARY INFECTIONS

A. Hydatid Disease

1. Caused by *Echinococcus granulosus,* it is endemic in the sheep-herding regions of the world (e.g., Australia, Argentina, Spain, Middle East, Greece, Turkey, and parts of Asia).
2. Renal hydatids are known to occur in 2 percent of cases.
3. Incubation occurs over a long period of time and symptoms depend on the size and location of the lesion. These include renal pain and pressure symptoms. Occasionally, cysts become quite large and rupture, giving rise to urinary and systemic symptoms. Sometimes the cysts involute and get calcified.
4. Casoni's test is a valuable skin test for diagnosis. Plain radiograghs and CT scans are also useful in the identification of disease.
5. Treatment includes simple surgical excision to various emergency surgical procedures for obstruction and abcess formation, including nephrectomy.

B. AMEBIASIS

1. This disease is quite prevalent in the developing countries with poor hygienic conditions.
2. Amebic infections uncommonly affect the kidneys.
3. Right kidney is more frequently involved, usually in association with liver abcess.
4. Amebic involvement of urethra and bladder is occasionally seen in association with fulminant amebic sepsis with multiorgan involvement.
5. Symptoms include fever, renal pain, and hematuria (sometimes seen in association with renal vein thrombosis).
6. Diagnosis usually is established on biopsy. Treatment aims to contain and control amebic systemic infection, which is often lethal. Drugs include: metronidazole, ornidazole, tinidazole, and chloroquine.
7. Surgery must be undertaken after control of infection has been achieved.

V. GENITOURINARY FUNGAL INFECTIONS

A. General Considerations

1. Fungal infections have been known to occur since the days of Hippocrates. Scmorl first described renal involvement

with Candida in 1890. Rafin first described bladder involvement with Candida infections in 1927.

2. There are two types of fungal infections.
   a. Primary fungal infections (blastomycosis, coccidioidomycosis, histoplasmosis).
   b. Opportunistic fungal infections (aspergillosis. cryptococcosis, candidiasis, torulopsosis). *Candida albicans, Candida tropicalis, Candida parapsilosis* and *Toruplosis glabrata* account for the the majority of opportunistic fungal infections. Of these, Candida is the most prevalent of the fungi, affecting the GU tract, accounting for almost 90 percent of all the fungal infections. *Candida albicans* is the most common among the Candida species. Candidiasis is described in detail.

VI. CANDIDIASIS

Normally inhabitants of mucocutaneous body surfaces, Candidas will overgrow and invade tissues when permitted by alterations in the host defenses. Virulence is related to this species ability to transform in tissues into the mycelial phase, a form more resistant to the cellular defenses of the host than the yeast phase.

A. Pathogenesis and Clinical Manifestations

1. Predisposing factors include extended use of broad-spectrum antibiotics, diabetes mellitus, corticosteroids, indwelling catheters, immunosuppressive and antineoplastic drugs, and an immunocompromised host.
2. Bladder involvement may be asymptomatic or present with urgency, hematuria, frequency, nocturia, severe dysuria, and suprapubic pain.
3. Upper tract involvement may be signaled by symptoms and signs of pyelonephritis, perinephric abcess, or obstruction from fungus balls.
4. Systemic candidiasis usually involves lungs or kidneys and presents with fever, shaking, chills, hypotension, lethargy, petechiae, and embolic phenomena. Candidemia, when associated with bacterimia, portends a poor prognosis for the patient.

B. Diagnosis

1. Blood and urine cultures must be evaluated in the context of clinical setting, as candidemia and candiduria may occur as transient phenomena.
2. Diagnosis of fungal cystitis is based on clinical presentation of irritative bladder symptoms, history of predisposing factors, positive urinary fungal cultures (greater than

104 CFU/mL, however, in presence of an indwelling catheters, these counts cannot be used to differentiate colonization from true infections), negative bacterial and acid-fast cultures, cystoscopy and bladder biopsy to rule out tumor, and tissue cultures.

3. Blood cultures, opthalmologic examination, and serum agglutinin titers may help to diagnose systemic involvement. Fungal infections are a difficult diagnostic problem, however, recent advances in molecular biology particularly, the polymerase chain reaction test, promise to detect *Candida* accurately and promises to be a valuable diagnostic tool of the future.

4. IVU may show calyceal defects and ureteral obstruction (fungal masses or bezoars).

C. Treatment

1. Asymptomatic candiduria implies a colonization of the urinary tract without tissue invasion.
   a. It will usually disappear when predisposing factors (antibiotics, indwelling catheters) are removed.
   b. Urinary alkalinization with sodium bicarbonate to a pH of 7.5 is helpful.

2. Symptomatic or intractable vesical candidiasis (higher than 15,000/CFU) can be treated with systemic (see treatment of systemic infections) and /or intravesical antifungal agents. Various intravesical irrigations agents have been used with success such as amphotericin B (50 mg in 1000 mL of 5% dextrose water solution per 24 hr as a continuous drip) and miconazole (50 mg/l000 mL of normal saline/day) is an alternative bladder irrigant. Local therapies must be undertaken after the obstructive disease has been corrected and an invasive disease has been excluded.

3. *Renal and systemic involvement.* Three major drugs commonly used for GU candidiasis are fluconazole, flucytosine, and amphotericin B.
   a. *Fluconazole (Diflucan).* Administered orally and intravenously. It can also be used for bladder irrigations quite effectively. Usual PO dose is 150 mg/day × 7 days for superficial bladder infections. It has excellent clinical efficacy in systemic candidiasis and comparable success rates with amphotericin B in the treatment of candidemia. Adverse effects include nausea, headache, skin rash, and hepatotoxicity.
   b. *Flucytosine (5-FC, Ancobon).* Oral agent. Interferes with fungal synthesis of DNA. Toxicity includes nausea and vomiting, rash, diarrhea, hepatic dysfunction, and bone marrow suppression. May be used alone in

urinary candidiasis; used with amphotericin B in systemic disease.

c. *Amphotericin B (Fungizone).* Intravenously administered macrolide antibiotic, combines with sterols in cell membranes. Mainstay of treatment in the critically ill patient with disseminated infection. Toxicity is quite common and noted in more than 85 percent of patients. It includes fever, hypotension, dyspnea, and nephrotoxicity. Synergistic with flucytosine.

d. *Surgical therapy.* Ureteroscopy, percutaneous nephrostomy along with irrigation and removal of fungal bezoars and placement of drains and stents may be required to rid the patient of fungus. This may be followed by continuous irrigation with an antifungal agent.

VII. OTHER OPPORTUNISTIC FUNGAL INFECTIONS

1. Causative organisms *Torulopsis* glagrata, Aspergillosis and cryptococcosis are uncommon GU infections but are seen with increasing incidence of AIDS. These infections are becoming more frequent and the clinician must have a high index of suspicion for these infections in patients who are immunocompromised.

2. *T. glabarata* is known to cause perirenal and pelvic abcesses. It has a similar course of disease as described in candidiasis and responds to the same chemotherapy.

3. Aspergillosis is known to cause renal mass or pseudotumor in immunocompromised patients such as those with renal transplants or AIDS. Occasional prostate and scrotal infections are encountered. It responds well to 5-FC and amphtericin B treatment.

4. *Cryptococcus neoformans* is a common opportunistic pathogen in the lung and CNS and occasionally involves the GU system in immunocompromised patients. It is also commonly seen in association with AIDS. It can cause infection in the kidney, adrenal, prostate, and penis. 5-FC and amphotericin B are effective in treatment of this disease.

VIII. PRIMARY FUNGAL INFECTIONS

1. Blastomycosis, coccidiodomycosis, and histoplasmosis are rare and primary fungal infections of the GU tract. These are seen with increasing frequency due to AIDS, transplants, and advancing intensive care techniques.

2. Kidney, adrenals, genitalia, and prostate are the target organs.

3. All these patients respond well to amphotericin B therapy and ketoconazole and/or itraconazole.

IX. FOURNIER'S GANGRENE
A. General Considerations

1. In 1883, Fournier, a French venereologist, described a rapid, fulminating gangrene of the genitalia in young male patients. Currently, the eponym Fournier's gangrene is applied to any large fulminating penoscrotal and perineal gangrenous processes, also known as necrotizing fascitis (Fig. 31-1).

2. There is no predilection for race. This condition has been described in all ages, although the mean age tends to be between 20 to 50 years.

3. Clinical presentation is that of irritation, itching, and erythema of the scrotum, which rapidly progresses to necrosis within a matter of hours. Crepitence may be felt with clostridial infections. Systemic symptoms such as fever, malaise, chills, or sweats have been described. Usually genital discomfort is out of proportion with the physical appearance.

4. Diabetes is the most commonly associated condition. There may be a GU history of urethral stricture or fistula or a GI history of anorectal processes such as fistulae, fissures, or an abscess. Other factors include local trauma and paraphimosis and urinary extravasation. Often, no etiologic source is found.

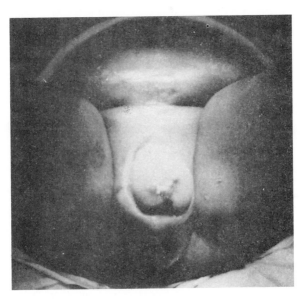

Figure 31-1 Fournier's gangrene.

B. **Pathogenesis**

1. *Source.* The source of infection is either the GU or GI tract. Once the inflammation sets in, there is a decreasing oxygen tension in the tissues, promoting the growth of anaerobic and facultative anaerobic organisms.

2. *Microbiology.* Multiple organisms are involved. such as gram-positive (*Strep* and *Staph*) cocci (12 to 25 percent), gram-negative (*Enterobacteriacae*) rods (25 to 50 percent), and anaerobic (*Bacteroides, Clostridia, Strep*) organisms (50 percent).

C. **Diagnosis**

1. A high index of suspicion is critical. A young diabetic patient with scrotal discomfort and systemic toxicity out of proportion with the physical signs with rapidly advancing erythema, edema, bronzing of skin, bleb formation, or a foul-smelling discharge should warn the urologist of a fulminant and rapidly progressive process. In advanced presentation, the patient may be septic and hemodynamically unstable.

2. Urine, tissue, and blood cultures are mandatory.

3. Serum creatinine, BUN, electrolytes, hematologic and coagulation studies, and arterial blood gas analysis are recommended.

4. A KUB is recommended and, if indicated, a retrograde urethrogram, cystoscopy, and proctoscopic examinations are done.

D. **Therapy**

1. Prompt and aggressive therapy is required. This includes rapid assessment and stabilization of the patient and administration of broad-spectrum antibiotics.

2. *Antibiotics.* Triple antibiotic therapy that includes an aminoglycoside and an anaerobic cover is recommended.
   a. Gentamicin (3 to 5 mg/kg per day) for gram-negative organisms.
   b. Clindamicin (600 mg every 4 hours) for adequate anaerobic coverage. Metronidazole can be used alternatively.
   c. A third-generation cephalosporin such as ceftriaxone should be used. Penicillin G (3 to 5 million U every 6 hours) for Clostridia is also useful. An infectious disease consult and input is often useful.

3. *Surgical therapy.* A wide excision and debridement of all devitalized tissues is recommended. A suprapubic catheter may be needed for urinary diversion. The patient is monitored carefully postoperatively and further de-

bridements are done as needed. Often, this leaves large denuded areas between the lower abdomen and upper thighs and may require the testicles to be placed in the upper medial thigh pouches. Postoperative hyperbaric oxygen therapy has been found to enhance wound healing. A wide variety of scrotal reconstruction is done once the patient is stable and the wound looks clean and granulating. In spite of the current advances, mortality is high and approaches 25 percent.

BIBLIOGRAPHY

Al-Ghorab MM: Schistosomiasis of bladder. In: Kaufman, IJ, ed. *Current Urologic Therapy.* Philadelphia, Saunders, 1986, pp. 248–251.

Antony SJ, Lopez PO: Genital amebiasis: Historical perspective of an unusual disease presentation. *Urology* 54:952–955, 1999.

Barrett-Connor E: Drugs for treatment of parasitic infections. *Med Clin North Am* 66:245–255, 1982.

Baskin LS, Carroll PR, Cattollica EV, Tanagho EA: Necrotizing soft tissue infections of the perineum and genitalia. *Br J Urol* 65:524–529, 1990.

Cohen MS: Fournier's gangrene. *AUA Update Series,* vol. 5, lesson 6: 1986.

Devasia A, Ponnaiya J, Gopalkrishnan G: Filarial cystitis with urertral obstruction. *J Urol* 159, 1637–1638, 1998.

Elert A, Von Knobloch R, Nusser R, Heidenreich A, Hofmann R: Isolated candidal prostatitis. *J. Urol* 163:244, 2000.

Gow JG: The current management of patients with genitourinarinary tuberculosis. *AUA Update Series,* vol. 11, lesson 26:202–208. 1992.

Grange JM, Stanford MD: Dogma and innovation in global control of tuberculosis: Discussion paper. *J R Soc Med* 49:537–539, 1994.

Hamory BH, Wenzel RP: Hospital associated candiduria: Predisposing factors and review of literature. *J Urol* 120: 444–448, 1978.

Hejase MJ, Bihrle R, Castillo, G : Amebiasis of the penis. *Urology.* 48:151–154, 1996.

Kan VL: Polymerase chain reaction for diagnosis of candidemia. *J Inf Dis* 168:779–783, 1993.

Kazura J: Filarial infections. In: Edberg SC, Bergger SA, eds. *Antibiotics and Infection.* New York, Churchill Livingstone, 1983, pp 110–112.

Kottasz S, Siller G, Brousil E: Fournier's gangrene: Experiencc in the treatment of gangrenous inflammation of the male genitals. *Int Urol Nephrol* 20:505–511, 1988.

Michigan S: Genitourinary fungal infections. *J Urol* 116:390–397, 1976.

Ottese EA: Filariasis now. *Am J Trop Aled Hyg* 41(suppl):8, 1989.

Powell CR, Allshouse M, Bethel K, Mevorach R: Invasive aspergillosis of scrotum. *J Urol* 159:1306–1308, 1998.

Spirnak JP: Fournier's gangrene: A true urologic emergency. *Contemp Urol* 4:46–52, 1992.

Walsh PC, Retik AB, Darracott Vaughn, Jr, E, Wein AJ, eds. *Campbells Urology,* 7th ed. Philadelphia, Saunders, 1998.

Weiner DM, Lowe FC: Gangrene of the genitalia *AUA Update Series,* vol. 17, lesson 6:41–48, 1998.

Weller TH: Schistosomiasis. In: Hoepvich PD ed. *Infectious Diseases.* Hagerstown, MD, Harper and Row, 1977, pp 658–665.

Wise GJ: Genitourinary candidal infections. *AUA Update Series* vol. 8, lesson 25:197, 1989.

Wong-Beringer A, Jacobs RA, Guglielmo J: Treatment of funguria. *JAMA* 267:2780–2785, 1992.

SELF-ASSESSMENT QUESTIONS

1. Is renal TB a primary infection of the kidney?
2. In renal TB does the severity of symptoms correlate with the degree of involvement?
3. How long is the treatment for renal TB usually required?
4. Is the incidence of schistosomiasis on the decrease?
5. Which organism is commonly involved with GU filariasis?
6. What is the drug of choice for all species of schistosomes?
7. What is most common cause of opportunistic GU fungal infections?
8. What are the commonly used drugs in the treatment of GU candidiasis?
9. In the case of necrotizing fascitis, are the signs proportionate to the severity of the disease?
10. What antibiotics are commonly used in the treatment of Fournier's gangrene?

Index

Page numbers in *italics* denote figures; those followed by "t" denote tables.

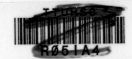

Date Due

ISBN 0-07-136201-0